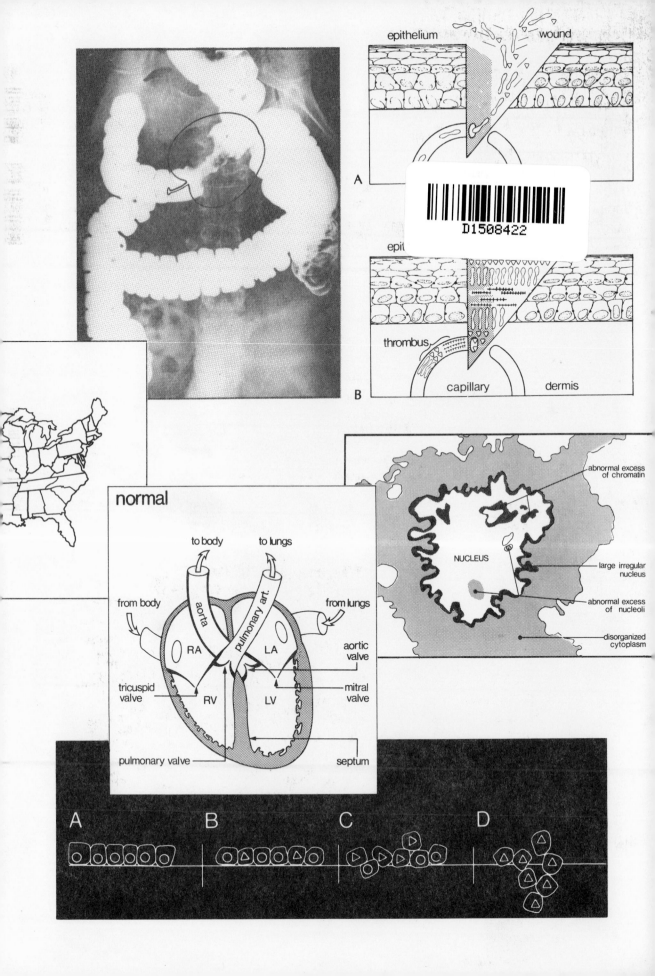

epithelium   wound

A

epith...

thrombus

B   capillary   dermis

abnormal excess
of chromatin

NUCLEUS

large irregular
nucleus

abnormal excess
of nucleoli

disorganized
cytoplasm

D1508422

normal

to body   to lungs

from body   from lungs

from body   aorta   pulmonary art.

RA   LA   aortic
                                        valve

tricuspid
valve   RV   LV   mitral
                                        valve

pulmonary valve   septum

A   B   C   D

Introduction to the Study of Disease

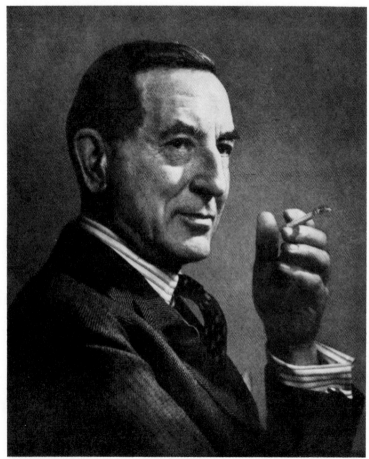

WILLIAM BOYD
1885–1979

Forty-three years ago this text was conceived with pleasure and nurtured with love by Dr. William Boyd. It has been through seven editions, twenty-five reprintings, and translated into Spanish and Japanese. Dr. Boyd died in 1979. His inspiration, guidance, instruction, and entertainment of generations of students of medicine at all levels is a legend. He will be missed particularly by those fortunate enough to have worked with him in the preparation of this text.

Introduction to the Study of Disease

William Boyd, C.C., M.D.

Late Professor Emeritus of Pathology, The University of Toronto;
Formerly Professor of Pathology, The University of Manitoba and
The University of British Columbia.

Huntington Sheldon, M.D., F.R.C.P.(C.)

Strathcona Professor of Pathology,
McGill University, Montreal

Eighth Edition

Lea & Febiger   1980   Philadelphia

Cover (front and back)

The cover shows a multiple-gated acquisition cardiac scan (MGA) of a normal heart. The scintillation camera is synchronized to the electrocardiogram and interfaced with a computer system. A photograph is made of the computer screen with a Polaroid camera. The patient's red blood cells are prelabeled with radioactive material. This is the only invasive procedure necessary.

The first of 16 frames shown is taken coincident with the R wave of the electrocardiogram. Using this computer program one cardiac cycle of contraction is divided into 16 parts. The fifth frame shows the maximal contraction of the left ventricle (the small, round red image). Since the scintillation camera is positioned in the oblique position, the right atrium and ventricle are shown as the large red image on the left of the small, round red image. With this technique, the volume of each systolic ejection fraction and the cardiac output can be calculated. Moreover, the movement of ventricular muscle during systole and diastole can be visualized in attempts to show areas of disease. This technique eliminates the use of invasive procedures and can be used to study cardiac function before and after stress and after coronary artery operations. (Courtesy of Dr. R. Lisbona, Royal Victoria Hospital, Montreal.)

Spine

On the spine of the book is a multiple-gated nuclear scan of the left ventricle of the heart. This is taken from the left anterior oblique position and shows the cardiac cycle divided into 16 frames. It demonstrates the normal contraction of the left ventricle. The outer white line is the size of the left ventricle when it is relaxed (diastole), and the inner red line shows maximal contraction (systole). The black area in the center is proportional to the volume of the left ventricle. (Courtesy of Dr. R. Lisbona, Royal Victoria Hospital, Montreal.)

First Edition 1937
    Reprinted 1938, 1939
Second Edition 1941
    Reprinted 1942, 1944
Third Edition 1945
    Reprinted 1945, 1947,1948, 1949, 1950 (Twice)
Fourth Edition 1952
    Reprinted 1953, 1954, 1955, 1957, 1958, 1960
Fifth Edition 1962
    Reprinted 1963, 1965, 1967, 1969
Sixth Edition 1971
    Reprinted 1972, 1975, 1976
Seventh Edition 1977
    Reprinted 1979

Library of Congress Cataloging in Publication Data

Boyd, William, 1885–
    An introduction to the study of disease.

    Bibliography: p.
    Includes index.
    1. Pathology.   I. Sheldon, Huntington, joint author.   II. Title.
RB111.B58   1980   616   80–23487
ISBN 0–8121–0729–2

Published in Great Britain by Henry Kimpton Publishers, London

PRINTED IN THE UNITED STATES OF AMERICA

Print No.   6   5   4   3   2   1

Preface

Rapid changes in many areas of the health sciences are a stimulus to revise this text once more. The eighth edition is a complete revision that presents a contemporary view of disease, its etiology, pathophysiology, and modern techniques of diagnosis. This book is designed for students who wish an understanding of disease without a quantity of detail. I have attempted to illustrate the important principles of disease and, of necessity, have had to minimize some of the supporting evidence. More than 250 new illustrations, diagrams, and scans have been added. Every chapter has been revised and most have been rewritten and restructured, but the organization of the previous edition has been retained. I have added sections on cardiac, renal, hepatic, and respiratory failure to emphasize the correlation of physiologic changes with symptoms, signs, and morphologic alterations. Above all, I have attempted to capture some of the excitement of modern medicine and to indicate areas where our ignorance is as important as our knowledge.

Dr. Mary Senterman wrote the chapter on the female genitourinary system, and Dr. Paula Traktman the chapter on viruses. Dr. Simon Braun assembled the radiologic material from the collections of Drs. L.A. Stein, J. Toth, G.B. Skinner, D.R. Patton, R. Lisbona, R.E. Wilson, and R.E. Hanson of the Royal Victoria Hospital in Montreal and wrote the section on radiologic procedures. Material to illustrate the chapter on the central nervous system was organized by Dr. S. Horowitz from the collection of Dr. R. Ethier of the Montreal Neurological Institute. Alexander Bulzan prepared all the drawings and graphs.

Holly Lukens and Tom Colaiezzi of Lea & Febiger have prepared the manuscript for publication.

I would like to thank all of them and Elisabeth Cotton, who has edited this with me, and Irma Niemi, who painstakingly and with unfailing good humor typed and prepared the manuscript.

Montreal   HUNTINGTON SHELDON, M.D.

Contents

1 General Principles

2 The Organs and Their Diseases

General Principles

1

The Living Body

1

To see what is general in what is particular, and what is permanent in what is transitory is the aim of scientific thought. —A. N. Whitehead

If we are to study disease, we need to be capable of distinguishing between what is disease and what is not, and this requires some knowledge of the normal workings of the human body. In fact, much of our contemporary knowledge of normal function and structure has come from comparisons between normal and abnormal. In this introduction, we outline contemporary views of how the human body is structured, from molecule to man, and how these many parts function, sometimes independently, but always in relation to the whole. This particular chapter reviews anatomy and physiology at the cellular level, and outlines the mechanisms on which the living body depends for its normal function, such as circulation and digestion, and in which various disorders of function (disease) may occur, leading ultimately to failure of the whole (death).

The human body is composed of an extraordinarily large number of minute elements known as **cells**, which form definite structures or **tissues**; these again are grouped into **organs**. Certain cells with definite properties form muscle tissue, and others with quite different properties form nervous tissue; these and other tissues are combined to form organs such as the heart and stomach. By definition, a tissue consists of cells of the same kind and an organ is composed of tissues of

different kinds. To visualize the elements of cells and tissues we must use optical aids such as the light or electron microscope, for most cells are too small to be seen with the unaided eye. The study of tissues is called **histology** (Greek *histos*, tissue, and *logos*, the study of). The word tissue itself comes from the French term *tissu*, which means weave or texture. There are 4 general basic types of tissue: epithelial, connective, muscular, and nervous.

Epithelial tissue (Fig. 1–1) serves to protect, absorb, and/or secrete. It is anatomically effective for these cells to be arranged in sheets to cover the surface; this is called an epithelium. One modification of most epithelial layers is the down-growth of groups of cells into the underlying connective tissue to form the secretory structures known as glands. Thus epithelia can act as protective coverings for external surfaces (skin), absorptive linings for internal surfaces such as the intestine, or secretory structures such as salivary or sweat glands.

Connective tissue (Fig. 1–2) holds together, connects, and supports other tissues and cells. In addition to the connective tissue cells themselves, it is composed of a large amount of intercellular substance, which varies from one kind of connective tissue to another. Most of the intercellular substance is secreted by

3

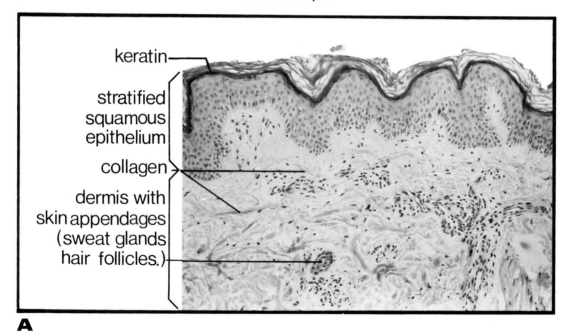

keratin

stratified
squamous
epithelium

collagen

dermis with
skin appendages
(sweat glands
hair follicles.)

A

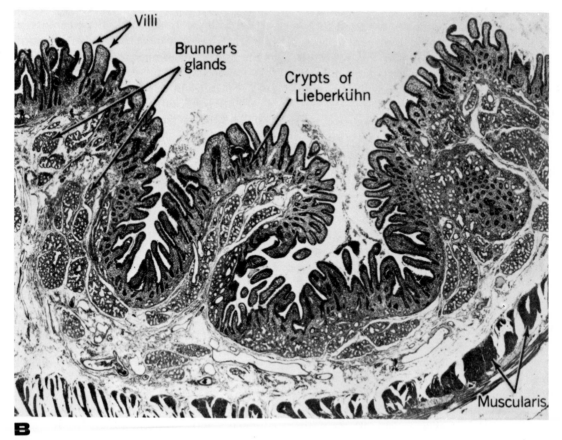

Villi

Brunner's
glands

Crypts of
Lieberkühn

Muscularis

B

Fig. 1–1. *A*, Photomicrograph of a section of skin shows the protective outer lining of stratified, squamous, keratinized epithelium, which lies over the dermis, the latter being composed principally of connective tissue. This epithelium serves as a natural defense to infectious organisms and prevents the body from drying by evaporation. *B*, Photomicrograph shows a section through the absorptive layer of the duodenum, where the epithelium is thrown up in many small folds and finger-like projections. This epithelium is specifically designed to increase the surface area. Microvilli at the surface of each cell serve the additional purpose of retaining extracellular enzymes to aid in absorption. (Courtesy of Dr. H. Mizoguchi.)

the connective tissue cells, whether they are cartilage cells, fibroblasts, or bone cells (osteoblasts). Depending on the type of connective tissue, the formed elements in the intercellular spaces will vary in appearance, so that we have collagen fibrils in the dermis, elastic fibers in tendons, and calcified collagen in bone.

Muscular tissue consists of cells whose chief characteristic is their ability to contract. Different types of muscle, such as in the heart, in the gut, and in the locomotor system, are composed of cells with varied amounts and different types of fibrils. The different types of muscle also function in various ways: automatically in the heart, voluntarily in the skeleton, and rhythmically in the gut.

Nervous tissue is highly specialized for the function of permitting quick reactions both automatically, such as a reflex, and voluntarily, as when we wish to lift a spoon to our mouths.

Thus there are general functions for each of these classes of tissue: epithelial cells cover, protect, secrete, absorb, and may be differentiated to perform special functions. Skin, gut, liver, and milk-secreting glands are all epithelial derivatives.

Connective tissue constitutes ligaments, tendons, joints, and bones, and it holds organs in place. Adipose tissue is a particular type of connective tissue.

Muscular tissue does the work in the heart, moves food along in the digestive system, and allows us to run, jump, and move about.

Nervous tissue is the responsive element that permits us to perceive the world about us, and to reflect on our being.

THE HEALTHY CELL

The word "cell" originally meant a small chamber, and it is still used in that sense in relation to a jail or a monastery. But it is a chamber holding a living inmate, actually the smallest unit of living matter. Some animals, such as the ameba and the malaria parasite, consist of a single cell and are therefore called unicellular organisms or protozoa. Although these elementary animals consist of only one cell, they breathe, digest, excrete, and move. One might recall that each of us started from the union of 2 cells, and recently it has been

shown that a fully developed higher animal can develop from a single cell that has been artificially provoked to undertake division and replication, a process called parthenogenesis. This development can even take place in an environment different from the natural one; ova can be transplanted in mammals, and a limited development can even occur in a test tube, as the popular press is only too happy to report. During the normal development of a mammal, for a short while, all cells of the embryo appear remarkably similar to one another. Despite 70 years of study of embryonic development, we are still not sure why some cells differentiate into muscle, others into skin, and still others into nerve or connective tissue cells.

A finished muscle cell, a finished nerve cell, and a finished liver cell are as far apart in visible structure as in what they do. Some cells pour out cement that binds them together, as in cartilage and bone. Some become as clear as glass, as in the cornea of the eye. Some develop into a system transmitting electrical signals. Each of the 70,000 billion cells in every human body specializes into something helpful to the whole. The differentiation of cells for different functions leaves us breathless—those functions we recognize in our own bodies as well as the incredible senses of "dumb animals," such as the vision of the eagle, the olfactory sense of the dog, the radar-like sense of the bat, and the sense of touch of the mollusc. This is the miracle of life and its specializations.

The human body was likened by Rudolf Virchow (1821 to 1902) to a "cell state" with a social organization and specialization of labor. This carries with it the hazard that one group of specialized cells becomes dependent on another group of specialists, and a strike on the part of a small group may paralyze or reduce to chaos the entire community. Thus, the normal, effective contractility of the heart depends on a small bundle of conducting fibers that synchronize the different chambers. If this is put out of business the heart may stop, and every function of the body ceases due to lack of oxygen. Death results. The ameba, consisting of only one cell, has no such hazards to fear. Specialization demands a price, in cells as well as in society.

There is a striking contrast between the

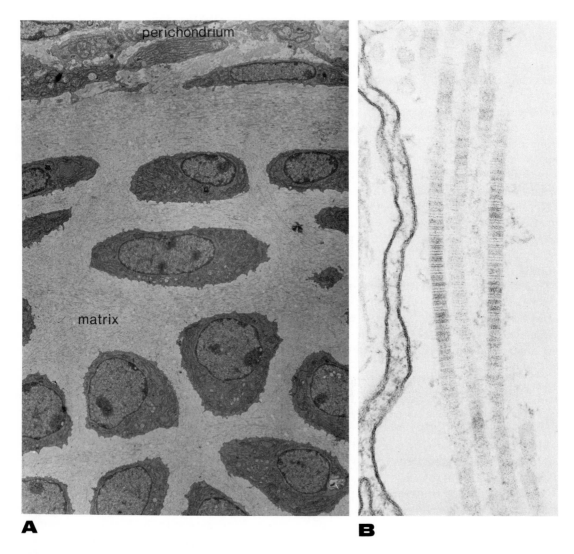

Fig. 1–2. *A*, Electron micrograph shows many cells in cartilage surrounded by their matrix. The perichondrium, or outer layer of the cartilage, is at the top of the field. Cartilage is an avascular tissue. All the constituents of this tissue enter by diffusion from the periphery. *B*, High-power electron micrograph shows collagen fibrils, which are identified by their characteristic repeated cross-striations. The other structures shown are portions of thin fibroblasts, limited by the bilaminar cell-surface membrane. *C*, High-power electron micrograph of soluble collagen shows the protofibrils and their arrangement as seen with negative staining. (From Prockop, D.J., et al.: The biosynthesis of collagen and its disorders. N. Engl. J. Med., *301*:13, 1979.)

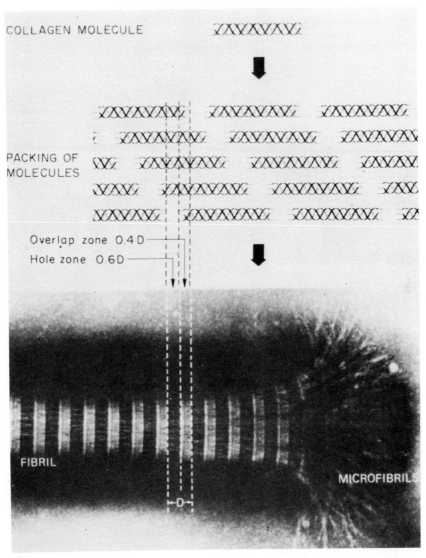

COLLAGEN MOLECULE

PACKING OF
MOLECULES

Overlap zone 0.4 D
Hole zone 0.6 D

FIBRIL

MICROFIBRILS

D

c

THE CELL

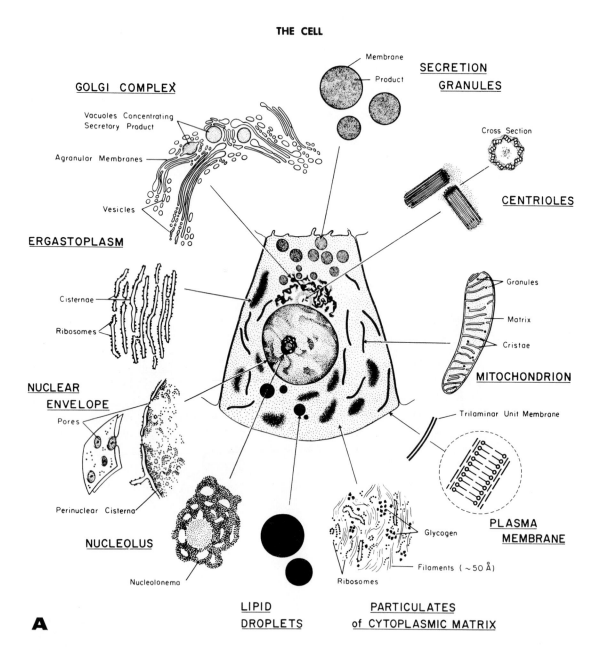

Fig. 1–3. *A,* Schematic representation of a secretory cell. Arranged around the cell are the various components that have been identified with the electron microscope. The significance of these components is discussed briefly in the text. (From Bloom, W., and Fawcett, D.W.: *A Textbook of Histology,* 9th Ed. Philadelphia, W. B. Saunders, 1968.)

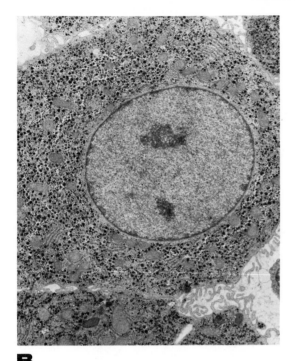

B

Fig. 1–3. *B,* Electron micrograph shows a liver cell in which the various components can be identified.

durability of our body and the transitory character of its elements. Man is composed of a soft matter than can disintegrate in a few hours, and yet he lasts longer than if made of steel. Moreover, he accommodates himself marvelously to the changing conditions of his environment. The body seems to mold itself on events. Instead of wearing out like a machine, it changes. In general terms, this characteristic of *adaptation* is one of the most important features of life at any level, whether it be of a cell, tissue, or organism. We shall say more about adaptability in both health and disease.

Just as the atom is a unit of physics, so **cells are the fundamental units of every living body,** whether it be animal or vegetable, and in the last analysis it is they that eat the food, drink the water, and breathe the air, all of which are necessary for the life of the body. The marvelous arrangements of structure (anatomy) and of function (physiology) are simply a complex mechanism to bring to the cells this food, water, and air, which are beyond their normal reach, as well as to per-

petuate the species to which the organism belongs.

Every cell, whether of an animal or a plant, consists of three principal constituents: **cell membrane, nucleus,** and **cytoplasm**. The nucleus contains: (1) the **chromosomes**, which are the carriers of the genes, the transmitters of hereditary characteristics, and (2) the **nucleolus**, which directs the cytoplasm and seems in turn to be the target for hormones. The cytoplasm contains a variety of structural constituents known as the **organelles**, or little organs. The cell is indeed a miniature universe (Fig. 1–3).

In recent years enormous advances have been made in our knowledge of the structure of the cell in health and, to a lesser degree, in disease. We owe these advances, in the main, to 2 new techniques: (1) The electron microscope, which gives us a magnification of 100,000 in place of one of 1,000, reveals a new wealth of structure. There are electron microscopes now being constructed at a cost of several million dollars that may make it possible for us actually to see the atom. (2) The development of new methods of cytochemistry, which demonstrate the sites of enzymes, not only in the intact cell, but also in subcellular particles such as mitochondria. These particles are obtained by disrupting the cell and then separating the organelles by means of the ultracentrifuge.

The techniques of cell fractionation have provided so much important information that it may be interesting to review some of the simple principles, methods, and results that have greatly contributed to our understanding of the cellular universe. DeDuve and his coworkers developed and refined centrifugation methods in the 1960's whereby a common soup (homogenate) could be separated into its component parts by the expedient of placing the soup in a centrifuge. If the soup, for example, were a simple pea soup, the heavy peas and their skins (pellet) would be driven to the bottom of the centrifuge tube, since they are more dense and larger than the broth that remains at the top (supernatant). In fact, it would even be possible to separate the peas from their skins if one placed some sort of screen in the tube as well, so that there might be three phases to the soup. Now the nourishment in the soup (protein) resides in the pellet of peas, and if one tested for the presence of an enzyme commonly found in peas (urease), this enzyme would be present in largest amounts not in the supernatant but in the green pellets at the

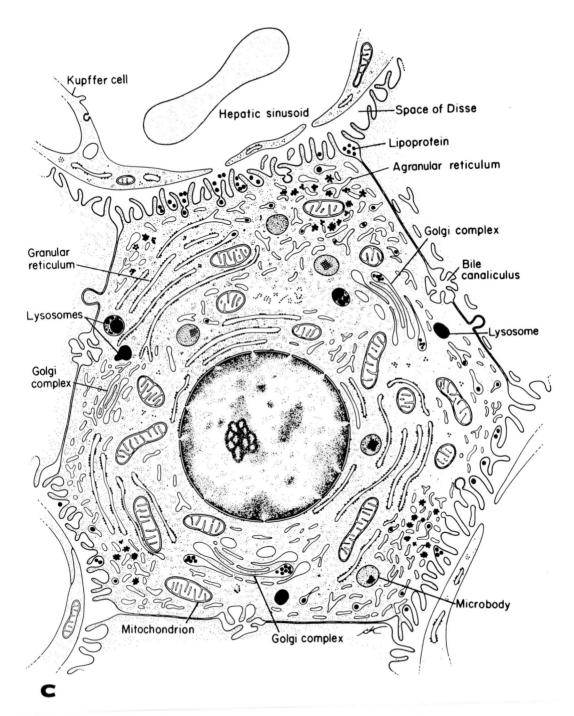

Fig. 1–3. *C,* Drawing interprets the electron micrograph. Labeled are various structures that have been discovered during the last 25 years. Not all of these structures can be identified in any single micrograph. For example, in Figure 1–3*B* no microbodies or lysosomes can be seen. (Drawing by Sylvia Colard Keene.)

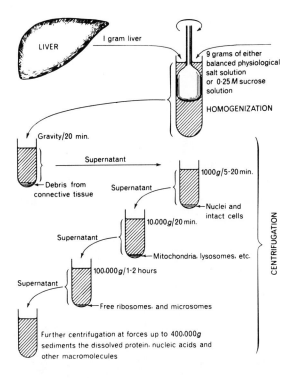

Fig. 1–4. This flow sheet shows the steps in preparing an homogenate for ultracentrifugal fractionation of liver. The preparation separates nuclei from mitochondria from the rough reticulum and the cell sap. (From Bloom, W., and Fawcett, D.W.: *A Textbook of Histology*, 9th Ed. Philadelphia, W. B. Saunders, 1968.)

bottom of the tube. The marker enzyme, which indicates where the nourishment is, would suggest that for camping trips only the precooked pellet be taken along and water added to reconstitute the soup.

DeDuve applied such differential centrifugation methods with marker enzymes to soups or homogenates made from liver and other tissues. He refined the sieving techniques by using sucrose of different densities so that he could separate particles that differed very slightly either in size or in density. Thus particles with differing shapes and surface-to-volume ratios behave differently in a gravitational field. The sedimentation coefficient of different molecules and particles (different from their density) has allowed them to be isolated and characterized enzymatically. Figure 1–4 illustrates the flow sheet of a conventional separation of tissues into the nuclear, mitochondrial, and membrane fractions. Figure 1–5 shows the appearance of each of the pellet preparations as seen with the electron microscope from a conventional, subcellular fractionation. Figure 1–6 illustrates the role of marker enzymes in discriminating among subcellular fractions.

Cell Membrane. The membrane or envelope of the cell is not evident with the light microscope, but it is well demonstrated by the electron microscope. Too little attention has been paid this membrane in the past, but it is now known to be a structure no less remarkable than the contents that it encloses. It is an all-important structure, for it regulates the internal environment of the cell, determining what goes in and what comes out. Thus it separates the high concentrations of potassium inside the cell from the high concentrations of sodium outside the cell, and it can push out processes to engulf harmful bacteria, which the cell then destroys, the process of phagocytosis. Water and all food particles must pass inward through the membrane freely, whereas metabolites must pass out. Virus particles are absorbed to the surface of the cell before penetrating to the interior. It is to the surface structure that many dyes and effective drugs become attached, and antigens are bound to the surface of the cell.

Contemporary views of the plasma membrane suggest that it is composed of lipid molecules arranged with their hydrophobic regions outward in the manner of a stockade, but interspersed among the palisades of lipids are protein molecules that may be visible from the outside of the cell only, or from the inside only, or that may extend in some areas the full thickness—60Å (Angstrom units)—and act as ports or channels. It is these protein molecules that confer the individuality of each cell; they allow cells to be recognized by one another and are the determinants of cellular specificity. This contemporary mosaic concept for the structure of the cell membrane has been developed by Singer and Nicolson as a general model (Fig. 1–7).

Nucleus. The nucleus may be regarded as the brain of the cell. When the nucleus dies, death of the cell will soon follow. There is a curious exception to this rule, for the erythrocyte (red blood cell) of man loses its nucleus when it enters the blood stream from the bone marrow, yet its life span is about 120 days. Perhaps its passive role of carrying oxygen from the lungs to the tissues makes the presence of the nucleus superfluous, although in some mammals such as the camel, and in

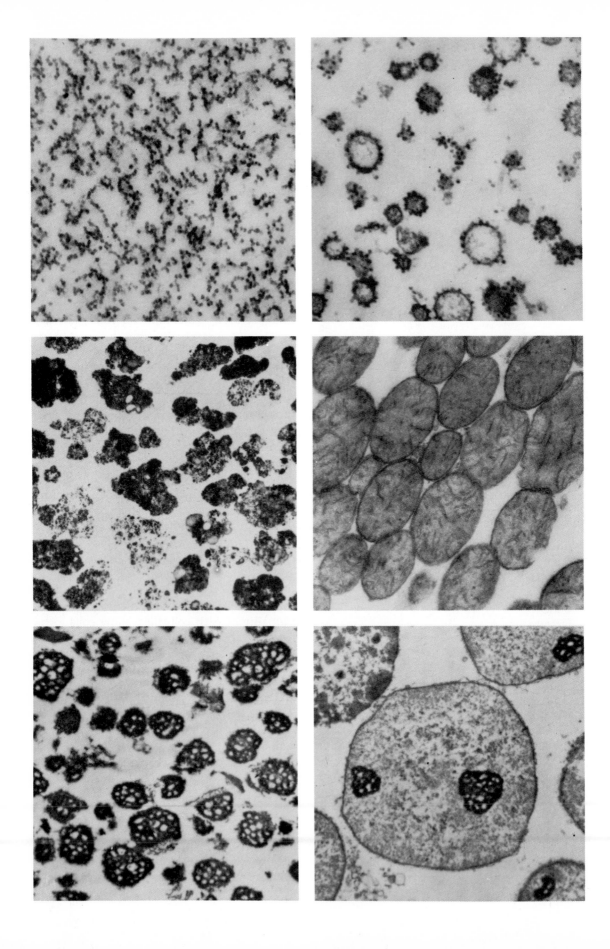

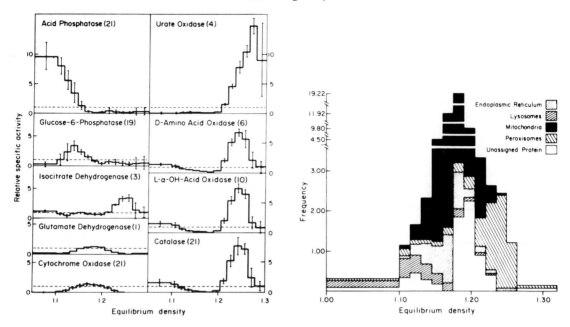

Fig. 1–6. These diagrams show the equilibrium density centrifugal pattern of mitochondria in the black pyramid, and the particular marker enzymes, such as cytochrome oxidase for mitochondria, acid phosphatase for lysosomes and catalase for peroxisomes. (From Leighton, F., et al.: The large-scale separation of peroxisomes, mitochondria, and lysosomes from the livers of rats injected with triton WR-1339. J. Cell Biol., 37:482, 1968.)

cold-blooded animals (frog), the nucleus is present in the erythrocyte. The nuclear material is sequestered from other cell components (cytoplasm) by the nuclear membrane. Thirty years ago electron microscopy of this interface between the two major compartments of the cell (nucleoplasm and cytoplasm) demonstrated curious and regular structures, which have been carefully studied and shown to be a kind of pore. So each nucleus is surrounded by a system of membranes, but there are pores in the membrane that permit the exchange of material and information between the nucleus and cytoplasm. This route is important because we know that many hormones must reach the nucleus of a cell to be effective. The control of cytoplasmic protein synthesis depends on information reaching the cytoplasm from the nucleus. Perhaps in the future we shall discover ways to control the ebb and flow of information through the nuclear pores.

Within the nucleus resides the DNA (deoxyribonucleic acid), the program for all cell activities. The DNA is complexed with other basic proteins in a diffuse structure known as chromatin. (These proteins are important for the structure of the total complex and probably serve a control function as well.) When the cell is resting (i.e., not dividing), the chromatin is dispersed throughout the nucleus and is barely visible. However, when the cell prepares for mitosis (cell division), the chromatin becomes condensed into long, thin structures known as chromosomes that can easily be seen with a light microscope. Each plant and animal cell has a species-specific number of chromosomes: man has 23 pairs (46

Fig. 1–5. This set of electron micrographs shows the appearance in the electron microscope of pellets from the respective fractions prepared in the previous picture. (From Bloom, W., and Fawcett, D.W.: A Textbook of Histology, 9th Ed. Philadelphia, W. B. Saunders, 1968.)

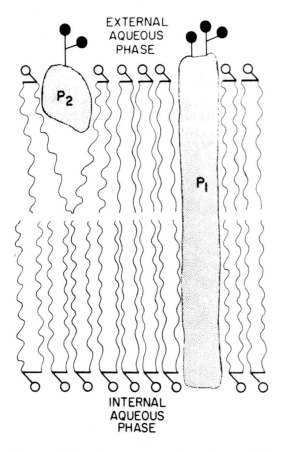

Fig. 1–7. Schematic representation of a small portion of the plasma membrane of a cell shows proteins at P_1 and P_2, which are an integral portion of the plasma membrane, but may extend the full thickness of the membrane or may reside simply at one layer. The membrane is thought of today as a fluid mosaic. (From Berlin, R.D., et al.: The cell surface. N. Engl. J. Med., 292:515, 1975.)

in all). Each pair consists of two nonidentical copies of chromosomes, one derived from each parent.

A gene is a segment of a chromatin strand; there may be 50,000 to 100,000 genes strung along one chromosome. The gene, not the chromosome, is the unit of heredity. A structural gene is now defined operationally as a functional unit of inheritance, situated on a chromosome and responsible for the synthesis of a specific polypeptide or protein. This synthesis results in the production of two general classes of proteins, namely, those concerned with the framework of cells (structure proteins), and those concerned with intermediary metabolism, or the rate of protein synthesis (regulatory proteins). Enzymes can

be considered as a subset of regulatory proteins. The genes, therefore, contain instructions for the design of both building blocks (structural proteins) and builders (regulatory proteins) of the living machine, as well as information about how that machine is to function. It is hardly too much to say that a man's biochemistry is as individual as his fingerprints, and that both are determined by his genes.

This general concept was enunciated more than 40 years ago in the dictum "one gene—one enzyme," which was subsequently amplified to "DNA makes RNA which makes protein." These ideas can be better understood by the following propositions. (1) All biochemical processes in all living organisms are under the control of genes. (2) Each biochemical reaction can be resolved into different steps, governed by the availability of substrate and enzyme. (3) Each step of any reaction is under the control of a different gene. (4) Mutations of single genes affect single steps of a reaction. (5) Mutations may affect either the structure of the product of a reaction, or the amount of the product of the reaction. Sickle cell anemia results from a single gene mutation that produces a structurally abnormal hemoglobin molecule. Other single gene mutations may result in an inborn error of metabolism, which sometimes manifests itself as disease.

Abnormalities can occur in chromosomes as well as in single genes. Often a chromosomal disorder results in the loss of thousands of genes and is lethal for the new embryo, which fails to develop completely and dies during the first few weeks after conception.

DNA (deoxyribonucleic acid) is a linear, unbranched molecule, whose sequence is determined by 4 component building blocks. Each building block consists of a deoxyribose sugar with a phosphate group (these are covalently linked and form the DNA backbone) with 1 of 4 sidegroups: adenine (A), guanine (G), cytosine (C), thymine (T). Each sugar-phosphate sidegroup complex is known as a nucleotide base. The key to the structure of DNA is that it is usually present as 2 intertwined strands, whose interaction is governed by strict rules of fit between the nucleotide bases (Fig. 1–8). Adenine and thymine form stable hydrogen bonds together, as do guanine and cytosine. Thus, in the 2 intertwined strands of the DNA molecule, an adenine of one strand always

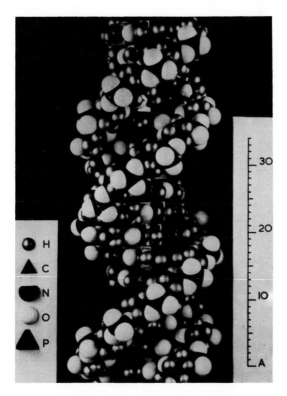

Fig. 1–8. This photograph of a molecular model of the double-helical DNA shows the arrangements and spacing of the component parts. The respective atoms of hydrogen, carbon, nitrogen, oxygen, and phosphorus are shown with their sizes as indicated on the left. (From Watson, J.D.: *Molecular Biology of the Gene*, 2nd Ed. Menlo Park, Calif., W. A. Benjamin, 1970.)

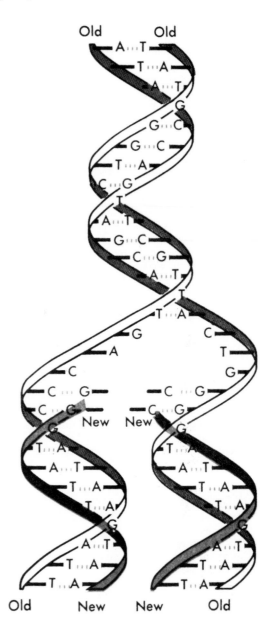

Fig. 1–9. The replication of DNA is illustrated in this drawing. (From Watson, J.D.: *Molecular Biology of the Gene*, 2nd Ed. Menlo Park, Calif., W. A. Benjamin, 1970.)

pairs up with a thymine of the other; guanine similarly pairs up with cytosine, and the resulting bonds connect the 2 strands tightly. The 2 strands complement each other: an ACGT sequence on one strand is always complemented by a TGCA sequence directly opposite it, on the other strand. This is the basis of DNA self-replication, which is the key to all life and reproduction. The 2 strands unwind, then enzymes (DNA polymerases) move along each strand, and base by base synthesize the complementary sequence (Fig. 1–9). The result is 2 DNA molecules, each containing a parent strand and a complementary new strand. The replication of DNA is an accurate process, especially as there are proofreading and repair enzymes that keep the genetic information correct.

DNA is the memory bank for the genetic program; it contains instructions for the design of protein molecules, as we have already stated. The question we now face is: How is the genetic program realized as the living individual? That is, how are the instructions followed to create this product? The answer is a complicated sequence of events, in which the main characters are DNA and a similar

molecule RNA, which perform 2 essential processes called transcription and translation.

RNA is chemically similar to DNA; the sugar is slightly different, and uracil replaces thymine as one of the 4 bases. When the time comes for the instructions in a gene to be carried out, the DNA strands of that gene temporarily separate. Then RNA polymerase enzymes move in to form an RNA strand, base by base, complementary to the DNA parent, as in DNA replication. This process is called transcription. There are sites on the DNA, known as promoters, where RNA polymerase binds and transcription begins. Similarly, there are termination signals, where transcription stops. The RNA molecule that performs this transcription process is called messenger RNA (or mRNA), to distinguish it from RNA molecules that serve different functions in this process. When the mRNA is completely transcribed, it is transported to the cytoplasm, where it lines up in a groove on the ribosomes (the complex molecule that consists of 2 parts held together by magnesium and that characteristically contains the 5 carbon sugar, ribose). It is now ready for translation into a protein.

A protein is a string of amino acids, joined together by peptide bonds. There are 20 different amino acids. How is the language of RNA, namely, nucleotide bases, translated into the language of protein, namely, amino acids? Obviously, 1 base cannot correspond to 1 amino acid. Instead, the RNA base sequence is read in triplets, and a triplet of bases is called a codon. The number of unique three-letter words (codons) that can come from a four-letter alphabet (the RNA bases A, U, C, G) is 64. Sixty-one of these words stand for specific amino acids. Three are stop signals. Since 20 amino acids are specified by 61 codons, there is "degeneracy" in the code, i.e., the same amino acid can be specified by a number of triplets.

In the ribosome, the mRNA is waiting to be translated. We now know that for each triplet of RNA base sequences, a single amino acid is intended; what remains is for these amino acids to be collected and assembled into the individual protein. This job is performed by another RNA molecule, known as transfer RNA (tRNA) and certain specific enzymes. A tRNA molecule is similar in design to an electric plug. One portion of it contains a loop that displays 3 nucleotide bases as accessibly as the prongs of the plug. This loop can be matched to or plugged into an mRNA at that position containing the complementary triplet. For example, the tRNA for the amino acid leucine has on its loop the triplet AAC, which will line up opposite the mRNA UUG. (Remember that the mRNA triplet UUG was originally transcribed from a DNA triplet reading AAC.) Another portion of the tRNA molecule has a combining site for a specific enzyme. The enzyme has 2 specific active sites, 1 for a specific tRNA, and 1 for a specific amino acid. Thus, as in the example of leucine, the enzyme catches a leucine molecule and becomes hooked onto a tRNA with AAC on its loop. This "charged" tRNA will then line up opposite a UUG codon on the mRNA. The leucine is then in a position to be enzymatically added to the growing protein. The process is then repeated for each codon (Fig. 1–10).

The ribosomes are structural units that allow for organized and efficient protein synthesis. The mRNA to be translated lines up in a groove on the ribosomes and is moved along

it as each successive triplet is read and as each successive amino acid is added to the growing protein chain. Many initiation, elongation, and termination factors are involved. In essence, however, the tRNA functions as an intermediary, an adaptor, between the nucleic acid code and the amino acid specified. The ribosome functions as a conveyor belt. It should be mentioned that the reading of the triplets occurs in a specified phase and in a given direction (polarity). One can see how a variety of mutations or errors in DNA would change the resultant protein. A change of base might cause a new triplet to specify a new amino acid, or perhaps even the stop signal. A loss or addition of a base would put the remainder of the sequence out of phase. Errors during RNA transcription would have a similar effect on protein synthesis, but these errors would not be inherited by the next generation of cells.

Proteins, once synthesized, go to work doing the business of the cell. They may be structural components, may work as catalyzing enzymes, or may be signal proteins such as hormones that direct a range of alterations in cellular behavior.

Cytoplasm. If the nucleus is the brain of the cell, concerned with such major problems as genetic constitution and cellular reproduction, it is the cytoplasm that does most of the everyday work. Just as the cells are specialized to do different kinds of work, such as the contraction of muscle, the secretion of digestive juices, the production of hormones, and the sending out of nervous impulses, it is natural that the shape and appearance of cytoplasm should vary correspondingly. An examination of the nucleus may indicate whether the cell is living or dead, but the appearance of the cytoplasm may tell the scientist looking down the microscope whether the cell has been sick and unable to work.

Every cell's cytoplasm contains a number of subcompartments known as *organelles*. These have been studied in detail by the modern methods already referred to: cell fractionation, high-speed centrifugation, and photography with the electron microscope. For expediency, we shall limit our discussion to 4 major cytoplasmic constituents—mito-

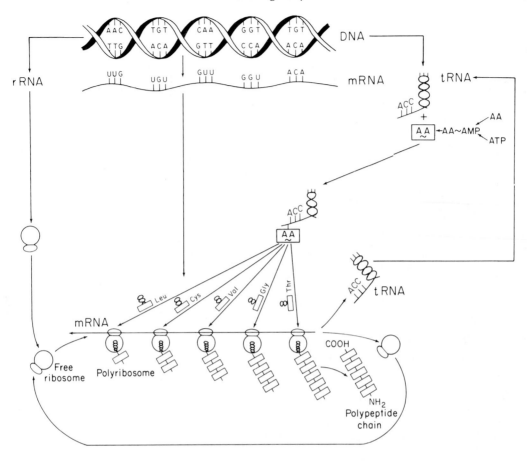

Fig. 1–10. The pattern of protein synthesis and the role of the various component parts are schematically displayed here. (From Bearn, A.G.: Genetic principles. In *Cecil Textbook of Medicine,* 15th Ed. Edited by P. B. Beeson, W. McDermott, and J. B. Wyngaarden. Philadelphia, W. B. Saunders, 1979.)

chondria, endoplasmic reticulum, lysosomes, and microtubules.

Mitochondria are thread-like bodies (Greek *mitos*, thread, and *chondrus*, granule) when viewed with the light microscope, but as seen with the electron microscope, they are rod-shaped or may look like a cucumber. Although they are not visible with conventional light microscopy, they are present in enormous numbers (2,500 per cell in the liver of the rat). They are surrounded with a paired membrane, so that each can be regarded as a separate chemical laboratory or membranous compartment; folds of the inner membrane project inward as shelves termed cristae (Fig. 1–11). It is on these shelves that the respiratory enzymes are arranged in an orderly way; these enzymes are responsible for the use of oxygen. Mitochondria are regarded as the

main power plants of the cell. It is of interest that organisms that do not depend on oxygen may or may not have mitochondria, depending on whether they are functioning anaerobically (without oxygen). In fact, yeast may be grown aerobically and will contain mitochondria, but the same yeast grown in the absence of oxygen will lose its mitochondria. Mitochondria also contain small amounts of DNA and some RNA. Isolated mitochondria respond to hormones such as thyroxine, but we now believe that they do not synthesize their specialized respiratory enzymes themselves, despite the presence of DNA and ribosomes, but rather that such enzymes as cytochrome oxidase are assembled in the mitochondria after synthesis by the endoplasmic reticulum.

The presence of these membrane-bound

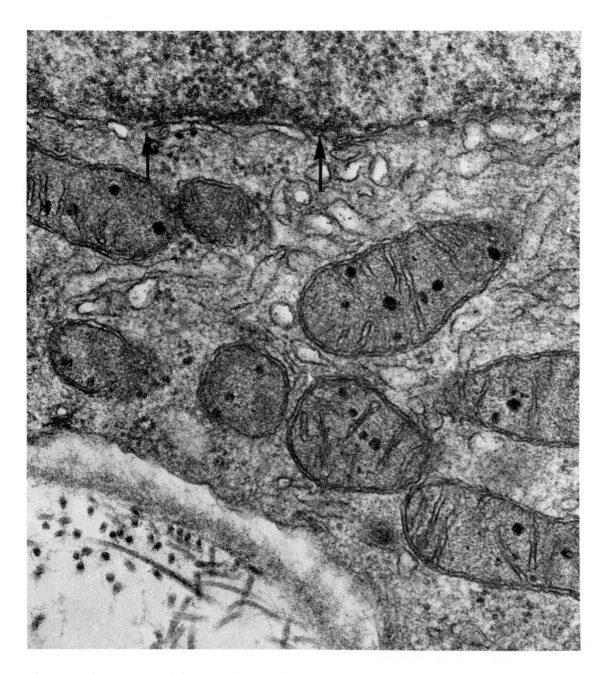

Fig. 1–11. Electron micrograph shows a small portion of a cell containing many mitochondria and bounded by a basement membrane. At the top of the field is the nucleus, and at the arrow is a nuclear pore. The mitochondria are surrounded by two parallel dense lines which constitute membranes enclosing the mitochondrial space from the cytoplasm. The mitochondria has a denser matrix than the surrounding cytoplasm and is divided into compartments by cristae. Within the mitochondria are dense aggregates that appear in this picture as black dots. Outside the border of the cell is a basement membrane. This area is seen at the bottom of the field. Extending into it are delicate fibrils of connective tissue.

cytoplasmic organelles (mitochondria) with even a little nucleic acid has suggested to some authors that mitochondria represent the symbiotic existence of prokaryotic (bacteria-like) forms, which at some remote time in evolution formed a useful alliance with nucleated cells. Whatever their origin, they are present in most living human cells and they exist in large numbers in those cells that require a large amount of energy to do their work. In fact, one may increase both the size and the number of mitochondria in skeletal muscle by aerobic training. Conversely, with disuse, these mitochondria decrease in number and in size. Such observations underscore the adaptability of living cells at all levels of organization.

The term *endoplasmic reticulum* has been given to the principal membranous component of the cytoplasm, a series of vesicles and intercommunicating canals, whose primary function is to separate the cell into different compartments, much as walls may delimit the kitchen from the bedroom or bathroom, where different functions are accomplished.

Endoplasmic reticulum is a collective term for cytoplasmic membranes; we recognize both the granular reticulum (that with RNA particles attached) (Fig. 1–12), and the agranular reticulum. The granular reticulum is a special group of cytoplasmic membranes, which appear in greatest abundance in cells that secrete protein for export, such as plasma cells (antibodies), pancreas cells (digestive

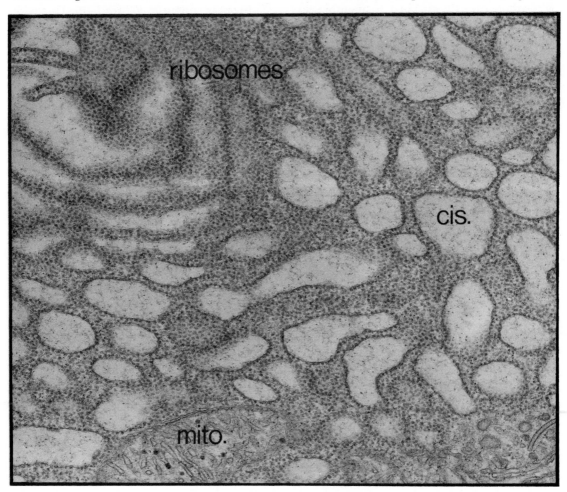

Fig. 1–12. Electron micrograph from an acinar cell of pancreas shows the granular reticulum arranged around small cavities that contain a delicately fibrillar material. The membranes of the cavities (cisternae) are studded with ribosomes. Hence the designation rough, or granular, reticulum. Mitochondria are seen at the left of the field. The endoplasmic reticulum divides the cell into compartments.

enzymes), osteoblasts (collagen), and liver cells (albumin, fibrinogen). The granular reticulum also exists in neurons and is called the Nissl substance. The granules on this system of membrane are attached polyribosomes, which synthesize specific proteins that are directly transferred across the membrane into the cavity called a cisterna. Here the newly synthesized proteins are sequestered from the general cytoplasmic compartment and are transported by a system of channels and vacuoles through the Golgi complex, which is a system of smooth membranes located near the nucleus, to the exterior of the cell, where they fulfill their appropriate destiny.

All cells contain ribosomes. However, as we have described, only some cells have their ribosomes directly attached to membranes, presumably for the express purpose of directing the synthesis of protein into a particular compartment. In most cells, ribosomes lie about in the cytoplasm until they are called to synthesize proteins. During this time they can be visualized as helical clusters or pearl-necklace arrangements along a messenger RNA molecule (Fig. 1–13). Their protein product is for cellular consumption as in the erythrocyte (hemoglobin) or the muscle cell (actin or myosin).

There is another part of the endoplasmic reticulum, those membranes without ribosomes, the so-called agranular reticulum. This system of smooth membranes (Fig. 1–14) is seen most obviously in tissues that synthe-

size steroid hormones and lipids, that are concerned with salt and water transportation, or that are involved in detoxification, as in liver cells. In each case, the type of the membranes, their arrangement, and their basic chemical structure may be different. In general, however, it is safe to say that whereas the granular reticulum is concerned with the synthesis of protein, usually designed for secretion, the agranular reticulum functions in a different way. The Golgi complex can be considered a special example of the agranular reticulum (Fig. 1–15).

The pathway for intracellular synthesis, secretion, and transport has been elucidated during the last 25 years, principally by Palade and his group. A scheme illustrating this pathway is shown in Figure 1–16. This pathway depends on energy derived from mitochondria and on direction derived from the genome (total gene complement) to achieve its goal. It also depends on the necessary substrates, such as amino acids, essential fatty acids, carbohydrates, and vitamins or coenzymes. A single perturbation in this elaborate network will destroy the normal sequence. The substitution of a single amino-acid analog for an essential amino acid will grossly distort the normal subcellular pattern as shown in the accompanying diagrams (Fig. 1–17).

LYSOSOMES. Membrane-bound bodies containing powerful digestive enzymes, lysosomes can be regarded as part of the digestive

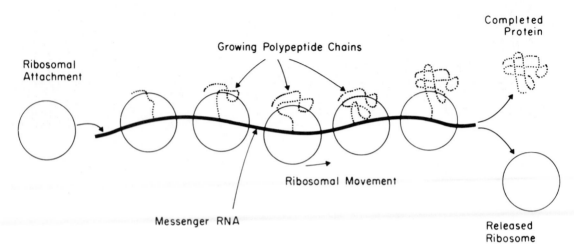

Fig. 1–13. This drawing shows a ribosome schematically attached to messenger RNA, and the nascent protein developing from the ribosome appears as a coiled set of small dots.

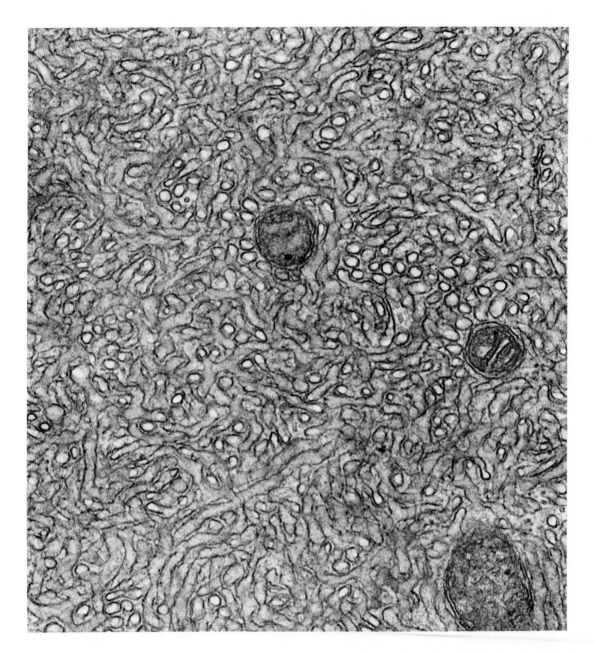

Fig. 1–14. Electron micrograph shows another type of membrane structure, the smooth reticulum, which has been associated with synthesis of steroid hormone, lipid metabolism, and detoxification of drugs and other metabolites. No RNP particles are seen in this field. Three small mitochondrial profiles are present.

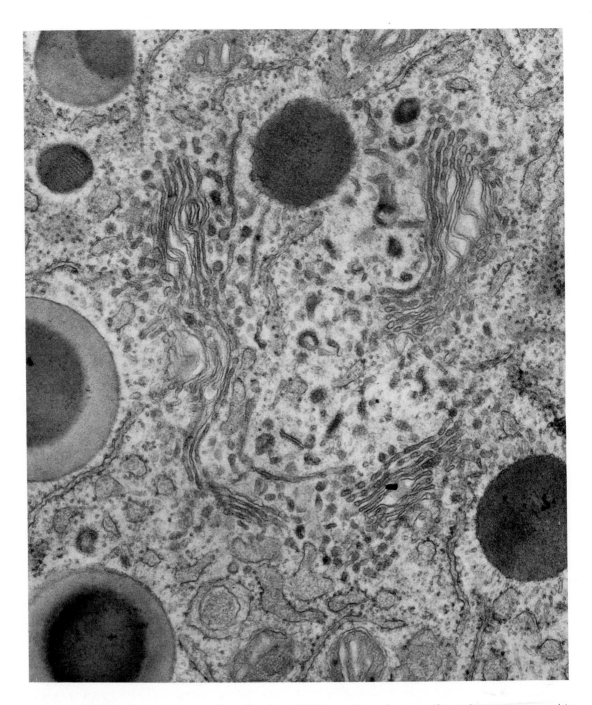

Fig. 1–15. Electron micrograph shows a horseshoe-shaped Golgi complex, where smooth membranes are arranged in parallel. The Golgi complex has been regarded as a packaging and shipping area for the segregation of materials that will be secreted by cells. The large dense granules contain enzymes in an inactive form.

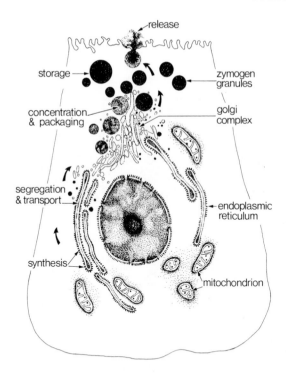

release

storage

concentration & packaging

segregation & transport

synthesis

zymogen granules

golgi complex

endoplasmic reticulum

mitochondrion

Fig. 1–16. This drawing illustrates the pathways of protein synthesis in the pancreatic acinar cell, and demonstrates the relationship between the different anatomical units and their function. (From Bloom, W., and Fawcett, D.W.: *A Textbook of Histology*, 10th Ed. Philadelphia, W. B. Saunders, 1975.)

to cross the membrane of the cell and thereby to enter into the cytoplasm proper.

MICROTUBULES. Another cytoplasmic organelle, microtubules, were not recognized until relatively recently as a part of most cells. These long, straight, thin structures appear most frequently in cells with asymmetrical shapes such as neurons (axons) or spermatozoa, and have been identified as the element responsible for movement in cilia and flagella. All cells during division have masses of microtubules, for they compose the mitotic apparatus. Microtubules may serve as a cellular skeletal apparatus, or they may perform a more dynamic role by providing a mechanism for motility. It seems likely that in the case of cilia, flagella, and the mitotic apparatus, **actin** (half of the energy-producing protein, actomyosin) is associated with the microtubules and provides the driving force for the sliding motion currently thought to be the mechanism by which this movement occurs.

Just as there may be abnormalities in mitochondria or in the endoplasmic reticulum, so there may be abnormalities in the microtubules of cells. One example discovered recently is an abnormal structure of cilia, which are responsible for clearing our airways of foreign particles, for propelling ova along the fallopian tubes, and for the motility of sperm.

Immotile but living spermatozoa were found in the semen of 4 men who were sterile. The sperm tail appeared as in rigor, that is, straight, stiff, and with no motility. Electron microscopy showed the spermatozoa to be relatively normal except that so-called dynein arms were not present (Fig. 1–18). Dynein arms are structures that form temporary cross bridges between adjacent ciliary filaments in normal cilia, flagella, and sperm tails, and are believed to be responsible for generating the movements of cilia or sperm tails.

Three of the 4 subjects had had, since childhood, chronic sinusitis and bronchitis, and frequent bouts of pneumonia, common cold, and ear infection.

Study of the tracheobronchial clearance in the three subjects revealed that there was no measurable mucociliary transport. Ordinary tracheobronchial clearance was nearly or totally absent, when no coughing occurred, but a reasonably good substitute for this clearance could be obtained by permitting the subjects to cough. Cilia from the respiratory tract also lacked the dynein arms.

system of the cell, just as the mitochondria represent the power plants. One view suggests they may be called the stomach of the cell.

Different types of cells have different numbers of lysosomes, which contain different populations of enzymes. The macrophage, a wandering scavenger, contains a rich and powerful store of lysosomes, as do polymorphonuclear leukocytes, for example.

Lysosomes are conventionally united with vacuoles that contain ingested particles. The original vacuole is called a phagosome; without the presence of appropriate digestive enzymes its role is limited to the suspension of the particle. When digestive enzymes from the lysosome join the vacuole and fusion of the membranes takes place, the phagosome then becomes a digestive vacuole. Most particulate matter that has been ingested into a phagosome must be broken down before it can be assimilated into particles small enough

	NUCLEUS	NUCLEOLUS	ERGASTOPLASM	GOLGI	MITOCHONDRIA	ZYMOGEN
STOCK DIET						
2 HRS.						
18 HRS.						
2 DAYS						
5-8 DAYS						
10 DAYS						

A

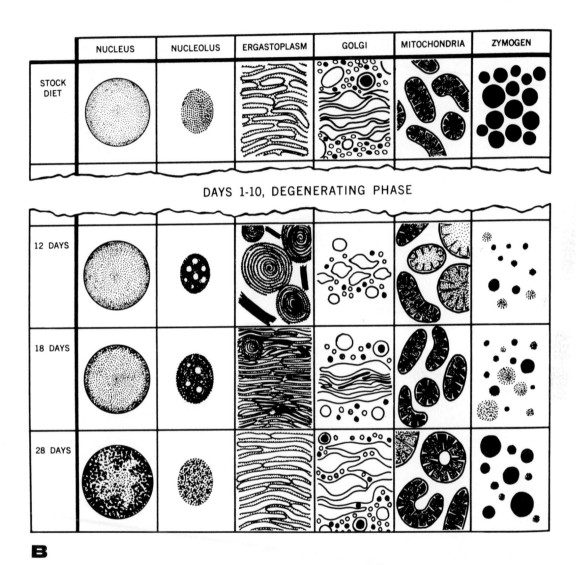

Fig. 1–17. *A* and *B,* These diagrams show the effect on the nucleus, nucleolus, rough endoplasmic reticulum, mitochondria, and cell products (zymogen granules), of the administration of ethionine, an amino acid analog of methionine, to guinea pigs. Over a period of days, the pancreas cells are unable to synthesize normal products. The cytoplasm and the nucleus reflect this inability. (*A,* From Herman, L., and Fitzgerald, P.: The degenerative changes in pancreatic acinar cells caused by DL-ethionine. J. Cell Biol., *12*:277, 1962. *B,* from Herman, L., and Fitzgerald, P.: Restitution of pancreatic acinar cells following ethionine. J. Cell Biol., *12*:297, 1962.)

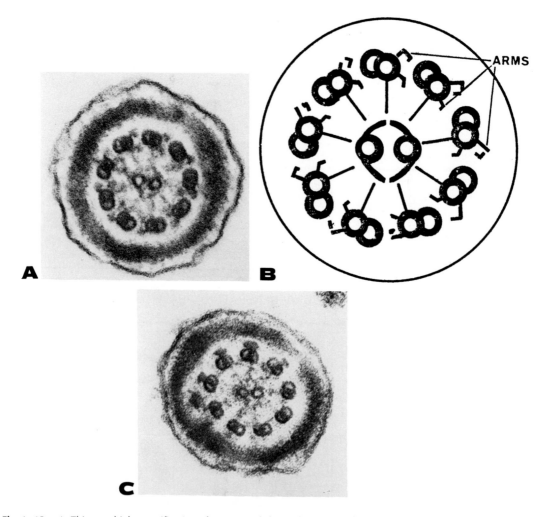

Fig. 1–18. *A,* This very high magnification of a sperm tail shows the normal microtubule structure and arms. The arms are better seen in the drawing, *B. C,* Section from a patient with immotile spermatozoa. The arms of the microtubules are not present. (From Afzelius, B.A.: A human syndrome caused by immotile cilia. Science, *193*:317, 1976.)

Three of the subjects had *situs inversus totalis* (their organs were placed in the reverse position in their bodies).

From these findings, 2 tentative conclusions are drawn. The cells of the 4 men cannot synthesize normal dynein arms, or if such dynein arms are formed, they cannot attach to the ciliary filaments; this causes immotility of spermatozoa and cilia. Visceral asymmetry is determined through the movements of cilia of some embryonic epithelial tissues.

The foregoing, then, illustrates how new observations on such a tiny structure as the cilia of a cell shed light on the reasons for infection, infertility, and even the mechanisms of development.

EXTRACELLULAR MATERIAL

The immediate environment of the cell is also of interest, for the ebb and flow of energy does not stop at the entrance to the cell. Just as one can reconstruct much of the life within a house by examination of the contents of its trash bin, so one should be aware of the materials that lie immediately adjacent to the cell. Epithelial cells sit on a basement membrane, and most of them are polarized with an outer surface and a basal surface. Along both sides they are usually attached to one another by junctions, across which they may communicate. Their secretory products are released at their apex either onto a free surface or into a duct.

Another class of cells, the connective tissue cell, is extremely important in repairing damage to tissue and in maintaining the integrity of the interstitial space. Its principal products are collagen and complex sugars (glycosaminoglycans), and we shall have more to say about this material in the chapter on the musculoskeletal system (Fig. 1–19).

Many kinds of enzymes are normally extruded by inflammatory cells, interstitial cells, and wandering cells into the extracellular or interstitial spaces.

Mitosis. Reference has already been made to the varying life span of cells. Some are short-lived, whereas others enjoy a long life. In either case, when they die they are replaced by new cells. (An important and sad exception to this rule is the cells of the brain and spinal cord; once these are destroyed, as in cerebral hemorrhage or poliomyelitis, they cannot be replaced, although in some instances their function can be learned by other cells.) In unicellular organisms, new cells are created by the division of the preexisting cell. In all the higher forms, new cells arise through mitosis or **mitotic division** (Fig. 1–20). A nucleus in the process of mitosis is referred to as a mitotic figure.

Mitotic figures are seldom seen in normal tissue because relatively few cells are dying and being replaced, but, as might be expected, they are common in the growing embryo. Cell division is frequent in the repair of wounds and in the replacement of excised tissue, especially in the liver. Examination of mitotic figures is of particular importance in the case of tumors, in which mitotic figures are not only numerous, but often atypical in

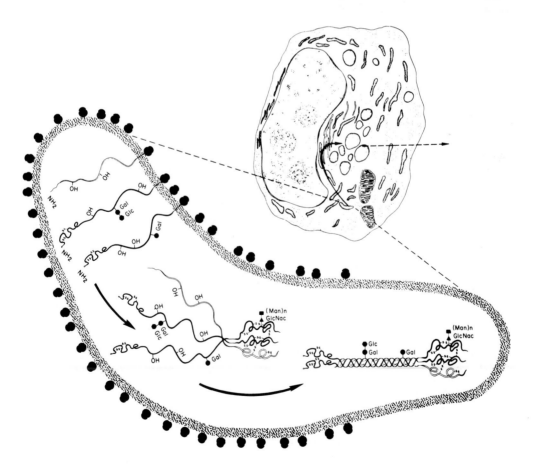

Fig. 1–19. This drawing illustrates the biosynthesis of collagen in the rough endoplasmic reticulum (ER) showing the vectorial transfer of a new protein into the compartment of the rough endoplasmic reticulum. (From Prockop, D.J., et al.: The biosynthesis of collagen and its disorders. N. Engl. J. Med., *301*:13, 1979.)

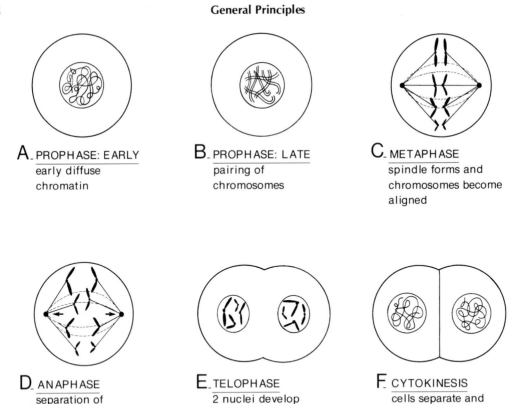

A. PROPHASE: EARLY
early diffuse
chromatin

B. PROPHASE: LATE
pairing of
chromosomes

C. METAPHASE
spindle forms and
chromosomes become
aligned

D. ANAPHASE
separation of
chromosomes

E. TELOPHASE
2 nuclei develop

F. CYTOKINESIS
cells separate and
chromosomes diffuse

Fig. 1-20.   These drawings illustrate different phases in mitosis.

appearance. This may enable the pathologist to decide whether he or she is examining a benign tumor or a malignant one.

THE INJURED CELL

The complex and delicate structure and function of the cell may be damaged by a variety of influences, of which chemical poisons and bacterial toxins are obvious examples. The cell becomes injured, so that it does not function perfectly. This injury is reflected in changes in the microscopic appearance of the cytoplasm and later of the nucleus. These morphologic changes can be regarded as the fingerprints of disease; when the damage is slight, the prints can be erased. Although morphologic changes are of importance to the pathologist, they are of little interest to the reader of this book, and they will only be mentioned so that the reader will recognize the names when they are discussed. It is important to recognize that a cell may be

sick without showing any morphologic change. We are now coming to think of disease in terms of molecular alterations, not merely in terms of the cell. The work of the cell depends chiefly on the integrity and availability of enzymes. An altered enzyme may escape detection by the physician. A person who dies in the convulsions of tetanus (lockjaw) has a morphologically normal nervous system, although we know that it is profoundly, indeed fatally, abnormal.

Perhaps we should state here an important concept which is that although changes in function and structure are intimately related, and although we conventionally think that the functional change depends on change in morphology (heart failure can be shown to be due to a diseased valve), it is more likely that the earliest indications of disordered function show no disordered structure even with sophisticated modern methods.

We can also introduce the idea that, up to a point, injury to any organ, tissue, or cell may be entirely **reversible**, so that when ischemia (loss of blood supply) occurs, provided blood flow and oxygenation are restored within a few minutes, the tissue and cells will not die. However, when injury is severe (burns) and enzymes of a cell are denatured, **irreversible injury** is done, which results in an entirely different situation. We shall now consider some of the irreversible changes.

Necrosis, as the name implies (Greek *nekros*, corpse), is the local death of cells. The cellular changes characteristic of necrosis are changes that the cell undergoes after it has died while still remaining in the body, and are due to the action of enzymes contained within those cells (in lysosomes). These enzymes turn their energies on the framework of the cell itself, a process known as **autolysis**. Death of the cell may be due to (1) chemical poisons, (2) bacterial toxins, (3) physical agents such as irradiation, and (4) most commonly, loss of blood supply due to closure of an artery by thrombosis. This last phenomenon is known as an **infarct**; cellular death in this instance is caused by the sudden cutting off of the supply of oxygen to the cell, that is to say, **anoxia**. Over a period of many hours or a few days the nucleus breaks up and disappears, and the cytoplasm becomes indistinct and fades away, with eventual **liquefaction necrosis**. In the case of some bacterial infections such as tuberculosis, the structural outlines of the affected part are wiped out. This process is known as caseation necrosis because the gross appearance of the material is

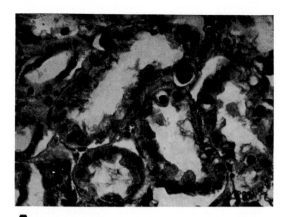

A

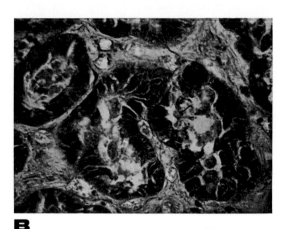

B

Fig. 1–21. *A*, Normal renal tubules. *B*, Tubules from an infarcted area showing coagulation necrosis. Note absence of nuclei and homogeneous cytoplasm. Photomicrograph. (From Bell: *Textbook of Pathology*, Philadelphia, Lea & Febiger.)

Table 1–1.   Types of Necrosis

TYPE	CAUSE	APPEARANCE	DISEASE
Coagulative	Ischemic cell death followed by denaturation of proteins	Basic outline of cells preserved for a period of time Loss of nuclei Increased eosinophilia of tissue	Infarcts in most tissue except brain
Liquefactive	Digestion of cells by intracellular and leukocytic enzymes	"Pus"	Brain infarcts Focal bacterial lesions (abscess)
Caseous	Tubercle bacillus inciting granulomatous inflammation with destruction of tissue	White, cheesy, "putty"	Tuberculosis
Fat	Abnormal release of pancreatic enzymes	Chalky, white flecks	Acute pancreatic necrosis

cheesy, or caseous. In an infarct, on the other hand, the general outline of microscopic structure can still be recognized, such as the tubules and glomeruli in the kidney, and the muscle fibers in the heart. The difference between the necrosis of an infarct and caseation is the difference between the site of ancient Pompeii, in which the outline of the streets can still be recognized, and the site of the destruction of Hiroshima (Fig. 1–21). Different types of necrosis are outlined in Table 1–1.

Somatic death is death of the body as a whole. It occurs when respiration and the heart's action cease, although individual cells and even tissues may continue to live for short periods. Soon characteristic changes begin to make their appearance in the dead body. The most striking of these are: (1) loss of response to stimuli; (2) cessation of the circulation, which can be seen with an ophthalmoscope in the small blood vessels of the retina; (3) gradual approach to the temperature of the environment (algor mortis); (4) muscular rigidity due to chemical changes in the muscle (rigor mortis), the stiffness beginning in 4 hours or more and passing off in about 3 days; (5) a reddish discoloration of the dependent parts of the body (livor mortis) due to the sinking of the blood from gravity combined with a breaking down (hemolysis) of the red blood cells; (6) postmortem clotting of the blood. The doctor or the detective in the story book can tell to within a few minutes how long the body has been dead, but so many factors, such as fever, high external temperature, and violent exercise at the time of death may influence the speed of the postmortem changes that anything approaching accuracy is out of the question. A note of these changes, however, may be useful in making a rough estimate of the time of death for medicolegal purposes.

We may conclude our necessarily brief study of that remarkable structure, the living cell, with the vivid words of Osgood in an address to the American Society of Medical Technologists: "In summary, can you imagine a mobile, self-reproducing factory, which selects its own raw materials, manufactures not one but many products, rebuilds and repairs itself constantly, provides its own power supply, has automatic local and remote controls, transports its fuels, products and waste products with great efficiency, which may be versatile or specialized, but is integrated by efficient communication systems with the needs of the community, and always provides reserves for emergencies? Such a factory is the cell."

We have considered the cell, together with the body fluids and metabolism, which make the life of the cell possible and give it meaning as the basic unit in the living body. Let us now turn our attention to a brief discussion of the systems that bring nutrients and oxygen to the cell, prepare the food for absorption, excrete waste products, make intercommunication between the cells and organs possible, and, finally, meet the supreme challenge of reproduction. All of these will be discussed in greater detail when we study the diseases of these system in Part 2 of this book.

BODY FLUIDS

In addition to considering the cells of the body we must recognize the importance of their environment, the interstitial spaces and fluids which surround them. After all, the nutrients on which they depend must diffuse across a few microns of interstitial space before they can be used, and the waste products of cellular metabolism must be carried away from the cells, which would otherwise drown in their own by-products.

Body fluids are of 3 kinds: tissue fluid, blood, and lymph. (1) **Tissue fluid**, or interstitial fluid, surrounds and bathes the cells; it is placid, a lake, not a stream. (2) **Blood** is contained in the blood vessels, and nowhere comes in direct contact with the tissues except in the spleen. It is carried to an organ in arteries. These break up into a vast network of capillaries, through whose infinitely thin walls the fluid of the blood (plasma or serum) is able to pass, mixing with the tissue fluid and carrying into it nutrients and oxygen that the waiting cells absorb. On the return voyage, such metabolic by-products as lactic acid and CO_2 are carried in the capillaries to the venules and veins back to the heart. Since tissue fluid continually increases in amount, it is obvious that there must be some means of escape. This is provided by (3) **lymph**, which, like the blood, is contained in a set of vessels, the lymphatics. The tissue fluid laden with waste products from the living cells passes through the thin walls of the lymphatics and is carried away as lymph. This is a round-about way of getting back into the veins, for all the lymphatics eventually form 1 or 2 main ducts, which open into the large veins in the neck. The advantage of this method is that the lymph has to pass through a series of filters, known as **lymph nodes**, in which bacteria and other injurious agents that may have gained access to the tissue fluid are strained out and are usually destroyed. A significant proportion of the tissue fluid passes directly back through the walls of the vessels into the blood stream.

It is possible to estimate the rate of passage of water from the vessels into the tissue spaces by injecting some traceable substance, such as a radioactive isotope, into a vein and noting the rapidity with which it disappears from the blood. The rate of exchange shown by this method is incredibly fast, for **more than 70% of the water of the blood is exchanged with extravascular water every minute.** The walls of the smaller capillaries appear to be veritable sieves with regard to water.

The principal mechanism by which this exchange is achieved was elucidated by the great English physiologist, Starling, who hypothesized that small molecules and water under the influence of the hydrostatic pressure at the arteriolar end of the capillary leave this delicate vessel, but large molecules such as the proteins, albumin, and fibrinogen cannot. At the venular end of the capillary the small molecules and water are attracted by the

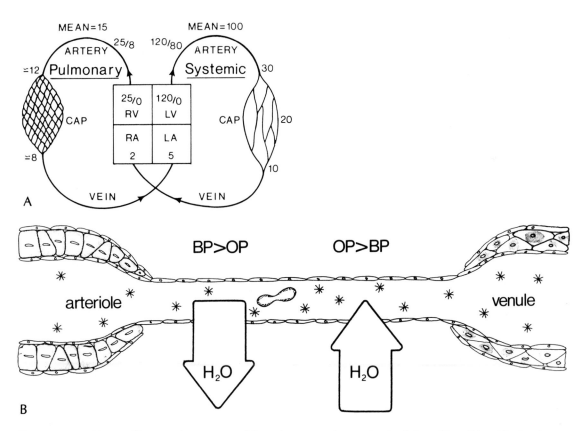

Fig. 1–22. A, Diagram illustrates the pressures of the pulmonary and systemic circulations. (From West, J.B.: *Respiratory Physiology.* Baltimore, Williams & Wilkins, 1974.); B, This drawing illustrates the equilibrium for exchange at the level of the capillary. The arteriole is shown at the left and protein is represented by stars within the capillary lumen. The large arrow shows the net transfer of water and small molecules out at the arteriolar end, and the transfer of water in at the venular end. The osmotic value of the serum proteins exceeds that of the intracapillary pressure at the venular end, thereby attracting fluids back in and maintaining the circulation's integrity.

high osmotic value of the intracapillary protein, and so water returns across the capillary cell to the blood. The pressure relationships in the circulatory systems are illustrated in the accompanying diagrams (Fig. 1–22).

It is important to recognize that if there are alterations in the pressure relationships, in the protein quantity, or in the nature of the capillary cells, there may be a disequilibrium that leads to **edema**, which is discussed in the following section. The different mechanisms that lead to an increased interstitial fluid accumulation can now be explained.

Water and Salt. The most important single constituent of the body is water, for water is the sustenance of everything that lives. Hunger can be endured for days or weeks, but thirst is unendurable; the cells of the whole body cry out for water, not merely the parched mouth. Life started in the water in the dim and distant past, for the sea is the original home of all life on the globe; even vertebrate life first appeared as a marine form. We still live in a watery environment, not, as we fondly imagine, in the air. For the surface of the body in contact with the air is either dead (the horny layers of the skin) or is separated from the air by a layer of water (eyes, nose, and mouth). After all, we are completely immersed in water during the first 9 months of life before birth. The baby consists mostly of water, whereas the old man or woman

shrivels up like a wilted plant (Fig. 1–23). In the salt content of the blood plasma and in the film of salt water through which we look on the outside world we carry the memory of the remote, ancient ocean in which we originated. Still more do we carry this modified salt water in the interstitial fluid, which constitutes what the great French physiologist Claude Bernard, more than 100 years ago, called the internal environment.

The water of the body, together with the salts or electrolytes (substances decomposed in solution by electricity) that are dissolved in it, is contained in two major compartments: (1) intracellular, and (2) extracellular. The **intracellular fluid** makes up nearly 30% of the body weight, the bulk of it being contained in muscle. The **extracellular fluid** is mainly represented by the interstitial fluid, with a much smaller amount in the blood plasma. It is the fluid in the interstitial space that constitutes the real internal environment, and the freest communication exists through the cell membrane between the water in this compartment and the water inside the cells. The passage of fluids or solutions through a membrane is known as osmosis; this is the passage from the less concentrated to the more concentrated side of the membrane. Osmolality represents the osmotic concentration of a solute. Thus for each cell in the body the same conditions prevail as for the single-celled creatures fixed on the bed of a flowing stream that brings to them their food and oxygen and carries away their waste products. The cells are bathed in salty fluids; without that fluid they cannot live. They are indeed islands in the interstitial sea. In many diseases, such as cholera, this fluid is drained away from the body, the tissues become dehydrated, and they will die unless the water is replaced.

It is the delicate balance of electrolytes and water that serves to maintain the constancy of the internal environment, the importance of which Bernard was the first to emphasize. For the preservation of this constancy the mechanism of **homeostasis** has been evolved. Important instruments in the homeostatic orchestra are the kidney, which modulates the salt and water music; the lung, which also modifies the pH of the body, the pituitary and adrenal, which dictate obligato passages for

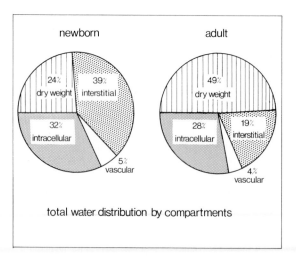

total water distribution by compartments

Fig. 1–23. This diagram shows the relative distribution of water by compartments in both the newborn and the adult human being.

salt and water; and the liver, which provides a bass by means of albumin synthesis. When the autoregulatory system breaks down we see the clinical picture that we call disease, a breakdown which, if sufficiently profound and prolonged, results in death due to acidosis, hyperkalemia (high serum potassium), or other fatal disorders.

The subject of the internal environment has become more important in the present day than in bygone years, not only to the physician, but also to other members of the health team, partly because of the strong likelihood of its being changed when the patient— especially the surgically treated patient—is placed in a hospital bed and fluids begin to flow into his veins, and partly because the physician, and still more the surgeon and the pediatrician, can do so much to correct disturbances of this environment, and to safeguard health and life itself in the process.

We have seen that an adequate and constant supply of tissue fluid is necessary for the health of the body cells. If this supply is insufficient, or if the fluid is withdrawn too quickly, a condition of **dehydration** develops, which can be recognized by the sunken appearance of the face and by the wrinkled condition of the skin. This may develop quickly, as after a night of hard drinking, or in acute diseases associated with severe vomiting or profuse diarrhea. Dehydration and loss of salt may be the result of excessive sweating, as is seen in the tropics or the desert and in men working under conditions of great heat. When the heat of Arabia comes out like a drawn sword and strikes you speechless, you realize that water comes before everything. In such cases it is important to drink amounts of fluid to which salt has been added. On the other hand, tissue fluid may accumulate in excessive amounts, so that the part becomes waterlogged, a condition known as **edema**. This can be recognized by the fact that when a finger is pressed into the swollen part, a temporary pit is formed, owing to the fluid's being forced away into the surrounding tissues. Edema may be caused in many ways. (1) In **inflammation,** the walls of the capillaries become unduly permeable and too much fluid passes from the blood into the tissue spaces. (2) In heart and kidney disease, edema is an important symptom; it may be caused by **fluid retention, albumin loss,** or by **increased hydrostatic pressure** in the veins and in the capillaries. (3) **Pressure on the lymphatics** by a tumor will also be accompanied by edema.

Derangements of the body fluids are discussed further in Chapter 4.

The following review of the normal physiologic processes may provide readers with a common framework to support the ideas and descriptions presented in the remainder of the text.

METABOLISM

The sum total of the chemical reactions that proceed in that remarkable laboratory, the living cell, is called metabolism. There are many cellular laboratories that do different kinds of work, and each individual laboratory can do various kinds of work. Intermediary metabolism is the chemical transformation of foodstuffs in the body so that they can be used. The essence of metabolism is change (Greek *metabole,* change), and the change may be a breaking down (catabolism), or a building up (anabolism). The 3 main constituents of food are proteins, carbohydrates, and fats. All contain carbon, hydrogen, and oxygen, but proteins are also distinguished by their content of nitrogen, which has to be built into the cells to make up for the loss that occurs in the wear and tear of activity. Proteins are made up of a large number of small units differing from one another; these units are the **amino acids**. Speaking generally, proteins are used for body building, whereas carbohydrates and fats are used for the production of energy. Carbohydrates and fats have been compared with gasoline and oil in an automobile, but it is protein that replaces worn parts. We usually picture the protein of meat being built up into body protein, and so on with the other food stuffs. It is now known that the derivatives of the ingested protein, carbohydrate, and fat of the diet pass into a common metabolic pool, in which one basic foodstuff can be converted into another according to need before being built into the tissues. The essential purpose of this disintegration is to provide energy, some of which is used to perform mechanical work, some to support metabolic processes, the remainder appearing as heat. All living systems require an external source of energy for growth and activity. Plants obtain their energy directly from the sun by virtue of the photosynthesis effected by their chlorophyll. By means of photosynthesis, plants build simple substances (carbon dioxide of the air and water) into more complex ones (starch, sugar, cellulose). In all other organisms energy originally comes from the sun by way of the plants. Thus it is that animals and plants must depend on each other. When we regard a plate of beefsteak with a liberal helping of vegetables, we are really looking at a plateful of energy. Pyruvic acid is a key substance in intermediary metabolism, as it represents a stage reached by all the foodstuffs, not only carbohydrate, but also protein and fat. The various complex steps by which pyruvic acid is broken down with the liberation of energy is known as the Krebs cycle. (For his work Krebs received the Nobel prize.) The energy is trapped or bound as "energy-rich phosphate bonds," more particularly adenosine triphosphate, for convenience known as ATP. This trapped energy can suddenly be released like the combustion of gunpowder when the call comes. What brings about these dramatic changes?

Enzymes. The profound importance of the biologic catalysts known as enzymes in every phase of metabolism has now come to be fully recognized. A catalyst is a substance that can enormously speed up a reaction without itself becoming altered or forming a part of the product of that reaction, so that it can be used over and over again an almost infinite number of times. Enzymes bring about reactions that, without them, would require great heat and strong chemicals. Enzymes are protein molecules, and over 600 of them have been isolated. They are remarkably specific for all kinds of proteins, carbohydrates, and fats—specialists in the true sense of the word. Indeed the specificity is so precise that it may be likened to the fit of a key for a lock, as if to make sure that the right chemicals undergo the right reactions at the right time. The substance on which a specific enzyme acts is known as the substrate. Many enzymes are inactive unless united with a nonprotein organic molecule, known as a coenzyme, which is therefore as important as the enzyme itself. Many vitamins are coenzymes.

Enzymes may pass out of the cell and take part in the digestion of food, as is the case in the enzymes of the saliva, the gastric juice, and the secretion of the pancreas, which is poured into the intestine. Or they may act inside the cell. It is customary to name enzymes by adding the suffix "-ase" to the name of the substrate, as in maltase and lipase. Some, however, retain their original names in popular usage, such as pepsin in gastric juice, and trypsin in pancreatic juice. The cellular enzymes may spill over into the blood when produced in excess, and their detection in the blood stream may be of great diagnostic value. Thus the presence of acid phosphatase may confirm a suspicion of cancer of the prostate, and the same is true of creatine phosphokinase in the case of myocardial infarction caused by coronary artery occlusion.

Enzymes belong to 2 great groups as regards their action on the substrate; they may be (1) hydrolytic or (2) oxidizing. The hydrolytic enzymes are those concerned more particularly with the digestion of food, and are therefore found in the mouth, the stomach, and the intestine. Hydrolysis involves the decomposition of a substance owing to the incorporation of water, followed by a splitting into simpler compounds with smaller molecules that are able to pass through the intestinal mucosa into the blood stream. Thus protein is split into amino acids (acids containing one or more amino or NH_2 groups), and the hydrolytic enzymes then recombine the products of digestion to build up complex tissue, proteins, carbohydrates, and fats.

The oxidizing enzymes are concerned more particularly with the metabolism of carbohydrates and the intracellular production of energy. All the activities of the cell require energy, and this energy is derived from the oxidation of carbohydrates and, to a lesser degree, of fats and proteins. As a result of the oxidation of carbohydrate, carbon is converted to carbon dioxide (CO_2) and the hydrogen to water (H_2O), while energy is released. The body may be compared to a gasoline engine, which also burns carbon and hydrogen. In an engine, heat represents a source of energy, but in the body it is a waste product representing energy the cells have failed to use and expressed as calories.

It becomes evident that respiration is not basically a matter of breathing air into and out of the lungs, but rather an interchange of oxygen in the course of intermediate metabolism within the cell, known as cellular respiration. The oxidative enzymes of the Krebs cycle have been pictured as arranged in an orderly manner on the shelves of the cristae of the mitochondria, the ultimate purpose of the mechanism being the synthesis of adenosine triphosphate (ATP). With this picture in mind, we can visualize how a poisonous compound such as carbon tetrachloride may play havoc with the physiology (functioning) of the liver cells by penetrating them, attacking the mitochondria, paralyzing their enzymes, and thus disrupting the Krebs cycle and the production of ATP. The cyanides and hydrocyanic acid (prussic acid) are deadly poisons because they damage the respiratory enzymes that normally transfer oxygen from the hemoglobin of the red blood cells to the cells of the tissue. Thus all the tissues immediately suffer from lack of oxygen (anoxia), although the blood cells remain oxygenated and therefore bright red. It may be noted in passing that cancer cells appear to have fewer mitochondria than normal, perhaps because these cells are more concerned with reproduction (mitotic division) than with functional activity.

CIRCULATION

The **circulatory system** is the mechanism by which fresh material is sent to the tissue fluid and waste material is removed from it. The fresh material is of 2 kinds, food and oxygen. The food is contained in the blood from the intestine, the oxygen in the blood from the lungs. Because the blood has to circulate from the intestine and lungs to the tissue fluid and back again, a pump is required. This pump is the **heart**, which is simply a hollow muscle. Contraction of the body muscles helps to force the lymph through the lymphatics, and when this is interfered with as the result of disease, massage may take its place. The blood from the tissues contains waste products, in the form of solid material in solution, and gas (carbon dioxide), also in solution. The solid material in solution is excreted, mainly by the kidneys, but also by the skin. If the kidneys go on strike, the skin may be stimulated to do at least part of the work through increased perspiration. The carbon dioxide in the blood is given off in the lungs and expired. At the same time oxygen is breathed in and taken up by the blood, as a result of which the color of the blood becomes a much brighter red. The system of blood vessels with the blood they contain (vascular system) is comparable to a system of roads and railways by means of which intercommunication between different parts of the cell state is maintained.

The tissues contain abundant reserves of water, salts, proteins, carbohydrates, and fat. These reserves can be used when the need arises. Unfortunately, oxygen is not stored anywhere; it must be unceasingly supplied to the body by the lungs, for the blood contains only a three-minute supply at any given moment. This is why the absence of oxygen or anoxia can only be tolerated for the shortest time, and is rapidly fatal to a tissue such as heart muscle or to the nervous system.

An organ is like a pond completely filled with aquatic plants and fed by a small brook. The water in the pond is nearly stagnant, and is polluted by waste products of the plants. The degree of stagnation and pollution depends on the volume and rapidity of the stream. This is the reason why the health of every organ suffers in the condition of prolonged heart disease known as congestive heart failure.

Blood from the body is carried to the heart by veins and is then sent by the pulmonary artery to the lungs to be oxygenated. The blood from the lungs is also carried to the heart by another set of veins, the pulmonary veins. It is evident that if these 2 kinds of blood were allowed to mix in the heart, the whole object of the circulation would be defeated. The cavity of the heart is therefore divided by a longitudinal septum or partition into 2 sides, right and left. The right side receives the deoxygenated blood from the body and sends it to the lungs. The left side receives the oxygenated blood from the lungs and sends it throughout the body in the arteries. Like any other pump, the heart is provided with valves, so that the blood will always move in one direction. If these are diseased, the blood may leak back through the valves, with great disturbance to the circulation. The names and arrangement of the valves and of the various

chambers of the heart will be considered in connection with diseases of that organ.

RESPIRATION

The **respiratory system** is designed to bring air, or rather oxygen, from the outside to the cells in the innermost recesses of the body. The air is inhaled through the trachea or windpipe into the lungs, where it is brought into intimate contact with a vast network of capillaries through the thin walls of which the oxygen is able to pass. It is seized on by the hemoglobin of the red blood corpuscles and is carried throughout the body. When the capillaries of the tissues are reached, the oxygen leaves the red blood cells, passes through the capillary walls, enters the tissue fluid, and is taken up by the cells. The energy of cells is obtained from the oxidation of food, particularly carbohydrates. At the same time the tissues give off one of their waste products in the form of a gas, carbon dioxide. The carbon dioxide passes into the venous blood, the plasma carrying 3 times as much as the red cells, and is taken up by the disengaged red blood corpuscles, carried back to the lungs, discharged into the air spaces of those organs, and exhaled into the outside air (Chap. 15). Tissue or cellular respiration is therefore the real meaning and reason for the rising and falling of the chest that we commonly call respiration.

DIGESTION

The **digestive system** is concerned with preparing the food that is to be carried by the blood to the tissue fluid for the nourishment of the cells. The tissue fluid must receive its food in the simplest form for conversion into the building stones of the body and the fuel that drives the engine. A beefsteak would be out of place in the tissue spaces; the cells would not know what to do with it. The work of preparing the food so that it may be used by the tissues is performed by the alimentary canal and by certain digestive glands, which are derived from the alimentary canal and pour their digestive juices into it. The alimentary canal consists of the **mouth**, where the food is broken by the teeth and acted on by the saliva; the esophagus or gullet, which is a mere passageway; the **stomach**, where the food is retained for some hours and is acted on by the gastric juice; the **small intestine**, where it is further digested and liquefied and from which it is absorbed; and the **large intestine**, which conducts the indigestible part of the food to the exterior. The food is converted into a soluble absorbable form by digestive juices, which are produced by collections of cells that form glands. The glands line the interior of the stomach and intestine and are also collected to form a most important digestive organ, the **pancreas**, which pours its digestive juice into the very beginning of the intestine. Bile from the liver also enters the bowel at the same point and assists in the digestion of fats.

The **liver** plays a much more important role in the use of foodstuffs than the mere production of bile, which in many respects is simply a waste product. The 3 main constituents of food are proteins, carbohydrates, and fats. We have already seen that all 3 contain carbon, hydrogen, and oxygen, and that protein in addition possesses nitrogen.

The complex **proteins** of the food are broken down in the intestine into their simplest elements, the amino acids or building stones of the body, still characterized by the possession of nitrogen. The amino acids and carbohydrates are absorbed into capillaries in the wall of the small intestine and carried to the liver by the portal vein. In the liver the portal vein breaks up into fine capillaries, which come into intimate contact with the liver cells, each of which is a little chemical factory filled with hardworking enzymes. Some of the amino acids pass on to the heart and are distributed to the tissues, where they serve the important function of body building. The rest of the amino acids lose their nitrogen in the liver, where it is converted into urea, a waste product that reaches the kidneys by the blood stream and is excreted in the urine as nonprotein nitrogen. The valuable non-nitrogenous portion (carbon and hydrogen) of these amino acids reaches the tissue cells, where it is used in the production of energy. This process of breaking down the protein of food into its constituents (catabolism) and of rebuilding these into the tissues of the body (anabolism) is graphically portrayed by Best and Taylor (*The Living Body*) in the following passage: "The utilization of protein in the construction of body tissue may be compared to the building of a number of houses of different types from materials derived from the wrecking of other structures. Each brick and stone in the old buildings must be separated and then sorted and carted to the new sites. Some of this building material will be more suitable for one type of house, some more suitable for other types. Other materials again will not be utilizable at all, and will therefore be discarded as refuse. The new buildings, though constructed from materials taken from the old, will be quite different in structure and in general plan."

The **carbohydrates** of the food are converted in the intestine into glucose or other sugars. From the intestine, glucose is absorbed into the capillaries and carried by the portal vein to the liver, where most of it is changed into a storage form known as glycogen and retained temporarily in the liver cells. Glucose is one of the important fuels of the body, necessary for muscular action and heat production. When fuel consumption is rapid, the carbohydrate depot, the liver, is called on to convert some of its glycogen into readily available glucose and to give it back to the blood for transportation to the muscles.

Some of the **fats** are carried to the liver by the portal vein; here they are converted into a form more readily available for use. The rest of the fat is absorbed into lymphatic vessels known as lacteals, and is carried by the thoracic duct to the great veins of the neck, where it enters the general circulation and is stored in the fat depots of the body.

It will be seen that the journey of the blood stream from the intestine to the tissues is somewhat in the nature of a cafeteria, various additions to the tray being made on the way. Denatured amino acids, now freed from their nitrogen and therefore no longer deserving of their name, are added by the liver; glycogen is converted into glucose when the storehouse in the liver is called on by the tissues; oxygen is added as the blood passes through the lungs; and fat is poured into the veins at the root of the neck.

EXCRETION

The **excretory system** is concerned with the removal of waste products from the body. This is brought about by the cooperation of a number of organs, i.e., the intestine, kidneys, skin, and lungs. The **intestine** offers the simplest example of an excretory organ. Food contains elements that are indigestible and cannot be used. These are passed on into the lower part of the bowel, the large intestine, from which they are discharged periodically as feces or stools. The **kidney** is a complex structure, the details of which will be considered in a later chapter, but the essential arrangement is not unlike that of the lung, except that fluid instead of gas leaves the blood. The arteries to the kidneys break up into fine capillaries, through the walls of which pass fluid from the blood together with waste substances in solution. The fluid or urine passes into tubules that open into a duct, the ureter; this duct carries the urine to the bladder, from which it is periodically discharged. The excretory function of the **lungs** has already been indicated. Here the waste product is carbon dioxide, which passes through the capillary walls into the air spaces or alveoli of the lungs and is breathed out through the trachea. The **skin** is an excretory organ by virtue of its sweat glands, which remove waste substances from the blood and pour them out on the surface in the fluid form of sweat. If the kidneys are not working properly, the sweating function of the skin can be stimulated by heat, and thereby relieve the kidneys of part of their load. The skin is a remarkable structure. Despite its thinness, it effectively protects the delicate internal structures and fluids against the unceasing variations of external conditions. It is moist, supple, elastic, and durable. Its durability is due to its being composed of several layers of cells that continually multiply.

These cells die while remaining united to one another like slates on a roof, slates that are continually blown away by the wind and continually replaced by new ones. All the openings in the skin except the nostrils are closed by elastic and contractile rings known as sphincters. Thus it is the almost perfectly fortified frontier of a closed world.

COMMUNICATIONS

From what has already been said, it is evident that the various highly specialized parts of the body are brought to work together for the common good. The runner breathes faster because his muscles need more oxygen; glycogen is converted into glucose when they need more sugar for energy; the rectum, the terminal portion of the large intestine, contracts (or should contract) so as to empty itself when it becomes full of feces; the eye is closed when threatened by a flying object; the foot is raised when its owner wishes to walk. What are the integrating influences that make the organs members of one another? They are of 2 kinds. One is telephonic or telegraphic in type, urgent in character, demanding instantaneous response; the messengers are **nervous impulses**, electrical in nature, and they are transmitted by the nervous system. The other may be compared to a special delivery service, slower but more detailed in character; the messengers are the **hormones**, chemical instead of electrical in nature, produced by the endocrine or ductless glands, and carried by the blood stream.

Nervous System. This system is singularly like a gigantic telephone organization, with a central exchange, an infinite number of wires, and receivers at the ends of these wires. The exchange is the brain and spinal cord, known collectively as the **central nervous system**, whereas the wires are represented by the nerves that form the **peripheral nervous sytem**. Some parts of the system act like automatic telephones without any conscious control; purely automatic messages are concerned in such functions as the beating of the heart, the contraction or dilation of the blood vessels, the swallowing of food, the movement of food along the intestine, the process of childbirth. The automatic messages are carried for the most part by a special set of nerves known as **autonomic** or sympathetic, which form the involuntary nervous system, although reflex action also plays some part in automatic responses.

The greater part of the nervous system is operated on the principle of a nonautomatic telephone exchange. On the surface of the body as well as in its interior there are myriads of receivers that, when stimulated, transmit sensations of various kinds to the spinal cord and thence to the brain, or directly to the brain. These receivers are known as receptors, some of which are specialized for the reception of sensations of sight, sound, taste, etc. (the special senses), whereas others respond to stimulation by giving rise to sensations of touch,

pain, heat, and cold. These varied sensations are carried to the central nervous system by afferent or sensory nerves, where they are sorted out and analyzed by the nerve cells of the brain. The sensory nerves form part of the voluntary nervous system, the other part of which is constituted by efferent or motor nerves. These nerves carry electrical messages from the nerve cells of the brain to the muscles, in response to which muscular contraction occurs. The actual stimulus that acts on the muscle fibers is apparently chemical in nature, for chemical substances of various kinds are liberated at the nerve endings when the nerves are stimulated. The structure of the nervous system is described in greater detail in Chapter 24.

Endocrine Glands. The other means by which intercommunication between organs is established is through the agency of the chemical messengers, the **hormones.** These are produced by the **endocrine** or ductless glands. Ordinary glands such as the salivary glands and pancreas pour out their secretion into the mouth or intestine through ducts. The endocrine glands have no ducts, and so discharge their secretion directly into the blood vessels with which they are in contact. These glands are among the most important structures in the body, for they control metabolism and regulate personality. In addition, they influence growth and reproduction. The effect that the ductless glands exert on the mind is equally striking, and the difference between endocrine health and disease may mean the difference between the finest mental power and imbecility. The principal endocrine glands are the pituitary at the base of the brain, the thyroid and parathyroids in the neck, the adrenals, the islets of Langerhans in the pancreas, and the gonads.

It would be absurd to attempt even to outline the complex functions of the endocrine organs in this place, but it may be noted that not only do they regulate the behavior of many of the tissues (e.g., the parathyroids determine the amount of calcium salts in the bones), but they also influence one another so as to act in harmony. They are like the instruments of a string quartet noted for its perfect ensemble, and the leader of the glandular orchestra is the pituitary, the master gland of the body. The pituitary produces hormones that influence the activity of the thyroid, the adrenals, and the ovaries, as well as other organs and glands.

The endocrines are stimulated to activity not only by hormones from other endocrine glands, but also by nervous stimuli. One simple example of this remarkable interrelationship must suffice. When a person is intensely activated by great rage or great fear, he is impelled to immediate muscular activity for purposes of either attack or flight. The muscles are called on to contract to the utmost of their ability, and therefore require a maximum supply of carbohydrate fuel in the shape of glucose. This is lying stored in the liver in the form of glycogen. A nervous stimulus passes from the brain along the nerves to the adrenal glands, and causes them to pour out their hormone, adrenalin (epinephrine). This is carried by the blood to the liver, where it causes the conversion of inert glycogen into active glucose. The glucose is carried by the blood to the muscles, supplying them with the fuel necessary for intense and immediate activity.

REPRODUCTION

The most complex of the mechanisms of the body is reproduction, but it is essentially simple in its elements. In the lowest forms of life, as in such a unicelluar organism as the ameba, reproduction is asexual. A line of division is formed along the middle of the cell, and the cellular constituents, first the nucleus and then the cytoplasm, divide into 2, one set passing to one-half of the cell, the other set to the other half. Finally, the line of division becomes complete and two new individuals are formed. This is called reproduction by fission. As both cells go on living, indeed need never die, they seem to enjoy the fountain of youth and can be regarded as immortal.

In all the higher forms of life reproduction is sexual in type, and is brought about by the union of two cells specially set aside for the purpose. They are known as the male and female **gametes** or germ cells, as distinguished from the body or **somatic cells**. The sex cells are produced by the male and female sex glands or gonads, the **testicle** with its tubules lined by germinal epithelium in the male, the **ovary** in the female. The male sex cells are the **spermatozoa** or sperm, the female sex cells are the **ova**. The sperm is a highly specialized cell with an oval flattened head and a long tail-like process, which, by violent lashing movements, propels the cell with great speed. In the human female, an ovum is liberated very month from the ovary and passes along a duct, the **fallopian tube**, to reach the **uterus** or womb, from which it is soon discharged in a flow of blood known as menstruation (Latin *mensis*, month). If impregnation is to occur, the male elements, the spermatozoa, ejected by the **penis** into the **vagina**, must pass through the uterus and enter the fallopian tube. (We are apt to think that fertilization of the ovum depends on sexual intercourse, but this is not necessarily so. For instance, the female salmon lays her eggs in a quiet pool, after which the male salmon comes along and fertilizes the eggs with his sperm.) It is breath-taking to learn that as many as 300,000,000 spermatozoa start the race for parenthood in mammals, but only a few hundred thousand get as far as the mouth of the cervix, probably because of dilution in the vagina and its acidic environment. A further obstacle awaits them, for many of the survivors enter the wrong tube, as only one tube contains the ovum. When the leading spermatozoon in the race encounters the ovum in the tube, its head, carrying the paternal chromosomes and genes,

penetrates the tough envelope of the ovum by means of an enzyme, hyaluronidase, its lashing tail is left behind because it is no longer needed, and impregnation has occurred. The sperm's remarkable journey has taken about twelve hours. A change at once occurs in the ovum's envelope, which renders it impermeable to any subsequent sperm that might wish to enter. When the male nucleus merges with that of the female, **fertilization** has taken place, and the result is **conception** and the creation of a new life. It is hard to believe, but the fertilized ovum, which is to produce all the mysteries of the human body in the course of a few months, is only the size of a grain of sand. The fertilized ovum continues on its way down the tube and enters the uterus. This time, however, it is not discharged, so that menstruation does not occur for the duration of the pregnancy. In the uterus it develops into an **embryo**, the original single fertilized cell at once beginning to divide and multiply, the resulting cells not separating from one another but becoming differentiated and arranged to form the infinitely varied tissues and organs, until in the fullness of time, 9 months in the case of the human being, a child is born.

There is one fundamental fallacy in the above account that the discerning reader will not fail to detect. We have seen previously that when a somatic cell divides, the chromosomes split longitudinally, one-half passing to each of the new cells, which therefore possess the correct number. How is it that the fertilized ovum, which is a combination of 2 cells, male and female, does not come to have twice the number of chromosomes that it ought to? The reason is that the germ cells, while still in their respective gonads, have undergone a process of **maturation** in anticipation of the impending fertilization. This is effected by a reduction division or meiosis. In the mitosis of somatic cells, each chromosome splits longitudinally and each pair separates into 2, so that each daughter cell contains the original number of 46. Since these consist of 23 pairs, somatic cells are said to have a **diploid** (Greek *diplous*, double) number of chromosomes. In the maturing germ cell there is no splitting of chromosomes, so that when division occurs each daughter cell contains only 23 chromosomes, which are said to be **haploid** (Greek *haplous*, single) in number. **The new germ cells, both male and female, contain only half the number of chromosomes and genes.** Fusion of the 2 gametes after fertilization results in a restoration of the chromosomes to their original number, but now one-half are maternal and one-half paternal in origin.

DETERMINATION OF SEX

The wish is sometimes expressed that something could be done to determine or to influence the sex of the unborn baby. This is particularly true in the case of farm animals. It also used to be true in the days when a king needed a male heir. It is felt that modern science, which can work other wonders, should be able to perform this miracle. The truth is that the sex of the newly created embryo has been determined at the moment of conception, and that nothing more can be done about it. To understand this we must take a second look at the chromosomes. These are divided into 44 **autosomes**, which are the ordinary chromosomes, and 2 **sex chromosomes**, which determine the future sex. In the immature female sex cell both sex chromosomes, known as **X chromosomes**, are alike and equal in size, so that when the cell matures and undergoes reduction division, each daughter cell has one X chromosome, which can be regarded as the hallmark of femaleness. In the immature male sex cell, on the other hand, one of the sex chromosomes is similar to the X chromosome of the female, but the other, known as the **Y chromosome**, is much smaller, and may be regarded as indicating maleness. It is evident that after reduction division of the male gamete, half of the sperm cells will receive an X chromosome and the other half a Y chromosome. If, now, the ovum containing one X chromosome should be fertilized by a sperm containing an X chromosome, a female (XX) will be produced, but if the sperm contains a Y chromosome, the result will be an XY individual, in other words a male. The result is pure chance and incapable of control.

Sex Chromatin. Unfortunately the matter is not always as simple as has just been suggested. When the gonads develop, the testicular or ovarian hormones that they produce profoundly influence what are called secondary sex characters, by which one is accustomed to distinguish a boy from a girl. Occasionally, owing to some defect in the genes, this development is not normal, and we are confronted with the tragic problem of **intersex**, when the child shares both male and female characteristics. In such cases a test for sex chromatin is of the greatest value. Thanks to the work of Murray Barr and his associates in 1949 at the University of Western Ontario, we now know that the cells of the body carry the fingerprints of their genetic sex, which may not correspond with the apparent somatic sex of the person. Barr has shown that a small mass of chromatin, the **sex chromatin**, lies against the nuclear membrane in about 85% of the cells of normal females, but in less than 10% of the cells of normal males. This chromatin mass, now known as the Barr body, is easy to see if you know what you are looking for, but no one before Barr realized its significance. The female cells are said to be **chromatin-positive**, and the male cells **chromatin-negative**. The most convenient source of cells is a smear made from the mucous membrane of the mouth. It would appear, as suggested by Mary Lyon, that in the somatic cells of the female one of the two chromosomes (one inherited from each parent) is genetically inactivated, be-

comes tightly coiled, and forms the sex chromatin or Barr body. There is at present no explanation for the occurrence of sex chromatin in a small proportion of male cells, unless it is related to the XY sex chromosome complex. With regard to the relation of sex to disease, nearly all the serious organic ailments are more common in the male, with the notable exception of disease of the gallbladder and, to a lesser degree, mitral stenosis. There appears to be an inherent weakness in the male, a sex-linked inferiority, so that by comparison with the female he is a weakling at all periods of life from conception to death. In the investigation of sterility, if the sex chromatin test reveals a discrepancy between apparent sex and chromosomal sex, the chances of fertility are practically nil. The question of sex reversal and other sex anomalies will be discussed again in Chapter 12, Inherited Disease.

In this chapter we have reviewed the structure and function of the living body at different levels of organization; they range from man to molecule. This range can be encompassed also in the concepts of disease. We recognize diseases of the whole individual (perhaps best expressed in psychiatric disor-

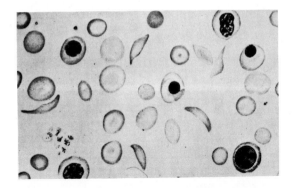

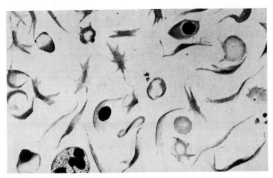

Fig. 1–24. This pair of photographs shows the appearance of the normal erythrocyte on the left and of sickle form cells from a case of homozygous sickle cell hemoglobinopathy on the right. (From Herrick, J.B.: Peculiar elongated and sickle-shaped red corpuscles in a case of severe anemia. Arch. Intern. Med., 6:517, 1910.)

ders such as the psychoses, or in a systemic disease like diabetes mellitus), diseases of a given organ (such as an infarct of the brain or heart), diseases of cells (perhaps best represented by cancer of different cell types), and finally, diseases at the molecular level where there is frequently an inborn error that results in the accumulation of glycogen or in the synthesis of an abnormal hemoglobin.

Sickle cell hemoglobinemia (hemoglobin S) is a prototype of **molecular disease**. The particular effect of the presence of abnormal hemoglobin S is exerted at each of the levels, molecular, cellular, tissue, organ, and host. When the abnormal, genetically determined sickle cell hemoglobin is subject to a lowered oxygen tension in the circulation, hemoglobin molecules form protein rods within the erythrocyte. This is seen, for example, in the drop of blood taken from the fingertip after 3 or 4 minutes of occluding venous circulation by a rubber band in a child with sickle cell homozygous disease. The erythrocytes, instead of being biconcave discs, assume a pointed, star shape (Fig. 1–24). These cells now cannot flow normally through the capil-

lary bed and often are stopped in the microcirculation. Frequently these capillary thromboses, which is what they are called, precipitate more anoxia in the neighboring tissue. The neighboring capillaries and veins share the lowered oxygen tension, multiplying the anoxic effects to wider areas.

The result of this anoxia is often thrombosis and occlusion of larger, more important blood vessels that supply critical areas of the brain or kidney. The effect causes ischemia and tissue necrosis, otherwise known as an infarct. The result of the infarct is the loss of function of the particular area. Whereas necrosis in small areas, such as the bowel, spleen, or bone marrow, may not cause anything more severe than pain, thrombosis and necrosis of the central nervous system, for example, usually result in a deficit of motor or intellectual function. This condition will often affect critical areas and cause death.

Thus one can consider the pathogenesis of disease at each level, ranging from the integrated action of the central nervous system, to the structural integrity of the single molecule of hemoglobin in an erythrocyte.

SYNOPSIS

The hierarchy of organization of living things is: whole organisms, organ systems, tissues, cells, organelles, macromolecular aggregates, and molecular structures. Cells are the units of life.

Subcellular structures: plasma membrane, mitochondria, rough and smooth reticulum, lysosomes, microtubules, nucleus, each may be abnormal, just as there may be lesions in the brain, or lung, or other organ systems.

Structural and functional relationships are inextricably connected, and morphologic changes can be looked on as fingerprints of disease. However, serious disorders of function may occur without any visible change from normal structure.

Injuries may be reversible or irreversible, and types of injury can be classified even if poorly understood at all levels.

The structure and function of the circulatory, respiratory, digestive, excretory, nervous, and reproductive systems are reviewed briefly.

Terms

Cells	Lysosome	tRNA
Tissues	Anoxia	mRNA
Organs	Chromosome	Transcription
Lesions	Homeostasis	Translation
Necrosis	Collagen	Replication
Infarct	Ribosomes	

FURTHER READING

Berlin, R.D., et al.: The cell surface. N. Engl. J. Med., 292:515, 1975.

Best, C.H., and Taylor, N.B.: *The Living Body*, 4th Ed. New York, H. Holt & Co., 1963.

Bloom, W., and Fawcett, D.W.: *A Textbook of Histology*, 10th Ed. Philadelphia, W. B. Saunders, 1975.

Dustin, P.: *Microtubules*. Berlin, Springer-Verlag, 1978.

Eliasson, R., et al.: The immotile cilia syndrome. N. Engl. J. Med., 297:1, 1977.

Fawcett, D.W.: What makes cilia and sperm tails beat? (Editorial) N. Engl. J. Med., 297:46, 1977.

Gelehrter, T.D.: Enzyme induction. N. Engl. J. Med., 294:522, 1976.

Ham, A.W.: *Histology*, 6th Ed. Philadelphia, J. B. Lippincott, 1969.

Judson, H.F.: *The Eighth Day of Creation*. New York, Simon & Schuster, 1979.

McConnell, H.M.: *Relation of Lateral Molecular Motion in Membranes and Immune Response*. (The Harvey Lectures, Series 72.) New York, Academic Press, 1978.

Palade, G.E.: Intracellular aspects of the process of protein synthesis. Science, 189:347, 1975.

Porter, K.R., and Bonneville, M.A.: *An Introduction to the Fine Structures of Cells and Tissues*, 4th Ed. Philadelphia, Lea & Febiger, 1973.

Rhodin, J.A.: *Histology: A Text and Atlas*. New York, Oxford University Press, 1975.

Rubinstein, N., et al.: Use of type-specific antimyosins to demonstrate the transformation of individual fibers in chronically stimulated rabbit fast muscles. J. Cell. Biol., 79:252, 1978.

Soifer, D. (Ed.): The biology of cytoplasmic microtubules. Ann. N. Y. Acad. Sci., 253, 1975.

Thomas, L.: *The Lives of a Cell*. New York, Viking Press, 1974.

Watson, J.D.: *Double Helix: Being a Personal Account of the Discovery of the Structure of DNA*. New York, Atheneum, 1968.

Watson, J.D.: *Molecular Biology of the Gene*. Menlo Park, Calif. Benjamin-Cummings, 1976.

Historical
Outline

2

History never embraces more than a small part of reality.—La Rochefaucauld

As the practice of medicine is an art based on a science, let us briefly review the development of that science. It will simplify matters for us if we divide this outline roughly into 4 periods: **primitive medicine, ancient medicine, the Middle Ages, and Renaissance medicine.** We may further subdivide Renaissance medicine into the sixteenth century with Vesalius; the seventeenth century with Harvey, Sydenham, and Malpighi; the eighteenth century with Morgagni, Hunter, and Jenner (the last named rather out of his proper era); the nineteenth century, which we must divide into before and after 1840; and modern medicine of the twentieth century. Of these various periods the most significant and revolutionary was the latter part of the nineteenth century.

PRIMITIVE MEDICINE

When we look back into the dim and distant past, we see primitive man terrified by the world around him and ascribing disease, as well as his other misfortunes, to supernatural malevolent forces, to the influence of spirits to be placated by sacrifice. It was the age of the witch doctor, the medicine man, the fetish and amulet, an age that perhaps has not yet

passed away for some. As a matter of fact, the medicine man represents the oldest professional class of which we have record. Guthrie, in his *History of Medicine*, remarks that primitive man at the present day, in whatever part of the world he is found, still does not admit the existence of disease from what we call natural causes. Death was and is a punishment for man's disobedience. The oldest surgical operation of which we have evidence is trephining or trepanning, which consisted in opening the skull with a sharp stone instrument for the purpose of letting out the evil spirit. If the patient died as the result of the operation, it could always be blamed on the invading demon, which refused to leave by the opening provided.

ANCIENT MEDICINE

The old civilizations of Egypt and Babylon had their medicine, and developed a knowledge of drugs and methods of embalming. The practice of medicine in Babylon must have demanded care, for we read that if a physician treats a severe wound successfully with a bronze lancet, or opens an abscess of the eye and cures the eye, "he shall take ten shekels of silver"; but if the patient dies of his wound or loses his eye, "one shall cut off his (the physician's) hands." Such a practice would at least encourage conservative methods of treatment.

Jewish medicine developed about the same time as that of Assyria. It was remarkable for its regulations for the prevention of disease and contagion, its hygiene of menstruation and the puerperium, and the establishment of social hygiene, details of which can be read in the Book of Leviticus.

Scientific medicine was born in Greece in the fifth century B.C.; it died in Rome 600 years later; it was resurrected after nearly 1,500 years in the Renaissance or rebirth of learning. **Hippocrates** (Fig. 2–1), born in 460 B.C.,

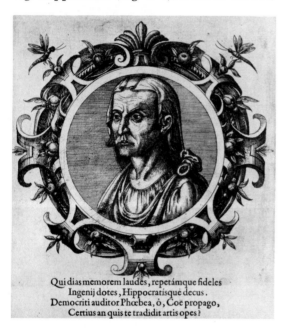

Qui dias memorem laudes, repetámque fideles
Ingenij dotes, Hippocratisque decus.
Democriti auditor Phœbea, ó, Coë propago,
Certius an quis te tradidit artis opes?

Fig. 2–1. Hippocrates. "Life is short, and the Art long; the occasion fleeting; experience fallacious, and judgment difficult. The physician must not only be prepared to do what is right himself, but also to make the patient, the attendants and the externals cooperate." Thus runs the first aphorism of Hippocrates on whom history has bestowed the title of "Father of Medicine." His countrymen believed he was descended from Aesculapius, the God of Healing, and most of the stories we possess concerning his life are legends and not historical facts. He was born about 460 B.C. on the island of Cos and had as contemporaries some of the greatest men of all time: Pericles the statesman; the poets Aeschylus, Sophocles, Euripides, Aristophanes, and Pindar; the philosophers Socrates and Plato; the historians Herodotus, Xenophon, and Thucydides; and that unrivalled sculptor Phidias. Hippocrates died in Thessaly, circa 375 B.C. (From Major, R.H.: *Classic Descriptions of Disease.* Springfield, Ill., Charles C Thomas.)

was its father, for he separated medicine from mystery and magic, relieved the gods of their responsibility for the prevention and treatment of disease, and laid that burden on the shoulders of man, its proper place. Hippocrates was the first and one of the greatest physicians, because he threw aside all the demonology of the priests and looked on disease as part of the order of nature, having a natural cause. The rise of rational medicine dates from Hippocrates. Dawson remarks with truth about Hippocrates that "probably no character in all history has through a single principle exerted so great an influence on civilization, upon the conditions of humans, as did he whom we revere as the father of modern medicine." He developed a system of thorough history-taking. His methods of physical examination are still used. He advocated clean hands and nails, and boiled water for operations. He preferred the "vis medicatrix naturae," the healing power of nature, to drugs. He was severely handicapped by a complete ignorance of anatomy and pathology, due to the fact that no dissections or autopsies were permitted, because the human body after death was regarded as sacred by the Greeks, an idea that was perpetuated later by the Church of Rome for many centuries.

One of the great contributions of this era was the application of some early philosophic concepts to medicine, such as the concept of harmony, arising from an appropriate balance in the individual between different temperaments. Even before Aristotle it had been held that "humors" were responsible for both good and bad health. These humors were blood, phlegm, yellow bile, and black bile. We shall see that these humors have arisen again throughout the ages as an opposite pole to the atomistic interpretation of disease. During the Renaissance, as organs were discovered, disease was attributed to failure of a given organ, then later the cell became the center of illness, and finally, in the second half of the twentieth century, the molecule is considered to cause the disease. At each stage there is another view that repudiates this splintering of the seats of illness and attempts to describe disease in "humoral" or "holistic" terms.

With the decline of Greece, due in part to the prevalence of malaria, the candle of learning continued to burn feebly in Rome. Here, progress was marked by practical organization rather than by originality. The outstanding contribution of Roman medicine was sanitation: clean streets, pure water, public baths, sewage disposal—all necessary to public health. The only great figure to emerge from Roman medicine was **Galen**, who lived in the second century A.D. He was the real originator of experimental methods in medicine, but he was dogmatic to a fault, and made facts fit his theories, instead of making theories fit the facts.

Galen's knowledge of anatomy was learned entirely from dissections on animals, but he was regarded as infallible. For a thousand years after his death no man doubted his work. The brilliance of his rhetoric had the effect of inhibiting subsequent generations from exploring the structure of the human body or from questioning the causes of disease. Without this healthy skepticism no progress is possible.

MIDDLE AGES

Galen died in 200 A.D., and in 410 A.D. the German barbarians under Alaric entered Rome. Then the dark night of the Middle Ages fell on Europe. All of science, including medicine, again became mystery and magic. Life itself was too precarious to allow for development. Even when there were periods of relative quiet between wars and turmoil, the authority of the Church did not encourage research in medicine, for the clerics were far more interested in the immortal soul than in the frail and mortal body. When men become slaves to authority they lose the power of independent thought, in medicine as in other things. And so the clear stream of scientific medicine was lost in the morass of the Dark Ages. In Osler's words: "Following the glory that was Greece and the grandeur that was Rome, desolation came upon the civilized world in which the light of learning burnt low, flickering almost to extinction."

The flame was kept alight by Arab medicine, many of the Greek and Roman texts being translated into Arabic, but it was not until the revival of learning and the founding of universities that this knowledge became available to western Europe. Perhaps the most important distinction between European and Arab medicine at this period was that the early Christian church regarded disease largely as a punishment for sin rather than as a result of natural causes, whereas the Arabs carried on the teachings of Hippocrates and the Greek school of thought, adding many drugs, such as opium, which has lasted to the present day. Perhaps the three greatest names were **Rhazes**, a Persian, who was the first to distinguish between measles and smallpox; **Avicenna**, another Persian, who was known as the Prince of Physicians; and **Maimonides**, a Jew, who has been called the William Osler of Medieval Arabic and Hebrew Medicine. Avicenna, the most famous physician of the Arab world, was not handicapped by undue modesty. In his autobiography, which covers only the first 21 years of his life, this passage appears: "Medicine is not a difficult subject, and in a short space of time, of course, I excelled in it, so that the masters of physic came to read with me, and I began to visit the sick. I was then about 16 years of age."

RENAISSANCE MEDICINE

It is not easy to know what period of time should be included under this heading. Taking a long view, we propose to review the advances made in the centuries that have elapsed from the Dark Ages to the present day. It will be convenient to consider the advances in separate centuries until 1840; after that date the advance becomes explosive.

Sixteenth Century. This century saw the rebirth of rational medicine, for in 1543 **Vesalius,** a young Belgian who became professor of anatomy at Padua at the age of 22 years, published a textbook, *On the Fabric of the Human Body*, in which he recorded what he saw and not what authority said he should see. Osler regarded this work as the greatest medical book ever written. Vesalius made his own dissections, begged all the doctors for their fatal cases, and even made friends with the judges, so that they would arrange executions to suit him, that is to say, not too many at one time. No one represents the true spirit of the Revival of Learning in medicine better than Vesalius. To pass from the writings of Galen and his followers to those of Vesalius is like passing from darkness into sunlight, for he shattered the idol of authority in the science of anatomy and dared to show that Galen was often wrong. Without an experience of normal structures it was impossible to interpret the anatomic effects of disease. Vesalius provided an essential background for the development of anatomic-pathologic correlations and for the later development of insights into the proper function of the different organ systems. His dissections are still a model of patient and elegant work and observation.

Ambroise Paré (Fig. 2–2), the great French military surgeon, whose life span covered the greater part of the sixteenth century, made surgery a practical art. Paré introduced the use of ligatures, the truss in hernia, massage, artificial eyes, and other innovations. His most famous aphorism: ''I dressed the wound; God healed it.''

Seventeenth Century. If the sixteenth century saw the birth of anatomy, the seventeenth witnessed the arrival of physiology in one of the greatest advances in the whole history of medical science, the discovery of the circulation of the blood by **William Harvey**, an English physician, in 1628 (Fig. 2–3). It is

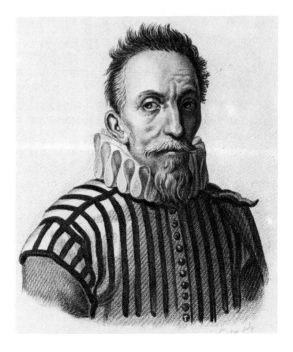

Fig. 2–2. Ambroise Paré was born in 1510. On the death of Charles IX, he became surgeon to Henry III and was also appointed ''valet de chambre du roi.'' In 1575 Paré published the first collected edition of his works, written in French and dedicated to the King. Paré died in 1590 at the age of eighty. His contributions to surgery were of capital importance. He devised many new surgical instruments, reintroduced the ligature, introduced massage, artificial limbs, and artificial eyes. One of his frequent and oft quoted remarks ''Je le pansay, Dieu le guarist'' (I dress him, God cures him) expressed his belief in the boundless healing powers of nature. (From Major, R.H.: *Classic Descriptions of Disease.* Springfield, Ill., Charles C Thomas.)

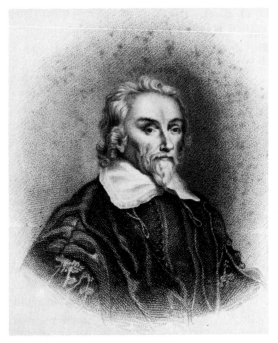

Fig. 2–3. William Harvey, who can be considered the founder of modern physiology, was born in Kent, England, on April 1, 1578. He showed experimentally that blood does not oscillate back and forth in blood vessels (as Galen believed), but travels in one direction only, and calculated that in one hour the heart pumps a quantity of blood equal to three times the weight of a man. He concluded that blood flows in a continuous stream through a closed circulatory system, moving from heart through arteries into veins and back to the heart. Although he was unable to find the connection between the arteries and veins which his theory demanded, he postulated correctly that these connections (capillaries) are too small to be seen by the naked eye. He became interested in generation and embryology and was one of the first since Aristotle to study carefully the stages of developing chick embryo. He died in London on June 3, 1657. (From *World Who's Who in Science, From Antiquity to Present.* Marquis Who's Who, Chicago.)

difficult to picture medical thought without this vital information. The function of respiration, diseases of the heart, hemorrhage, embolism, the spread of infection, the distribution of tumor metastases by the blood stream, and a host of other phenomena would be unintelligible without the magic words of Harvey: "I began to think whether there might not be a movement as it were in a circle." As usual, the epoch-making discovery was greeted with ridicule and abuse. In reality it formed the beginning of modern medical science. There was one serious gap in Harvey's demonstration and argument. He failed to show by what means the blood passed from the arteries to the corresponding veins. The gap was filled by the work of an Italian, **Marcello Malpighi**, born in the year that Harvey's book was published. Malpighi was the father of histology, the first man to apply the microscope to the minute structure of the body, although the instrument, which at that time was 1-1/2 feet long, had been invented half a century earlier. The microscope was as essential to advances in biology as the discovery of the wheel was to mechanical progress. Malpighi must also be regarded as a great physiologist, for form and function are merely two aspects of the same truth. Soon after his appointment to the chair of medicine at Bologna, he wrote a letter to a friend describing the minute vascular network joining the endings of the smallest arteries and the beginnings of the smallest veins. Thus he had found the missing link in the chain of Harvey's discovery. The great practitioner of this century was **Thomas Sydenham**, who has been called the English Hippocrates. He was not interested in theories or experiment, but if you fell sick in those days with one of the infectious fevers, you would do better with Sydenham than with Harvey as your doctor.

Eighteenth Century. In Europe at this time, there was little of the stirring of spirit and uprush of new ideas that had characterized the seventeenth century. This was a period of consolidation, an age of criticism rather than of discovery in medicine, of philosophers and philosophizing, culminating in the French Revolution. But it witnessed the birth of pathology in the limited sense of morbid anatomy. **Giovanni Battista Morgagni** of

Padua, at the age of 79 in 1761, published a book entitled *The Seats and Causes of Disease,* which at once rendered obsolete all others dealing with the diseased body. Before Morgagni, disease was considered as a general thing. Doctors speculated as to the nature of the process, built up a hypothesis no matter how fantastic, and gave it a name. Strangely enough, they did not inquire as to the seat of the disease. It was Morgagni who was the first to correlate the symptoms of the patient during life with the changes in the organs found at autopsy. He showed that it was not true that dead men tell no tales. Dead men have for centuries been telling doctors the story of how they got sick and why they died. For the first time we could think of liver disease, kidney disease, and heart disease, and have a mental picture of the clinical condition in relation to the lesions in the organs responsible for that condition. Morgagni made few real discoveries, nor did he revolutionize pathology as did Virchow in the coming century; his great service to pathology was his emphasis on detail and thoroughness.

The direction taken by medical thought at this time was away from a holistic (or single-cause) explanation of disease and toward an explanation of disease that related the pain in the chest and subsequent death to a particular organ or group of cells, such as the heart, which might show a large pale soft area (infarct). This ascription of particular symptoms and signs to anatomic changes in particular organs has formed the cornerstone of rational medicine for the past 200 years. It is only recently being questioned, as newer understandings of the interdependence of special systems (cardiovascular, respiratory, nervous) push the pendulum of thought back toward a more holistic or humoral way of looking at disease.

Many gifted clinical observers were born at the end of this century, **Laennec** in France, **Addison, Bright,** and **Hodgkin** in England. Early pathologists were merely medical men who performed autopsies as a sideline. But two men of this period stand out from the others as imbued with the spirit of inquiry. These are **John Hunter** (Fig. 2–4) and **Edward Jenner,** who was Hunter's pupil. We have seen that Paré, in the sixteenth century, made

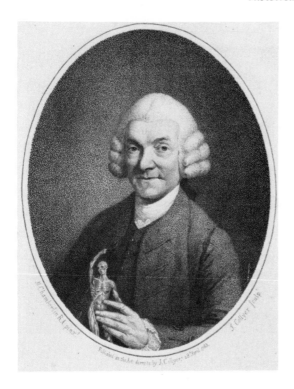

Fig. 2–4. William Hunter, the Father of Modern English Anatomy, was born in Lanarkshire on May 23, 1718. He studied medicine in Scotland, practiced surgery and obstetrics in England, and become physician extraordinary to Queen Charlotte. In 1768 he became the first Professor of Anatomy at the Royal Academy. He wrote several books on anatomy and was the first to describe the retroversion of the uterus. In 1774 he discovered the separate nature of the fetal and maternal circulations. From 1748 until 1760 he was associated with his brother, John Hunter. William Hunter died in London in 1783. (From *World Who's Who in Science, From Antiquity to Present.* Marquis Who's Who, Chicago.)

surgery an art. Two hundred years later, Hunter, an extraordinary and turbulent personality, made it a science. He correlated surgery for the first time with physiology and with pathology, and introduced a spirit of scientific inquiry that had been entirely lacking in surgical practice. So great was his influence that it is no exaggeration to say that surgery may be divided into two periods, before Hunter and after Hunter; but the surgery was still only the surgery of the surface of the body and the extremities. Jenner, by introducing vaccination against smallpox, was the founder of preventive medicine, as well as one of the greatest benefactors of mankind. Some idea of the ravages and prevalence of the disease that he did so much to eradicate

may be gained from the old saying "mothers counted their children only after they had had the smallpox."

Nineteenth Century. The dawn of this century did not indicate the stupendous and revolutionary discoveries that were in store. Until the nineteenth century, the history of medicine is largely a catalog of the follies of medical mankind. As late as the end of the eighteenth century, the kings and queens of England and France still "touched for the King's Evil," i.e., laid their healing hands on those suffering from scrofula (tuberculous glands in the neck)! In the eighteenth century all doctors were general practitioners. The surgeon could not open the abdomen, so he had plenty of time to practice medicine. In the first half of the nineteenth century, hospitals were little more than a refuge for sick poor, who died of mysterious infections. It was only after the conquest of surgical infection that the teaching hospital become a medical scientific center and that the age of specialization began, with the eventual development of intracranial, intrathoracic, and now cardiovascular surgery. The first 40 years were quiet, but in the remaining years of the century, medicine advanced further than in the entire course of recorded history. It was a triumph for the application of experimental methods to medical problems. Time now has to be reckoned not in centuries but in decades.

1840 TO 1850. In 1846 **Morton** demonstrated to an audience of Boston doctors that ether would abolish the pain of a surgical operation. In the following year **Sir James Young Simpson** of Edinburgh introduced chloroform to relieve the pain of childbirth as well as that of general surgery. For the first time in the world's history it was possible for a surgeon to operate without inflicting terrible anguish on his patient.

1850 TO 1860. **Nursing** is as old as the human race, but in this decade **Florence Nightingale** organized it and made it a profession for trained gentlewomen. It is easy to forget that only 100 years ago there were no nurses and no nursing as we know it today. Between the seventeenth and nineteenth centuries, nursing, as a career, had sunk to a very low level. This was a time when no respectable woman earned her living in that profession, and there was no longer much religious motivation behind hospital work. Florence Nightingale completely revolutionized nursing service by insisting that it was a highly satisfying profession requiring intelligence, education, and adequate compensation. She had the statistics to prove the value of her nursing service; due to her efforts the mortality rate of the hospitals she organized fell from over 40 to 2%. In this same decade some of the most valued medical instruments of precision were invented. Darwin's *Origin of the Species* was published in 1859, and in 1858, Virchow's *Cellular Pathology*.

Rudolf Virchow (Fig. 2–5) is the father of modern pathology as we know it; he showed for the first time that the structural changes in disease are to be found, not in the organ as a whole, but in the cellular elements of which the organ is composed; what the molecule is to the chemist and the electron to the physicist, the diseased cell has been to the pathologist since Virchow. He bestrode the world of scientific medicine like a colossus, contributing to our knowledge in an endless variety of fields. He was the first to demonstrate the occurrence of pulmonary embolism and the first to describe leukemia. But Virchow was much more than the supreme student of disease. He was also Germany's leading anthropologist, leading archeologist, and leading liberal statesman in opposition to Bismarck. We may ask how all this was possible? Perhaps an answer may be found in part in the title of his graduation thesis on leaving high school at the age of eighteen: "A Life Full of Work and Toil is not a Burden but a Benediction."

We must not make the mistake of thinking that the structural changes connoted by the term morbid or pathologic anatomy are the essence of disease, although they are certainly the easiest to recognize and to demonstrate. In the last analysis it is function that makes life possible, and it is disordered function that constitutes what we regard as disease. Physiology constitutes the study of function, and in the middle of the nineteenth century the figure of **Claude Bernard,** the French physiologist, ranks equal with Virchow, the German pathologist. It was Bernard who was the first to recognize that the pancreas was by

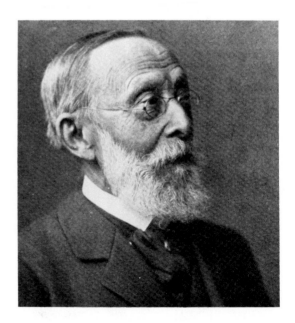

Fig. 2–5. Rudolf Virchow was born in Pomerania in 1821 and attended the gymnasium at Koslin. In 1839 he began the study of medicine at the Kaiser Wilhelm Akademie and received his degree at the University of Berlin in 1843. He became at once an assistant at the Charite Hospital and two years later became Prosector of Anatomy and Assistant in Froriep's clinic. In 1847 he became Privatdozent in Pathology and entered upon the great work of his life. From this period onward, Virchow seems to have been interested in only two things—the study of pathology and the study of economic and social problems. In 1848 Virchow was sent to investigate an epidemic of typhus in Silesia. His report contained not only a severe criticism of the hygienic regulations in that province, but also a harsh indictment of the prevalent social injustices. Virchow's report and his continued agitation for reforms caused trouble with the Prussian government, and he was dismissed from his position at Berlin. His fame as a pathologist, however, was already established, and he was immediately called to Wurzburg as Professor of Pathology and director of their newly founded pathologic institute. Virchow remained at Wurzburg seven years and while there completed the work that formed the basis of his cellular theory. In 1858 he returned to Berlin. His life there was one of unparalleled activity. He collected an amazing museum of pathology, was very active in teaching and research, and found time to enter political life, serving in the Reichstag for thirteen years. Here he was the leader of the Radical party and an active, outspoken, and persistent opponent of Bismarck. Students flocked from all over the world to attend his lectures and every year brought new honors and fresh testimonials of esteem. On his seventieth birthday he was presented with a gold medal by the Emperor, and his eightieth birthday took on the character of a national holiday, with delegates from all over the world assembling in Berlin to do him honor. Virchow died the following year, 1902. (From Major, R.H.: *Classic Descriptions of Disease.* Springfield, Ill., Charles C Thomas.)

far the most important digestive gland in the body, producing enzymes that act on proteins, carbohydrates, and fats. Of equal importance was his discovery of the glycogenic function of the liver. Before that time the only function of the liver was thought to be the production of bile. Bernard showed that the sugars of the intestinal food are changed to glucose, which is carried to the liver and there converted by enzymes to a substance he called glycogen. This is the storage form of sugar, which can be reconverted into glucose as the need arises and as the metabolic fire demands more fuel. Another great achievement was his demonstration of the existence of the vasomotor nerves, which control both the constriction and dilatation of blood vessels. From his experience he generated the concept of **the constancy of the internal environment as a biologic law** as the condition of free and independent life, to which reference has been made in the preceding chapter. His character and moral worth were so outstanding that at his death all Paris wept, and he was the first man of science to be laid to rest with a state funeral in the cathedral of Notre Dame.

1860 TO 1870. Up to this time the ideas of causal agents and disease had been slow to find concrete support. Observations tended to provide correlations of anatomic change with symptoms of disease, but true cause-and-effect relationships were hard to establish. In this decade comes the first unequivocal evidence that shows that a particular disease and its anatomic traces can be credited to an external agent: a bacterium. The existence of bacteria had been fairly well known in the seventeenth century, but it was not known then that they could cause disease. Fortunately, at this time the efforts of 3 men—Pasteur, Lister and Koch—led to the discovery of this relationship.

Louis Pasteur, a Frenchman, was a chemist, not a physician, but he became interested in the problem of why wine spoils, and he came to the conclusion that the fermentation of wine and beer was due to the action of living bacterial agents. From this he was led to the study of putrefaction, i.e., the decomposition of meat and other dead organic material. This was again found to be due to the same living agents, and the process could be prevented by

heating organic fluids, such as milk, to a temperature below the boiling point, the procedure now known as **pasteurization**. At this time the English surgeon, **Joseph Lister**, was pondering the problem of wound infection following surgical operations, which rendered the most brilliant operation worse than useless, and gave origin to the popular gibe ''the operation was successful but the patient died,'' when he came across Pasteur's work. At this time the mortality rate from operations, now frequently performed owing to the use of anesthetics, was appalling. At least 45% of amputations resulted in death from septicemia, infection, and gangrene. Lister had previously realized that putrefaction of dead organic material and infection of wounds were intimately related, and now he saw in one lightning flash that if putrefaction was bacterial in origin, so also was wound infection. Destruction of bacteria in infected wounds (antisepsis), and later exclusion of bacteria from the field of operation (asepsis), wrought a revolution in surgery so far-reaching, so overwhelming, that surgery as we know it today is essentially the gift of Lister to humanity. His work alone made possible the surgery of the abdomen, chest, brain, and joints, as well as rendering a hundredfold safer operations on the limbs and the practice of obstetrics.

1870 TO 1880. This is the decade of bacteriologic advance. Pasteur and Koch are the two most eminent figures. **Robert Koch** (Fig. 2–6), at first a German country practitioner, must share with Pasteur the title of the founder of modern bacteriology, for he introduced the methods of bacteriologic investigation, such as the use of pure cultures and special stains and reproduction of the disease by animal inoculation, which are employed at the present day. In addition he demonstrated the bacterial cause of many infections such as anthrax, cholera, and above all tuberculosis. In this decade a large number of infectious diseases (as opposed to wound infections) were shown to be due to specific bacteria. Pasteur also introduced the idea of ultramicroscopic filterable viruses, agents of disease so small that they could not be seen with the microscope and were able to pass through the finest filter, although ordinary bacteria were

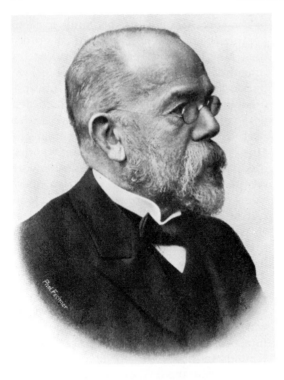

Fig. 2–6. Robert Koch, a physician and pioneer bacteriologist, was born in Hanover on December 11, 1843. He received the Nobel Prize for physiology and medicine in 1905. He introduced the method of making bacterial smears and fixing them with heat, was the first to isolate and obtain pure culture of anthrax bacillus, identified comma bacillus as the cause of Asiatic cholera, and discovered the organism responsible for Egyptian ophthalmia. He produced tuberculin and erroneously thought it to be the cure for TB, and later showed it to be of value in diagnosing the disease. He studied the rinderpest in South Africa and developed a means of vaccinating against it. He investigated the bubonic plague in India and malaria and sleeping sickness in Africa and discovered the methods of transmission. He elaborated general methods of bacteriologic research and developed a method of disinfection. He also developed a means of cultivating bacteria in liquid and solid media and laid the foundation for a rational system of bacterial culturing. He established rules for properly identifying causative agents of various diseases. Robert Koch died in Baden-Baden on March 27, 1910. (From *World Who's Who in Science, From Antiquity to Present.* Marquis Who's Who, Chicago.)

held back by such a filter. It should be added that at the present day the electron microscope, with its enormously increased power of magnification, has brought even the smallest viruses into view, so that they no longer deserve the term ultramicroscopic.

1880 TO 1890. The two outstanding discoveries of this period were preventive inoculation against disease, and the knowledge that the microscopic animal parasites known as protozoa may cause widespread epidemics. Jenner's discovery in 1798 of the value of vaccination against smallpox (now known to be a viral disease) was an isolated miracle that led to further advances. Pasteur now introduced the principle of preventive inoculation by means of "vaccines" against bacterial and virus disease. The modern development of protection against poliomyelitis by virus inoculation need only be mentioned here. The discovery of protozoa as agents of disease was of special importance in the case of malaria, the most widespread disabling and killing disease in the world. It was **Laveran**, a French army doctor, who first discovered the malaria parasite.

1890 TO 1900. The nineteenth century ends with a tremendous burst of activity in scientific medicine, but only three outstanding achievements can be mentioned here. These are: (1) the discovery of x rays (Roentgen) and radium (Marie and Pierre Curie) and their application to medicine; (2) the treatment of infectious disease by antitoxins; and (3) the discovery of the insect transmission of disease. The use of x rays has revolutionized diagnosis in every region of the body, and radiations either of this type or those of radium constitute the greatest recent advance in the treatment of many forms of cancer. The first and most successful of the antitoxins was against diphtheria, but the other antitoxins have been replaced by antibiotics. The demonstration that infection can be carried by insects was one of the most important contributions ever made to preventive medicine. It was **Sir Patrick Manson** who was the first to show in 1877 that the embryos of the minute worm filaria, the cause of elephantiasis, were present in the blood at night and transmitted by the culex mosquito, and **Sir Ronald Ross** who proved in 1897 that malaria was spread in the same way. We now know that the anopheles mosquito carries malaria and yellow fever, the flea bubonic plague, the louse typhus, the tsetse fly sleeping sickness, and so on. Haggard, in his delightful little book, *Mystery, Magic, and Medicine,* sums up the effect of these discoveries as follows: "Six hundred years ago men believed that disease was due to the wrath of the gods; they prayed—and died. Three hundred years ago they believed it due to meteorological disturbances and contaminated air; they closed their windows at night and burned coal and powder in the streets—and died. Today we turn from such omniscient powers as the gods and the weather to prosaic matters such as the exterminating of the mosquito, the killing of the rat and its fleas, and the delousing of the traveller—and we live free from plague, malaria, and yellow fever."

Twentieth Century. Now the emphasis is directed to disturbed function rather than to the description of structural changes, so that physiology and biochemistry have come to assume front rank. It is for this reason that the work of the medical technologist in the laboratory has come to be of such commanding importance. The most striking achievements of medical science in the twentieth century so far may be considered under the following headings: chemotherapy, nutrition, medical genetics, immunology, and the diagnostic techniques that have permitted entirely new approaches to organic disease. The great advances in what may be called social medicine lie outside the scope of this review.

Chemotherapy made its debut in the first decade of the twentieth century in the treatment of syphilis. At that time the cause of the disease was unknown, accurate diagnosis was difficult and often impossible, and treatment was unsatisfactory and inefficient. Incredible though it may appear, these 3 problems were solved in the space of 5 years. In 1905 **Schaudinn** discovered the cause of syphilis (*Treponema pallidum*, formerly called *Spirochaeta pallida*); in 1906 **Wassermann** introduced his famous blood test; and in 1910 **Ehrlich** demonstrated that arsenic preparations provide a specific treatment against the disease.

The concept of antisepsis dawned with Lister in the late nineteenth century and was followed by vaccination as a natural step, once the germ theory became accepted. The idea of an antibacterial agent, a drug or chemical that might specifically destroy the infectious agent while not harming the infected patient, arose gradually during the first half of the twentieth century, culminating in the development of the sulfa drugs and then of penicillin. Prior to this time heavy metals like mercury, arsenic, and bismuth, had been used, particularly for such diseases as syphilis, but too frequently their effect on the patient was as toxic as the disease itself. The ideas of a specific antibacterial agent, of a dose-response curve, of uptake, excretion, and toxicity were slowly evolved as men began to manufacture and to take chemicals in increasing amounts, some for specific diseases, and others for reasons less well-established.

Seeing that some of these preparations had a direct action on the treponema of syphilis, it was hoped that other chemicals would soon be found that would have a similar action on other bacteria. The story of Fleming's discovery of penicillin is well related in his biography and provides an example of serendipity.

Penicillin is a substance naturally produced by one of the common green molds growing in nature, called *Penicillium notatum*. Since it prevents the growth of gram-positive bacteria, it is known as an antimicrobial. The discovery of penicillin in 1928 by **Alexander Fleming** was followed by that of streptomycin, which acts on another group of bacteria, and later by that of aureomycin, terramycin, chloromycetin, and many others. All of these antibiotics have their particular uses, which will be described later. Some are bacteriostatic rather than bactericidal, that is to say they inhibit the growth of the bacteria, thus leaving them an easy prey to the defensive forces of the body. These dramatic and epoch-making therapeutic advances due to the entry of chemistry into medicine were one of the most important features of twentieth-century progress.

Dietetics, or the science of nutrition, is largely a twentieth-century product, although scurvy, that scourge of armies and navies, had already been conquered by fruit juice. Knowledge of vitamins and the mineral requirements of food is extremely recent. It is of importance in the prevention rather than the cure of disease, and will go far to the future physical betterment of animal life.

Medical genetics really originated with the studies of **Gregor Mendel** in 1866 on the inheritance of color in sweet peas and the transmission of characteristics from one generation to another. The ability to separate and study the chromosomes carrying their cargo of genes composed of DNA is recent, and has thrown a flood of light on such mysteries as sex anomalies and sex reversal as well as on the complex problems of inherited disease. The implications of asexual reproduction or "cloning" are currently of interest, but have not become a practical consideration for man, although the possibilities are provocative. Can you imagine the situation in which a single germ cell is removed from each newborn child and kept until such time as the person needed a replica?

Immunology, the science of how our body recognizes itself, and how it produces soluble and cellular defenses, has developed rapidly in the last 30 years. This subject is covered in the chapter on immune mechanisms, and, of course, has directly affected the success of efforts to manage diseases by transplantation.

Diagnostic techniques today include everything from a therapeutic trial with a particular drug to see if the patient improves to the use of computerized scanning equipment. (In 1980 there are 1,200 scanners in the United States, i.e., one per 150,000 to 160,000 persons. The cost of each scanner is between $750,000 and $1,000,000). The diagnosis of infectious disease by culture methods, of tumors by biopsy, of heart disease by catheterization, or of gastrointestinal disease by glass fiber optical instruments are all routine procedures even in the office of the local physician. Lasers, radioisotopes, ultrasound, and most modern technologic innovations have been applied to problems in medicine, but no modern machine has replaced the physician's experience, nor human reason, in attempting to solve the medical problems of an individual patient.

The most exciting recent developments in human biology are in newer understandings of the interrelationships of various sympathetic amines and their role in the function of the central nervous system, particularly the hypothalamus. These discoveries have already begun to explain some of the mechanisms which have been observed in the pharmacologic management of mental illness

and promise to explain some of the controls over hormone secretion. This area of new knowledge alone is responsible for a trend away from the atomism of cellular theory and toward a holistic or humoral understanding of human health and disease.

In this lightning review of the development of medical science, far more has been omitted than has been mentioned. Only a few scientists and a few outstanding achievements have been selected. The aim has been to show the different position of the sick person now compared with that in bygone days. What once seemed impossible and then miraculous is now almost commonplace. Perhaps the three biggest steps in the past have been: (1) **the development of dissection** of the human body, (2) **the use of the microscope** in the examination of pathologic tissue, and (3) **the introduction of chemistry and biochemistry** in the investigation and treatment of disease.

Two final thoughts are important in considering disease in the context of our history. First, it is clear that the prevalence of different diseases and their economic, social, and personal significance change with time. As shown in Figure 2–7, in the first half of this century there has been a marked change in the number of deaths due to tuberculosis, and to all infections. This is due in part to the discovery and use of antibiotics, but mainly to changes in our social and economic conditions; the significance of typhoid fever has been altered by our handling of sewage and food, as well as by immunization and the availability of antibiotics.

Despite all the advances in the technology of medicine, it is important to recognize that the changes in life expectancy and survival are not the product of modern surgery or chemotherapy, but are rather the result of the changes in our environment. Clean water, sewage disposal, better housing, pasteurization of milk, and vaccinations are responsible for our general increased life span.

A second important idea is the distinction between **morbidity** and **mortality**, which our experience with disease in a textbook does not always recognize. Morbidity refers to those diseases that are not fatal, although they may be disabling. Examples of this are the common cold, and a disease that causes pain

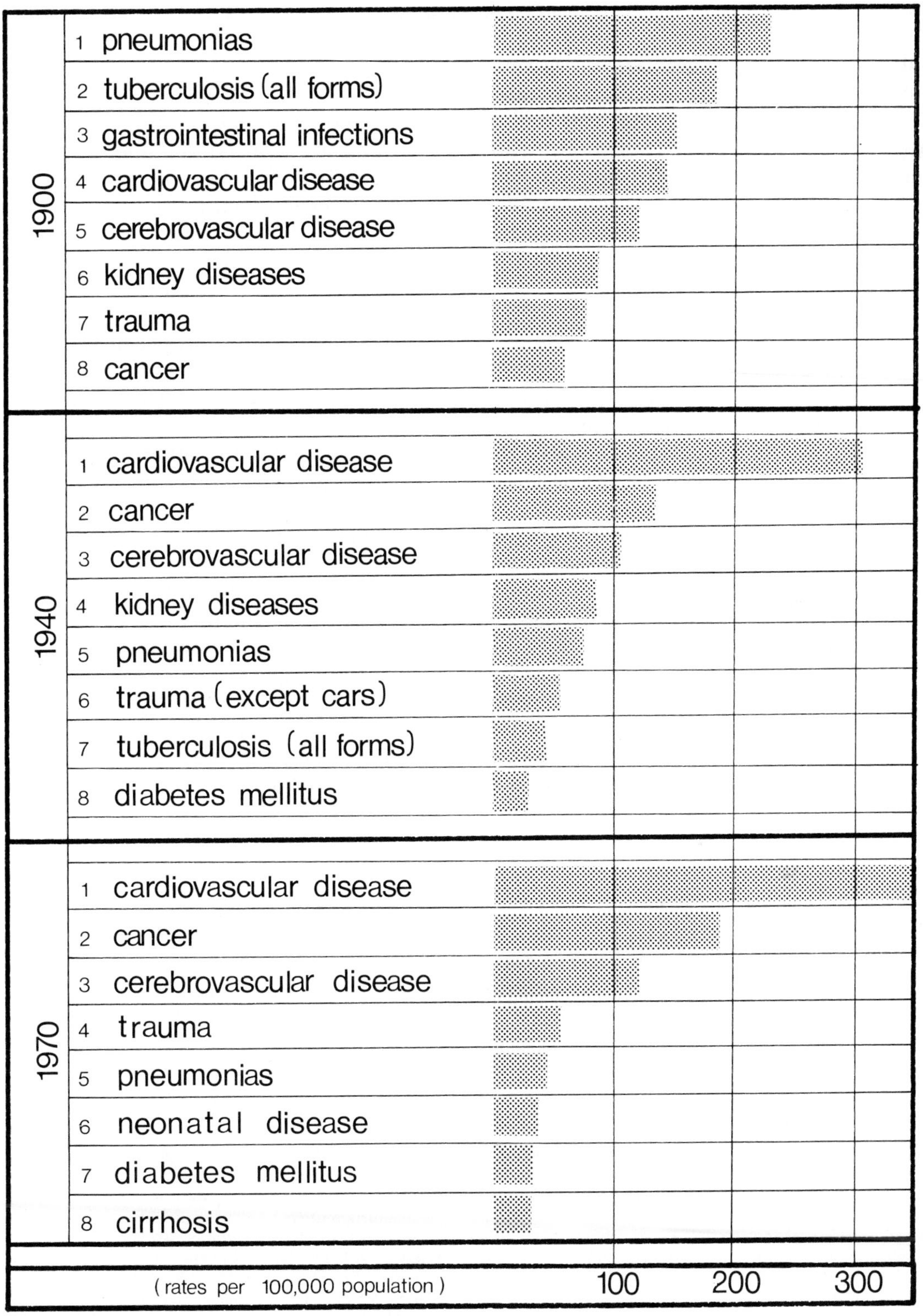

1900

1 pneumonias
2 tuberculosis (all forms)
3 gastrointestinal infections
4 cardiovascular disease
5 cerebrovascular disease
6 kidney diseases
7 trauma
8 cancer

1940

1 cardiovascular disease
2 cancer
3 cerebrovascular disease
4 kidney diseases
5 pneumonias
6 trauma (except cars)
7 tuberculosis (all forms)
8 diabetes mellitus

1970

1 cardiovascular disease
2 cancer
3 cerebrovascular disease
4 trauma
5 pneumonias
6 neonatal disease
7 diabetes mellitus
8 cirrhosis

(rates per 100,000 population)   100   200   300

Fig. 2–7. Vital statistics provide an additional vantage point for perceiving and classifying the ills of man. The bar charts, for example, list the 8 leading causes of death in the United States for the years 1900, 1940, and 1970 in order of decreasing death rates. Certain changes in terminology occurred during this interval. For example, "intracranial lesions of vascular origin" (1940) corresponds to "cerebrovascular diseases" (1970). Concurrently with the changes depicted in his table, the average life expectancy at birth in the United States increased from 47 years in 1900 to 71 years in 1970. (Adapted from Dingle, J.M.: The ills of man. Sci. Am., 229:82, 1973.)

in the joints (arthritis) and lasts for decades but is not life-threatening. On the other hand, there are many disorders that may take only a short while to cause death. A myocardial infarct, an intracerebral hemorrhage, a pulmonary embolism—all may be immediate causes of death and contribute to our "mortality rate," whereas the common cold and arthritis contribute to the "morbidity rate." The distinction between the duration, discomfort, severity, and seriousness of different diseases also changes with time as we gain new techniques for dealing with disease.

SYNOPSIS

The "magical" causes of disease were displaced by the beginnings of science in Greek times.

Renaissance medicine began with the study of anatomy and the understanding of the function of different organs.

The concept of disease as arising in a specific organ or system, rather than as a "humor," is based on the correlation of the patient's signs and symptoms with the findings at autopsy.

The fact that biologic agents cause disease was established only after the development of techniques for microscopy and culture of organisms.

Modern medicine begins in the twentieth century with the application of chemotherapy, radiation , genetic knowledge, biochemical technology, and modern surgical and invasive techniques to the study and management of the sick person.

Disease changes with time.

The understanding of disease depends both on the technologic development of the era and on the cultural and intellectual attitudes to the problem.

Disease results from the failure of an oganism to adapt successfully to genetic variations, to invasion by biologic agents, to repair of trauma, or to complications of aging.

Disease is perceived as a change from the normal or "steady state" and is expressed by the organism's reaction pattern. Disease need not be physical or "organic."

Terms

William Harvey	*Robert Koch*	*Immunology*
Giovanni Battista Morgagni	*Chemotherapy*	*Morbidity*
Florence Nightingale	*Antibiotic*	*Mortality*
Rudolph Virchow	*Dietetics*	

FURTHER READINGS

Castiglioni, A.: *A History of Medicine*. New York, Knopf, 1947.

Fabrega, H.: Concepts of disease: logical features and social implications. Perspect. Biol. Med., *15*:583, 1972.

Major, R.H.: *Classic ·Descriptions of Disease*, 3rd Ed. Springfield, Ill., Charles C Thomas, 1948.

McNeill, W.H.: *Plagues and People*. Garden City, N. Y., Anchor Books, 1976.

Murphy, E.A.: A scientific viewpoint on normalcy. Perspect. Biol. Med., *9*:333, 1965.

Osler, Sir William: *The Evolution of Modern Medicine*. New Haven, Yale University Press, 1921.

Rosenberg, C.E.: The therapeutic revolution: medicine, meaning and social change in 19th century America. Perspect. Biol. Med., *20*:485, 1977.

Science, Vol. 200, No. 4344, May 26, 1978.

Scientific American, Vol. 229, No. 3, September, 1973.

Sontag, S.: *Illness as Metaphor*. New York, Farrar, Straus and Giroux, 1978.

Causes
of Disease

3

To talk of disease is a sort of Arabian Nights entertainment. —OSLER

WHAT IS DISEASE?

Before beginning a discussion of the possible causes of disease, it may be well to ask, "What is disease?" This is a question that is easier to ask than to answer. To the patient it means discomfort, dis-ease, dis-harmony with his environment; to the physician or surgeon it may be revealed by a variety of symptoms and signs; and to the pathologist it may be represented in one or more structural changes (lesions), which may be gross, i.e., seen with the naked eye, or microscopic, only made visible with the light or the electron microscope. The study of lesions forms a part of the science of pathology. Pathology itself can be defined as that branch of medicine that deals with the nature of disease.

But to return to the question, What is disease? Perhaps the best answer we can give is that **disease is the pattern of response of a living organism to some form of injury.** In order for disease to be present there is usually some alteration in normal function. This broad definition must include disease as a response to all kinds of injury, ranging from infection with a virus to stress from crowding or depression from loss.

Pathology was originally an investigation into structural changes revealed in the autopsy room. At first only gross changes (naked eye) and later (from 1850) microscopic findings were demonstrated. From the very beginning the aim was to explain the patient's signs and symptoms. In 1483 Leonardo da Vinci dissected an old man in Florence "to see the cause of such a quiet death." When the investigation of disease moved from the autopsy room to the bedside of the living patient, the study was called clinical pathology, or in recent years, because so much of this work is done in the laboratories, the term laboratory medicine has gained in popularity. Our knowledge of the processes and patterns of disease and the techniques for investigating them has continued to grow at an increasing rate. It is now obvious to everyone that the practice of medicine without adequate laboratory facilities denies the patient some important advantages. The diagnostic laboratory is no longer run by a single individual, but rather by a team of experts in various fields—medical, scientific, and technical. The amount of work required from clinical laboratories has led to the introduction of automation, which in turn has resulted in an enormous increase in the volume of work that can be done. But we must not forget that the object of the whole exercise is the care of the patient, a matter to which we shall return in the final chapter.

Anatomic or histologic lesions in tissue may bear an obvious relation to the symptoms, as in the case of acute appendicitis or poliomyelitis. But there may be lesions without symptoms, as in early cancer or pulmonary tuberculosis. Finally, there may be symptoms without anatomic lesions, as in the psychosomatic (Greek *psyche*, spirit and *soma*, body) diseases and the various psychoses. As we have already seen, it is possible that future research may reveal hitherto-unsuspected biochemical lesions in these cases also. For disease itself is merely life under abnormal conditions. The presence of lesions distinguishes organic disease, in which there are observable gross or microscopic changes in an organ, from so-called "functional disease," in which there is some disturbance of function without any observable organic change. Although it is true that at the present time diagnosis consists largely in the naming of lesions (e.g., cancer of the lung, coronary artery thrombosis), **disease should be viewed as disordered function rather than only as altered structure**.

It has been popular to think of disease as arising in disorders of cellular function since the time of Virchow (1858), and recently it has been appropriate to talk of molecular disease (Pauling, 1952), but it seems wise now to recognize that this trend to "atomism" in the study of disease may be less illuminating than fashionable. In fact, as suggested in an earlier chapter, new knowledge about hormonal control mechanisms suggests that there is a greater interdependence of the different organ systems than has been suspected.

We may classify disease in anatomic or physiologic terms, e.g., "diseases of the heart or nervous system," or "diseases of the endocrines or circulatory system." We may also think of disease according to its causative organism, so we can talk of tuberculosis (caused by the tubercle bacteria), or talk of viral diseases. Or we can consider disease in terms of the reaction patterns to the injury, e.g.,

pneumoconioses (lung damage in persons who have inhaled various kinds of dust). None of these methods of classifying disease is exclusively right or wrong, and all help to organize the ways in which we try to cope with the incomplete understanding we have.

One point, however, seems clear: patterns emerge to show us that some illnesses are confined exclusively or principally to a single anatomic compartment and that others involve many systems or the whole host, so we have come to talk also about **systemic diseases**. That is not to say that an infection is always local, as in an abscess, because we all know that infections may spread, but some diseases involve many organ systems, in fact the whole body, and exact their toll because of this. An example is diabetes mellitus, in which there may be lesions in blood vessels of the eye and kidney, as well as heart and aorta, all related in some poorly understood way to disordered metabolism of glucose.

Fortunately, there is a natural tendency to recover from disease, more especially from acute illnesses. Perhaps the best example is the spontaneous healing of a clean wound, which we all take for granted. This healing power, however, presents us with great difficulties in assessing the value of new therapeutic measures, especially new drugs. Is the happy outcome merely a natural event thanks to mother nature, or is it the result of the therapy?

One important point in the understanding of disease is knowing what happens in most cases when there is no therapeutic intervention or attempt at modifying the disease by medical or surgical or other means. This knowledge of the "natural history" of a disease is sadly lacking in many instances because, simply, it would be unethical not to offer some help to an afflicted person. However, there are always cases in which a person denies or fails to seek assistance for a pain, or a mass, or a recurrent problem, for whatever reason, until the process is far advanced. Through such anecdotal experiences we have accumulated some knowledge of the natural history of various diseases.

It is interesting, for example, to know that there is a recent study of patients who acquired primary syphilis but who were not treated either with penicillin or with any other drug. After 25 years, only about one-quarter of these untreated persons developed any of the legendary and debilitating signs or symptoms of tertiary syphilis that may affect the central nervous system (general paresis), dorsal columns of the spinal cord (tabes), or cardiovascular system (aortic aneurysm, aortic valvular insufficiency, or coronary artery ostial narrowing). This suggests that the natural history of the disease syphilis is more benign than previous generations, in a more prudish era, were wont to believe. But these observations, that only about one-quarter of those affected by the spirochete become seriously incapacitated, still suggest that to go without treatment is a type of Russian roulette that has little appeal when one considers the unpleasant outcomes of tertiary syphilis.

It is often said that the nature of disease is changing, that we hear much more about people dying of heart failure and cancer than used to be the case. This does not mean that these diseases have become actually more common, although more people do die from them. Long ago, Addison, in the *Vision of Myrza*, drew a picture of great masses of mankind walking over the bridge of life that spans the dark river of death. In the bridge there were many hidden trapdoors through which the unwary travelers dropped into the flood below. Their numbers became ever fewer as they approached the far side, but none succeeded in completing the journey. The trapdoors represent diseases. At the near end of the bridge there are many trapdoors—infantile mortality, typhoid, malaria, smallpox—that have been so securely closed by medical science that they seldom open now. But at the far end there are a few wide trapdoors—cancer, heart failure, cerebral hemorrhage—and great numbers must fall through these into the dark flood of oblivion.

The outcome of disease varies between the extremes of complete recovery and death. The prediction of this outcome is called prognosis; it is a forecast of what may be expected to happen. If one knows the pattern of disease and if the patient's disease conforms to the pattern, then one can forecast or anticipate what may occur and thereby offer a prognosis. Clinical diagnosis is the art of recogniz-ing the pattern from only pieces of the puzzle. Diagnosis is often difficult, but accurate prognosis is much more difficult and requires a complete knowledge of the various patterns that may develop from the pieces of this puzzle. It is largely the result of experience and judgment, and depends to a great extent on a complete comprehension of the natural history of the disease in question. That is what is likely to happen in the way of interaction between the injury process and the host response.

ETIOLOGY

The study of causation of a pathologic process is known as the **etiology** (Fig. 3–1). **Pathogenesis**, a term easily confused with etiology, is the process of production and de-

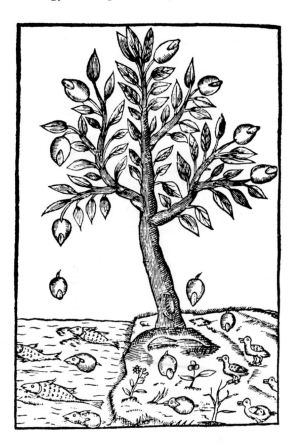

Fig. 3–1. This fifteenth-century woodcut of the tree of life shows leaves falling into the sea and onto the land. The interpretation that the genesis of animal life comes from such sources is clearly at variance with our modern knowledge. It is important to recognize that simple association is not the same as causality.

velopment of the lesion. It might be supposed that the relation of etiologic agent to disease, of cause to effect, was a relatively simple matter. Often the reverse is the case. Perhaps we are misled into imagining that only one cause is responsible. We say that the cause of tuberculosis is the tubercle bacillus, but we know that many people may inhale these bacilli yet only one may develop the disease, and that the bacilli may lurk in the body for years and only become active as the result of an intercurrent infection, prolonged stress, or starvation. In fact, Rich derived an equation to describe the development of disease in which he proposed that the occurrence of disease is directly proportional to the number and virulence of organisms and inversely proportional to the native and acquired resistance of the host (constitutional factors).

Obviously, the pathologist who investigates the causation of a disease must consider such elements as heredity, sex, age, environment, immunity, allergy, nutrition, and previous exposure to injury. It becomes evident, then, that there is no simple answer to such questions as, what is the cause of cancer or of arteriosclerosis?

The following classification may prove helpful in our attempts to cope with the infinitely large number of diseases to be identified now and in the future.

CLASSIFICATION OF DISEASES

Hereditary	Vascular
Congenital	Metabolic
Traumatic	Nutritional
Physical	Psychologic
Chemical	Iatrogenic
Infectious	Idiopathic
Inflammatory	Tumors

HEREDITY AND CONSTITUTION

Heredity. During the last 2 decades it has become increasingly clear that heritable disorders of structure and function may explain many diseases that have been poorly understood. Often the inherited abnormalities are subtle and their contribution to signs and symptoms of disease are debated. On the other hand, we have known since the time of Garrod (1909) of the relationship between the inborn error of metabolism and how it causes a failure of function. The field of medical genetics has advanced with exponential speed. It is based on several technologies: cytogenetics and the recognition of karyotypic or chromosomal abnormalities, human population studies and pedigree analysis, and modern biochemical methodologies that permit refined analytic procedures to distinguish small differences in serum, blood, urine, and cells of human beings—differences not detectable heretofore.

It is important to recognize that whereas hereditary disease implies a genetic basis for the disease, mutations do occur in persons. It is also important to recognize that all hereditary diseases do not appear or become identifiable at birth. It may well be that some heritable diseases that only appear at age 30 or 40 such as Huntington's chorea, a disease of the central nervous system that results in loss of motor control, may become detectable in the childhood period with more modern methods.

In addition, one must be aware that not all abnormalities seen in the newborn have their origin in genetic disorders. We now recognize that the fetus is unusually susceptible to a variety of influences during uterine life and not only the infectious diseases such as German measles, but the diet and drugs of the mother may directly affect the development of the fetus. Thus we distinguish between *congenital* disease (appearing at birth) and genetic disease, and between *genetic* disease that is heritable and that occurring spontaneously, due to a mutation.

Constitution comprises those features of the mind and body that a man derives from both heredity and environment. It is the sum total of his being. There can be little doubt that nutrition is a factor of great importance, especially in the early formative years of life. Every hour the cells of the body take up elements from the food, including vitamins, and if these are deficient in quantity or quality, the constitution as a whole cannot fail to suffer. It has been said, with what truth we are unable to tell, that if all the diseases in the textbooks could be removed by the wave of a wand, doctors would still be left with 80% of their patients. Their ill health would be due not so much to any known disease as to the failure of the constitution to adapt itself to the life the patient is leading. A good constitution is not to be confused with a good physique; it is something more and something more valuable. Those who have it seem able to do whatever they wish without impairing it in any way. When it is poor, small causes may impair health or even endanger life. The athlete with the most perfect physique may be prostrated by every infection that he encounters.

We now have available to us several different methods of finding information about a person's genetic makeup. There are various substances in the body whose presence, absence, or variations provide this information. Three groups of substances can be isolated and examined in the pursuit of genetic information: chromosomes, red blood cell antigens, and white blood cell antigens or HLA (human leukocyte antigens). These are called **markers** because their presence, absence, or variations are visible manifestations of the genes in the same way that blue eyes or dark skin are manifestations of the genes. Looking at skin color provides information about one genetically determined category, namely race. Looking at red blood cell antigens also yields information about genetic categories, namely, blood type (A, B, AB, O).

Examination of bands on chromosomes and the chromosomes themselves (a process called karyotyping) provides a picture of the shape, size, and number of chromosomes as well as (recently) location of bands on chromosomes. Certain human characteristics have been linked with these chromosome traits, for example, normal female sex is associated with two X chromosomes of a certain size and shape. Thus, in the case where a child's sex is not clear, the chromosomes are useful markers or indicators of the true genetic situation.

Red blood cell antigens were discovered after disastrous attempts at blood transfusion. Certain individuals were discovered to be (genetically) so different that their blood could not be exchanged. The donor and recipient must be of genetically compatible types, and the A, B, AB, O, groups serve as markers or indicators of who the compatible individuals are.

More recently, there have been some disas-

trous attempts at tissue transplantation, and it has been discovered that the red blood cell marker system does not provide sufficient information about compatibility. It seems that white blood cells also have surface antigens that must be matched if graft rejection is to be minimized. HLA, then, serve as markers of different genetically determined groups.

HLA have been found to have other uses outside of tissue transplantation. Not only are they markers of tissue compatibility; they have also been associated with various diseases. In this case, groups of persons suffering from the same disease appear to have the same combination of HLA antigens. (Each HLA antigen has been designated by a specific letter and number; hence HLA B27, HLA W6.) Investigators noticed that all sufferers of ankylosing spondylitis (a form of arthritis) had HLA B27, although not all persons with HLA B 27 either have or get ankylosing spondylitis. Current theory describes the presence of HLA B27 as a marker or indication that the person may be susceptible to ankylosing spondylitis, although given the right environmental conditions, he or she may never contract the disease. Thus the HLA marker system provides us with information about disease susceptibility; it allows us to distinguish between those who are most likely and those who are unlikely to contract the disease, and that is all. It provides us with no certainties, because it appears that other probable, nongenetic factors are crucial to the onset of the disease.

The following story provides an example of this concept. In June 1962, the United States Navy cruiser *Little Rock* departed from Trieste, Italy. Two days later, 602 of the 1,276 crew members came down with dysentery caused by the Shigella bacteria. Two weeks afterwards, 10 of the sailors who had been infected showed symptoms of Reiter's syndrome—swollen joints and skin infections— although no cases of this developed in the uninfected sailors. (Reiter's syndrome has been known to follow a Shigella infection.) Years later, 6 of the 10 sailors were located for HLA testing and it was discovered that 5 of them had HLA B27. (The sixth had had a much milder form of the disease.) Thus it appears that some people are born with a genetic susceptibility to Reiter's syndrome, a susceptibility that can be identified by the presence of HLA B27, but these persons will probably not develop the disease unless they encounter a triggering environmental factor, the Shigella.

Table 3–1.   HLA Antigens and Disease

DISEASE	HLA ANTIGEN SHOWING CHANGE IN FREQUENCY
Ankylosing spondylitis	↑ B27
Reiter's syndrome	↑ B27
Juvenile rheumatoid arthritis	↑ B27
Adult celiac disease	↑ B8, D3
Addison's disease	↑ B8, D3
Chronic active hepatitis	↑ B8, D3
Graves' disease	↑ B8, D3
Juvenile diabetes	↑ B8; ↑ B15; ↑ D3; ↑ D4
Myasthenia gravis	↑ B8, D3 (♀<35 yrs.)
Hodgkin's disease (>5-year survival)	↑ A3; ↑ A11
Multiple sclerosis	↑ D2

(Courtesy of Dr. R. D. Guttmann)

Many other diseases have since been linked with HLA antigens. Most of these have long been recognized as hereditary to some extent, but now there is a way to pinpoint who in a family is most susceptible, and who runs no risk. Eventually, we may be able to state that all disease is hereditary, meaning that we are all born with our own set of susceptibilities, and sooner or later the right environmental conditions will trigger development of the disease (Table 3–1).

TRAUMA

Trauma or mechanical injury may damage a part to such an extent that the tissues may be killed. It may take the form of a blow, a wound, a fracture of bone, or a sprain of a joint. Mechanical injury may act as a predisposing cause of a nontraumatic disease. One of the best examples is acute osteomyelitis, an acute inflammation of bone and bone marrow caused by microorganisms, usually staphylococci, which settle in the bone often at the site of a traumatic injury. It is the possibility that the disease may be predisposed or precipitated by trauma that makes Worker's Compensation cases so difficult to decide. Trauma may injure a bone, causing a fracture, or it may injure the soft parts, with a resulting wound or bruise.

An injury of the soft parts associated with rupture of the skin is known as a **wound**. It is obvious that there can be a great variety of wounds. The wound may be clean or infected, incised, punctured, penetrating, and so on. Trauma may injure the soft tissues even though the skin is not broken. The finer vessels, especially the capillaries, are ruptured, so that there is bleeding into the tissue spaces. The result is a **bruise** or **contusion**, which is at first red, then greenish or yellow before it fades. This is the basis of the so-called "black eye." The changes in color are caused by changes that the red blood cells undergo after the blood has been trapped in the interstitial spaces where the blood vessels have been ruptured (hematoma).

PHYSICAL AGENTS

Trauma, as described above, is the most obvious physical agent causing injury. Other physical agents that may prove dangerous are unusually high or low temperatures, irradiation, and increased or decreased atmospheric pressure.

Temperature. A high temperature may produce local or general damage. Local damage takes the form of **burns**. The burn may be first degree (slight reddening of skin), second degree (blistering), or third degree (destruction of whole thickness of skin). The threat to life depends as much on the size of the area burned as on the severity of the burn, because of the leakage of fluid and the concomitant shock.

Heat stroke may be caused by direct exposure to the sun (sunstroke), or to a high temperature. The heat-regulating mechanism of the body seems to be paralyzed, so that the temperature shoots up to an alarming degree, collapse and unconsciousness develop, and death may result; this is particularly true for temperatures above 42°C.

A low temperature may cause **frostbite**, which usually involves exposed parts such as the ears, the tip of the nose, the hands, and the feet. The fluid in the cells becomes converted into ice crystals, a change that ruptures cells. The result varies, as in the case of burns, from mild blistering to necrosis and gangrene.

Electrical Hazards. The enormous grid of power lines and the ready availability of electricity in the western world is taken for granted, but few of us recognize the hazards to life this provides until an accident occurs. Summer thunderstorms with lightning, and hospital or household hazards, are usually thought of, but the important concept is that very small currents (200 micro amps) may be sufficient to cause ventricular fibrillation when the normal protection of dry skin is altered, as in incisions or wetness. We have heard of one freak occurrence where a person found it necessary to empty his bladder in a place where the stream of urine fell on a live circuit, and the current was conducted through the stream to the bladder, alternately closing the urethral sphincter with electricity and temporarily paralyzing the victim. Fortunately, the sparks-stream episode was short-lived, but many other instances of human exposure to electrical current have had fatal results.

Radiation Injury. Different tissues differ widely in their sensitivity to radiation. Different kinds of animals also vary in a similar and, at present, inexplicable manner. In general terms it may be said that those cells are especially radiosensitive that normally continue to multiply throughout life, owing to their own short life span. Such are the cells of the lymphatic and hematopoietic or blood-forming systems, and the germinal cells of the gonads. We could expect a lymphocyte, with its life span of a few hours, to be more sensitive to radiation than a nerve cell that never divides.

CANCER CELLS. The cells of a neoplasm, like the normal cells from which they originate, differ widely in their response to irradiation. (Irradiation is the deliberate or therapeutic use of radiation.) Rapidly dividing cells may be expected to respond well, but the radiotherapist must beware of generalizations and know the peculiarities of individual tumors. Thus such tumors as malignant melanoma and osteogenic sarcoma may be teeming with mitoses and yet be quite radioresistant. Lymphosarcoma, composed of short-lived lymphocytes, is particularly radiosensitive, and may melt away as quickly as the proverbial snowball in hell. Unfortunately, there is a profound difference between radiosensitivity and radiocurability, for even the most radiosensitive of tumors have often a small

proportion of cells that survive and transmit the property of resistance to their progeny, so that eventually the entire mass may be radioresistant. We shall see the same thing happening in the case of antibiotics and bacteria.

There never has been a time when the question of radiation hazards was of graver concern or closer to the hearts of men than it is at present. These hazards are of 3 kinds, which in their order of importance may be termed diagnostic, therapeutic, and fallout hazards. **Diagnostic radiation**, when used with judgment (Fig. 3–2A), presents so small a hazard to health that it is completely outweighed by the potential for good. If overdone and repeated too frequently, it may be a source of danger. **Therapeutic radiation** obviously involves greater hazard, because the radiotherapist's object is to disable or kill cancer or other undesirable cells, and in the process the normal tissue may easily be injured. In some cases the injury may be much more serious and devastating than that inflicted by the surgeon's knife. The effect of radiation depends on (1) size of dose and (2) sensitivity of tissue, to which must be added the area involved in the radiation. The dosage is expressed as roentgens or r, in honor of Roentgen, who first observed the rays or radiations from the vacuum cathode tube. **Fallout radiation**, which gives rise to total body radiation (Fig. 3–2B), may be the result of atomic or hydrogen bomb bursts in war, of atomic weapon tests, or of accidental leakage from atomic energy installations. A dose of 400 r over the total body surface is believed to be enough to kill half of a given human population.

SKIN. The skin is most frequently involved, because all therapeutic external radiations must pass through the skin. **Acute radiodermatitis** is really a burn of the skin, but one that takes many days or a week or two to develop. It is equally slow in healing, and scarring may go on for many months, causing marked deformity. **Chronic radiodermatitis** is likely to be the result of frequent small doses. It was a common lesion on the hands of radiologists before the danger was realized and efficient screening was practiced. The epidermis is thinned and devitalized, so that minor injury may result in localized areas of necrosis that often take months to heal. The surrounding capillaries are dilated, so that the skin is red. Finally, carcinoma may develop, often after an interval of many years since the last exposure to radiation.

LYMPHOID AND HEMATOPOIETIC TISSUES. These are the most sensitive to radiation. Damage to these tissues is most likely to be seen in total body radiation. As the life span of the lymphocyte is only a few hours, extensive injury to lymphoid tissue is immediately followed by a marked drop in the number of lymphocytes in the circulating blood. The hematopoietic cells of the bone marrow are even more sensitive than the lymphocytes. There is

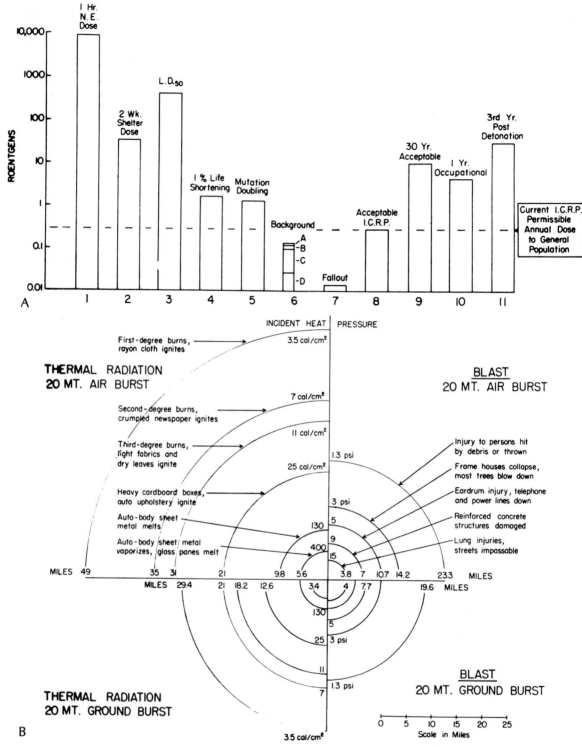

Fig. 3–2. *A,* The normal background of man-made radiation, such as x rays, luminous watch dials, and television screens is shown in column 6 at *A,* internal emitters such as potassium 42, calcium 45, and radon at *B,* gamma rays from radium thorium and granite at *C,* and cosmic rays at sea level at *D.* The estimated total global fallout from atomic testing through the year 1961 is shown in column *7,* and the annual dose suggested by the International Commission on Radiological Protection as the maximum permissible dose for the general population from all sources is shown in column *8.* Compare this with the doses that would be received in the vicinity of atomic explosion shown in columns *1* and *2.* The estimated level of exposure that doubles the mutation rate in mammalian germ cells is shown in column *5. B,* This diagram shows the effect of radiation at different distances from the center of an atomic blast. (*A* and *B* from Ervin, F.R., et al.: Human and ecologic effects in Massachusetts of an assumed thermonuclear attack on the United States. N. Engl. J. Med., 266:1127, 1962.)

a striking drop in the number of circulating granular leukocytes and blood platelets, the maximum effect being seen about the end of the first week of total body radiation. By that time the bone marrow is almost acellular. If the patient survives, he is sure to suffer from recurring infections due to the lack of leukocytes as well as failure in antibody formation owing to the loss of lymphocytes, and from frequent hemorrhages due to the lack of platelets. Long-continued exposure to small doses of ionizing radiation may cause neoplasia rather than destruction of the marrow cells, which results in leukemia, an occupational hazard of radiologists before this danger was recognized. Leukemia is also liable to develop in patients receiving long-continued heavy radiation for the disabling disease of the spine, ankylosing spondylitis.

GASTROINTESTINAL TRACT. The epithelium of the stomach and intestine is continually being renewed, so that it is highly radiosensitive, but the deep location of these structures serves to protect them against external radiation of moderate intensity. When radium is implanted for the treatment of carcinoma of the cervix, the mucosa of the rectum and colon may be seriously injured, with changes comparable with the lesion of radiodermatitis. In about 2% of presumably oversensitive persons inflammatory lesions with ulceration may develop in the anterior wall of the rectum from 6 months to several years after completion of the treatment. These ulcers are painful and the partitions between the rectum, bladder, and vagina may break down with distressing results. Even if the lesions heal, there may be extensive scarring with stricture (narrowing) of the rectum.

GERM CELLS. The germinal cells of the ovary and testis are highly radiosensitive, so that these organs have to be shielded with particular care in persons liable to be exposed to radiation, more especially workers with radioactive material. The testicles are naturally more exposed than the deeply situated ovaries. If the cells are killed, sterility is the result. If, on the other hand, one of the chromosomes or even one of its genes is damaged, the result may be a mutation, which becomes hereditary, transmitted to future generations. This is the basis of the genetic hazard of fallout radiation resulting from the atomic bomb explosions or tests.

ACUTE RADIATION SYNDROME. This syndrome, caused by whole body radiation due to atomic fallout from the air, must be distinguished from **radiation sickness**, the result of intensive local radiotherapy, which is characterized by loss of appetite and nausea, but rarely by vomiting. The essential lesion of total body radiation is cell depletion. This applies particularly to the intestine, the bone marrow, and the testes, but with a marked difference in the time element. After a single small total body exposure, the maximum damage to the small bowel occurs within a few days, to the granulocytes of the marrow in 3 to 5 weeks, while the sperm cells reach their minimum number in about a year. In the low dose range (100 r) death is due to depression of the bone marrow; in the middle-dose range (500 r) it is due to damage to the gastrointestinal tract; in the high-dose range (2,000 r) it is the result of failure of the central nervous system. There is a wide variation in individual susceptibility both in the experimental animal and in man. There were many thousands of survivors of the Hiroshima and Nagasaki blasts who resumed their previous occupations with full vigor. Of these we hear little.

The **clinical picture** is as follows. Within 2 hours of exposure there is a sudden onset of anorexia (loss of appetite), nausea, fatigue, malaise, and drowsiness. By the third day the patient feels well. Some 3 weeks later he begins to suffer from chills, fever, malaise, and shortness of breath. These are followed in a day or so by (1) diarrhea and other evidence of ulceration of the bowel, (2) hemorrhages into the skin and from the mucous membranes due to destruction of the megakaryocytes in the bone marrow which make the blood platelets, (3) severe infections in the mouth and elsewhere due to the disappearance of the polymorphonuclear leukocytes and of the lymphocytes which make antibodies, and finally (4) severe anemia due to destruction of the blood-forming cells of the marrow.

A moving account of the development of the acute radiation syndrome in an entire community representing the last survivors of a world war fought with atomic weapons will be found in Nevil Shute's novel, *On the Beach.*

In addition to the foregoing account of radiation effects, three other types of hazard deserve mention. First, those exposed in an atomic blast run the risk of developing later cataracts, leukemia, and possibly a variety of neoplasms. Second, there is a danger that radioactive isotope strontium-90, formed during the blast, will be incorporated into vegetation, and eventually into milk, and then into the bones of mammals such as man. Finally, we must not forget that we are all constantly exposed to other forms of radiation such as microwaves from television sets and microwave towers. Prolonged exposure to microwaves produces headaches, a general feeling of malaise, a reduced white blood cell count, and possibly more change in our physiology and cellular function than we have detected to date.

Atmospheric Pressure. As in the case of temperature, the pressure of the atmosphere may be too high or too low.

INCREASED PRESSURE. People so affected are those involved in construction of piers under water (when caissons are used), in construction of tunnels under rivers, and in deep-sea diving. Additional pressure of 2 or 3 atmospheres may be experienced, which results in additional air becoming dissolved in the blood plasma. When a person passes too rapidly from a high to a normal atmospheric pressure, the dissolved air is released as bubbles in the blood. The oxygen is absorbed, but the nitrogen may form bubbles or emboli in the small arteries to the brain with resulting damage. Pains develop in various parts of the body (the bends), and there may be temporary or even permanent paralysis. The condition in general is known as **caisson disease**.

DECREASED PRESSURE. Effects of decreased pressure may be experienced by aviators flying at altitudes over 30,000 feet unless the plane is pressurized. The gases in the body cavities such as the intestine expand, causing marked discomfort, and gas bubbles are released in the blood and cause air embolism, with results similar to those of caisson disease.

CHEMICAL POISONS

The subject of poisoning, or toxicology, is a large and specialized one that need not detain us long. Poisonous chemicals may be introduced into the body under 4 different circumstances: (1) by **accident**, especially in the case of young children, (2) for **suicide,** (3) for **homicide,** (4) as an **industrial hazard.** In these days, when every industry seems to use a new and different chemical, the last-named has become of particular importance. Strong acids and alkalis burn and kill the skin or the mucous membrane of the mouth and stomach if taken internally. Lead poisoning (plumbism) deserves special mention, because it belongs to both the first and fourth groups. Children are apt to put painted objects in their mouths and repeatedly swallow small amounts of the lead in the paint. Lead is used in many industries—painting, glass making, lacquering, among others. In these occupations it is particularly important to wash the hands well before eating. Poisons such as lead, mercury, arsenic, and phosphorus interfere with the working of some of the cell enzymes, thus producing sickness and even death.

INFECTIONS

Biologic agents are the cause of infections. They may be minute and exist only as nucleic acid (viruses), or gigantic and complex, as are some intestinal parasites (nematodes, cestodes). Basically, one can think of infectious diseases as a form of parasitism, in which man is the host and the parasite is more or less successful, depending on the nature of the response that it elicits in man. Disease is the product of the interaction between the agent and the host; thus we may be visited by many bacteria, without developing any signs or symptoms, but at other times the same organisms may elicit a strong response that causes destruction and loss of function in various parts of our body. The most successful agents are not those that cause death of the host quickly. In fact, a virulent organism will prevent itself from becoming disseminated should it destroy the host: viruses, bacteria, fungi, and parasites are more successful if they create a symbiotic relationship.

By far the most common cause of disease is **bacteria**. Finally there are **filterable viruses**, forms of living matter so minute that they pass through the pores of filters fine enough to hold back bacteria, so tiny that they cannot be seen with the most powerful light microscope.

Bacteria (commonly called microorganisms or germs) can be divided into 3 main groups: (1) **cocci**, which are round, (2) **bacilli**, which are rod-shaped and (3) **spirilla**, or spirochetes, which are spiral like a corkscrew. They cause disease either by their presence in the tissues or by producing toxins (poisons), which either act on the surrounding structures or are carried by the blood stream to distant organs; in both instances they cause inflammation and degeneration.

It would be useless to list here the bacteria that cause disease, for it would be merely a list of names with little meaning. Some of these are considered in Chapter 7, and others in connection with the organs that they are most prone to attack.

INFLAMMATION

Whereas most infections produce inflammation in the host, not all inflammation is due to infectious agents. The body responds to any injury such as wounding or burns with inflammation: heat, swelling, redness, pain.

Recently, another type of injury has been

identified as responsible for arousing the fever, chills, and leukocytosis that herald inflammation. We now know that there are many instances in which our bodies elaborate and circulate antibodies in response to an injury or exposure to an antigen, e.g., response to poison ivy or a bee sting. This type of inflammation can cause just as serious a disability as an infection with a bacterium. In fact, we now believe that many chronic and a few acute diseases (rheumatoid arthritis, glomerulonephritis, serum sickness) are diseases in which inflammation is the only part of the disease that we really comprehend; the exact mechanism of injury and the nature of the antigenic stimulus are still unclear. Some of these diseases respond dramatically to anti-inflammatory agents such as cortisone or aspirin, but these drugs are palliative and do not cure the disease. In our classification of diseases, therefore, we should distinguish inflammation from infection. It is important to keep this in mind as we read on, because there are even instances in which the inciting agent may be some tissue or altered tissue of the body itself, leading to the concept of **autoimmune** diseases.

VASCULAR DISEASE

Perhaps the commonest disease of the civilized world is atherosclerosis or arteriosclerosis. It is not clear whether this disease of blood vessels is acquired or has a hereditary factor, but it is clear that occlusion of branches of the arterial tree causes untimely death in more than 500,000 North Americans each year. It is most convenient at present to consider it as a multifactorial disease that has an increased incidence in those who have hypertension, hypercholesterolemia, or diabetes mellitus, in those who are overweight, or in those who smoke. There is increasing evidence to support the idea that a sedentary life accelerates the process and that exercise may ameliorate or delay the onset of arteriosclerosis. We also believe, from experiments in baboons, that atherosclerosis is reversible to some degree, but of course this is difficult to study in man.

Loss of blood supply to a part is called **ischemia**. This is a local loss of blood supply in contrast to anemia, which is a general condition of bloodlessness affecting the entire body. The result is **anoxia** or loss of oxygen to the part. As the food and oxygen are carried by the blood, it is evident that if the supply of blood is diminished by narrowing of the lumen of an artery, the part of the body deprived of its blood supply will suffer and become diseased. An example of this is seen in arteriosclerosis of the vessels supplying the leg; the tissues of the foot will finally die, a condition formerly known as **gangrene**. An even more important example of ischemia is blockage of the coronary arteries to the heart muscle, either by arteriosclerosis or by thrombosis, resulting in sudden death, in arrhythmias, or in permanent damage to the heart (infarction).

METABOLIC DISEASES

Diseases of this type can be thought of as those in which disorders in the production of enzymes, hormones, or secreting products can be identified. These diseases commonly are hereditary, such as the glycogen storage diseases, and have been found for all kinds of metabolism whether it is an amino aciduria, hypertriglyceridemia, or defect in mucopolysaccharide synthesis. But some metabolic diseases are acquired later in life, perhaps due to changes in the function of an organ or organ system caused by viral infection, or by destruction by such forces as the presence of tumor in a vital organ, or by necrosis of an endocrine gland due to infarction, presence of a cyst, or inflammation.

This heading is a catchall because it depends on your point of view whether you wish to include diabetes mellitus here or under, for example, hereditary diseases. In fact, as we gain newer knowledge, diseases may be shunted around like boxcars in a railyard in our classification. Recently there has been some evidence that diabetes mellitus occurs in young people following a viral infection. So is diabetes mellitus a metabolic, an hereditary, or an infectious disease?

This does not really damage the validity of the pigeonhole, because there are many diseases in the same category. For example, is atherosclerosis a metabolic or a vascular disease? Clearly, the use of any classification system is simply to aid you in organizing the information that comes your way. Diseases of the endocrine system can be cataloged under metabolism, along with disorders of fluids and electrolytes, such as shock and dehydration.

NUTRITIONAL DISEASES

The idea that disease may be due to something lacking, rather than to some positive hostile factor such as bacteria, injury, or poison, is a sophisticated one, but enormously important and far-reaching. It has always been recognized that starvation will affect the health of the body and will eventually result in death. But there may be an insufficient supply of some particular element in the food, such as a particular amino acid or essential lipid. Perhaps more important as a cause of disease is an inadequate supply of **minerals** and of the essential coenzymes known as **vitamins.** Even though actual disease may not be present, perfect health is impossible if there are deficiencies in the food. This is particularly true of the growing period of life.

With every year that passes, the importance of nutritional deficiencies is becoming more apparent. It is the quality rather than the quantity of the food that is essential (Fig. 3–3). During starvation, the demands of the body are so much lowered that true deficiency disease may not become apparent. However, if the food is abundant in carbohydrates, but deficient in minerals or vitamins, the health of the cells is impaired and evidence of disease becomes manifest.

The most common worldwide cause of disease attributable to nutrition may be inadequate caloric intake, as in many parts of Asia today; in North America there is a malnutrition of a different kind. Large populations eat carbohydrates exclusively; on the other hand, some eat an expensive, high-protein, high-fat diet that they do not need. Eating is a cultural and social activity, and most people do not understand or consider the rationale of eating. Although most of this section on nutritional disease will be devoted to deficiencies, it is worth mentioning that

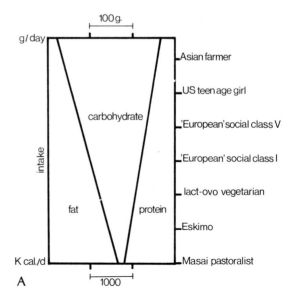

Fig. 3–3. *A,* This graph shows the relative proportions in the diet of different persons of fat, carbohydrate, and protein. At the top the chart is shown in grams. The Asian farmer subsists on a principally carbohydrate diet, whereas the Eskimo lives on a diet rich in fat and protein. (From Thorn, G.W., et al. (Eds.): *Harrison's Principles of Internal Medicine,* 8th Ed. New York, McGraw-Hill, 1977.)

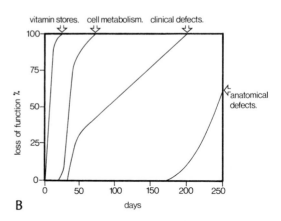

B, This graph shows the time span related to the loss of function before anatomical defects occur in vitamin deficiencies. Clearly, cell metabolism and clinical defects occur first. (Adapted from Marks, J.: *The Vitamins in Health and Disease.* Boston, Little, Brown, 1968.)

problems also arise at the other end of the spectrum, where too much food rather than too little is the problem. Obesity is a major health problem in many countries. For example, in Karelia, Northern Finland, there is the highest incidence of death from heart attacks in the world. This population is well nourished and also has a high incidence of hypertension. In general, obese persons run a greater risk of developing hypertension, cardiovascular disease, diabetes, and gallstones. The mortality rate is higher than for people of normal weight. Each pound of fat has been estimated to add as much as a kilometer of blood vessels that increase the work of the heart, to say nothing of the load added weight places on the joints of the skeleton. To complicate matters further, each pound of additional adipose tissue is a living thing, not an inert brick of lard, and like all living things it requires energy, usually in the form of glucose. Thus, once you have transformed 25 or 30% of your body into adipose tissue, you have acquired a hungry population of cells which continually cry for more nourishment. Most obese people feel they have to eat because the hypoglycemia (low blood sugar) they experience is a very real part of being fat; this vicious cycle is hard to break. Excess adipose tissue uses glucose, makes you hungry, you eat more, you make more adipose tissue, you continue to eat to feed the adipose parasite. It's a little like spending all your electricity budget to keep your freezer cold when you are eating fresh vegetables.

The most obvious method of production of nutritional deficiency is lack in certain elements in the diet. But the same result may be brought about in a number of other ways. If a patient suffers from persistent vomiting, he cannot assimilate his food, no matter how excellent it may be. Conditions such as gastric ulcer and diabetes may necessitate the long-continued use of diets that may be deficient in particular food elements. Widespread disease of the intestine, commonly associated with diarrhea, may interfere so seriously with the absorption of food that deficiency must result. Even when satisfactory absorption has occurred, such an important organ as the liver may be unable to deal with the food elements owing to cirrhosis, for example, and once again symptoms of deficiency may appear. This discussion, which could be expanded considerably, indicates how readily a condition of dietary deficiency may arise.

Resistance to infection appears to depend to some extent on the food supply and particularly on proteins, for it is from proteins that antibodies to bacteria are manufactured.

Chronic starvation is associated with a greatly lowered resistance to such infections as tuberculosis. A tragic demonstration of this fact is provided by the high incidence of tuberculosis and other serious infections among the peoples of Europe impoverished by a great war. Although this association between starvation and infection has frequently been noted, it has not yet been firmly established.

The earlier work on nutritional deficiency, particularly vitamin deficiency, was concerned with what may be termed full-blown diseases such as scurvy, rickets, and beriberi. It is now realized that minor manifestations of deficiency are much more common, although they have been overlooked in the past. In certain localities where, for geographic reasons, there is a grave lack of such essential foods as milk and fresh vegetables, a large proportion of the population may exhibit symptoms and signs of deficiency disease, although they may be unconscious of the fact.

Mineral Deficiency. Among the important minerals that may be deficient in the food are calcium, iron, and iodine. **Calcium** is necessary both for the formation and the continued health of bone. If it is deficient in the diet during early childhood, there is danger that rickets may develop; the bones that are deficient in calcium are soft and easily bent, so that bowlegs and other deformities develop. In adult life calcium deficiency may also lead to softening of the bone or osteomalacia (the same thing in Greek). **Iron** is absolutely necessary for the synthesis of hemoglobin, and when it is deficient in the diet, anemia inevitably develops. Normal adults have 2 to 6 gms of iron, of which 80% is in the hemoglobin of the erythrocytes, and 20% is in stores in the liver, spleen, or in cellular enzymes (cytochrome), or myoglobin. Normally, adults lose about 1 mg per day in the urine, stool, or sweat, and this is matched by absorption from the small bowel from dietary sources. Menstruation increases this loss to 30 mg for each period, and in pregnancy, 500 mg of iron goes to the fetus. With extra exercise (marathon training) there is an increased loss, just as there is with hemolysis (breakdown of red blood cells) whatever the cause. As will be seen when diseases of the blood are studied, anemias are now divided into iron-deficiency anemias and other forms of anemia. It is of interest to note that the most important member of the latter group, pernicious anemia, is also a deficiency disease. **Iodine** is essential to the proper functioning of the thyroid gland, and when it is deficient, one form of goiter develops. Although minerals are essential for the health of the body, the actual amounts needed are extraordinarily minute. For instance, the amount of iodine needed to prevent the development of goiter is only 10 to 20 mg a year.

Potassium deficiency has come to assume a position of special importance. The deficiency of the mineral is due to loss from the body, not to an insufficient supply in the food. We owe the realization of the importance of potassium in the body's economy to an advance in medical technology, for the use of the flame photometer has made it possible to estimate the potassium content of body fluids and tissues. At least 98% of the potassium of the body is located in the intracellular fluid, mainly in the muscle cells, in contrast with sodium, which is mainly in the extracellular fluid. Potassium deficiency (hypokalemia) may develop from a variety of causes, of which the most important are: (1) stress, usually the result of surgical trauma, the cells of the postoperative patient leaking potassium into the extracellular fluid and thence at once into the urine, and the leak being activated by aldosterone liberated as part of the reaction of the adrenal cortex to stress; (2) vomiting and diarrhea, when severe and prolonged; (3) deficiency caused by therapy, especially the continued intravenous administration of salt and glucose solutions, or the use of modern antihypertensive drugs that may lower the serum potassium level to a dangerous degree. The muscles suffer most, with lack of tone, weakness, and finally, paralysis. The abdominal distention so common in the postoperative patient is caused by lack of tone of the muscular wall of the intestine due to potassium depletion caused by stress. Cardiac dilatation and myocardial failure with marked changes in the electrocardiogram are among the most serious of its effects.

There is a curious relationship between mineral metabolism and the ductless glands, which will be discussed in more detail when diseases of these organs are considered. Iodine metabolism is regulated by the thyroid gland, and as we have just seen, lack of iodine causes disturbed iodine metabolism. The parathyroid glands bear the same relation to calcium metabolism, and the adrenals govern the metabolism of sodium chloride.

Other minerals or trace elements that are important in man include zinc (Zn^+), which plays a role in the healing of surgical incisions and any injury; magnesium (Mg^{++}), which is essential for protein synthesis; phosphorus (PO_4^{++}), which is fundamental to energy production and to the normal development of bone; and, naturally, sodium and chloride.

Vitamin Deficiency. An adequate supply of protein, carbohydrate, fat, and mineral salts is not sufficient for the needs of the living body. Certain "accessory food factors" are also necessary for life. These are called vitamins. They are formed or synthesized by plants, not by animals. Man's supply therefore comes directly from plants, or from animals (including fish) that have eaten the plants and have stored the vitamins—unless these happen to be bought at the corner drugstore. They need only be present in minute amounts, but their absence (avitaminosis) leads to profound pathologic changes. Some deficiency diseases, such as rickets and scurvy, have been known for centuries. Although it was not recognized that they were due to a simple deficiency in diet, empiric methods of treatment were successfully employed. The old explorers recognized the value of fresh fruit in the prevention of scurvy, and cod liver oil has been used in the treatment of rickets for more than 100 years.

The original list of 4 vitamins (A, B, C, D) has been greatly extended, and the end is not in sight. Moreover, vitamin B, a complex, has been separated into a number of distinct chemicals. With such complexity, the alphabetic system of names has broken down, and the chemical names have come into general use. Vitamins are organic catalysts of exogenous origin, which are intimately related to the enzyme systems. They play the part of coenzymes in the chemical mechanism of the cell by which foodstuffs are metabolized. In many respects they resemble hormones, the chief distinction being that hormones are endogenous in origin, whereas vitamins are exogenous, the body being unable to synthesize them.

It is customary to divide the vitamins into 2 groups, the fat-soluble and the water-soluble. The **fat-soluble vitamins** are A, D, E, and K, and the **water-soluble** ones are B and C.

Avitaminosis or vitamin deficiency may be due to 2 different conditions. (1) The supply of the food factor may be inadequate. This is known as primary deficiency, and is exogenous in origin. This is no longer of great importance in developed countries, except among food faddists and other health cranks, but it is widely prevalent in underdeveloped countries, particularly in Africa and in the Orient. (2) The supply is adequate, but for various reasons it cannot be used properly. This is secondary conditioned deficiency. Conditioning factors may be: (1) **reduced intake**, as may occur in prolonged vomiting, esophageal obstruction, and loss of appetite; (2) **malabsorption**, such as occurs in chronic inflammation of the pancreas and small intestine; (3) **excessive demand**, seen especially in infancy and puberty, but also during pregnancy and lactation; (4) **reduced storage facilities**, the best example being cirrhosis of the liver in the chronic alcoholic. Before proceeding to a consideration of the various vitamin deficiencies, it should be pointed out that man seldom shows the picture of pure vitamin deficiency seen in the experimental animal, and that the administration of a single vitamin in a chemically pure state may not serve to correct the condition. We now know enough, however, to prevent the 5 major vitamin-deficiency diseases, namely **beriberi** (vitamin B complex—thiamin), **pellagra** (vitamin B complex—niacin), **scurvy** (vitamin C), **rickets** (vitamin D), and **keratomalacia** (vitamin A).

Vitamin A. This fat-soluble vitamin is found in butter, cream, egg yolk, and fish liver oils, as well as in yellow and green vegetables such as carrots, spinach, peas, and beans. The plants do not really contain vitamin A, but a yellow pigment called **carotene** that is converted by the liver into the vitamin. The vitamin A content of milk and butter depends on the carotene content of the plants the animal eats. Even the vitamin in fish liver oil comes

from marine plants (plankton). Minute invertebrates feed on the plants; they are devoured later by small fish; these in turn serve as food to large fish in whose livers the vitamin is stored.

Lack of vitamin A in the diet leads to change in the epithelium lining the mucous membranes in the respiratory and digestive tracts as well as in certain glands such as the lachrymal and salivary. These mucous surfaces are especially susceptible to infection. In children, in whom the deficiency is most likely to develop, drying of the cornea, known as xerophthalmia (Greek *xeros*, dry) may occur owing to lack of secretion of the lachrymal glands. Bronchopneumonia in children may be caused by the changes in the mucous membrane of the bronchial tree. A peculiar symptom is night blindness, or inability to see in a dim light. This is due to deficiency in the visual purple of the retina, a substance necessary for vision in poor light.

Under ordinary conditions of life, vitamin A deficiency is seldom seen in Europe and North America, although it is common in India, China, and other countries where the diet is often of low quality. When war brings restriction in diet, however, night blindness and xerophthalmia may become common, the former being particularly dangerous during blackouts. Governments have recognized this to such an extent that they have added vitamin A to bread when necessary.

Vitamin B Complex. One of the earliest discoveries regarding vitamins was that beriberi, a disease of the Orient, was due to eating "polished" rice, i.e., rice from which the outer covering and the germ had been removed in the milling process. The vitamin responsible was called vitamin B. It is now known that what was thought to be a single vitamin is really a complex, from which a number of components have been separated. The 3 best known of these are thiamin, niacin, and riboflavin. This group of vitamins is one of the most widely distributed, being present in all natural foodstuffs. The various members of the group are water-soluble, so that they are readily absorbed, but they pay a penalty, because much is lost in the process of refining and of converting natural into artificial foods, as in the case of white bread and polished rice. Fortunately, most of the B complex vitamins used by the body are produced by the bacteria in the intestine.

Thiamin (formerly vitamin B_1) is the antiberiberi factor. The principal features of beriberi are peripheral neuritis (marked by weakness of the limbs), widespread edema, and myocardial weakness. When rice is polished, the skin and the germ, which contain the vitamin, are removed, so that in rice-eating countries such as China, beriberi is a common disease. Thiamin is now added to enriched wheat flour, to restore what is lost from the whole wheat in milling.

Riboflavin (formerly vitamin B_2) is also desirable for the enrichment of bread, but the supply is still inadequate. Mild symptoms of its absence (ariboflavinosis) are not uncommon among the under-nourished and among those women who subsist on absurdly inadequate diets with the object of improving their figures. Severe manifestations are seen principally in the southern United States and in Newfoundland. There may be fissured lesions at the corners of the mouth (cheilosis) and erosions around the eyes and the sides of the nose. The tongue may acquire a characteristic magenta color. The most serious disturbances are those involving the eye. In persons whose occupation exposes them to bright light, including workers with the microscope, there may be eyestrain and redness of the conjunctiva and the lower lids. In advanced cases there is invasion of the cornea by capillaries. In the past, these ocular symptoms were never attributed to the real cause, namely, vitamin deficiency. The principal source of riboflavin is milk.

Niacin (formerly nicotinic acid) is the pellagra-preventing vitamin. **Pellagra** is a disease common in Italy and the southern United States, but it is not confined to these regions. It is characterized by reddening and scaling of the skin on the exposed parts of the body, as well as by gastrointestinal, nervous, and mental disorders. The tongue may become smooth and fiery red. Although a deficiency disease, it is also in some way connected with eating diseased maize.

Vitamin B$_{12}$ is a growth factor in the maturation of red blood cells in the bone marrow. It is derived from the food, but it is absorbed from the intestine only in the presence of an "intrinsic factor" secreted by the stomach. Absence of this factor leads to the development of pernicious anemia, in which the progenitors of the red blood cells in the marrow do not develop into adult erythrocytes, but enter the blood stream as abnormally large red cells (macrocytes), which have a shortened life span, even though the bowel is full of vitamin. Vitamin B$_{12}$ deficiency is therefore an excellent example of a conditioned deficiency, depending on absence of the gastric intrinsic factor.

VITAMIN C (ASCORBIC ACID). This is the antiscorbutic vitamin, which prevents scurvy or scorbutus. It occurs in fruits and fresh vegetables rather than in fats. It is particularly abundant in tomato, orange, lemon and grapefruit. It is destroyed by heat and drying, so that preserved foods and fruits are lacking it. In vitamin C deficiency, the level of ascorbic acid is low in the urine and very low in the blood. By estimation of this level, deficiency of the vitamin can be readily detected. Linus Pauling, Nobel Prize Winner, believes that taking large doses of vitamin C in the form of powdered ascorbic acid leads to increased vigor, increased protection against infections, and increased rate of healing of wounds.

When ascorbic acid is lacking, the cement substance, which holds together the endothelial cells lining the capillaries, becomes deficient. The vessels thus develop leaks through which bleeding occurs into the tissues. The health of the ground substance of the connective tissue in general also suffers.

Scurvy is the manifestation of vitamin C deficiency. It used to be a common disease among sailors, soldiers, arctic explorers, and others deprived of fresh fruit and vegetables. The old Elizabethan seaman, Captain Hawkins, called it "the plague of the sea and the spoil of mariners," adding that "the sea is natural for fishes and the land for men." That was all changed by Captain Cook's discovery that limes and lime juice would prevent the disease, and now even that is not necessary, for the vitamin can be put up as tablets of ascorbic acid.

Hemorrhage occurs owing to lack of cement substance in the capillaries. The gums are soft, spongy, bleed readily, and are heavily invaded by bacteria, while the teeth fall out, so that the condition of the mouth becomes foul and distressing. The skin presents numerous small hemorrhages (petechiae). There is hemorrhage into the joints and the internal organs. Owing to the deficient ground substance of connective tissue, there is delayed healing of wounds. After healing they tend to break down under strain. If the scorbutic condition is not relieved, it may end fatally, and in the past it frequently did so.

VITAMIN D. Much of the romance of the vitamins centers around this member of the group. Several factors are concerned in the action of this vitamin, and the unraveling of these might easily have taken half a century, but the whole problem was cleared up in little more than half a dozen years by workers in many widely separated countries.

Vitamin D is the antirachitic vitamin; it prevents rickets. It does this by controlling calcium metabolism. It is a fat-soluble vitamin, and so, as might be expected, it is found in milk, butter, egg yolk, and other fats, but by far the most abundant supply is in cod liver oil.

One of the remarkable discoveries was that the vitamin is formed by the action of ultraviolet light on certain waxy compounds known as sterols, particularly ergosterol, found in yeast, and cholesterol, present in the skin. When the skin is exposed to abundant sunlight, a sufficient amount of the vitamin is formed from the cholesterol. In dark and gloomy climates, however, and in the slums of cities, there is not enough light to form the vitamin. It is prepared commercially by irradiating yeast, which is rich in ergosterol, by the mercury vapor lamp, and is then called viosterol. The vitamin has been synthesized in the laboratory; it is a yellow, crystalline substance, which has been named calciferol, because of its influence on calcification.

Without a sufficient supply of vitamin D, the proper calcification of bone in the child cannot take place, and rickets is the result. It is also required for the formation of normal teeth in the growing child. Marked deficiency of the vitamin is rare in adults, but when present it may produce osteomalacia.

This disease is more likely to be seen in countries such as India and China, where the diet is deficient. It is most common in women, who are not often exposed to sunlight in those countries.

Rickets is a disease of young children. The bones are not properly formed, owing to insufficient deposition of both calcium and phosphorus. The bones are therefore soft and bend easily, so that deformities (e.g., bowlegs) result. (These deformities are described in more detail in connection with disease of bones.) The disease occurs usually in bottle-fed babies, and in young children brought up in the slums of smoky cities in northern latitudes. It is unknown in the tropics. As we have seen, it may be due to one of two factors, or often to a combination of the two: (1) insufficient vitamin D in the diet; (2) insufficient sunlight (ultraviolet), which could produce the vitamin by activating the cholesterol in the skin. There are also rare causes of rickets that may be inherited. Treatment of rickets is more successful if the correct cause is established.

There have also been tragic instances in which excessive amounts of vitamin D have been administered on the basis of "where a little is good, a lot is better." Excess vitamin D can lead to calcification in the brain and other organs.

VITAMIN E. This vitamin is necessary for normal reproduction, and so it has been called the antisterility vitamin. The chief sources are the germ of various cereals and green vegetable foods. Wheat germ oil contains a large amount of the vitamin. Knowledge of its actions is limited to animals. Deficiency in female rats causes the embryo to die early, and in males spermatozoa are not produced because of degenerative changes in the testes. This has not been established for human beings.

VITAMIN K. The story of vitamin K is as remarkable as that of vitamin D. In 1930 a Danish observer, Dam, noticed that chicks fed on a deficient diet developed hemorrhage, and that this was prevented when they were given alfalfa. There was evidently some factor in the alfalfa that was necessary for the coagulation of the blood and without which hemorrhage would occur. Soon this factor was extracted and crystallized. It was called Koagulations vitamin, being German for the vitamin that promotes coagulation; this became shortened to vitamin K.

The **prothrombin** of the blood must be at a normal level if the coagulation of blood, which is necessary to stop hemorrhage, is to occur normally. It was soon found that animals deficient in vitamin K were also deficient in prothrombin, and so it became apparent that vitamin K is necessary for the formation of prothrombin. The mere presence of a sufficient amount of vitamin K in the food is not enough; it has to be absorbed before it can be used for the manufacture of prothrombin.

The next discovery was that the vitamin is not absorbed unless bile is present in the intestine. It had long been known that operations on jaundiced patients were apt to be followed by hemorrhage, often fatal, at the site of operation. In jaundice, the bile is unable to reach the intestine. Now it was clear that the reason for the bleeding tendency in jaundice was lack of vitamin K, that lack being due to failure in absorption, which in turn was due to absence of bile in the bowel. The prothrombin in the blood was found to be low in cases of jaundice, as was to be expected.

This was a discovery of great practical importance, because now it is possible to raise the prothrombin in the blood of jaundiced patients before operation. This is done by administering bile, or rather bile salts, combined with vitamin K. The vitamin is absorbed, the prothrombin rises to normal, and the operation can be performed without the danger of hemorrhage.

Another condition in which the prothrombin is low is hemorrhagic disease of the newborn. Shortly after birth the baby may show a tendency to bleeding, and if there has been any birth injury to the head, there may be fatal intracranial hemorrhage. This is due to vitamin K deficiency in the baby, and can readily be prevented by administering the vitamin to the mother before delivery.

Table 3–2 is a summary of some of the principal clinical features of the vitamin deficiencies in man.

The various vitamins are necessary for perfect health. Deficiency in any one of them may lead to disease. It is important, however, to remember the following facts, which are apt to be overlooked in view of the flood of articles on vitamins in the press and periodicals, not to mention the persuasive pamphlets from the pharmaceutic houses. (1) Under modern conditions, outspoken deficiency disease is uncommon except in a few, less-favored localities, in Oriental countries, or as the result of war, although minor degrees of deficiency are far from rare. (2) An average mixed diet including fresh fruit and green vegetables contains an ample supply of vita-

Table 3–2. Vitamin Deficiency Diseases

Vitamin A	Night blindness, xerophthalmia, keratomalacia
Thiamin (B_1)	Beriberi
Riboflavin (B_2)	Cheilosis, eye lesions
Niacin (nicotinic acid)	Pellagra (skin, alimentary canal, central nervous system)
Vitamin B_{12}	Pernicious anemia
Vitamin C	Scurvy
Vitamin D	Rickets, osteomalacia
Vitamin K	Hypoprothrombinemia, tendency to bleeding

mins. (3) Whereas pure vitamin deficiency can be produced in the experimental animal, in human cases an inadequate diet is likely to be lacking in more than one vitamin, so that the clinical picture will tend to be mixed. (4) More than $100,000,000 are spent annually by the United States public in buying vitamins. (5) It is better and infinitely cheaper to get your vitamins from the grocery store, where they have been manufactured by nature, than from the drugstore, where they have been manufactured by man. Although this is true for healthy persons, it may not be true for those suffering from avitaminosis. When the condition is of long duration, it may be necessary to administer artificially prepared vitamins for a correspondingly long period before the needs of the tissues are fully satisfied and the normal balance of vitamins is restored. Finally, it must be borne in mind that vitamins, although essential to life, are no substitute for food. They provide no energy, calories, or body-building materials, and are merely accessory to diet.

DRUGS

The causes of disease are endless, and it is sad to implicate man as the agent of his own ills. There is nothing better than drugs for both the prevention and cure of disease. But,

as we have already seen, what is powerful for good may also be potent for evil. The picture of disease is changing before our very eyes, and while old diseases are passing away as the result of modern therapy, new diseases are taking their place, and many of these new diseases are due to drugs, which are a two-edged sword. These are usually drugs used by the general public, but they may be drugs prescribed by the doctor (Fig. 3–4). In these days when tranquilizers take the place of baby-sitters, blood transfusions are given indiscriminately and often needlessly, antibiotics are regarded as the cure-all for the most minor infections, and steroid therapy is a panacea, it is small wonder that old maladies are replaced by new, man-made ones.

There has never been a period in human history when such a deluge of new drugs has been poured forth. The public press daily reports a quota of miracle drugs, which the public demands. No drug is completely safe. One person may have an allergy to such a harmless drug as aspirin. If the reader will consult the table of contents of Spain's *The Complications of Modern Medical Practices*, he will see the truth of this statement. A most tragic example is, of course, thalidomide given to pregnant women with results that we all know. The use of oral contraceptives involves a distinct danger of thromboembolism, stroke, and hypertension.

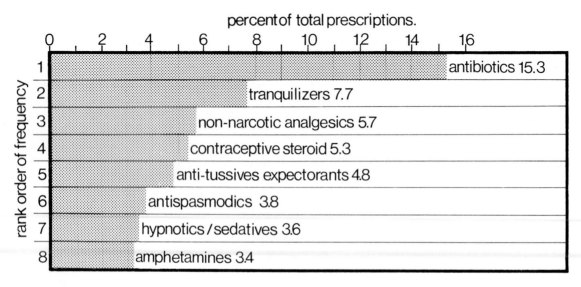

Fig. 3–4. This set of bar graphs shows the percentage of total prescriptions ordered in the 1970's for North America. (From Stolley, P.D., et al.: Drug prescribing and use in an American community. Ann. Intern. Med., 76:537, 1972.)

PSYCHOGENIC DISEASE

Clearly, it is possible to identify situations in which, by their reaction pattern or attitude, subconscious or otherwise, people become incapacitated and are unable to enjoy a normal life. In other words, they become ill. The death of a loved one may lead to depression, which in turn takes away the appetite not only for life, but for simple sustenance. This self-imposed starvation resulting from depression can have real consequences. Selye has popularized the interface between organic and functional disease. It goes beyond the scope of this introduction. However, psychologic causes for disordered health are real and common.

IATROGENIC DISEASE

We alluded previously to diseases caused by the medical profession (Greek *iatros*, doctor), and we shall come back to the subject frequently. This cause ranks as one of the most important in western medicine today.

IDIOPATHIC DISEASE

This heading for disease simply covers our ignorance; it refers to those diseases of unknown cause. We recognize many patterns of disease for which we can relate the anatomic lesions and physiologic dysfunctions to a causative agent. Thus we speak of tuberculosis of the lung as a disease caused by the tubercle bacillus (infectious etiology). Some disease processes are so poorly understood that we can only accept at present that we do not know their etiology, although we may collect cases in which the same pattern repeats itself in many people. Cancer is of unknown etiology, as are sarcoidosis and systemic lupus erythematosus, although in each instance we have theories as to the possible causes of these processes. Thus we may classify the processes, if we wish, under the heading Idiopathic.

TUMORS

One cause of disease is the presence of abnormal growth. Normally in the adult, cell

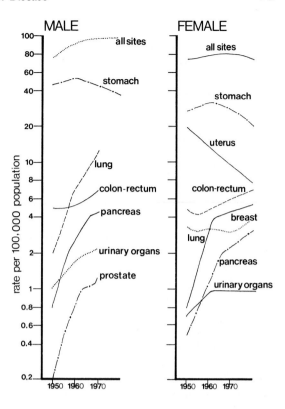

Fig. 3–5. This set of graphs shows the frequency of different types of cancer in men and women in North America in 1950, 1960, and 1970. Note the decline in cancer of the stomach in men and women; the decline in carcinoma of the uterus in women, which includes the carcinoma of the cervix in this graph; and the extraordinary rise in carcinoma of the lung for both sexes. Naturally, some of this change is due to better methods of detection. (From Hirayama, T.: Changing patterns of cancer in Japan with special reference to the decrease in stomach cancer mortality. In *Origins of Human Cancer, Book* A. Edited by H. H. Hiatt, et al. New York, Cold Spring Harbor Laboratory, 1977.)

replication constitutes an adaptive response; for example, replacement of old or damaged cells. However, in some instances a group of cells will proliferate as if out of control, without regard for the health or survival of the body. This process is called neoplasia and results in a tumor (Fig. 3–5).

Tumors interfere with body functioning in several ways. First, they occupy space, and in doing so they may obstruct essential pathways or compress essential structures, and thereby destroy normal tissue. Second, some tumors have been found to secrete substances that act like hormones and thereby interfere with endocrine function. They can be benign or malignant, but the extent of damage to the body depends on additional important factors, such as location. A benign tumor in the pituitary will have far-reaching consequences through uncontrolled hormone production, whereas a malignant tumor in the abdominal cavity can grow to the size of a basketball without killing the patient.

MAKING THE DIAGNOSIS

Although every patient who visits a physician does so with good reason, every physician is faced first with the question, "What is the cause of this patient's discomfort or disease?" To make a diagnosis of a particular disease is often not easy, and the increasingly sophisticated techniques available today are expensive and sometimes time consuming as well. They are also subject to error, if not of a technical sort, then of interpretation. This section outlines both traditional and newer methods used to determine the pattern that we recognize as disease.

Clinical Methods. By this term we mean the deductive and inductive reasoning that relates the presence of certain symptoms or signs in a patient to the patterns of disease we have learned about in other patients. Clearly, there are situations in which the difficulties in medicine are complicated by the appearance of a new disease (e.g., Lassa fever) or by new manifestations of a known disease to such an extent that it cannot be identified, but these are rare. **Symptoms** include the complaints of the patient, either voluntary or elicited by careful cross-examination. It is often possible to make a correct diagnosis from the symptoms alone. Thus the agonizing pain in the chest in coronary thrombosis, or the digestive distress and pain relieved by taking food, so characteristic of ulcer of the stomach, may tell the doctor in clear and unmistakable language the disease from which the patient is suffering. In the majority of diseases, there is a close relationship between the symptoms of the patient and the lesions that the pathologist may be able to demonstrate. Thus if the air spaces of the lung are filled with inflammatory material in pneumonia, it is only natural that the patient should be severely short of breath. This close relationship of lesions to symptoms is one of the chief reasons why a knowledge of pathology is of value to the doctor. Unfortunately, the number of symptoms of which a patient can complain are unlimited, and pain, shortness of breath, fever, and loss of strength can be caused by many different diseases. On this account the doctor has to turn to physical signs for further help.

Physical signs are elicited by physical examination of the patient. By listening to the heart a murmur may be heard, palpation of the kidney may show it to be enlarged, and pressure over the appendix may elicit tenderness even though the patient has not complained of pain. These signs are of the greatest help in diagnosis.

Simple visual inspection of the patient may tell the doctor or the nurse all that needs to be known. The patient with pneumonia can be recognized by reason of the rapid respiration, cough, and flushed feverish appearance. In chronic heart failure there is shortness of breath (dyspnea), swelling of the legs, and the bluish tinge of cyanosis. In an acute heart attack, such as that of coronary thrombosis, the face is clammy and ashen in color, the expression that of deep anxiety, and there is a strange immobility, as if the patient feared to move a muscle. In nephritis, the face and eyelids are swollen and the skin presents a typical pallor. Acute intestinal obstruction can be suspected from the sunken appearance of the eyes due to extreme loss of fluid (dehydration), the leaden skin, and the board-like rigidity of the abdomen. The wasted and emaciated appearance (cachexia) of the cancer patient is only too readily recognized. Among the most characteristic of clinical pictures are those of certain diseases of the endocrine glands, as illustrated by the pigmentation of the skin in Addison's disease associated with destruction of the cortex of the adrenals, and the striking contrasts presented by Graves's disease due to hyperactivity of the thyroid and by myxedema due to hypoactivity of the same gland.

What may be called the "**scopes**" can be included in a discussion of physical signs. The scopes in use today range from short metal specula used for rectal or vaginal exams to the long, flexible, fiber optic scope that can visualize the ampulla of Vater, nearly 100 cm from the mouth of the patient. The laryngoscope reveals the interior of the larynx, the bronchoscope the interior of the bronchial tree, the gastroscope the interior of the stomach, the sigmoidoscope the interior of the colon (sigmoid), the cystoscope the interior of the bladder, and so on. In the case of the ophthalmoscope, a beam of light is directed into the eye, the interior of which is illuminated and can be studied.

Laboratory Methods. These comprise tests that cannot be done at the bedside, but require the use of laboratory apparatus such as the microscope and the test tube with all its complicated extensions. It must be emphasized that laboratory tests, with which must be included x-ray examination, do not provide the doctor with a ready-made diagnosis; they merely give him additional information, which, taken in conjunction with the clinical evidence (history of the illness, symptoms, and signs), enables him to arrive at a correct conclusion—we hope.

These tests constitute what has now become the specialty of **clinical pathology**, and comprise the examination of fluids (including blood) and cells taken from the patient during life.

Laboratory tests are numerous and complex. Indeed entire books are devoted to them. Only a few of the more important will be mentioned here. In what follows we have kept to the barest outline, intended as a preview of some more detailed accounts in the second part of this book.

Urinalysis is the commonest of all laboratory tests. Examination of the urine serves not only to give indirect evidence of kidney function, but may also reveal disease of the bladder and urethra. Other diseases not connected with the urinary tract may be detected by urinalysis, e.g., the presence of sugar in the urine in diabetes. As a matter of fact, the urine represents the main route by which abnormal substances are eliminated from the blood. It is obvious how many of these substances, such as minerals and hormones, may be revealed by skillful urinalysis.

Examination of stomach contents and **feces** give valuable information as to the presence of disease in the stomach and intestine.

A **blood count** shows the number and con-

dition of both the red blood cells and the leukocytes. The red cells are diminished in number or are altered in size or shape in various forms of anemia. The number of the leukocytes is increased in acute infections (appendicitis, pneumonia), and in the blood disease leukemia.

Blood chemistry is of ever-increasing importance. Thus the blood sugar is increased in diabetes, the urea nitrogen is increased in renal failure, the phosphorus may be abnormal in rickets, and various enzymes may be increased in amount, whereas others not normally present may make their appearance.

The **cerebrospinal fluid** shows changes in many diseases of the nervous system. Thus the diagnosis of acute meningitis is made by finding large numbers of leukocytes in this fluid, together with the bacteria causing the infection. The fluid, which is obtained by means of lumbar puncture, is a mirror in which is reflected disease of the brain and spinal cord.

Bacteriologic examination is of the greatest importance in the diagnosis of many of the infectious diseases such as diphtheria, pneumonia, and tuberculosis. A blood culture may show the presence of streptococci, and other organisms in the circulating blood.

Serology consists in the examination of the blood serum for substances that indicate the presence of bacterial infection. Examples of such tests are the Widal test for typhoid fever and the Wassermann test for syphilis. It must be understood that these are not tests for the bacteria, but for substances produced by the body in response to the infection.

Tissue diagnosis is the microscopic examination of pieces of tissue. When such a piece is removed during life for the purpose of diagnosis, the procedure is called a **biopsy**, in contrast to the examination of tissues at autopsy. It is usually done to determine whether a tumor is malignant.

The **electrocardiogram** is an electrical record of the contractions of the heart. All contracting muscles produce an electric current, and such a current is produced by the contractions of the auricles and ventricles. The current is made to write a permanent tracing (electrocardiogram), which is of one pattern when the heart muscle is healthy, but of a different pattern when the muscle is diseased. These fingerprints of the heart's action are of great value to the heart specialist.

Radiography. The radiologist provides invaluable assistance to the clinician in search of a diagnosis. X rays have the power of passing through solid objects and affecting a photographic film on the other side of that object. But their use is limited by the fact that they can only show differences in density. An opaque object, such as a bullet, will stand out clearly; large solid organs can be seen on the film, but the outlines of hollow structures, such as the stomach, intestine, gallbladder, and bronchi, are indistinguishable. It is these outlines, however, that are most likely to be altered in disease.

DIAGNOSTIC IMAGING—RADIOLOGY, ULTRASOUND, AND NUCLEAR MEDICINE

X rays are high-energy, electromagnetic waves with the ability to penetrate solid objects. The penetrance, and thus the transmission, is related to the energy of the wave and thickness, density, and relative atomic number of the object being exposed. These are collectively referred to as the attenuation characteristics. X rays are conventionally generated by a tube external to the portion of the anatomy being radiographed (Fig. 3–6). The waves then pass into the object, where they may be absorbed, scattered, or transmitted. Those that are transmitted are routinely recorded on radiographic film, a photographic emulsion in which the degree of blackening is proportional to the degree of transmission. For many newer techniques, such as CT scanning (Fig. 3–7), the transmitted waves stimulate detectors similar to a Geiger counter. The output signals may be integrated and a visual image transmitted to a screen. Thus not all radiographic techniques use film in the conventional sense. Four major densities are described in radiology—air, fat, water, and metal. Air is the least dense and exhibits the greatest transmission. Fat is denser and transmits less; water is next, followed by metal, which is the densest and transmits least. This is why the normal air-filled lung appears black, and normal calcium-containing bone appears white.

Most of the body tissues, however, have approximately the density of water. Different organs may be identified from others by the air within them (bowel), or by the fat around them (kidney). It is difficult at times to separate one organ from another. Therefore, radiologists administer different contrast agents to outline particular organs in a selective fashion. Barium, a heavy metal, is a positive contrast agent denser than the tissues it out-

Conventional Radiology:

AP film

LAT film

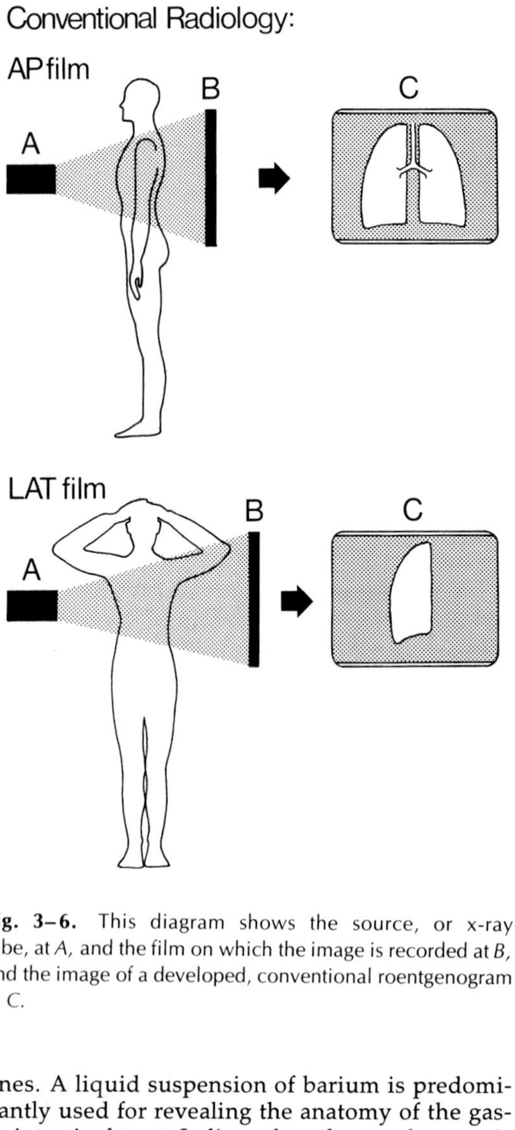

Fig. 3–6. This diagram shows the source, or x-ray tube, at *A*, and the film on which the image is recorded at *B*, and the image of a developed, conventional roentgenogram at *C*.

lines. A liquid suspension of barium is predominantly used for revealing the anatomy of the gastrointestinal tract. Iodine, also a heavy element, is used in a wider variety of examinations. Iodinated agents administered either orally or intravenously may outline the biliary tree (cholangiography, oral cholecystography), thereby enabling the radiologist to determine function as well as structure. Iodine may also be administered intravenously to demonstrate the kidneys, ureters, and bladder (intravenous urography). Some insight into the function of the organs is also provided because of the rate at which the contrast agent is taken up and excreted. Iodinated agents may also be administered directly, by catheter into blood vessels (angiography) (Fig. 3–8), into the urinary bladder and/or ureters (retrograde urography), into the pancreas (endoscopic retrograde pancreatography), into the lungs (bronchography), or by direct needle puncture into the liver (percutaneous transhepatic cholangiography), into the spinal canal (myelography), and by other techniques into

Computerized Tomography:

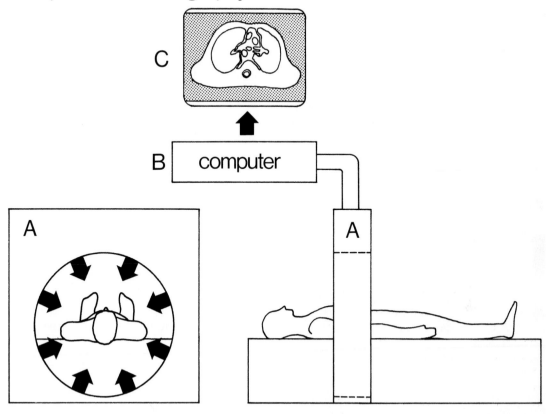

Fig. 3–7. This diagram illustrates at *A* the position of a patient inside the net of x-ray tubes, which are represented by black arrows. The images are interpreted by the computer and are reconstructed in cross-section representation as shown at C. Several images of CT scanning are shown in the chapter on the Central Nervous System.

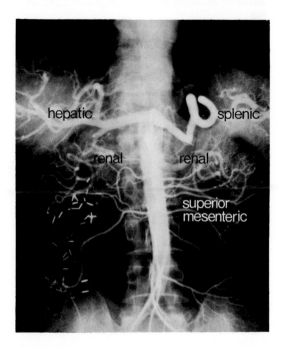

Fig. 3–8. This roentgenogram shows the presence of iodinated, radiopaque material in the arterial tree of a patient, outlining the hepatic, renal and splenic arteries as well as the aorta. This is called an arteriogram and the technique is called angiography.

Ultrasound:

A

B

POST.

cystic mass

cephalad

collecting system

kidney cortex

caudad

C   ANT.

other organs. These studies demonstrate structure but not function. Air (a negative contrast agent) has been used, for example, to outline the ventricular system of the brain (pneumoencephalography), which is used less and less because of the efficacy of the CT scanner.

Many of these examinations are performed under fluoroscopy. The fluoroscope is basically a screen that emits an image on stimulation by x rays. Fluoroscopy allows the radiologist to visualize what is happening directly as it happens, rather than "after-the-fact" static images. The radiologist may record what he or she sees by cineradiographic film or on videotape, and is able to evaluate the moment-to-moment activity of a particular organ, such as the beating heart, the contracting bowel, or the moving diaphragm. Fluoroscopy may be used in conjunction with other procedures. For example, needle biopsies have been performed under fluoroscopic guidance, drugs may be delivered to specific parts of the body, catheters may be specifically placed under fluoroscopic control, and calculi have been removed from the biliary tree with the aid of fluoroscopy.

Another technique of great importance is laminography, or tomography, which focuses on a particular section of the body by blurring out structures in front of and behind the plane of interest. This too can be used with contrast agents.

Until recently, radiologists have been able to obtain radiographs in planes longitudinal to the long axis of the body only. The recent development of computerized tomography (CT) has allowed the radiologist to visualize structures in a transverse plane. This device is sensitive to the attenuation characteristics of various structures. It employs computer technology to reconstruct transverse images on the basis of information fed into the computer by a series of detectors that are stimulated by x rays transmitted in the transverse section.

Ultrasound, like CT scanning, enables one to see body section cuts in planes other than longitudinal. Ultrasound employs high-frequency sound waves rather than x rays. The image depends primarily on the reflection of these waves, not their transmission. Waves are reflected at the interface of 2 objects of different acoustic density. A uniform cystic structure reflects waves at its front and back walls, but the uniform fluid in between is "echolucent" (Fig. 3–9). However, a solid, nonuniform structure has many internal interfaces, and is therefore "echogenic." The sound waves are gen-

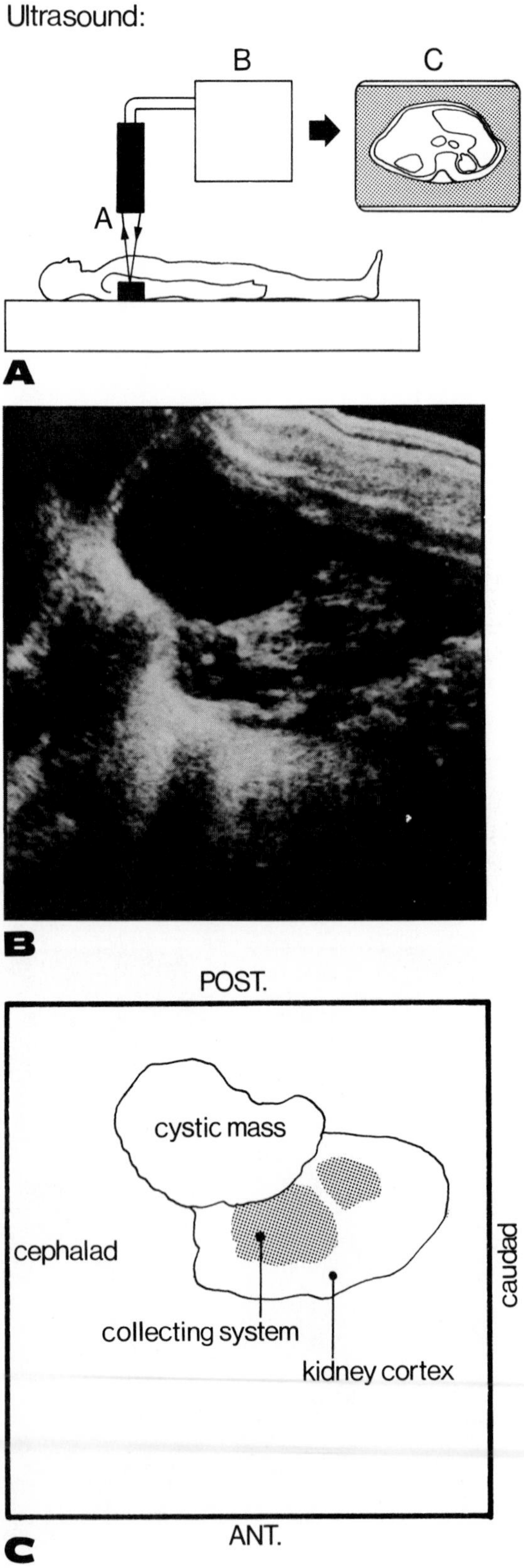

←

Fig. 3–9. *A,* This drawing shows the patient in relationship to the ultrasound emitter (*B*) and transducer (*A*), and shows the image that is created (*C*). *B,* This film shows an ultrasound image of the kidney. An interpretive drawing of the cystic mass is shown on the right.

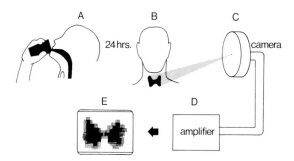

Fig. 3–10. This drawing shows the administration of a radioactive substance at *A*, the delay of 24 hours and the concentration of this radioactive iodine in the thyroid at *B*, and the scintillation counter at *C*, which records the uptake of the emissions and projects them, *D*. The result is the computer-aided image at *E*.

erated, and the reflected waves detected, by the same device, a piezoelectric transducer. Only waves reflected from surfaces perpendicular to the angle of the beam are received by the transducer. The return signal from the transducer is fed into the electronic circuitry of the ultrasound machine, and an image is produced. The recorded image may be static (B mode), it may detail motion on a strip recording (M mode), as in echocardiography, or it may demonstrate active motion on a "real time" scanning device, as in fluoroscopy. Ultrasound, like fluoroscopy, has also been used to guide needle biopsies, for the puncture of cysts, for the placement of needles for amniocentesis, and as a guide to the obstetrician.

Nuclear medicine as a diagnostic tool employs radionuclides, that is, elements that emit gamma rays and/or other charged particles. The best-known examination in nuclear medicine is the thyroid scan, which involves the uptake of radioactive iodine by gland tissue (Fig. 3–10). Gamma rays, like x rays, are electromagnetic waves with similar properties. However, unlike x rays, which are generated in the electron orbits of an atom, gamma rays originate in the nucleus of an atom by a radioactive decay of the nucleus. In addition, rather than being generated by an external source and recording an image by transmission, gamma rays are emitted from within organs in which radionuclides have accumulated. Emission, like transmission, is affected by wave energy and by the attenuation characteristics of the organs involved. These emitted rays do not expose films directly, as do x rays, but rather stimulate light-emitting crystals or other types of radiation detectors in devices known as scanners or gamma cameras. The output of these detectors is then fed through electronic amplification circuitry and an image is produced.

Radionuclides may be administered orally or intravenously, and their accumulation within an organ depends on the carrier to which they are attached and on the function of the organ involved. Therefore, function takes precedence over anatomic detail. The nuclides most commonly used are Tc99m and I131, although I123, I125, Ga67, thallium, and others are available. Carriers include such compounds as methylene diphosphonate, a calcium-seeking agent that localizes in areas of active calcium hydroxyapatite turnover (bone) (Fig. 3–11); sulfur colloid, which is taken up by the reticuloendothelial system of the liver, spleen, and bone marrow; hepatoiminodiacetic acid, which is taken up and excreted by liver cells (Fig. 3–12); hippuran, which undergoes active secretion by the renal tubules (Fig. 3–13); and albumin macroaggregates, which embolize the microvasculature of the lung. Gallium is actively taken up by white blood cells and therefore accumulates in areas of inflammation.

Moreover, there is a therapeutic side to nuclear medicine. Radioactive iodine, an emitter of *beta* particles as well as of gamma rays, given in appropriate doses, is used to treat hyperthyroidism and either local or metastatic thyroid carcinoma.

Newer techniques involve the labeling of radionuclides to antibodies of tumor-marker antigens such as carcinoembryonic antigen (CEA), or other specific endogenous proteins, for example parathyroid hormone, so that those proteins may be quantitated or identified; the use of computers to study the active function of the heart; and the use of radioactive blood-soluble gases to measure regional blood flow. Newer short-lived lower-dose nuclides are also being developed.

Although some of these techniques have supplanted others, these examinations are generally used in a complementary fashion. However, with benefits provided by new investigational techniques come risks. The CT scan of the thorax, for example, is noninvasive and shows the anatomy in great detail, but the dose of radiation is higher than with the equally noninvasive routine chest roentgenogram. Ultrasound avoids the use of damaging ionizing radiation; however, the long-term effects of high-frequency sound waves are not known. Contrast agents such as iodine are invaluable in defining anatomy, but they run the risk of allergic reactions. Ionizing radiation in general has deleterious effects on actively growing cells. However, when in the hands of persons skilled in its proper use and aware of its dangers, its long-term benefits far outweigh its risks.

The imaginative use of gamma cameras and computer analysis has made possible the visualization and localization of small amounts of isotopes in organs of the body. For example, when visual cells in the brain are working, reading a signal, their metabolism increases and they consume more oxygen and glucose than when the eyes are closed. If, in

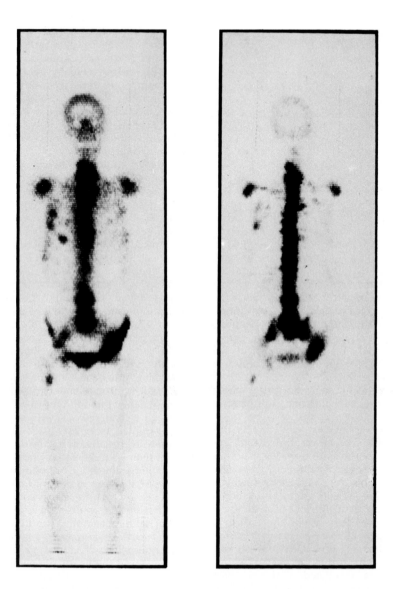

Fig. 3–11. These two pictures are nuclear scans that show the appearance of bone-seeking agents concentrated at sites of metastases, where new bone formation is taking place. The dense areas show multiple sites of active bone formation.

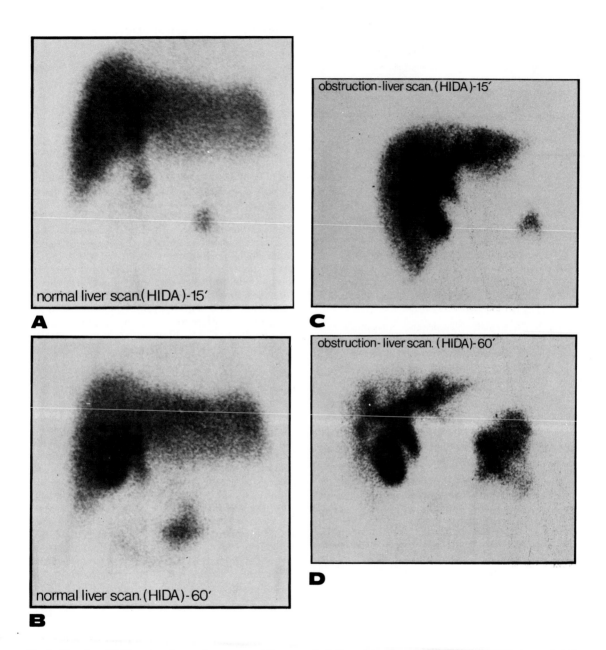

Fig. 3–12. *A* and *B,* These two figures show a normal liver scan. In *A,* the uptake of a radioactive material that is concentrated in liver cells is shown 15 minutes after injection. A normal liver scan shown 60 minutes after injection is on the right at *B. C* and *D,* These two figures show by comparison the pattern of uptake in a liver where there is obstruction and where the liver cells themselves are not normal metabolically. Compare the 60-minute HIDA scan in the obstructed liver with that of the normal liver.

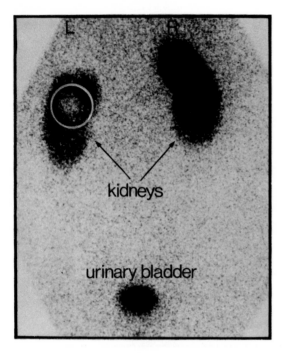

Fig. 3–13. This scan shows the presence of a normal kidney on the right, and the absence of uniform scanning on the left. Such an area could be due to a cyst or to the presence of a tumor or an abscess, for example.

an experimental situation, radioactively labeled glucose is injected into the arteries of the brain, and the eye is opened to a strong, visual image, a gamma computer can show the increased concentration of the isotope in the part of the brain that is working to read the image. This scintillation imaging holds real promise, not only to understand normal function, but possibly also to localize tumors when they are small enough that they can be easily removed, before they invade and destroy tissue and the host.

These new chemical and mechanical diagnostic techniques have become so much a part of modern diagnosis that we forget that there was a time when they did not exist. Even today, in other parts of the world, accurate diagnoses are made without these machines, depending only on human knowledge, skill, and senses. Richard Selzer, in his book *Mortal Lessons*, describes the diagnostic techniques of the personal physician to the Dalai Lama, Yeshi Dhonden, who once visited the United States. His methods are virtually incom-

prehensible to us, yet they are successful, as can be seen in the following passage:

He bows in greeting while his young interpreter makes the introduction. Yeshi Dhonden, we are told, will examine a patient selected by a member of the staff. The diagnosis is as unknown to Yeshi Dhonden as it is to us. The examination of the patient will take place in our presence, after which we will reconvene in the conference room where Yeshi Dhonden will discuss the case. We are further informed that for the past two hours Yeshi Dhonden has purified himself by bathing, fasting, and prayer. I, having breakfasted well, performed only the most desultory of ablutions, and given no thought at all to my soul, glance furtively at my fellows. Suddenly, we seem a soiled, uncouth lot.

The patient had been awakened early and told that she was to be examined by a foreign doctor, and had been asked to produce a fresh specimen of urine, so when we enter her room, the woman shows no surprise. . . . Yeshi Dhonden steps to the bedside while the rest stand apart, watching. For a long time he gazes at the woman, favoring no part of her body with his eyes, but seeming to fix his glance at a place just above her supine form. I, too, study her. No physical sign nor obvious symptom gives a clue to the nature of her disease.

At last he takes her hand, raising it in both of his own. Now he bends over the bed in a kind of crouching stance, his head drawn down into the collar of his robe. His eyes are closed as he feels for her pulse. In a moment he has found the spot, and for the next half hour he remains thus, suspended above the patient like some exotic golden bird with folded wings, holding the pulse of the woman beneath his fingers, cradling her hand in his. . . . It is palpation of the pulse raised to the state of ritual. . . .

At last Yeshi Dhonden straightens, gently places the woman's hand upon the bed, and steps back. The interpreter produces a small wooden bowl and two sticks. Yeshi Dhonden pours a portion of the urine specimen into the bowl and proceeds to whip the liquid with the two sticks. This he does for several minutes until a foam is raised. Then, bowing above the bowl, he inhales the odor three times. He sets down the bowl and turns to leave.

We are seated once more in the conference room. Yeshi Dhonden speaks now for the first time, in soft Tibetan sounds that I have never heard before. He has barely begun when the young interpreter begins to translate, the two voices continuing in tandem—a bilingual fugue, the one chasing the other. It is like the chanting of monks. He speaks of winds coursing through the body of the woman, currents that break against barriers, eddying. These vortices are in her blood, he says. The last spendings of an imperfect heart. Between the chambers of her heart, long, long before she was born, a wind had come and blown open a deep gate that must never be opened. Through it charge the

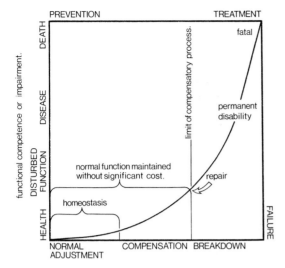

Fig. 3–14. This graph shows the range of adaptation from health through to death.

full waters of her river, as the mountain stream cascades in the springtime, battering, knocking loose the land, and flooding her breath. Thus he speaks, and is silent.

"May we now have the diagnosis?" a professor asks.

The host of these rounds, the man who knows, answers.

"Congenital heart disease," he says. "Interventricular septal defect, with resultant heart failure."

A gateway in the heart, I think. That must not be opened. Through it charge the full waters that flood her breath. So! Here then is the doctor listening to the sounds of the body to which the rest of us are deaf.

To conclude our discussion of disease, it may be useful to regard diseases in the light of the failure of the organism to adapt to whatever changes are wrought in its external and internal existence. This can be illustrated in the form of a graph, as shown in Figure 3–14. The natural result of failure of adaptation is death.

DEATH

We have been discussing various causes of disease and how to circumvent them. There remains the fact that for every living being there is an end to life, whatever the cause. That end we call death.

If we consider the termination of life of each of our cells, we die a thousand million deaths,

but in most parts of the world it is the cessation of the heartbeat that has been used as the criterion of death. As everyone knows today, the heartbeat may often be restored by prompt medical attempts to convert the fibrillation or to restore the rhythm. From the biologic point of view, death is a process, not just a particular moment, and we are all partaking of that process unwittingly all the time.

It would seem simple to say that when the heart has ceased to beat, the lungs to breathe, or the brain to think, that a man is dead, but we know there is a wide variation in the ability of different tissues to survive the loss of their essential circulation. Muscle cells, particularly smooth muscle, may be reanimated after days of anoxia. Liver and kidney cells can repopulate large areas that have been destroyed, and these organs can be restored to normal function after hours of anoxia. However, the neurons of the brain are incapable of regeneration and rarely survive more than 15 minutes without normal oxygen and glucose.

It is not strange to redirect our definition of death from the heart and respiratory functions to the essential features of a particular person, his personality, attitudes, emotions, and intellect, which compose his character. These are all manifestations of his cerebral functions and depend on the integrity of these self-same susceptible neurons.

Today, the most accepted definitions of death consider that when the normal signs of responsiveness are absent, and when the brainstem and spinal reflexes are also gone, death has occurred. Electrical activity of the central nervous system as shown by electroencephalography demonstrates only flat waves. This observation should be repeated at least once in 24 hours. When these findings have been confirmed by a second physician, the patient can be considered biologically and medically dead.

At this point, the question of continuing supportive medical measures becomes a consideration. Much debate surrounds the suitability of such active intervention, or on the other hand, the decision to withdraw such support, once started. These decisions differ in every case and are beyond the scope of this chapter.

The knowledge that dialysis for renal failure and transplantation of kidneys have altered the hopeless prognosis of thousands of patients 3 decades ago underscores the important question of who is to give and who is to receive in these circumstances. Hundreds of successful renal transplantations and scores of cardiac transplantations as well as some successful liver transplantations all testify to the importance of these efforts. One outcome of this has been to cause us to define death in a new and more complex way.

We might conclude this section on the causes of disease with the thought that when all the natural frailties are considered, it seems strange that a harp with so many strings should stay in tune so long.

SYNOPSIS

Disease is the pattern of response of a living organism to some form of injury.

The pattern of disease is as much determined by the reaction of the host as it is by the nature of the injury.

The morphologic manifestations of disease (lesions) are no more or less important than the disorders of function. The symptoms of disease (subjective) are as significant as the signs (objective).

Our ideas of the causes of disease are changing and reflect the scientific knowledge of biology of the time and our cultural paradigms.

Classification of disease is an arbitrary but useful way to systematize our knowledge. It does not matter what the basis of the taxonomy is, so long as it is used in a rational way.

Techniques for establishing a specific diagnosis include history taking, physical examination, routine laboratory examinations, special laboratory examinations, radiologic methods, and invasive techniques such as biopsy.

The principle of causality in our understanding of disease may be misleading. The association between 2 phenomena does not imply a causal relation.

Terms

Lesion	*Ischemia*	*Idiopathic*
Prognosis	*Anoxia*	*Dyspnea*
Etiology	*Infarction*	*Cachexia*
Pathogenesis	*Iatrogenic*	*Death*
Inflammation		

FURTHER READING

Abrams, H.L., and McNeil, B.J.: Medical implications of computed tomography. N. Engl. J. Med., 298:255, 1978.

Barrett-Connor, E.: The etiology of pellagra and its significance for modern medicine. Am. J. Med., 42:859, 1967.

Black, P. McL.: Brain death. N. Engl. J. Med., 299:393, 1978.

Boyd, W.L.: Cause and effect. Can. Med. Assoc. J., 92:868, 1965.

Bruner, J.M.R.: Hazards of electrical apparatus. Anesthesiology, 28:396, 1967.

Burkitt, D.P.: Relationship as a clue to causation. Lancet, 2:1237, 1970.

Burnet, F.M.: A modern basis for pathology. Lancet, 1:1383, 1968.

Copeland, D.D.: Concepts of disease and diagnosis. Perspect. Biol. Med., 20:528, 1977.

Dean, J., and Schechter, A.N.: Sickle cell anemia: molecular and cellular bases of therapeutic approaches. N. Engl. J. Med., 299:752, 1978.

Dick, Heather M.: HLA and disease. Br. Med. Bull., 34:271, 1978.

Doll, J.R.R.: The pattern of disease in the post-infection era: national trends. Proc. R. Soc. Lond. [Biol.], 205:47, 1980.

Dubos, R.J.: Infection into disease. Perspect. Biol. Med., 1:425, 1957.

Engel, G.L.: The need for a new medical model: a challenge for biomedicine. Science, 196:129, 1977.

Feinstein, A.R.: Boolean algebra and clinical taxonomy. N. Engl. J. Med., 269:929, 1963.

Galen, R.S.,and Gambino, S.R.: *Beyond Normality: The Predictive Value and Efficiency of Medical Diagnoses.* New York, John Wiley & Sons, 1975.

Goldenberg, D.M., et al.: Use of radiolabeled antibodies to carcinoembryonic antigen for the detection and localization of diverse cancers by external photoscanning. N. Engl. J. Med., *298*:1384, 1978.

Lasagna, L.: The diseases drugs cause. Perspect. Biol. Med., *7*:457, 1963.

Mann, G.V.: The influence of obesity on health. N. Engl. J. Med., *291*:178, 1974.

Moss, N.H., and Mayer, J.: Food and nutrition in health and disease. Ann. N.Y. Acad. Sci., *300*, 1977.

Pace, N.: Weightlessness: a matter of gravity. N. Engl. J. Med., *297*:32, 1977.

Petersen, P.: A perspective of infection and infectious disease. Perspect. Biol. Med., *23*:255, 1980.

Potkin, S.G., et al.: Are paranoid schizophrenics biologically different from other schizophrenics? N. Engl. J. Med., *298*:61, 1978.

Roueché, B.: *Eleven Blue Men and Other Tales of Medical Detection.* Boston, Little, Brown, 1954.

Scrimshaw, N.S., and Behar, M.: Malnutrition in underdeveloped countries. N. Engl. J. Med., *272*:137, 193, 1965.

Selzer, R.: Mortal Lessons, Notes in the Art of Surgery. New York, Simon & Schuster, 1976.

Shute, N.: On the Beach. New York, Morrow, 1957.

Spain, D.M.: The Complications of Modern Medical Practices. New York, Grune and Stratton, 1963.

Taussig, H.B.: Death from lightning and the possibility of living again. Ann. Intern. Med., *68*:1345, 1968.

Disturbances of Blood Flow and Derangements of Body Fluids

4

Education is the acquisition of the art of the utilization of knowledge—A. N. WHITEHEAD

NORMAL FLUID EXCHANGE

Before we consider abnormal or pathologic changes in blood and body fluid, let us review the forces in the circulatory system that provide nourishment to all our tissues and that keep the "vital juices flowing." The central pump, the heart, provides energy with each contraction (systole) sufficient to move the plasma and blood cells around the arterial, capillary, and venous circuit, so that no cell is without oxygen or glucose or chokes in its own waste for more than a few seconds during the 70 or more years of a normal human life. How does this miniature irrigation system achieve this goal? The English physiologist, Starling, was perplexed by this problem. Although he understood that the pressure of 150 mm mercury in the aorta was sufficient at the time of each ventricular contraction to provide a reservoir of energy to pump blood through the circulation, he could

not see how fluid from the small capillaries, if it moved into the interstitial space, moved back into the capillary bed. If the circulation was to continue to function, there had to be some mechanism to return fluids from the tissue spaces to the vascular compartment, to keep the blood volume constant. The lymphatic circulation certainly did not accumulate all this material. Starling proposed that one of the forces at work in the microcirculation was the hydrostatic pressure at the arteriolar end of the capillary bed, the net effect of which was to move water, salts, and small organic molecules across the capillary wall to the neighboring cells, to which they provided nourishment. At the same time, at the venous end of the capillary, small molecules, salts, and water, had to return to the vascular lumen. This could happen if there were an equal and opposite force to the hydrostatic pressure to attract the small molecules back into the circulation, and Starling proposed that the

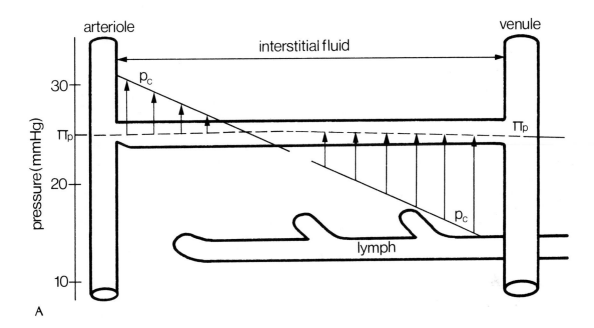

Fig. 4–1. *A,* This diagram illustrates the gradient of pressures from the arteriolar to the venular end in the capillary bed. Joining the arteriole and venule is the capillary, the arrows indicating the relative forces moving fluids into the interstitial space and into the lymph. (After Landis, E.M., and Pappenheimer, J.R.: Exchange of substances through the capillary walls. In *Handbook of Physiology.* Section 2: Circulation, Vol. II. Edited by Hamilton and Dow. Washington, D.C., American Physiological Society, 1963.)

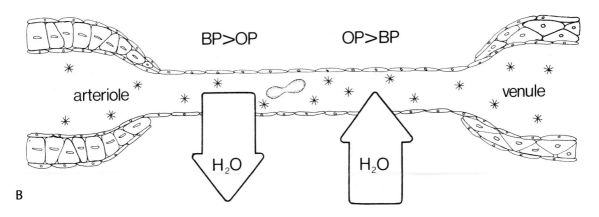

Fig. 4–1. *B,* This diagram demonstrates the cellular nature of the arteriolar capillary and venular bed and illustrates diagrammatically the red blood cells and proteins (shown as stars).

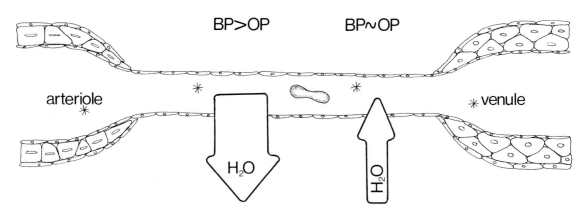

Fig. 4–2. The protein most responsible for the osmotic pressure gradient is albumin (symbolized by the stars within the capillary lumen). If the body loses albumin (e.g., by excretion through a diseased kidney), or if it has a problem in production (e.g., a diseased liver), hypoalbuminemia will result. Here, the level of albumin in the blood is too low to produce a sufficient osmotic pressure gradient across the capillary wall, and flow cannot return as normal, symbolized by the smaller, unequal arrow on the right side of the diagram and the notation that the blood pressure (BP) is equal to the osmotic pressure (OP) (unlike the normal situation shown in Figure 4–1), resulting in edema.

osmotic pressure of the plasma proteins was just such a force. This is shown in Figure 4–1. Large molecules such as albumin, fibrinogen, and prothrombin cannot normally move across the capillary wall.

This microcirculation, then, provides for a constant exchange between the vascular and interstitial compartments, bringing oxygen, glucose, calcium, sodium, and fatty and amino acids to the cells, while at the same time returning lactate, carbon dioxide, urea, and other conventional waste products to the general circulation.

Simple perturbations in this scheme can be imagined. If there are inadequate numbers of protein molecules (hypoalbuminemia), free water will not return to the vascular compartment (Fig. 4–2). If the hydrostatic pressure is raised at the venular end, water will not return to the capillary (edema) (Fig. 4–3). If the capillary walls become indiscriminately permeable, the whole system fails because there is no maintenance of the vascular volume (shock) (Fig. 4–4). We shall consider these changes under appropriate headings.

EDEMA

An abnormal collection of fluid in tissue spaces (extravascular compartment) is called

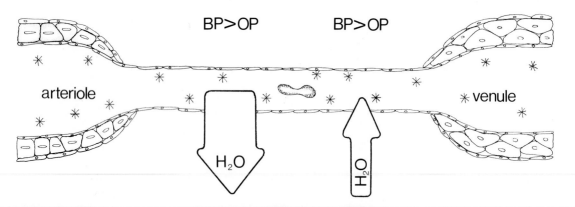

Fig. 4–3. This diagram illustrates what happens to the equilibrium at the capillary bed when the venous pressure is raised. Here the hydrostatic pressure is raised either because of an obstruction (e.g., tumor), or because of congestive heart failure. Raised hydrostatic pressure at the venous end interferes with the normal gradient and fluid cannot return to the capillary. Excess fluid in the interstitial space is called edema.

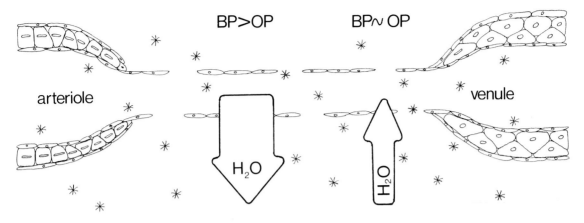

Fig. 4–4. Owing to inflammation, the capillary may become abnormally leaky. Protein (and cells) leak out into the tissue, which causes local edema (as in the swelling of an infected finger). Because of this change in permeability, the normal gradients for exchange cannot be maintained and there is a net loss of fluid to the interstitial space that results in edema. These diagrams (Figs. 4–1 to 4–4) thus illustrate three mechanisms that result in edema: hypoalbuminemia, increased hydrostatic pressure, and increased capillary permeability.

edema. This may be local, for example when the lymphatic or venous drainage in a person's leg has been partially blocked. Edema may also be generalized in all the dependent portions of the body, as when venous pressure is raised because of congestive heart failure. It may also occur in the pulmonary circulation. This last situation is perhaps the most common emergency in an acute myocardial infarct in which the left ventricle fails and the venous pressure rises, leading to pulmonary edema and extreme shortness of breath. When edema fluid accumulates in the interstitial tissues of the leg or the hand, one may displace the fluid by pressure in the same way that one might leave a fingerprint on an over-ripe melon. However, when there is edema in the lung, one cannot see or feel the interstitial fluid externally; nevertheless, it is often possible to hear, with the stethoscope, moisture in the alveoli that sounds like tissue paper rustling or, in extreme cases, like bubbles with each breath. These are called rales and are a clinical sign of pulmonary edema of which anxiety and breathlessness are symptoms. Rales constitute a medical emergency, whether the cause is high altitude, sickness, or acute heart failure (Fig. 4–5).

There are 3 general causes of edema. The first of these, and perhaps the easiest to understand, is the **general or systemic loss of selective permeability of the capillary wall.**

This may occur in anoxia, shock, or severe allergic response. This permeability permits all contents of the capillary (large and small molecules) to escape into the interstitial space, and it effectually brings about a major loss of blood volume, thereby precipitating a state of shock because of the lack of tissue perfusion. The loss of the selective permeability, which normally retains plasma proteins within the capillary bed, occurs locally in inflammation and is responsible for the local production of increased tissue fluid. When this fluid accumulates in a compartment, such as the pericardial sac or pleural space, it is often referred to as an **effusion** (Fig. 4–6). Collections of fluid can be readily aspirated and examined for their specific characteristics, which merely suggest the mechanism that has caused their accumulation. If the fluid accumulates in the peritoneal cavity, it is referred to as **ascites.**

Thus it is that one may well find in the same patient both the presence of pulmonary edema and a pleural effusion. This brings us to a second major general cause of the displacement of vascular equilibrium that leads to edema. **Any increase in pressure at the venous end of the capillary bed, or increase in venous pressure anywhere,** whether it is right heart failure or a small benign pelvic tumor pressing on an ovarian vein, **decreases the ease with which interstitial fluid returns to**

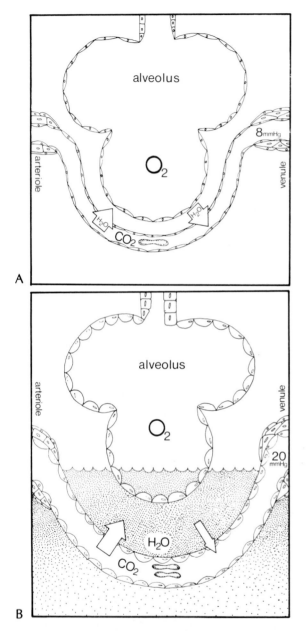

Fig. 4–5. This figure illustrates the normal and edematous lung. In *A*, venous pressure is normal, as is fluid exchange between capillary and tissue space. In *B*, venous pressure is raised as in left heart failure. This increased pressure interferes with fluid exchange; water and small molecules pass out of the capillary under normal arteriolar pressure, but are then prevented from returning by the high venous pressure. Thus fluid accumulates in the interstitial space and interferes with gas exchange, because the distance between capillary and alveolus is increased. Eventually fluid passes into the alveolus, where it may be perceived as bubbling rales on auscultation of the chest.

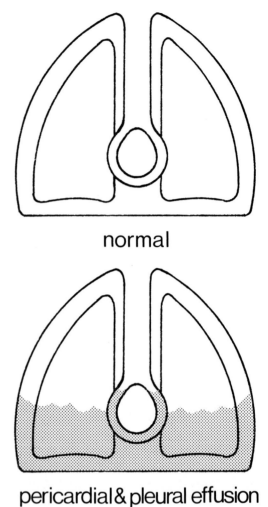

normal

pericardial & pleural effusion

Fig. 4–6. This drawing shows the presence of a pleural effusion in schematic diagram. It also shows a pericardial effusion caused either by increased hydrostatic pressure or by disequilibrium of the normal distribution of fluid between the circulation and the tissue spaces. The normal relationships show the heart in the center of the drawing lying within its sac (pericardium) and the lungs on either side, lying in the pleural spaces.

the capillary at the venular end. The fluid that has passed out of the normal capillary (small molecules and water) remains in the interstitial space. Eventually it may find its way back to the circulation. Such a fluid without any protein (or only small amounts) is called a **transudate** to distinguish it from the protein-rich fluid (greater than 3 gm per 100 ml) that is generally referred to as an **exudate**. Thus the pleural effusion (and the edema fluid in the lung) in congestive heart failure are typically clear and have a low specific gravity, whereas the effusion seen with pneumonia (an inflammation) may have a higher specific gravity, may even form fibrin threads because of the protein (fibrinogen) present, and may show the presence of white blood cells. All of these characteristics testify to the loss of selective permeabiltiy that is characteristic of an exudate. If the fluid in the pleural space contains enough white blood cells to be considered as pus, we speak of a purulent exudate, and if there is a great amount of fibrin, we talk about fibrinopurulent exudate, but we are getting ahead of ourselves and beginning to talk about aspects of inflammation.

The third general cause of increased interstitial or tissue space fluid (edema) is any **decrease in the osmotic pressure of plasma proteins.** As we have said, the principal serum protein responsible for osmotic pressure is serum albumin, synthesized in the liver. The pool of serum albumin so essential to maintaining the vascular equilibrium can be reduced in several ways. It may simply be lost by the body more rapidly than it is made, as happens with the kidney disease, glomerulonephritis. This renal loss is referred to as proteinuria, or more specifically as albuminuria, and is detected routinely on urinalysis. We shall discuss this further in the chapter on kidney disease.

A second reason for the fall of serum albumin (hypoalbuminemia) is the failure of the liver to synthesize adequate amounts of albumin. One reason may be simply starvation, in which the ingredients for albumin synthesis (protein) are not available in the diet (amino acids). With the prolonged loss of albumin, one of the tissue compartments, the peritoneal cavity, may accumulate vast amounts of watery fluid (ascites) to produce a bloated belly, as seen in the prison camps of World War II and in the starving populations of poor countries. Another cause of hypoalbuminemia is the failure of liver cells to function, because they themselves have been poisoned or injured, such as in toxic or viral (hepatitis) injury to the liver. Here again, the dramatic accumulations of edema fluid in the peritoneal cavity (transudate) may reach 10 or more liters.

Sometimes there are local accumulations of fluid following surgical explorations or operations. Occasionally this happens to the arm on the side from which a breast tumor has been removed. This form of edema may be attributed to interference with another circulation, namely that of the lymphatics. If the lymphatic drainage system is blocked, fluid accumulates. We can distinguish between lymphedema and edema caused by venous obstruction, but in the end, because the lymphatics drain through the thoracic duct into the venous system, one might consider the disorder to follow the same general principle as its cause, namely, interference with the hydrostatic forces normally at play.

HEMORRHAGE

When a vessel ruptures, blood escapes naturally into the surrounding tissue or onto a free surface. The hemorrhage may be large and form a swelling known as a **hematoma.** Or the hemorrhages may be as small as a pin's head and are then called **petechiae.** The significance of bleeding depends on the size and the site of the hemorrhage. If it occurs into a muscle, it does little damage, but if it takes place in the brain or on a free surface such as the interior of the stomach, where it cannot be arrested, it may cause death. Rupture of an artery or vein may be produced in several ways: (1) The most common cause is **trauma**, a

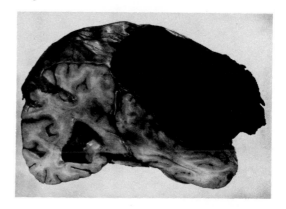

Fig. 4–7. This large black mass is an extradural hemorrhage that occurred following traumatic injury to the head. The skull fracture led to arterial bleeding, and the hematoma has compressed the underlying brain substance, as can be seen immediately beneath the extradural hematoma. (McGill University, Department of Pathology Museum.)

wound or bruise (Fig. 4–7). (2) An ulcer or a cancer in the neighborhood of a large vessel may finally perforate the wall and give rise to profuse hemorrhage; this may happen in the esophagus or the stomach (Fig. 4–8), or in a tuberculous cavity in the lung. (3) The wall of the vessel may be weakened by a condition such as **atherosclerosis,** and finally give way under the pressure of the blood; this is what often happens in cerebral hemorrhage (Fig. 4–9). Sometimes this is preceded by a localized bulging of the vessel wall, known as an **aneurysm.**

The remarkable thing about hemorrhage is not that it should occur, but that it should ever stop. If a hole is made in a pipe through which water is passing, the water will flow out until the pipe is empty. It is true that if we fill the pipe with a glue-like material too thick to pass through a small hole, none will escape, but such a material would never be able to flow through the small arteries and the minute capillaries. The wonder in the case of hemorrhage is how a fluid thin enough to pass through the finest channels ceases after a short time to flow through a comparatively large opening in the vessel wall.

The arrest of hemorrhage is brought about by the **coagulation** or clotting of the blood. As long as the blood is inside the vessel, it does not clot, but when it escapes into the surrounding tissue or onto the surface of the

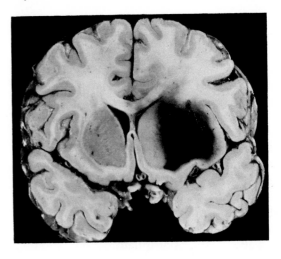

Fig. 4–9.   The cross section of brain shows an intracerebral hemorrhage (dark area) which has occurred in the thalamus of the brain and has shifted structures across the midline. This hemorrhage occurred in a patient who had hypertension and was attributed to rupture of an arteriosclerotic blood vessel. (McGill University, Department of Pathology Museum.)

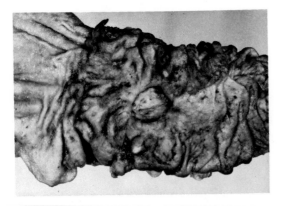

Fig. 4–8.   The circular structure in the center of the photograph is an ulcer in the first portion of the duodenum. At the base of this ulcer can be seen a small dark dot, which is an eroded artery. This peptic duodenal ulcer eroded into a blood vessel and caused a massive hemorrhage into the gastrointestinal tract (McGill University, Department of Pathology Museum.)

skin, it begins at once to coagulate. Soon the clot is able to plug the hole in the vessel, unless that hole is much too large. The clotting of blood is due to the interaction of substances in the plasma such as **fibrinogen** and **thrombin.** Thrombin is formed by the interaction of prothrombin and calcium. Prothrombin is a substance of great importance; it is formed from vitamin K; when a person suffers from vitamin K deficiency, his prothrombin is low and the blood loses the power of clotting. Heparin (antithrombin) prevents this mechanism from making the blood clot in the vessels of a normal person; it acts by preventing prothrombin and calcium from uniting to form thrombin. Heparin is present in minute quantities in the blood. It was first obtained from the liver, hence its name (Greek *hepar,* liver), but it is also present in large amounts in the lung and intestine. When blood is shed, blood platelets are activated and liberate thromboplastin, which neutralizes heparin, and when it is eliminated, the whole complex machinery of clotting is set in motion. A clot is formed of interlacing threads of **fibrin.** These threads seal over the opening in the vessel in much the same way as the threads of a spider's web might do. This plug is greatly reinforced by the blood platelets, particles that float in the plasma and aggregate to form

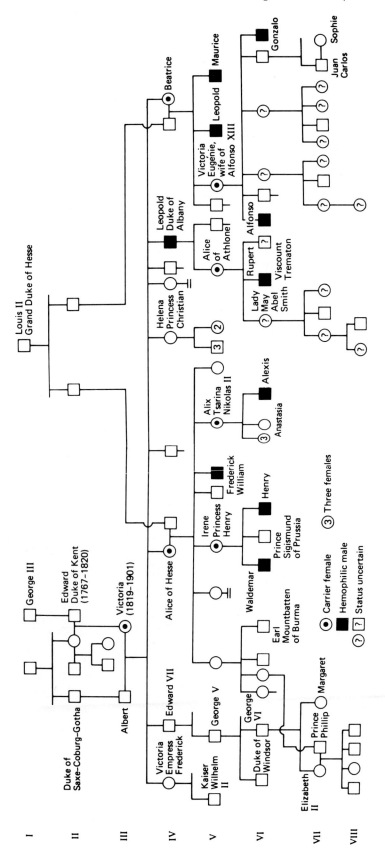

Fig. 4-10. Pedigree of the descendants of Queen Victoria showing carriers and afflicted males possessing the X-linked gene conferring the disease hemophilia. (McKusick, V.: *Human Genetics*, 2nd Ed. Englewood Cliffs, N.J., Prentice Hall, 1969.)

a sticky mass that effectually seals up the hole in the vessel wall. In time this emergency plug is converted into fibrous or scar tissue, just as an inflammatory exudate becomes changed into scar tissue, and the opening is closed permanently. The coagulation mechanism is more complex than is outlined here, and the reader is referred to the chapter entitled "Blood and Lymph Nodes."

Occasionally, although fortunately rarely, the mechanism for the temporary arrest of hemorrhage is defective, so that the blood continues to flow out of the vessel. This condition is most marked in the hereditary disease called **hemophilia,** sufferers from which are known as "bleeders" who may die of hemorrhage from a trivial wound, cut, or tooth extraction. Their essential defect is a lack of a globulin fraction of the plasma known as the antihemophilic factor (AHF). When this factor is added to hemophilic blood, it causes coagulation to occur, and when it is injected into the patient, clotting time is reduced. Prothrombin seems not to be used properly in the hemophiliac. Hemophilia is a good example of sex-linked heredity; only the males of a family exhibit the disease, and only the females transmit it (Fig. 4–10). Most readers are familiar with the story of the Czar of Russia's only son, so well told in *Nicolas and Alexandra* by R. Massie.

THROMBOSIS

Speaking teleologically, clotting of the blood should occur when the blood escapes from the vessel, but not when it is flowing through the lumen of the vessel. Should this occur, it is called thrombosis; the clot within the vessel is known as a thrombus. It consists mainly of platelets that adhere to the vessel wall, fibrin, and red blood cells trapped in the mesh, which gradually form a mass that may finally close the lumen of the vessel and stop the flow of blood through it. A thrombus may be defined as **a mass formed from constituents of the blood on the inner surface of the heart or a blood vessel.** The difference between a clot formed postmortem or in a test tube, and one that forms in the flowing stream of an artery, vein, or chamber of the heart, is that in a tube or after death the heaviest ele-

ments, the red blood cells, gravitate to the bottom and the lighter fibrin forms a jelly-like clear layer on top, whereas during life thrombosis occurs in layers. First, a layer of platelets attaches to the injured vessel, then some fibrin forms and snares some red blood cells. The process then repeats itself. These layers were described and are referred to as the lines of Zahn, after their discoverer. It has been said with some truth that throughout his entire existence man is almost constantly hemorrhaging or thrombosing.

The causes of thrombosis are threefold, as Virchow stated over 100 years ago (Virchow's triad). They are: (1) **slowing of the blood stream;** (2) **changes in the vessel wall,** and (3) **changes in the blood itself.** As the first of these factors is more common in veins than in arteries, it is natural that thrombosis usually should occur in veins. The normal vessel has an exquisitely smooth lining known as the

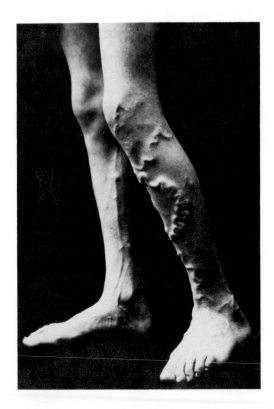

Fig. 4–11. Varicose veins. While these are dramatic and aesthetically unpleasing, they are infrequently a cause of thrombophlebitis and pulmonary embolism. The deep femoral veins are the most likely source of pulmonary emboli. (The Evans Collection, Osler Library, McGill University.)

endothelium. When this is destroyed by injury or inflammation, platelets adhere to the rough spot and gradually build up a thrombus from the blood as it flows past. The slower the flow, the more likely are the platelets to fall out of the stream and to adhere to the vessel wall, so that thrombosis is associated with varicose (dilated and tortuous) veins (Fig. 4–11) and a slowed circulation. Thrombosis frequently follows abdominal operations, particularly on the pelvic organs. Closely related to this is the thrombosis that may occur in the puerperium, the period following childbirth. This phenomenon is due to the unusual dilatation and stasis in the pelvic veins caused by the growing uterus. When the child has been delivered, the veins cannot involute so rapidly and remain a site for stasis, thrombosis, and potential embolization.

Stasis is the name given to slowing of the circulation. It occurs most frequently in inactive or immobilized persons. In addition to inactivity, any impairment of cardiovascular function (heart failure) may also lead to slowing of the blood stream.

Changes in the vessel wall can occur acutely or with chronic disease. After any surgical intervention, there may have been local pressure from a retractor or an anoxic injury due to transient ischemia that would affect the venous or arterial endothelium. This local acute injury sets the scene for thrombosis. On a long-term basis, there may be loss of the endothelium with the progression of atherosclerosis in the arterial tree. This loss also predisposes a patient to thrombus formation, particularly in the abdominal aorta, and occasionally in smaller vessels such as the coronary arteries or the circle of Willis at the base of the brain.

Changes in the blood itself can occur with lesions that result in deoxygenation, such as intracardiac shunts due to congenital heart disease. The body makes up for the deoxygenation by a compensatory increase in red blood cell numbers (polycythemia). When the blood cell number increases, the circulating blood itself (plasma and cells) becomes more viscous. This viscosity often precipitates thrombus formation. Thus cerebral thromboses are a complication of congenital,

cyanotic heart disease. There are changes in the clotting and fibrinolytic mechanisms that may alter the blood's predisposition either to remain liquid and free-flowing or to form thrombi in the arterial or venous system.

The principal sites of thrombosis are the veins and the heart. Thrombosis may also occur in arteries, particularly in the coronary arteries, the cerebral arteries, and the arteries to the leg in old persons. In all of these cases there may be preliminary narrowing of the lumen by arteriosclerosis. The veins of the leg are frequently affected because of the tendency for postoperative and puerperal thrombosis to involve these veins. Thrombosis of the veins of the leg is also common in chronic heart failure, owing to the sluggish circulation, particularly when a patient is confined to bed for some time. A number of cases of thrombosis in the legs followed by fatal pulmonary embolism occurred during World War II in London air raid shelters in elderly persons who sat all night in deck chairs, the wooden supports of which pressed continuously on their thighs. The leg is swollen owing to interference with the return of blood, and the thrombosed vein may be felt as a hard tender cord. In the heart, a common site of thrombus formation is an inflamed valve, on which the platelets are deposited as the blood flows past, until they form a large thrombus that, in this situation, is known as a vegetation. Even more common is thrombus formation in one of the atria, particularly in the part called the atrial appendage, a kind of cul-de-sac in which the blood is apt to stagnate.

Thrombosis may be a serious complication of surgical operations, particularly in operations on large blood vessels such as arteries. This can now be anticipated by the use of heparin, which prevents the platelets from sticking together and to the vessel wall, so that a thrombus is not formed. Heparin has also been used to prevent thrombosis in the veins of the leg after an operation. The action of the substance dicumarol resembles that of heparin in prolonging the coagulation time, but it has the advantage over heparin of a much more prolonged action, and it can be taken by mouth instead of by injection.

The subsequent history of a thrombus var-

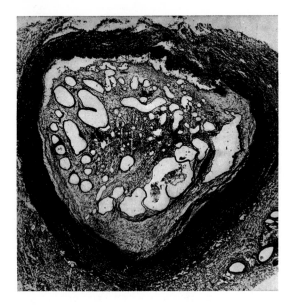

Fig. 4–12. An arterial thrombus showing canalization. Photomicrograph. (Bell: *Textbook of Pathology.* Philadelphia, Lea & Febiger.)

ies: (1) The thrombus may become converted into fibrous tissue with permanent closure of the vessel. (2) It may contract or become canalized so that blood can flow through the lumen once again (Fig. 4–12). (3) Finally, parts or all of the thrombus may become detached from the vessel wall and enter the blood stream as a floating body known as an **embolus**, a catastrophic occurrence, as we shall see in the next section. This detachment of the thrombus is particularly likely to occur when there is sepsis at the site of thrombosis as the infection predisposes the thrombus to break down and become loosened (Fig. 4–13).

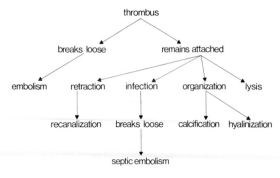

Fig. 4–13. This figure illustrates the possible fates of a thrombus. (Adapted from Walter, J.B.: *An Introduction to the Principles of Disease.* Philadelphia, W. B. Saunders, 1977.)

Another factor may be rough handling of the part. It is evident that a thrombosed leg has to be treated with the greatest care, and that anything in the nature of massage must be avoided.

Fibrinolysis. Blood clots are not necessarily permanent structures, and Nature tries to remove an obstructing thrombus by means of fibrinolytic enzymes in the blood. One enzyme, called plasmin, or fibrinolysin, is a globulin. It exists in the form of a precursor, plasminogen, and it digests the fibrin of the thrombus. Unfortunately, Nature is often far from successful in its efforts, although it must be admitted that myocardial infarction associated with thrombotic occlusion of the coronary arteries is accompanied by the production of fibrinolysis. In view of the serious damage that a thrombus can do in obstructing such arteries as the coronaries and cerebrals, not to mention the veins, great efforts have been made to find some substance that would dissolve the thrombus. These efforts have been much more successful in the test tube than in the living body, and the work is still in an experimental stage.

EMBOLISM

An embolus may be a thrombus that has become detached and has entered the blood stream. As it is most commonly a vein that is the site of the thrombus, and as the veins become larger as the heart is approached, it follows that the embolus will meet with no obstruction in its voyage to the heart. But no sooner has it passed through the right side of the heart and entered the pulmonary artery that carries the blood to the lungs than the chances of arrest of the embolus increase with every millimeter the embolus travels, for the arteries become narrower the farther they pass from the heart. Finally, the embolus will lodge in one of the arteries of the lung. The vessel blocked depends entirely on the size of the embolus. Indeed, the main pulmonary artery may be blocked if the embolus is sufficiently large.

Embolism refers to occlusion of some part of the cardiovascular system by impaction of a foreign mass transported to the site through the blood stream. An embolus may originate

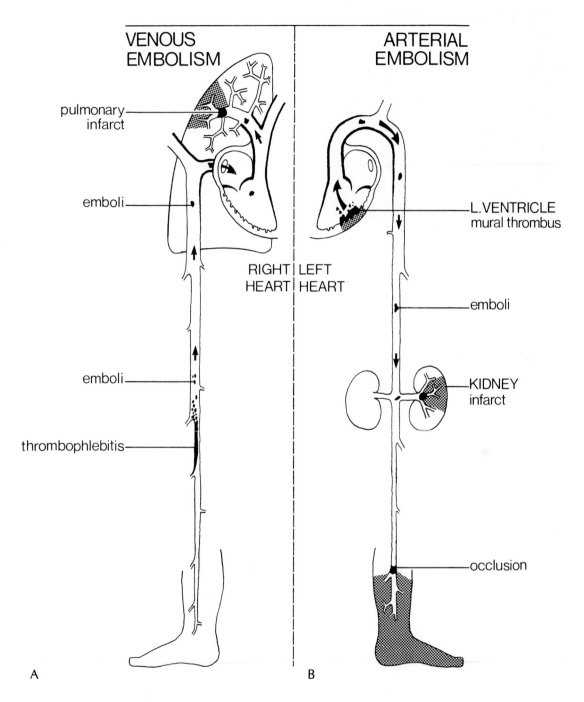

Fig. 4–14.   This set of diagrams illustrates the complications and eventual fates of embolism. In *A,* a venous embolism arises in thrombophlebitis in a leg vein. It may pass through the inferior vena cava into the right heart and out to the pulmonary artery, causing pulmonary infarcts. Arterial embolism, shown in *B,* arises on a mural thrombus in the left ventricle, possibly arresting in a branch of the cerebral blood vessels, causing kidney infarcts, or occluding peripheral vessels.

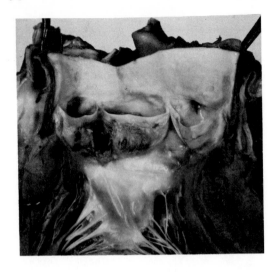

Fig. 4–15. This figure shows the aortic valve with the two coronary artery ostia arising above the valve cusps. Just below the free margin of the valve cusps is an irregular fibrinous material which is gray and shaggy. This is an area of endocarditis from which platelet and bacterial emboli were liberated into the arterial blood stream. These may lodge in the brain, kidneys, spleen, or terminal branches of the arterial tree. Occasionally they may even find their way into those coronary arteries. (McGill University, Department of Pathology Museum.)

in the heart instead of in a vein, usually on the left side of the heart (Fig. 4–14). The original thrombus may have been a vegetation on a valve (Fig. 4–15), as has already been described, or it may be formed in one of the chambers of the heart, usually the left atrium. In either case the destination of the embolus is now different, for it enters the aorta, the great vessel that leaves the left side of the heart, and passes not to the lungs but to the brain, kidneys, and other organs.

There are other types of emboli besides those that originate as a thrombus. The most important of these are fat emboli, air emboli, septic emboli, and tumor emboli. **Fat embolism** occurs as the result of crushing injuries to bones, which allow the fat in the bone marrow to enter the veins in that substance in the form of globules. Fat embolism may be the cause of death in such injuries as car accidents, in which the blood loss, shock, and mechanical injuries can be managed, but the pulmonary and cerebral emboli cannot.

Air embolism is due to the entrance of air into the veins either during a surgical operation or because of the injection of air into the uterus in an attempt to produce a criminal abortion. An air embolus is a bubble too large to dissolve that may eventually occlude a small vessel. The oxygen in the bubble is useless to the cells in the area because they can only use dissolved oxygen.

Septic emboli occur in bacterial endocarditis and when bacterial colonies either are growing in veins or gain access to the circulation.

Tumor emboli are groups of cancer cells that have invaded a vein, become detached, and are then carried to the lungs or other organs. It is by this means that cancer is disseminated throughout the body, with the formation of secondary growths known as **metastases.**

Effects of Embolism. When an embolus lodges in an artery, it blocks the lumen and cuts off the blood supply to the organ or part supplied by that artery. The effect depends on the size of the embolus and on the circulatory arrangements of the part. It is obvious that if an embolus is large enough to block the main artery to an organ or a limb, the effect will be as disastrous as the cutting off of the main water supply to a city. In the case of a smaller embolus, the question of the vascular connections is all-important. In most parts of the body there is what is called a **collateral circulation,** a communication between two sets of arteries (Fig. 4–16). The blood to the hand is carried by two main arteries, one on each side of the wrist, and between the branches of these there pass numerous small communicating vessels (Fig. 4–17). Should one of the main arteries be blocked by an embolus or be ligatured, the communications from the remaining artery become greatly dilated, so that sufficient blood can still reach the area supplied by the blocked vessel. Under these circumstances an embolus does little or no harm. The availability of collateral circulation determines the outcome of occlusion in the systemic circulation.

There is another consideration, namely, that organs such as the lung and liver have a double blood supply. Each segment of the lung is perfused by blood from both the pulmonary artery (pulmonary circulation) and the bronchial artery (systemic circulation)

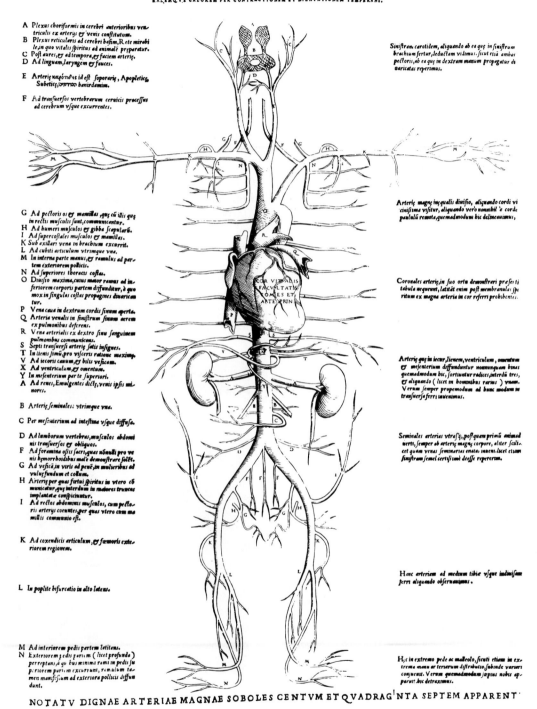

Fig. 4–16. This drawing from the fifteenth-century anatomist, Vesalius (Tabulae Sex), shows the heart and arterial tree. In many areas, such as the arm, one can see two arteries, which extend the length of the limb. There is obviously the possibility, if the circulation to one of these arteries is arrested, that the other may supply the extremity with adequate blood. (Saunders, J.B. de C.M., and O'Malley, C.D.: *The Illustrations From the Works of Andreas Vesalius.* Cleveland and New York, World Publishing Company, 1950.)

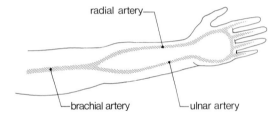
radial artery

brachial artery   ulnar artery

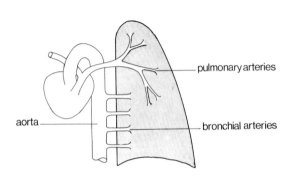
pulmonary arteries

aorta

bronchial arteries

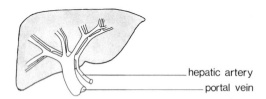
hepatic artery

portal vein

Fig. 4–18. These diagrams show the dual circulation to the lung and the liver. The lung receives venous blood from the right heart through the pulmonary arteries (one circulation). This blood is oxygenated in the lung, returns to the left heart, and is pumped out into the aorta. The bronchial arteries supply the lung with oxygenated blood from the aorta (the other circulation). The liver similarly receives both venous and arterial blood. The portal vein carries deoxygenated blood from the spleen, stomach, intestine, and other parts of the digestive system. The hepatic artery carries arterial blood from the aorta. One important advantage of a double circulation is a reduced susceptibility to infarcts. Both circulations must be impaired in order for the tissue to become ischemic.

(Fig. 4–18). This dual supply provides a safety factor, for if there is a small embolus to a small branch of the pulmonary artery, that part of the lung does not die, since it is also supplied by its respective bronchial artery. However, if there is a degree of heart failure present, the auxiliary circulation may be inadequate, and the embolism may cause an infarct despite the dual circulation.

Infarction. It is a different matter, however, if the main artery to a limb, such as the femoral artery in the thigh, is blocked. Here there can be no efficient collateral circulation, and the tissues are completely deprived of their blood supply and die. A similar state of affairs exists in a number of organs such as the brain, heart, kidney, and spleen. Each organ is supplied by arterial blood and drained by a system of veins. If the arterial supply is occluded by a thrombus or embolus, by mechanical means (traumatic injury), or even by surgical intervention (ligature or clamp), the organ thus deprived of blood may

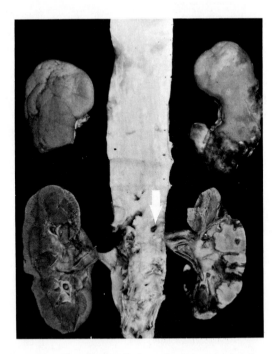

Fig. 4–19. This photograph shows the thoracic and abdominal aorta, the renal arteries, and the kidneys, as viewed from the posterior aspect. At the arrow is the right renal artery which is occluded. The right kidney shows a large area of recent infarction (the pale area with the dark border). This has been caused by occlusion of the renal artery by embolic material from a mural thrombus. (McGill University, Department of Pathology Museum.)

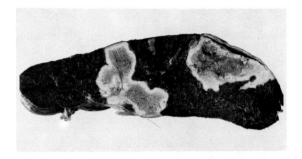

Fig. 4–20. This section of the spleen shows two large infarcts, one in the center of the picture, and one in the right hand corner. The infarcts are pale areas caused by arterial occlusions. (McGill University, Department of Pathology Museum.)

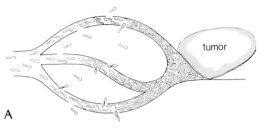

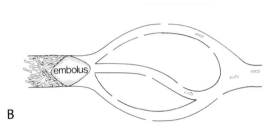

Fig. 4–21. *A* and *B*, These diagrams illustrate 2 mechanisms that cause infarcts. In *A*, occlusion of the outflow (venous) from an organ or a part of the circulation results in infarction because once the venous-capillary pressure equals arterial levels, no further oxygenated blood can perfuse the organ. This leads to anoxic death in an organ that is paradoxically suffused with erythrocytes. These infarcts look red (hemorrhagic) because the capillary walls are stuffed with red blood cells, but they also become permeable because of the anoxemia, and leak blood into the tissue space. *B* illustrates a more common situation, in which arterial occlusion (embolism, thrombosis) blocks perfusion of the organ leaving it bloodless and therefore anoxemic. These infarcts are pale or white. The capillaries, if they are subsequently perfused, will leak (reflow phenomenon).

undergo ischemic coagulative necrosis, provided the interruption lasts for a significant time. This is called ischemic (or anoxic) infarction, and is demonstrated in the kidney (Fig. 4–19) and the spleen (Fig. 4–20), where the infarcts appear as pale areas. The arterial blood does not reach parts of the organs and the cells become mummified following prolonged anoxemia (Fig. 4–21A).

Another cause of infarction is occlusion of the venous system (Fig. 4–21B). This may occur by simple thrombosis or by a thrombus initiated by compression from outside a vein (as in many cases of cancer). In cases of venous occlusion, arterial blood enters the organ and perfuses the tissue, but cannot leave because the vein is obstructed, much as a beaver dam may raise the water level in the forest and drown the trees. So, in the case of venous thrombosis, blood rich in oxygen reaches the tissue, but cannot leave, and anoxemia occurs in this stagnant area. Then the capillaries become permeable and congestion passes to hemorrhage. This lesion is an infarct, but its appearance is different; the tissue is suffused with blood and the infarct appears as a hemorrhagic area. A good example of this is thrombosis of a mesenteric vein (Fig. 4–22). Here the bowel becomes darkly hemorrhagic due to segmental occlusion of the venous return. This kind of ischemic necrosis used to be referred to as gangrene.

It is evident that infarction is the result of a sudden cutting off of the blood supply to part of an organ with an insufficient collateral circulation. An **infarct may be produced by thrombosis as well as by embolism.** Thus an infarct of cardiac muscle is nearly always caused by thrombosis of one of the coronary arteries; an infarct of the brain may be caused by either thrombosis or embolism of the cerebral arteries. The most frequent and important sites of infarction are the heart, lung, brain, spleen, kidney, and intestine.

Before leaving the subject we might recapitulate the importance of pulmonary embolism and infarction. The effect on the patient depends principally on the size of the embolus and collateral circulation and its competence. If the embolus is small, it will not be arrested until it reaches a correspondingly small arterial branch, and the area of the infarct produced will be equally small. The pa-

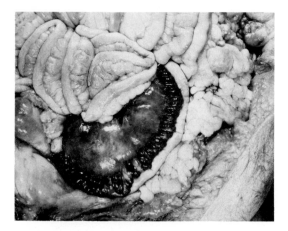

Fig. 4–22. This photograph shows small bowel (white) which is normal, and infarcted bowel (dark) caused by thrombosis of the mesenteric vein. (McGill University, Department of Pathology Museum.)

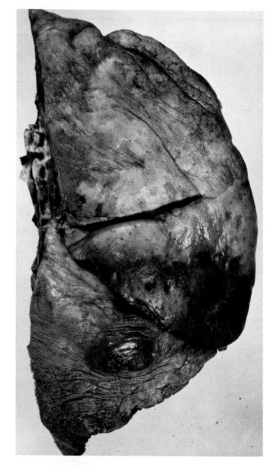

Fig. 4–23. This photograph of the external surface of the lung shows two large, dark areas in the center of the field. These areas are infarcts of the lung caused by recent pulmonary emboli. (McGill University, Department of Pathology Museum.)

tient will experience a sharp pain in the chest, and may cough up a little blood during the next few days, after which recovery will be complete (Fig. 4–23).

Of course, if there is a competent bronchial (systemic) circulation, there need not be any infarct. The course of events is tragically different when the embolus is large enough to block the main pulmonary artery or one of its principal branches. After an uneventful, postoperative convalescence, suddenly, almost out of a clear sky, there is strange restlessness, rapidly ensuing shock, air hunger, and collapse, and death usually in 2 to 15 minutes. The exact explanation of sudden death is not easy. We have suggested that the cause is the shock of the abrupt pulmonary ischemia. But when the surgeon ties off the main pulmonary artery before removing a lung for cancer, he does not expect the patient to die. Perhaps a more probable explanation is the release of **serotonin** from the blood platelets at the site of embolism. Serotonin is a vasoconstricting substance obtained from clotted blood as long ago as 1884, is stored in the platelets, readily released, and stimulates plain muscle, including that of the bronchi. The full tragedy of this accident is evident in those cases in which the embolism occurs about a week after an abdominal operation or after childbirth, when the patient is convalescing splendidly, but after sitting up in

bed suddenly feels faint, drops back on the pillow panting for breath, and is dead in the course of a few minutes. Often, however, embolism is a complication of medical rather than surgical cases, and it is particularly likely to complicate heart failure.

In all these cases the patient is confined to bed, and the condition (failing heart, childbirth, abdominal operation, immobility) tends to interfere with the flow of blood from the veins of the leg to the heart. It is in these veins that thrombosis occurs; the thrombus becomes dislodged by some sudden movement, and pulmonary embolism is the result. Precautions can be taken to prevent the stagnation of circulation that leads to thrombosis. Voluntary movements of the legs, frequent changes of position, and elevation of the foot of the bed all contribute to this end. In order to counteract the tendency to thrombosis, which is associated with prolonged rest in bed after pelvic operations and childbirth, it is becoming the fashion to make the patient get up, if only for a short time, at a much earlier date than in the past.

ISCHEMIA—ITS CAUSES AND EFFECTS

Ischemia is the condition in which the blood supply to a part is diminished or stopped. It is a local rather than a general bloodlessness. As blood is carried to the part by an artery, it is evident that ischemia will be caused by anything that narrows or closes the lumen of an artery, provided the collateral circulation is not sufficiently adequate to compensate fully for the primary loss of blood supply.

The closure of the artery may be sudden or slow, and the effect varies accordingly. We have already studied the effect of sudden closure of an artery, whether by the formation of a thrombus or by the lodgment of an embolus. If the collateral circulation is inadequate, the result will be an infarct. Slow closure is due to the degenerative disease of arteries known as arteriosclerosis or atherosclerosis, commonly called hardening of the arteries (Fig. 4–24). The exact cause of this condition is not known, a matter that is discussed in Chapter 14, but it is a common condition in advancing years, just as is graying of the hair. The blood vessels begin to feel the effect of the sharp tooth of time. The subject of atherosclerosis is currently of much interest, partly because autopsies on United States soldiers as young as age 19 who were killed in Vietnam showed atherosclerosis of their coronary arteries. This evidence suggests that the American way of life was creating lesions in apparently healthy young persons. On the other hand, there are many octogenarians who die of other causes and who appear to have little atherosclerosis at autopsy. The saying that "a man is as old as his arteries" is profoundly true. The essential change is a nodular thickening of the intima or inner coat of the artery, as a result of which the lumen slowly becomes narrowed, until finally a mere chink may be left through

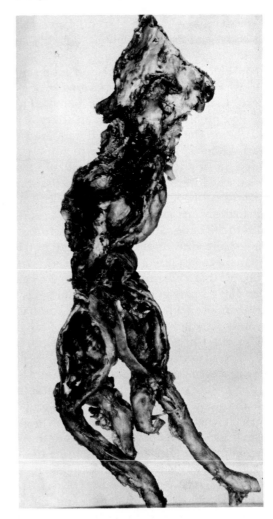

Fig. 4–24. This photograph of the abdominal aorta and iliac vessels shows a markedly deformed vessel with thrombosis of the wall with thrombi superimposed on the markedly atherosclerotic vessel. Compare the appearance of this aorta with that in Figure 4–19, where only below the renal arteries is there any evidence of arteriosclerosis. (McGill University, Department of Pathology Museum.)

which the blood can only trickle with difficulty. The smooth endothelium lining the vessel becomes lost in time where atherosclerosis exists, so that the inner surface is now roughened. Since the platelets tend to stick to the rough surfaces, a thrombus may form, which suddenly completes the closure of the already narrowed vessel. This is what happens in **coronary artery thrombosis**, one of the most common causes of sudden death in persons over 50 years of age. The coronary arteries are the vessels that supply blood to the heart muscle, the most essential muscle in the body, and if that supply is suddenly cut off, the heart will stop beating.

For some reason not understood at present, arteriosclerosis is not a general process affecting all the arteries in the body, but a selective process that picks out an artery here and there. The 3 principal sufferers are the heart, kidneys, and brain, to which may be added the arteries of the leg. Not all of these are attacked in the same person, so that one person may have symptoms pointing to injury to the heart, another to the kidneys, and a third to the brain. Strokes and "little strokes" are usually due to thrombosis and not to hemorrhage, as used to be believed. It is probable that a hereditary or inherited weakness plays a part in the selection, for several members of one family may die of coronary thrombosis at about the same age.

The effect of ischemia is gradual death of the specialized cells of the part, i.e., nerve cells in the brain, heart muscle cells, and so on, and their replacement by scar tissue, so that the organ loses the power to do its proper work. In the brain there is failure of recent memory and of the power of accurate thinking, and there may be actual softening of the part of the brain affected owing to degenerative processes.

Closure of the arteries in the leg and, rarely, in the arm may lead to death of the parts farthest from the heart, the toes or fingers, since in them the circulation is likely to be most sluggish. Here another change becomes evident, for bacteria invade the dead tissue through the skin and cause decomposition and putrefaction of the ischemic tissue. The necrotic part undergoes a series of color changes, becoming first green and finally black. The necrosis spreads slowly up the limb as the narrowing of the arteries becomes more extreme and widespread. Diabetes often leads to the occurrence of marked atheroma in the arteries of the leg, so that necrosis is a common complication in diabetic patients.

When a patient shows evidence of marked interference of the circulation in the leg, special care is necessary to prevent any injury, however trivial, that may start the process in the devitalized tissues, a process that may eventually require amputation of the affected foot. Additional care must be taken in cutting the nails, lest the toe be injured. Bandages must not be too tight, and the limb must be kept warm to encourage any circulation that may still remain in the collateral vessels. However, too much heat in the form of an electric foot warmer or a hot-water bottle is a particular source of danger.

ARTERIAL HYPERTENSION

Blood pressure in health is the result of a number of forces, the chief ones being the contractions of the heart and the peripheral resistance provided by the arterioles. In spite of rapid fluctuations in both the peripheral resistance and the cardiac output from minute to minute, depending on whether you sit or stand, are tranquil or excited, are drinking tea or eating cake, the systemic blood pressure remains remarkably constant in a normal person.

Hypertension or high blood pressure is defined by the life insurance companies as any elevation of the systolic pressure above 140 mm of mercury and of the diastolic pressure above 90 mm of mercury. This may be true statistically, but it does not follow that these figures can be applied to every person and thus label him as hypertensive. A rise in the diastolic pressure is much more important than a similar rise in the systolic pressure. **Hypertension** is at present divided into 2 forms, **primary** or essential, of which the cause is unknown, and which constitutes about 90% of all cases of hypertension, and **secondary,** in which there is some associated lesion, such as chronic nephritis or tumor of the adrenal cortex, that is proven to be responsible for the elevated blood pressure.

Essential Hypertension

This is the term commonly used for the primary variety. It is divided in turn into so-called benign and malignant forms. The **benign form** is characterized by a gradual onset and a long-continued course, often of many years. The **malignant form,** fortunately much less common, is frequently of abrupt onset and runs a course measured in months rather than years, so that it justifies its name. It often ends with renal failure (uremia) or cerebral hemorrhage.

Etiology. The very names primary and essential indicate our ignorance of the etiology of the condition, but that does not prevent us from speculating on the causes. There is considerable evidence, both experimental and human, to suggest that the kidney and the adrenal cortex exert a regulating effect on the blood pressure (Fig. 4–25). Over 100 years ago Richard Bright pointed out the association between **chronic nephritis** and hypertrophy of the left ventricle. When the arteries to both kidneys in the dog or one kidney in the rat are gradually constricted by a clamp, the resulting **renal ischemia** causes hypertension. The same thing happens in man when the main renal artery to one kidney is narrowed by disease. The **adrenal cortex** exerts its influence on blood pressure by regulating the salt content, and therefore the water content, in the walls of the smaller arteries, thus affecting their lumen. One of the most striking features of Addison's disease, which is caused by destruction of both adrenals, is low blood pressure. **It seems clear that both the kidney and the adrenal are associated in the control of blood pressure in health.**

A new family of chemicals, called prostaglandins, has an opposite effect, namely an ability to lower blood pressure in some circumstances. These chemicals are also synthesized partly in the kidney and have been implicated, although largely in a speculative way, in disorders of blood pressure. Perhaps an upset in this balance between pressor or vasoconstrictive agents and vasodilators is responsible for so-called essential hypertension.

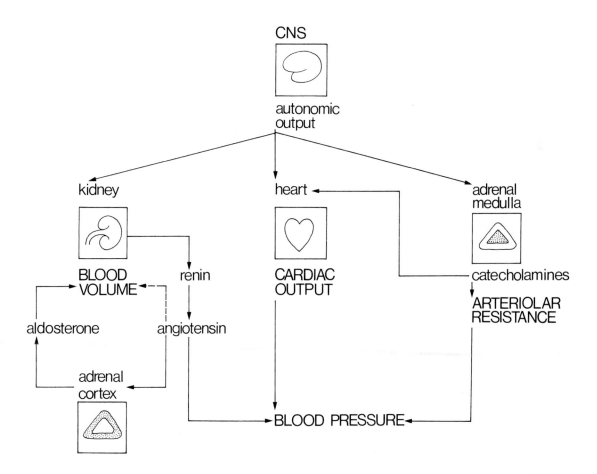

Fig. 4–25. This graph illustrates factors that affect blood pressure. In particular, the interrelationship between the kidney (renin) and the adrenal cortex (aldosterone) shown in the lower left corner has been of great diagnostic and therapeutic interest.

Clearly this is an oversimplification, because many other factors such as the central nervous system, cardiac contraction, and blood volume all play important roles in regulating the blood pressure. We shall discuss this further in chapters on the heart, the kidneys, and the endocrine system.

The difference between the essential and the secondary forms is that in the former no constant lesions can be demonstrated at autopsy either in the kidneys or in the adrenals. **Heredity** plays a part in determining whether or not a patient will develop essential hypertension.

Secondary Hypertension

Raised blood pressure may be associated with renal disease, endocrine tumors, and constriction of the arteries. **Renal lesions** may take the form of (1) **glomerulonephritis,** which causes diffuse glomerular ischemia, (2) **chronic pyelonephritis,** and (3) **stenosis of the main renal artery** on one or both sides by atheroma. **Endocrine tumors** may be (1) **pheochromocytoma of the adrenal medulla,** which produces vasoconstricting hormone, or (2) **adenoma of the adrenal cortex,** which produces excess salt-retaining hormone with resulting **aldosteronism. Constriction of the arteries** may take the form of **coarctation of the aorta,** in which the hypertension is naturally restricted to the upper part of the body and the upper limbs. This last is a cause of hypertension in childhood, and one readily cured by operation. The **arteriolar narrowing of age** is associated with hypertension, but which is cause and which effect is difficult to know.

DERANGEMENTS OF BODY FLUIDS

Millions of years ago, the first land animal crawled out of the sea where, with relatively little effort, he maintained an equilibrium. To float and move about in the sea is much easier than standing upright and running, or even crawling on all fours on your belly. The preservation of an internal aqueous environment on land requires work, too; to conserve water and to excrete wastes requires energy from cells of the kidney, lung, and skin. For each of us there is a brief but visible recapitulation of evolution in the months before our birth.

For a tadpole, who diffuses away ammonia into the pond water, to adapt successfully to terrestrial life, gills must be exchanged for lungs, a tail for feet, and osmotically important material (albumin) must be synthesized for the functioning of the circulation. New enzymes capable of excreting nitrogen in a relatively innocuous form (urea) are evoked during metamorphosis from the liver. In disease, some of the principal disorders of human beings are those of overly diminished body fluids, whether they circulate, are in the interstitial compartment, or are intracellular. Intoxication or depletion of the substances that are present in these various compartments is the source of many ills. This section will treat some of these disorders, such as water and electrolyte balance, acid-base balance, dehydration, and shock.

Water Balance

The importance of water has already been discussed in Chapter 1. Water comprises about 50% of the weight of the body, is present in the vessels (in the form of plasma), in the interstitial space, and in the cells. These may be regarded as 3 compartments, among which a continual exchange of fluid is taking place. Water lost from one compartment can be supplied from another compartment. Thus plasma that is lost may be replaced by fluid from the interstitial compartment. There is 12

Table 4–1. Body Water Distribution in an "Average" Normal Young Man

SOURCE	ml/kg of BODY WEIGHT	% OF TOTAL BODY WATER
Plasma	45	7.5
Interstitial lymph	120	20.0
Dense connective tissue and cartilage	45	7.5
Inaccessible bone water	45	7.5
Transcellular	15	2.5
Total extracellular	270	45.0
Total body water (D_2O)	600	100.0
Total intracellular	330	55.0

(From Perez-Tamayo, R.: *Mechanisms of Disease,* Philadelphia and London, W. B. Saunders, 1961.)

times as much water in the cells as in the blood, and 4 times as much in the interstitial space (Table 4–1). Water balance is the remarkably constant balance between the fluid in the vessels and the fluid in the tissues, both cellular and interstitial. It is in the cells themselves that the correct content of water is so important. The balance will be influenced by both the intake and the output of water. Water balance, for the most part, is regulated by water loss, which averages about 2,500 ml a day in the adult, and proportionately more in children, whose surface area is large in proportion to their weight. The loss takes place by 4 routes: (1) from the intestine, (2) from the lungs in expired air, (3) from the skin, and (4) from the kidneys. The kidneys are mainly responsible for removing excess fluid in health, although the large amount that may be lost in severe and continued diarrhea or in the profuse sweating brought about by natural or artificial heat is obvious. The renal glomeruli excrete water and sodium chloride, but these are reabsorbed by the renal tubules in quantities necessary to maintain the correct balance. The entire mechanism, called **homeostasis,** maintains the constancy of the internal environment.

It is this mechanism that serves to maintain the constancy of the acid-base balance, the osmotic pressure, the concentration of the different solutes or of ions, the blood sugar no matter how much glucose is consumed, the body temperature despite changes in the outside temperature, and the blood volume even after severe hemorrhage or copious intravenous fluid infusion. It is on the internal environment that the multiplicity of laboratory tests are now performed to determine the state of health of a person.

Electrolyte Balance

Some substances in body fluids are present in the form of salts, such as sodium chloride or calcium phosphate, which are **electrolytes**; that is when placed in water, they become dissociated into electrically charged particles called **ions.** This dissociation was first observed 150 years ago when an electric current was passed through a solution of inorganic compounds with the result that some elements passed to the negative pole and the adjacent fluid became alkaline, whereas others went to the positive pole and the fluid became acid. Ion is derived from the Greek word meaning to pass or go. The ions may be positively charged **cations,** so-called because they collect at the negative or cathode pole, the more important being sodium (Na^+), potassium (K^+), and calcium (Ca^{++}). The negatively charged ions are **anions,** which pass to the positive pole or anode, the chief being chlorine (Cl^-), carbonates, and phosphates. Substances are not electrolytes unless they become dissociated into charged particles. All the sodium and potassium and much of the calcium of the body are ionized. Cations include all the metals and hydrogen. Anions include the nonmetals, the acid radicals, and the hydroxyl (OH^-) ion. The ions of the electrolytes with their positive and negative charges and their consequent chemical combining power determine the constancy of the acid-base balance.

Electrolytes exert an important effect on the amount of water in the various compartments because of the osmotic pressure that they produce. (Osmosis is the passage of a fluid through a semipermeable membrane to that side that has the higher concentration of molecules.) A semipermeable membrane offers no obstacle to the passage of electrolytes, but does not permit the passage of large molecules, e.g., those of proteins such as albumin, prothrombin, fibrinogen, and globulins. The salt content in the cellular compartment is different from that in the interstitial and vascular compartments.

The normal figures for the principal electrolytes in the plasma, which vary within narrow limits, are given below, together with round or average figures, which are easier to remember:

Sodium	135 to 155 mEq/L	(150)
Chloride	97 to 105 mEq/L	(100)
Potassium	3.6 to 5.0 mEq/L	(4)
Bicarbonate	25 to 32 mEq/L	(30)

The equivalent weight of an electrolyte is the weight in grams that combines with or displaces 1 gram of hydrogen. Because the concentrations of electrolytes in body fluids are so low, we express them as milliequivalents per liter (mEq/L). This is in place of milligrams per 100 ml, as has been used in the past, and which must still be used for nonelectrolytes that cannot be dissociated into ions. The use of milliequivalents facilitates the expressions of the total amounts of cations and anions in body fluids. Thus plasma contains about 155 mEq/L of cations and an equal number of anions.

The electrolytes present may determine the amount of body fluid. Their relative proportions determine the reaction of that fluid and influence the action of nerve on muscle. The total electrolyte concentration is essentially the same in all 3 phases of body fluid, but the relative amounts of the different electrolytes vary widely. In the extracellular fluid (plasma and interstitial fluid), the important ions are **sodium, chloride,** and **bicarbonate,** of which sodium is the principal basic ion (cation), and chloride and bicarbonate are the chief acidic ions (anions). In the intracellular fluid, **potassium** is the chief cation and **organic phosphate** the corresponding anion.

Acid-Base Balance

In addition to changes in the volume of the fluids in the various compartments, we must consider changes in the ionic equilibrium that affect the reaction of the acid-base balance of the fluid. The **concentration of hydrogen ions** in the body fluids indicates their reaction, and this is expressed as the **negative** logarithm of this concentration. In practice this is abbreviated as pH. Thus 10^{-7} becomes pH 7.0, which is the hydrogen ion concentration of pure water, representing electroneutrality, and is taken as the reference point for expressing the ionic concentration of other solutions. The pH of normal serum is 7.4, and the normal limits of variation are narrow, between 7.35 and 7.45. An increased concentration of hydrogen ions, or a shift of pH toward 7, indicates acidosis, whereas a decreased concentration, toward 7.5, signifies alkalosis.

It is of extreme importance that the H^+ ion concentration be maintained within normal limits. The **regulation of the acid-base balance** depends on 3 principal factors: (1) buffer systems; (2) excretion of acid or alkali by the kidneys; (3) excretion of carbon dioxide by the lungs.

Buffer Systems. Body fluids contain substances known as buffers, which "soak-up" excess acid or alkali and thus minimize changes in hydrogen ion concentration. They convert strong acids and bases into weaker ones, so that the narrow limits of hydrogen ion concentration are not transgressed. Hydrochloric acid is a "strong" acid because in solution it is highly ionized, and as a result nearly all its hydrogen is present in the ionized form, whereas carbonic acid is a "weak" acid, because only a small number of dissociated ions are in solution. The chief buffers of the blood are carbonic acid (H_2CO_3), its bicarbonate salt ($NaHCO_3$), and hemoglobin, which is weakly acidic. **Sodium bicarbonate buffers strong acids, whereas carbonic acid buffers strong bases such as sodium hydroxide, converting it into sodium bicarbonate and water,** with only a few OH^- ions. Both plasma proteins and hemoglobin are buffer systems. Hemoglobin is the buffer for carbonic acid derived from carbon dioxide and changed into carbonate in the red cells as part of the mechanism of respiration.

Respiratory Control of pH. The respiratory center in the brain is extremely sensitive to changes in the H^+ concentration of the plasma. The amount of sodium bicarbonate present in the extracellular fluid available for the neutralization of acids stronger than carbonic acid is known as the **alkali reserve.** It is a measure of the degree of disturbance of the acid-base balance. The plasma bicarbonate is expressed as the **carbon dioxide combining power. The simplest measurement for the demonstration of acidosis or alkalosis is the estimation of this combining power,** which is done by a gas analysis test. The quantity of carbon dioxide normally present as bicarbonate is 55 to 75 volumes per cent. In moderate acidosis the carbon dioxide combining power is less than 40 volumes; in alkalosis it is above 80 volumes. As bicarbonate is continually being formed by tissue metabolism and as carbonic acid is readily eliminated as carbon dioxide, it is easy to appreciate the paramount importance of respiration in conjunction with bicarbonate in maintaining the acid-base balance.

Renal Control. **Although carbonic acid is regulated by respiration, all the other electrolyte components of the plasma structure are under the control of the kidneys.** There is a constant production of acid products such as sulfuric and phosphoric acids from protein metabolism, lactic acid from muscle activity, and ketone acids in high-fat diet when the carbohydrates are low. These acids must be eliminated without a loss of base, so that the alkali reserve will not be depleted. Urea is formed from the blood by the cells of the renal tubules; ammonia is formed in turn from the urea; and the ammonia thus formed combines with the acid phosphate and sulfate radicals to be excreted in the urine. Another renal device for conserving fixed base is the ability of the kidney to separate sodium from fixed acid salts in the tubules and return it to the blood, where it combines with bicarbonate while the acid radical is excreted in the urine in the form of free acid.

Acidosis. We have already seen that the alkali reserve of the blood is represented by bicarbonate. Any change in this reserve is reflected in the plasma carbon dioxide level. The buffer system $\dfrac{H_2CO_3}{NaHCO_3}$ has a normal ratio of 1/20. Four things may happen to upset this ratio. Acid may be increased if the numerator, carbonic acid, is increased, or if the denominator, sodium bicarbonate, is decreased; the reverse is true of alkali. A primary alkali deficit with resulting acidosis is the most important disturbance of the acid-base balance. The mechanism for the change may be metabolic or respiratory.

METABOLIC ACIDOSIS. This condition develops whenever the available alkali is diminished. Such a state of affairs may arrive in 1 of 3 ways: (1) An **excess of acid ions** may develop as the result of disease that uses up the bicarbonate. This may occur in diabetic acidosis or in the ketosis of starvation. (2) An **inadequate excretion of acids** due to renal failure. This is retention acidosis. (3) **Loss of sodium bicarbonate,** as in chronic diarrhea, the secretions of the bowel being alkaline. The ratio of carbonic acid to carbonate may fall from a normal of 1/20 to 1/10, with a fall in pH to as low as 7.1.

RESPIRATORY ACIDOSIS. When there is interference with the exchange of gases in the pulmonary alveoli, an insufficient amount of carbon dioxide is blown off. The retention of carbon dioxide leads to an increased carbonic acid concentration in the blood and acidosis. The carbonic acid-bicarbonate ratio may be only 1/15. The exchange of gases may be depressed by advanced chronic pulmonary disease such as fibrosis or emphysema, or by impairment of the respiratory muscles.

Alkalosis. It is only natural that alkalosis is not nearly so common as acidosis, nor does it have the same clinical significance. Again it may be metabolic or respiratory in character.

METABOLIC ALKALOSIS. Here there is a primary bicarbonate excess. Occasionally this is due to an increased intake of alkalis, as in overdone sodium bicarbonate therapy for duodenal ulcer. Much more important is the loss of fixed acids, as in the depletion of free hydrochloric acid in the vomiting of duodenal ulcer. When chloride is lost, its place is taken by bicarbonate.

RESPIRATORY ALKALOSIS. This is the result of a primary carbon dioxide deficit. The usual cause is the deep and rapid breathing that may accompany hysteria or fear. It may also result from the anoxia of heart disease or of high altitudes. The increased ventilation blows off such large volumes of carbon dioxide that the concentration of carbonic acid in the blood falls in relation to the bicarbonate, so that

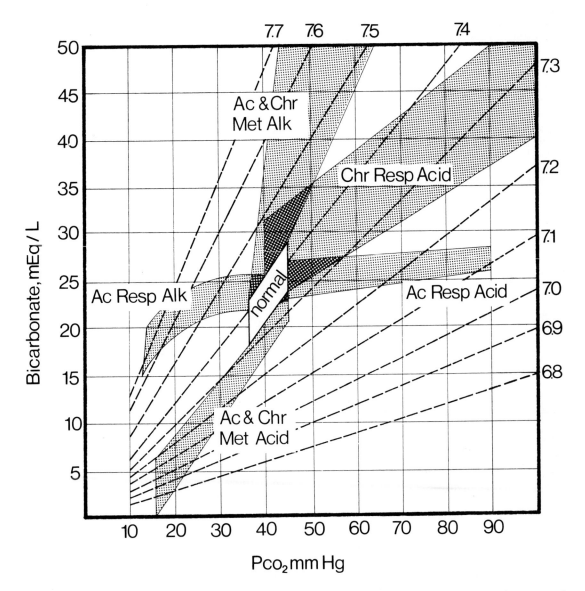

Fig. 4–26. This nomogram illustrates the range of normal pH, bicarbonate, and P_{CO_2}, and demonstrates the mean ± 2 standard deviations for the compensatory response of patients. (From Arbus, G.S.: An *in vivo* acid-base nomogram for clinical use. Can. Med. Assoc. J., *109*:291, 1973.)

a relative alkalosis results. If the pH is above 7.6, the spasmodic attacks known as **tetany** may occur, owing to increased neuromuscular irritability. These relations are all demonstrated in Figure 4–26.

Dehydration

Under normal conditions more water is taken in than is needed, and the excess excreted in the urine by the kidneys. If the **intake is insufficient,** the output due to evaporation from the skin and the lungs and the excretion in urine and feces results in a negative water balance and a state of **dehydration**. The same result is produced by **excessive loss** of water through the skin, lungs, kidneys, or gastrointestinal tract. A patient suffering from Asiatic cholera may become completely dehydrated in the space of 24 hours. Death occurs when the loss reaches 15% of the body weight. As this percentage is reached twice as quickly in an infant as in an adult, it is evident that the water in the tissues will be exhausted at twice the rate of those of an adult, and that the infant will die in half the time. **Dehydration is therefore a much more acute problem in infants and young children than in adults.**

From what has been said it is obvious that fluid balance depends not only on water but also on salt. If both water and salt are lost, as in vomiting and diarrhea, or even in profuse and continued sweating, such as occurs in the tropics or in persons working at blast furnaces, salt must be replenished as well as water. One of the hormones of the adrenal cortex, aldosterone, controls the excretion of sodium chloride by the kidneys. If this hormone is insufficient, excessive salt is lost in the urine, the salt content of the plasma falls, water is not retained in the tissues, and dehydration results. This is seen to a marked degree in Addison's disease, which is due to destruction of the adrenal cortex.

Decrease of body water from whatever cause is naturally first seen in the intravascular compartment, with a reduction in blood volume, carrying with it the possibility of shock. The regulating mechanism at once comes into play, withdrawing fluid from the interstitial compartment, and finally the intracellular fluid. This is significant, for cellular dehydration creates thirst that may become so intense as to be unendurable, and it interferes with cellular enzymes to a degree that may be fatal.

Disturbance in the water (and salt) balance may occur in a number of diseases, some of which will be discussed in this book. Examples are shock, acute intestinal obstruction, renal failure, and Addison's disease.

Shock

Shock may be defined as the **condition arising from a reduction in tissue perfusion.** When prolonged, it not only leads to interference with cellular function, but also may lead to death. The person in shock experiences many physiologic derangements, extremely disturbing and anxiety-producing. A few summers ago, while tending honey bees, I (Huntington Sheldon) had become sensitized to bee serum and was sufficiently stung to develop an acute anaphylactic reaction (see Chap. 6), which is usually accompanied by shock. The sweating, tachycardia, weakness, dizziness, and transient cerebral ischemia when my blood pressure fell to 80/40 was an awesome experience.

Without knowing the state of the circulation, the systolic or diastolic pressures, or the central venous pressure, it takes only one experience to recognize the outward signs of shock in a person. He or she looks pale and apprehensive, and beads of perspiration stand out on the skin. The patient in shock may either lie still or be restless. His responses to questions are abbreviated, as he conserves whatever energy remains. The skin, hands, and feet are blue and cool to the touch in the most common types of shock, and the pulse rate is increased over normal.

Shock is not a disease: it is a physiologic state that changes rapidly as the underlying cause and homeostatic reactions to it progress. It is important to emphasize here that although we may be able to recognize different types of shock, and in doing so to treat them differently, we do not completely understand the process. For example, in the past 25 years, we have gone from treating shock with vasopressor agents to increase the peripheral resistance, to using vasodilators to decrease the peripheral resistance and therefore the work of the heart in one particular type of shock.

For the purposes of this chapter, we can discuss 4 general causes of shock.

(1) Shock caused by a **loss of blood volume** (e.g., hemorrhage). This is called hypovolemic shock and is the type most commonly associated with traumatic injuries and obvious blood loss, or blood loss into some portion of a body cavity.

(2) Shock caused by **failure of the heart** to pump blood through the circulation (e.g., myocardial infarct). This is probably the most common cause of shock in the North Ameri-

can population, and we refer to it as cardiogenic shock.

(3) Shock caused by **vasodilatation,** in which the arteriolar bed and capillary branches fail to maintain their normal diameter or become leaky and allow blood to pool in the tissues of the body. This may occur in anaphylactic (severe allergic) shock, in which the various mechanisms result in a decreased venous return to the heart, or can be caused by specific interference with vasomotor nerves or by substantial tissue injury. In a few instances, a person who has received what appears to be superficial trauma may die with shock, and the cause may never become apparent anatomically. This type of shock is referred to as neurogenic or vasomotor shock.

(4) Shock that occurs in patients with severe infections, particularly those caused by gram-negative bacteria such as *E. coli,* is known as **septic shock**. The mechanisms that have been used to explain the cause of this shock include the production of a toxin by the organism, and also the overwhelming insult to the body by the presence of millions of bacteria.

The importance of these different general causes is that, if one mistakenly treats the shock caused by myocardial infarct with transfusion because the shock is thought to be caused by some hidden hemorrhage, the patient will not fare as well as if the correct diagnosis of the cause of the shock had been made. Treatment that increases cardiac output is in vain when the patient has an overwhelming bacterial sepsis. We shall now discuss some of the mechanisms whereby shock causes injury to the patient that may be reversed, or that may become irreversible and result in death.

First let us consider the final common path that makes shock such a life-threatening condition. Without regard for the initiating event (myocardial infarct, hemorrhage, anaphylaxis) the result of the reduction in tissue perfusion at the cellular level is the interference with the normal aerobic metabolism of all tissues. This cellular hypoxia is reversible for some time, as we have discussed in Chapter 1. However, an inevitable result is the increased production of lactate as the tissues attempt to survive without adequate oxygen and shift

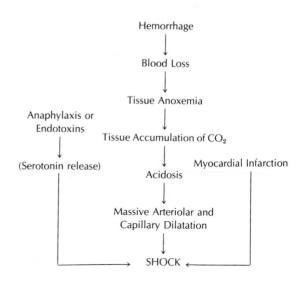

Fig. 4–27. This diagram shows the steps in the development of shock and illustrates the interrelationship of a variety of causes at the tissue level.

into anaerobic metabolic pathways. The increasing leakiness of all cells and the production of lactate progressively moves the pH of the blood away from the normal of 7.4 toward a more and more acidotic range. Metabolic acidosis itself compounds the injury to cells, and at some stage an irreversible phase is entered whereby the cells can no longer produce energy by any mechanism. For example, dogs that are bled and then retransfused within 2 hours have a 10% mortality rate, whereas those that are not retransfused until 4 hours later have only a 10% survival rate.

It is not difficult to understand that if there is a transient, sudden loss of blood pressure, the body in its wisdom perceives that something is wrong and takes immediate steps to restore the circulatory pressures to normal. Sometimes we experience this when we get up from a chair and feel dizzy, or "black out," which is due to the failure to keep the circulation to the brain at a normal pressure because there has been a pooling of blood in the lower limbs. When faced with a blackout, the heart may immediately beat more rapidly (increased cardiac output restores the cerebral circulation). Almost as quickly, there is a narrowing of the arterioles in the systemic circulatory bed, which increases peripheral resistance. A concomitant increase in the venous end of the microcirculation increases venous return of blood, which in turn allows the heart to fill more effectively, and thereby increases cardiac output. Some of these effects are mediated by reflex arcs; the baroreceptors in the carotid arteries inform the brain that the blood pressure is too low, and as a result the brain sends signals to the vagus nerve, which regulates the heart rate. Similar effects are mediated by chemical messengers or hormones; shock signals the adrenal medulla to release epinephrine and norepinephrine, which have a direct effect on the heart and the arteriolar bed.

Some responses to shock, such as the shift in major circulatory pathways, shunting blood from the gastrointestinal tract or peripheral musculature to the brain and heart, may take longer, and it is much longer still before major readjustments in the distribution of fluids between the vascular bed and the interstitial or cellular spaces become evident. A fall in hematocrit (see Chap. 23) that indicates major blood loss may not be evident for an hour or more, just as the readjustment to a minor loss of blood, as when one donates a pint for the Red Cross, may be delayed and not revealed in the hematocrit for several hours. When the kidneys are not perfused, whether because of a low cardiac output or because of pooling elsewhere, urine will not be made normally. This decrease in the amount of urine produced may not become apparent for several hours. Shock therefore is a complex, physiologic phenomenon.

Newer methods of diagnosing shock and of distinguishing between possible etiologies of shock have made the management of it simpler in some ways and more complex in others. We have talked about increased heart rate (pulse) and have indicated that it reflects a compensatory effort to increase the cardiac output. Blood pressure, shown in the accompanying diagram (Fig. 4–28), is many things; we conventionally speak of the pressure taken in the brachial artery as blood pressure, but changes in the venous pressure and in pressures in the pulmonary circulation are also important reflections of the state of the circulation and of its principal pump, the heart.

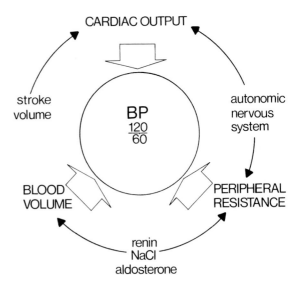

Fig. 4–28. This figure shows the major factors which affect the blood pressure.

Having established the nature of the peripheral arterial pressure, and determined that it is low, for the surgical patient, where the diagnosis is an issue and the prognosis of the patient is grave, it is relevant to obtain additional pressure measurements by the use of direct catheterizations. The **central venous pressure** (pressure in the superior vena cava) normally is 5 to 10 cm of water or less than 2 mm of mercury. Any change in this pressure must be explained. If the heart is failing, the central venous pressure will be raised. This is a direct reflection of failure of the right heart, which is one step removed from the left ventricle. If there is volume overload, the increased central venous pressure can be caused by excess intravenous therapy. Changes in the central venous pressure occur during therapeutic intervention with drugs and transfusions. Such changes serve to confirm the appropriateness of the diagnosis and therapy. However, these assessments reflect only indirectly the functions of the left heart, as we have stated, because the pulmonary circulation and right heart pressure are being read indirectly.

A more modern attempt to assess directly the function of the left ventricle is to insert a catheter into a branch of the pulmonary artery. This catheter, with a balloon at the tip, is inflated when it is in a branch of the pulmonary artery, and the measurements derived are called the pulmonary wedge pressure. This catheter is now much closer to the left ventricle and atrial pressures and is named after its inventors, Drs. Swan and Ganz. The pressures thus recorded reflect the left atrial pressure just as the central venous pressure reflects the right atrial pressure. Naturally, these invasive procedures have potential and real hazards: the catheter can introduce infections, precipitate thrombus formation and emboli, and may obstruct the blood vessels in which it is placed. Catheters may also cause reflex cardiac arrest or arrhythmia. Therefore they are used only when the data is important for the management of the patient's shock.

A final way to determine the extent, prognosis, and severity of shock is to measure blood gases. The PO_2, PCO_2, and blood pH all directly reflect the capacity of the circulation to maintain life. A progressive decrease in the PO_2 indicates that somewhere there is inadequate oxygenation, which may be due to respiratory disease at the outset, but which

may also reflect inadequate perfusion of the lung. A progressive rise in the PCO_2 again may be caused by inadequate ventilatory mechanisms. However, it may also be due to an inappropriate circulation through the lungs. A fall in the blood pH may be the result of the accumulation of retained acid products as in chronic renal failure, but such a fall in pH may rapidly occur when anaerobic metabolic events cause many tissues of the body to accumulate lactate. Thus changes in the PO_2, PCO_2, and arterial pH and a rise in blood lactate are all indicators of the shock syndrome.

We have come to recognize both the anatomic and the physiologic effects of reversible shock, in that specific organs such as the lungs and kidney may have impaired function for days and weeks in the patient who has survived the acute and critical episode. Therefore we talk about shock lung and shock kidney. Fortunate, indeed, is the patient who eventually recovers, because he has teetered on the edge of the precipice over which so many acutely ill patients have fallen.

SYNOPSIS

Edema may be caused by increased capillary permeability, decreased plasma proteins, or increased hydrostatic pressure in veins or lymphatics.

Thrombosis may be caused by stasis of the circulation, by injury to the endothelial lining of the vessel, or by changes in the character of the blood itself.

Emboli may arise anywhere in the circulation (heart, veins, arteries) and usually travel to where the vessel size limits their progress. Emboli may result in infarction or sudden death (pulmonary emboli), or may be asymptomatic.

Thrombosis and embolism may both cause and result from infarction.

Hypertension is of multifactorial etiology. There are known (renal, adrenal, coarctation of aorta) and unknown (essential) causes of hypertension.

Shock, a significant reduction in tissue perfusion, may be caused by blood loss, heart failure, or loss of peripheral resistance.

Terms

Anasarca	Exudate	Embolus
Edema	Hematoma	Infarction
Hemorrhage	Petechiae	Hypertension
Ascites	Aneurysm	Metabolic acidosis/alkalosis
Effusion	Fibrinolysis	Respiratory acidosis/alkalosis
Transudate	Thrombosis	Shock

FURTHER READING

Clagett, G.P., and Salzman, E.W.: Prevention of venous thromboembolism in surgical patients. N. Engl. J. Med., 290:93, 1974.

Clowes, G.H.A., Jr., and O'Donnell, T.F., Jr.: Heat stroke. N. Engl. J. Med., 291:564, 1974.

Dalen, J.E., and Alpert, J.S.: Natural history of pulmonary embolus. Prog. Cardiovasc. Dis., 27:259, 1975.

Deykin, D.: Emerging concepts of platelet function. N. Engl. J. Med., 290:144, 1974.

Gamble, J.L.: *Chemical Anatomy, Physiology and Pathology of Extracellular Fluid*, 6th Ed. Cambridge, Harvard University Press, 1954.

Goldstein, J.L., and Brown, M.S.: The LDL receptor locus and the genetics of familial hypercholesterolemia. Annu. Rev. Genet., 13:259, 1979.

LeQuesne, L.P.: Relation between deep vein thrombosis and pulmonary embolism in surgical patients. N. Engl. J. Med., 291:1292, 1974.

Light, R.W., et al.: Pleural effusions: the diagnostic separation of transudates and exudates. Ann. Intern. Med., 77:507, 1972.

Loeb, J.N.: The hyperosmolar state. N. Engl. J. Med., 290:1184, 1974.

Man, S.O., and Carroll, H.J.: The anion gap. N. Engl. J. Med., 297:814, 1977.

Massie, R.: *Nicolas and Alexandra*. New York, Atheneum, 1967.

Moore, F.D., et al.: *The Body Cell Mass and Its Supporting Environment*. Philadelphia, W. B. Saunders, 1963.

Parving, H.H., et al.: Mechanisms of edema formation in myxedema. N. Engl. J. Med., 301:460, 1979.

Relman, A.S.: Lactic acidosis and a possible new treatment. N. Engl. J. Med., 298:564, 1978.

Thompson, J.E.: Acute peripheral arterial occlusions. N. Engl. J. Med., 290:950, 1974.

Tremper, K.K.: Oncotic pressure and wedge pressure. N. Engl. J. Med., 297:616, 1977.

Inflammation and Repair

5

In science the credit goes to the man who convinces the world, not to the man to whom the idea first occurred—OSLER

INFLAMMATION

The reaction of living tissue to injury is called inflammation. It is a tapestry, woven of cells and their products, enzymes, soluble factors, of blood vessels and their contents; its texture and appearance changes with time. It is best viewed as a process that starts with an injury and that ends with what we call healing. Yet the boundaries between injury and inflammation, and between inflammation and healing, are indistinct. The process depends on a number of factors, including general features of the host, such as nutrition and age, and specific local and tissue factors, such as the blood supply and the presence of foreign bodies or bacteria in the injured area. The type of injury itself, whether a burn, an ischemic injury, or a surgical wound, and its size often determine the nature of the reactions that are collectively called inflammation. Inflammation has many different aspects; it can be recognized by the presence of redness, swelling, pain, heat, and a loss of function. These aspects of inflammation were recognized more than 2,000 years ago and were known in the ancient world by the Latin terms *rubor, tumor, dolor, calor,* and *functio laesa.*

An important concept is that inflammation is a defense reaction whose purpose is to protect the host. Having said that, it is important to recognize that this defense reaction also has some disadvantages. The ways in which we have come to understand inflammation have been from observations in man after injury and in disease states, and from studies on experimentally-induced inflammation, as in the capillary network of frogs and rabbits.

Inflammation, whatever its cause, is called by the suffix *itis* (as in appendicitis or cholecystitis, which mean, respectively, inflammation of the appendix and of the gallbladder). Inflammation is important in that its symptoms and signs such as pain, swelling, and fever, lead the person to inquire about its cause. Moreover, the cause of inflammation is not decided simply by describing its existence. The causes of inflammation in any organ may include obstruction, infection, injury, and a compromised vascular supply, as well as physical and chemical injury (Fig. 5–1). Biologic agents such as bacteria are often the inciting agent, but frostbite or sunburn may also initiate such inflammatory responses as heat and pain. Attempts to understand the general and specific reactions

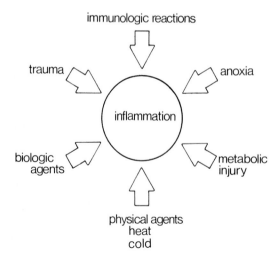

Fig. 5–1. This diagram illustrates some of the multiple causes of inflammation. Naturally, in many instances, more than one factor may be responsible for the inflammatory response.

to injury in living tissue have been made more difficult by the imperceptible transition from acute reaction, through more vigorous and obvious responses, to the melting away of the angry signs and the restoration of the tissue to normal, or healing. The lines between injury, inflammation, and healing are arbitrary at best, and should be considered only as a way of explaining what little we know of this complex process.

Before considering inflammation in more detail, it is useful to outline a classification of inflammation so that our descriptions and interpretations may be kept in perspective. Inflammation may occur in any tissue or in any organ, as we have already said, but there may be differences in the changes that take place in different tissues.

First, there are acute, limited areas of redness and painful swelling, which may disappear in a day or 2 at most. Because of its short duration, and because of the histology of the tissue and cellular responses, we call this response **acute inflammation.** Examples are insect bites, small abrasions or cuts, mild burns, or other injuries that are generally considered to be minor.

The prerequisite for inflammation is that it must happen in a living tissue. Where the nervous innervation has been changed, or where the blood supply curtailed, for

example by atherosclerosis, the traditional responses to injury may be lacking. It is also true that in the elderly, the very young, or the very sick, the normal inflammatory responses may not occur. Finally, in many cases where a patient is taking drugs that suppress the inflammatory response (steroids, aspirin), the usual signs may not occur.

One outcome of the host's reaction to minor injuries may be the continued evolution of this response, so that it lasts for many days or weeks and may spread to involve adjacent or distant tissues. The response may persist because of continued or repeated insults, and it may be considered **chronic** because of the length of its duration. It also may be considered chronic if one examines the tissue microscopically and finds a pattern of tissue and cell response that differs from the acute response. Acute inflammations characteristically show large numbers of polymorphonuclear leukocytes, whereas chronic inflammations consist of lymphocytes, monocytes, and plasma cells, collectively called "round cells" (Fig. 5–2).

There is a third type of inflammation that can be separated from the typical acute and chronic types; this is designated **granulomatous** inflammation. Granulomatous inflammation is a subset of chronic inflammation and is distinguished from simple chronic inflammatory responses by the broader range of

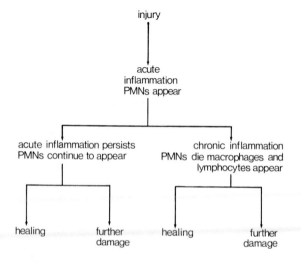

Fig. 5–2. This scheme outlines the alternative responses to injury in terms of acute inflammation on the left, and of chronic inflammation on the right.

cell types found in tissues. These include epithelioid cells, as well as mature monocytes, macrophages, and giant cells.

Having attempted to distinguish these 3 types of inflammation, let us consider a typical injury and discuss the sequence of responses in a normal adult human being.

Injury by bacteria is the commonest cause of inflammation. Everyone has had a boil or an abscess. The bacterium (a staphylococcus, for example), a normal contaminant of the skin, gains access to the host when the primary line of defense, the epithelium of the skin, has been breached by a splinter, a cut, or a wound. This bacterium is now able to cause local injury by the production of toxins and enzymes that may have a lethal effect on the cells of the host in the immediate vicinity of the bacterium. Cells of the host release, in their dying stages, proteins, enzymes, and peptides, many of which have general and specific designations, and have been shown to affect directly the neighboring tissues' components, such as the capillaries, venules, and arterioles. Bacteria that are able to multiply rapidly may increase the circle of injury and may recruit more of the host's tissue into the zone of destruction.

Capillaries in the tissue that surrounds the injured area become permeable to large and small molecules and to white blood cells that would normally stay within the circulation. These changes in the microcirculation, which can be seen with the light microscope, are responsible for the increasing redness of the inflamed area. The permeability of the capillaries allows fluid to accumulate in the injured area and causes the swelling that is so typical of all inflamed tissues.

The sequence of tissue response to injury is shown in Table 5–1. This sequence may also be outlined thus: The liberation of low-molecular-weight substances (vasoactive peptides, histamine, lymphokines) from injured tissue stimulates local nerve endings. The process causes pain and elicits a brief phase of vasoconstriction and blanching in the injured area. This axon reflex was described more than 50 years ago. Following the transient vasoconstriction, the blood vessels become dilated and blood flow slows in the injured area.

Stasis within the microcirculation has many results. Red blood cells clump together and the channels widen as more and more erythrocytes move sluggishly through this inflamed area. One reason for the apparent increase in the number of red blood cells is that the capillaries are no longer normally intact, but rather lose both high- and low-molecular-weight substances into the interstitial tissue. This permeability sets in motion the disequilibrium of Starling's forces, so that fluid is no longer returned at the venous end of the capillary circulation (Fig. 5–3). Naturally, this disequilibrium contributes to the turnover of the inflamed tissue.

Injury to the endothelial walls of the microcirculation renders the surface of the capillary cell sticky, which enables white blood cells that normally flow past to attach themselves to the wall. In an inflamed area, whole segments of capillaries may soon be covered by white blood cells, much as barnacles attach

Table 5–1. Bodily Changes in First Phase of Metabolic Response to Injury

CIRCULATORY	METABOLIC	BLOOD
Tachycardia	Hepatic glycogenolysis	Increase in platelets and fibrinogen
Increase in cardiac output	Hyperglycemia	Decrease in prothrombin time
Generalized vasoconstriction	Increase in O_2 consumption	Accelerated coagulation
Splenic contraction	Decrease in adrenal cholesterol and vitamin C	Leukocytosis
Hypertension	Increase in urinary corticoids	Accelerated sedimentation rate and rouleaux formation
		Hypoferremia
		Fibrinolysis
		Eosinopenia

(From Perez-Tamayo, R.: *Mechanisms of Disease.* Philadelphia and London, W. B. Saunders, 1961.)

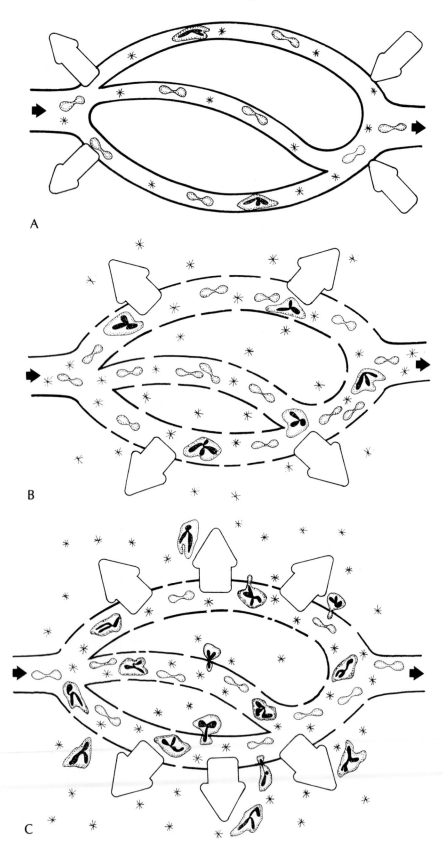

A

B

C

themselves to old pilings. This phenomenon is called pavementing and is regarded as an early stage in the sequence of the cellular phase of inflammation. These white blood cells also respond to the presence in neighboring tissues of foreign bacteria or antibody-antigen complexes.

The direct migration of the inflammatory cells toward an injured area is called **chemotaxis** (Fig. 5–4). This phenomenon has great value as a second line of defense in infections. The polymorphonuclear leukocytes are active, motile cells that contain large amounts of enzymes that are capable of degrading biologic materials, as well as of isolating them, and of removing the noxious effects of these materials from the host. We now know that there are congenital disorders of the polymorphonuclear leukocytes themselves, of their structure, of their complement of enzymes, and of their motility, and that many agents can interfere with their normal response to such chemotactic agents as the presence of complement and antigen/antibody macromolecular complexes. Nearly 100 years ago, Dr. Almoth Wright, in London, used early knowledge of phagocytosis in his attempts to treat infectious disease; he is caricatured by George Bernard Shaw in *The Doctor's Dilemma* as Sir Colenso Rigeon, whose battle cry is "Stimulate the phagocyte" as the panacea for all illness.

Accumulating evidence suggests that the importance of the polymorphonuclear leukocyte as a line of defense cannot be underestimated. There are many ways in which a loss of this phagocytic capability renders the host susceptible to acute and chronic illness. These ways are outlined in Table 5–2. When the white blood cell count falls below 2000 per cubic milliliter, patients are often put on protective isolation, and when the count falls

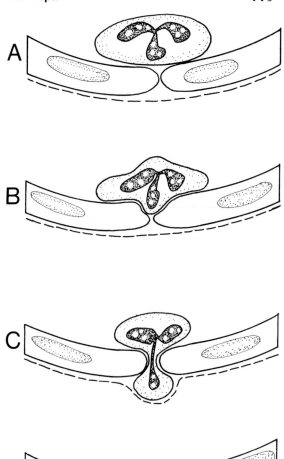

Fig. 5–4. *A, B, C,* and *D,* This diagram shows one mechanism whereby white blood cells may leave the microcirculation, crawling through or between the endothelial cells of the capillary. This process is known as diapedesis, and it occurs under the influence of chemotactic signals. (From Marchesi, V.T., and Gowans, J.L.: The migration of lymphocytes through the endothelium of venules in lymph nodes: an electron microscope study. Proc. R. Soc. Lond. [Biol.], *159*:283, 1964.)

←

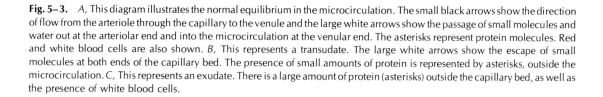

Fig. 5–3. *A,* This diagram illustrates the normal equilibrium in the microcirculation. The small black arrows show the direction of flow from the arteriole through the capillary to the venule and the large white arrows show the passage of small molecules and water out at the arteriolar end and into the microcirculation at the venular end. The asterisks represent protein molecules. Red and white blood cells are also shown. *B,* This represents a transudate. The large white arrows show the escape of small molecules at both ends of the capillary bed. The presence of small amounts of protein is represented by asterisks, outside the microcirculation. *C,* This represents an exudate. There is a large amount of protein (asterisks) outside the capillary bed, as well as the presence of white blood cells.

Table 5–2. Some Factors that Influence Phagocytosis

FACTORS FAVORING PHAGOCYTOSIS	FACTORS INHIBITING PHAGOCYTOSIS
Temperature (37° to 40°C)	Temperature (>40°C)
Mild ionizing radiation	Intense ionizing radiation
Opsonization	Capsular factors
Nervous stimuli	Leukemia
Hormones (ACTH, cortisone)	Acid pH (6.6)
Calcium ions	Gastric mucin
Good nutritional status	
Anemia (experimental)	

(From Perez-Tamayo, R.: *Mechanisms of Disease.* Philadelphia and London, W. B. Saunders, 1961.)

further (below 600), leukocyte transfusions are given.

We might now consider the normal protective barriers before we reconsider their role in inflammation and in healing.

The intact, functioning, mammalian host has a remarkable series of defense mechanisms against injury. They can be considered under several different headings, and, for simplicity's sake, we shall divide them into 3 categories. First, the external, epithelial, and mucosal barriers (skin, respiratory tract, bowel), which protect the *milieu intérieur* (Fig. 5–5). The second level of defense consists of the cellular and humoral apparatus, granulocytes, round cells, the microcirculation, and the "immune system," subject of a chapter of its own. The third category, which we designate as systemic defense mechanisms, includes fever, leukocytosis, and general humoral or adaptive responses to injury of any kind (Fig. 5–6).

Primary Defenses

Particularly in man, the mucosal barriers that protect us from injury have been well developed to provide a continuing, stable, internal environment where our imaginations, artistic sensibilities, and higher cortical centers may flourish. This environment is made possible by special adaptations of the epithelial boundaries that separate us from the external world. Whereas the skin and its specializations, at first glance, might seem as uncomplicated as a plastic poncho, serving only to keep the inner man from being washed away by the tempests of life, every square centimeter of our skin is adapted specially to keep us from drying out and to prevent the normal bacterial flora and fauna from having a free lunch. Specific, definitive adaptations are best seen in the eye, where this transparent area of skin is kept moist by tears,

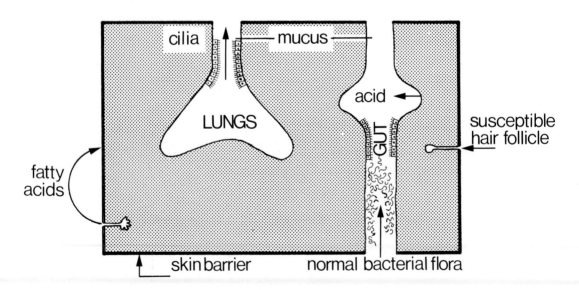

Fig. 5–5. This diagram shows the primary defense mechanisms of the body. The skin is a waterproof barrier covered with fatty acids. The respiratory tract is lined by mucus and cilia, and the gastrointestinal tract contains mucus as well. (From Roitt, I.: *Essential Immunology.* Oxford, Blackwell Scientific Publications, 1977.)

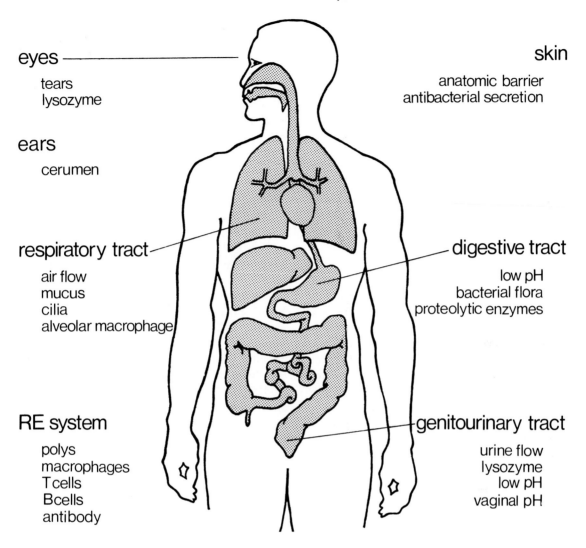

eyes
  tears
  lysozyme

ears
  cerumen

respiratory tract
  air flow
  mucus
  cilia
  alveolar macrophage

RE system
  polys
  macrophages
  T cells
  B cells
  antibody

skin
  anatomic barrier
  antibacterial secretion

digestive tract
  low pH
  bacterial flora
  proteolytic enzymes

genitourinary tract
  urine flow
  lysozyme
  low pH
  vaginal pH

defense mechanisms

Fig. 5–6. This drawing illustrates many adaptations of different parts of the human body that act as defense barriers. The reticuloendothelial (RE) system is distributed throughout the body. The other defense mechanisms are labeled in the figure. (Adapted from Barrett, J.T.: *Basic Immunology and Its Medical Application.* St. Louis, C. V. Mosby, 1976.)

a fluid in which there is significant antibacterial activity (lysozyme). This enzyme has the ability to lyse bacterial colonies in dilute solutions, and maintains a sterile film of transparent cells through which we view the world.

The respiratory tract, which is normally exposed with each breath to millions of potentially injurious agents each day, has the wonderful and effective external surface, mucus, that covers the epithelial cells and that serves as a trap for bacteria and microscopic particles of dust, smog, pollen, and soot, much as a flypaper catches flies. However, unlike the flypaper, which must be changed when it is covered, the mucus blanket is continuously renewed and, better yet, is constantly swept toward the mouth by the ciliated epithelial cells of the airways. This combination of mucus and cilia protects the underlying epithelial barrier from bacteria and the injury they cause. Cigarette smoke, alcohol, and chronic irritation from environmental toxins all interfere with the maintenance of this respiratory barrier. Viruses that infect the respiratory cells and kill the ciliated epithelium destroy the effectiveness of this barrier and permit bacterial overgrowth to occur. In fact, the danger from influenza epidemics in the past has not been from the tracheobronchitis caused by the viral infection, but rather from the superimposed bacterial pneumonias, once this defense mechanism has been destroyed.

The other extension of a mucosal barrier to infection is, of course, the oral cavity and the rest of the digestive tract. This tube is lined by millions of cells that are constantly renewed. Again, the rich mucous barrier throughout its length buffers the billions of bacteria that normally populate our colon. Seldom do these bacteria come into direct contact with the underlying epithelial cells, or penetrate further to cause disease. Peristalsis which is a rhythmic movement of the smooth intestinal muscle, moves the ingested contents sufficiently rapidly to forestall stasis under normal conditions. Only in blind pouches, such as the appendix or colonic diverticuli, do biologic agents linger sufficiently to injure the tissue locally.

Pain

We might say a word here about pain, as it is another component of our defense system, one that is easy to understand in the light of an injury such as a burn, but is nonetheless important to put in perspective because, most frequently, pain is accompanied by inflammation, and vice versa.

In the most general sense, pain is a response to injury. The mechanism by which it is induced is currently the focus of much interest. The subject is larger than we can encompass here, but a simple consideration of pain may draw attention to its relation to inflammation and may suggest some more important aspects of pain as a part of the picture of disease.

First, pain may be caused by direct stimulation of nerve endings, which are in some instances directly designed to respond to inflammation, just as other nerve endings respond to light, odor, or temperature. The skin, an organ in its own right, contains naked nerve endings that signal pain, just as others signal pressure or temperature change. Other organs, such as the gut, do not respond in exactly the same way, and the sensation of pain is perceived in the gastrointestinal tract only when there is stretching, as in overdistension of the stomach, or when the mucosa is removed and free nerve endings are exposed, as in an ulcer. Both ischemia and anoxia, in skeletal and cardiac muscle, signal pain, where traction of an artery may give pain when an arterial puncture is performed. Veins, however, are relatively insensitive, as anyone who has given blood can testify. However, all structures of the body, except perhaps the brain itself, respond to inflammation by signalling pain. The substances credited with this perception are polypeptides and substances of low molecular weight, such as histamine, acetylcholine, 5-hydroxytryptamine, bradykinin, all comprising a class known as mediators. These substances may be secreted by cells that are distributed through all tissues, such as mast cells, or they may be the product of dead or dying cells, or the result of interaction between the injured tissue and serum proteins in inflamed areas. These substances may be activated by a cascade of enzymatic reactions, and they leak, during inflammation, out of the microcirculation. Whatever its origin, pain is often the earliest and one of the most important signs that an injury has occurred.

It is of interest, because of the difficulty in deciding what the true cause of the pain may be, to recognize that pain that appears to come from one place does not necessarily arise in the tissues or organs underlying the apparent location. For example, pain during a myocardial infarction may be felt to radiate down the inner aspect of the left arm. This phenomenon is called referred pain, and several explanations have been offered, none of which is entirely satisfactory. Two existing theories are: (1) pain is referred between parts of the body that share the embryologic derivation and innervation, and (2) it is referred through connections in the spinal cord.

There is a large variation in the perception of pain in different persons. The awareness of pain can be dulled by drugs (morphine). Rage and fear may suppress pain, so that one may not even be aware of an extensive injury. Pain remains one of the commonest and most important signs of disease, and of all the processes in disease states, inflammation is one of the most common.

It is possible to spend many pages characterizing pain of different origins, its onset, duration, and factors that either alleviate or exacerbate it, and to relate these characteristics to different types of disease or organ systems, but that is beyond the scope of this chapter.

Humoral Responses to Injury

It has been known for more than 50 years that after an injury of any kind, there is a sequence of changes in the local vascular bed that have been described as a triple response: a red line that changes to a spreading flush, which is replaced by a pale wheal. The raised area then becomes pale and subsides after a period of up to an hour. Lewis described this change and the accompanying pain. We shall consider these vascular changes in the next section, but we shall first turn to the mediators of these responses that result in an abnormal increase in permeability of the local blood vessels.

Current views separate the substances that have been identified in inflammation; the principal ones are now described.

Histamine. This substance is a naturally occurring, labile, highly active derivative of histidine that probably is liberated from mast cells in all tissues. Mast cells are particularly abundant along the course of capillaries in all tissues. Histamine causes capillary dilatation and may either constrict or dilate arterioles and venules. Its effects on smooth muscle depend on the tissue and the animal species. The circumstantial evidence that supports histamine's importance in inflammation is

the suppression of its effect by the administration of histamine antagonists.

5-Hydroxytryptamine (serotonin). Widespread in tissues of the body, serotonin resides in silver-staining cells in most organs, especially the gut and respiratory system, and at strategic sites in the neck and pelvis. This substance is a powerful permeability factor and may also play other roles in the body, possibly as a transmitter substance both in the diffuse endocrine system and in the central nervous system.

As discussed in the chapter on the brain and in this section, the effects of serotonin are not limited to local effects on the permeability of the microcirculation. Serotonin may be the effector for producing fever; it is a thermogenic (heat-producing) amine in man, whereas norepinephrine is a thermolytic (heat-dissipating) amine in man and primates. In rodents, the role of the substances is reversed, curiously.

Kallikreins. This family of enzymes is able to hydrolyze peptide bonds and to break ester groups. There are kallikreins in saliva, sweat, tears, urine, and the gut, and also in plasma. In plasma, the enzyme circulates as a large molecule that may be activated during early injury, particularly if clotting is involved. The result of activation is the formation of rapidly inactivated fragments that are highly active permeability factors, lasting only for seconds. Bradykinin is a member of this family.

While our attention here is focused on the local effects of such substances, there is considerable evidence that such materials may play a greater role at the organic level. For example, following shock, there is evidence that heart muscle may fail to respond despite supportive measures, and a "depressant factor" has been postulated and sought. These kinins are likely candidates for many unexplained phenomena in the physiology of systemic circulatory failure.

The generic term "kinin" is traditionally applied to small polypeptides that cause vasodilatation, increase capillary permeability, provoke pain, stimulate smooth muscle, and are increased at sites of acute inflammation. The kinins are derived from plasma by the action of kallikrein or by granulocytes. Substances such as cortisone probably interfere with the activation of kinins, and also inhibit the chemotaxis of polymorphonuclear leukocytes. In passing, we know that cortisone, acting as an anti-inflammatory agent, also decreases the synthesis of interferon and inhibits the production of antibody (see Chap. 8).

Prostaglandins. These are newly discovered pharmacologic agents that affect the normal economy of the body in various ways. Their role in inflammation is being uncovered daily. There is abundant evidence that the injection of prostaglandins may mimic the early phases of inflammation and that they affect the microcirculation.

Complement. Another part of the humoral aspect of inflammation is the initiation of the whole complicated sequence of events by the mere presence of antigen and antibody. When a person who has circulating antibody, or antibody attached to his cells, is exposed to antigen, the reaction at the tissue and cellular level is as potentially explosive as the overheating of a nuclear reactor is to a community. The complex of antigen with antibody is accompanied by the consumption of a serum component that has many parts, but is designated generally as *complement*. It has been shown that the presence of antigen-antibody and complement initiates the early stages of the inflammatory response, and, in addition, that these macromolecular aggregates are chemotactic to white blood cells. They are specifically responsible for the evocation of polymorphonuclear leukocytes from the circulation to the site of reaction, just as the sirens of Greek mythology called Ulysses to the rocky shores of the Aegean Sea.

Additional aspects of the role of antibody in inflammation are discussed in the next chapter.

Fibrin. When inflammation occurs, one important molecule that normally circulates in the vascular compartment in a precursor form is able to escape into the interstitial spaces. Fibrinogen, a high-molecular-weight protein synthesized by the liver, is normally inactive and contributes to the intravascular osmotic pressure. When capillary permeability is increased, fibrinogen escapes from the lumen and is converted to fibrin by the inflammatory response. It turns into threads of fibrin that are woven into a mesh or network in the interstitial space. These threads act as a lattice on which polymorphonuclear leukocytes can gain a foothold. Lattice-building facilitates

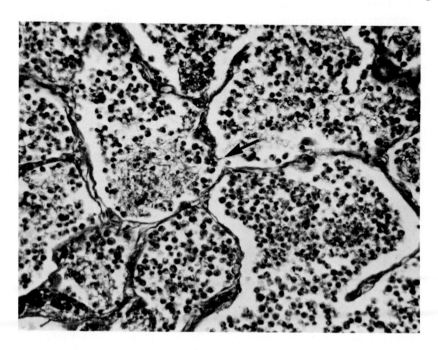

Fig. 5–7. This photomicrograph of the lung in lobar pneumonia shows abundant polymorphonuclear leukocytes, and, at the arrow, fibrin strands passing through the pores of Kohn between 2 alveoli.

the process of phagocytosis, particularly in the lung (Fig. 5–7). Fibrin meshworks also act in a manner similar to that of a gauze bandage, which delays the flow of vital juices by creating barriers around an inflamed area, barriers that may entrap antibody molecules and bacteria that may otherwise spread into neighboring tissues. Thus the role of fibrin to contain the spread of infection and inflammation is important.

There is increasing evidence that in inflammation there are changes in the normal coagulation and fibrinolytic systems, but the data are not yet conclusive. It would be only natural in man that injury and inflammation should elicit some response from these elemental defense mechanisms.

Cellular Responses to Injury

This is a good place to introduce the dramatis personae of the hematopoietic system, of whose many roles none is more important than that of the second line of defense to injury. Figure 5–8 lists the cells of this system and suggests their relationship to the progenitor stem cell. Here we shall not discuss the sequence of steps in maturation of the erythroid series, which culminates in the mature red blood cell, but rather we shall consider the white blood cell series, paying particular notice to those cells with granules. The "round cells" (lymphocytes, monocytes, plasma cells) are considered in more detail in the next chapter, but will be mentioned briefly here.

The myelocyte series can be recognized as large cells with granules and a nucleus without lobes. The next step in differentiation is the maturation of the nucleus, which becomes segmented, until in the most mature stage it has as many as 7 different segments. As the myelocyte becomes more differentiated, there are more granules that, in the mature cells, acquire a particular staining quality. These granules may be brilliant red (eosinophilic), bright blue (basophilic), neutrophilic, or azurophilic. The granules are modified lysosomes. In fact, granulocytes may contain 2 populations, each derived from the opposite side of the Golgi complex. These granules, which contain active enzymes that are occa-

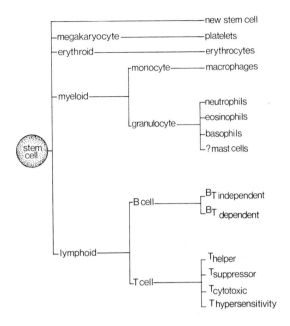

Fig. 5–8. This diagram illustrates the relationship of the lymphoid elements, the myeloid elements, and the erythroid elements in the blood, on the left, all arising from the stem cell, to the specific cells on the right. (From Roitt, I.: *Essential Immunology*. Oxford, Blackwell Scientific Publications, 1977.)

sionally secreted into the environment, are usually reserved for intracellular digestion. It is the staining quality of each type of granule that gives these cells their names (eosinophil, basophil, neutrophil). Each granulocyte seems to be associated with particular aspects of inflammation, yet they all act as a secondary defense line.

The neutrophil is better known as a **polymorphonuclear leukocyte,** the generic name for granulocytes in general (including the eosinophil and basophil). The life span of these cells after they are mature is short (4 to 6 days), and they are constantly liberated into the peripheral blood from the bone marrow in numbers that range around 5,000 to 6,000/ mm³. When the white blood cell count falls below 1,000 per mm³, there is a serious risk from infections, and if it falls below 100 per mm³, 70% of patients develop bacterial infections with a mortality rate that may reach 70%. It is estimated that the daily output in man is about 11×10^{10} cells. Their half-life in the circulation is estimated at 6 to 7 hours. The proportions of these cells normally is 60% neutrophils, 2% eosinophils, and 0.5%

basophils, if one counts 100 cells on a smear (differential count). These cells may appear in the peripheral blood in larger numbers and as immature forms (without many lobes to their nuclei) if there is more serious injury or if chemotactic substances are present in large amounts.

The importance of these cells to the host is best illustrated by the observation that the absence of polymorphonuclear leukocytes for only 3 hours increases the infectivity of bacteria in tissue as much as 100,000 times.

Patients with abnormal neutrophils, or absent neutrophils, suffer multiple, frequent, prolonged infections. There are examples of particular defects, such as the "lazy leukocyte syndrome," where the polymorphonuclear leukocytes are relatively immotile, failing to respond normally to chemotactic substances; however, these leukocytes have a normal complement of digestive enzymes. Other variations are polymorphonuclear leukocytes in which there are giant granules that seem to interfere with normal function. Equally rare conditions are those in which the polymorphonuclear leukocytes either do not migrate normally or fail to have adequate or normal digestive enzymes. In all these cases, the discovery of the defect has stemmed from thorough investigations to explain the reason for persistent and recurring infections in a particular person.

The second major group of white blood cells that must be considered whenever the inflammatory response is mentioned comprises those that have been called round cells to distinguish them from granulocytes. "Round cells" include lymphocytes, monocytes, macrophages, and plasma cells. They can be thought of as including both those cells found in the peripheral blood and those fixed in more or less specific tissue sites, such as the Kupffer cells of the liver. As a general idea, round cells have been considered to constitute a major part of the reticuloendothelial system, and are considered to be the constant warriors in disease states, because their presence is inevitable when recurring or constant injury takes place. These cells in general belong to 1 of 2 types.

The first is that family of cells principally concerned with phagocytosis; these are called monocytes or mononuclear phagocytes to distinguish them from the polymorphonuclear phagocytes (granulocytes). It has recently been discovered that these cells secrete at least 3 classes of substances into the immediate environment when they are activated. It might be expected that one of their principal products would be enzymes useful to the monocyte for its phagocytic digestive activity. Indeed, these enzymes have now been found in the immediate neighborhood of these cells. Some of these enzymes are active on the extracellular materials such as collagenase, elastase, and plasminogen activators. Other enzymes are principally concerned with the intracellular digestion, such as acid-activated lysosomal enzymes (phosphatase, sulfatase, and assorted nucleases). The former group of enzymes seem to be secreted in such large amounts that they may even be found in the interstitial space, perhaps when the cells have broken down.

A second group of substances that macrophages (phagocytic monocytes) secrete consists of those associated with the defense mechanisms, proteins such as interferons, lysozymes, and complement (Fig. 5-9). These materials clearly are not secreted without reason and the macrophage needs to have been stimulated for this to happen.

A third family of substances that macrophages may secrete comprises materials that affect the activities of cells in the immediate vicinity of the macrophage, much as in times of danger a fire alarm may be rung. These materials may inhibit cell growth, or they may fall into the category of lymphocyte-stimulating substances. These substances and the complex interactions between macrophages and lymphocytes will be considered in more detail in the chapter on immune mechanisms.

Each white blood cell can only attempt to isolate, ingest, and immobilize such threats as bacteria. In large numbers, leukocytes, in a contained space, can radically change the nature of the microenvironment. Their active metabolism consumes oxygen, glucose, and reduces the local pH, as they ingest the bacterial invaders. The liberation of large quantities of enzymes, including many nonspecific nucleases as well as hydrolytic

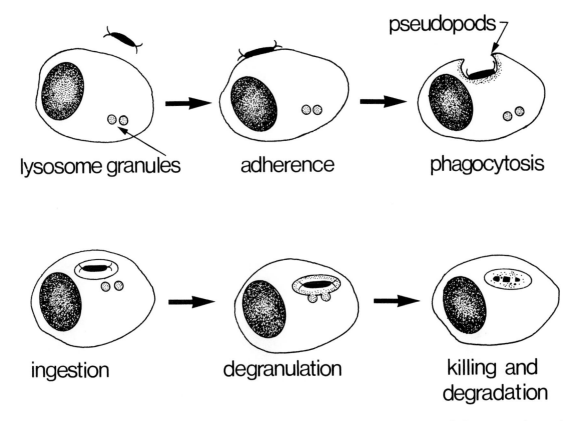

pseudopods

lysosome granules   adherence   phagocytosis

ingestion   degranulation   killing and degradation

Fig. 5–9. This scheme illustrates the role of lysosomes in phagocytosis and intracellular digestion. The bacterium at the top of the drawing is ingested in a vacuole that is subsequently joined by the lysosomes, which contain enzymes that aid in the killing and degradation of the bacteria. (From Pelczar, M. Jr., et al.: *Microbiology,* 4th Ed. New York, McGraw-Hill, 1977.)

and proteolytic enzymes that are often activated at low pH, limits the growth of microorganisms. If these organisms have not already been killed by intracellular digestion, they may be unable to withstand the hothouse climate that the short-lived polymorphonuclear leukocyte has created. This enzymatic soup is called pus. "Laudable pus" was recognized by the ancients as an attribute of infection, and its presence was regarded as a healthy and good sign. Pus is the result, in all acute infections, of the death of millions of leukocytes, whose primary function is to be the line of defense that isolates, ingests, and ideally digests bacterial invaders.

In some instances, the bacteria are hardier and survive both ingestion and the enzymatic attack of the specialized leukocyte lysosomes. Bacteria such as the waxy-coated tubercle bacillus and some other spore-forming bacteria are notoriously resistant to ingestion. In

fact, they can survive for many months in macrophages, outliving several generations of polymorphonuclear leukocytes.

A particular type of adaptive response to foreign material is the evolution of a population of cells that wall off the foreign material, whether it is silk suture, silica dust, or an indigestible biologic agent such as foreign vegetable matter, or, for that matter, bacteria such as we have just mentioned. These collections of chronic inflammatory cells appear as a halo about the object and may include cells with a dozen or more nuclei (giant cells) (Fig. 5–10). Such a cellular reaction, typical for chronic inflammations, is called a **granuloma.** The characteristic morphologic lesion always suggests persistent irritation. Sometimes the inciting agent is a biologic agent of moderate pathogenecity, such as a spirochete or a fungus. Special stains may reveal this organism within the boundaries of the granuloma. In other instances, no particular agent can be

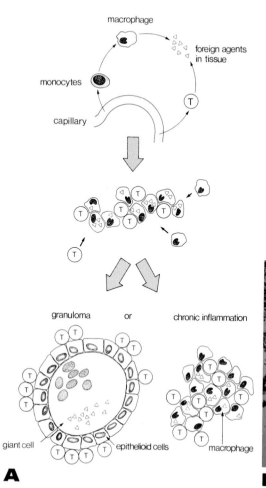

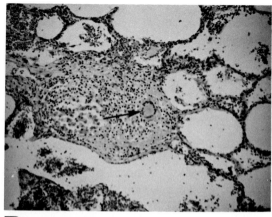

Fig. 5–10. *A,* This diagram shows the relationship of the monocyte-macrophage in the formation of a granuloma. The epithelioid cells are derivatives of monocytes. In *B,* one sees a microphotograph of this type of giant cell.

A

B

identified, and in another small group of cases, the pathologic process can be attributed to some types of hypersensitivity. The subtle variations in types of granulomas should not concern us here.

Systemic Defense Mechanisms

Under this umbrella we consider fever, leukocytosis, and some less-well-understood changes that accompany major stress.

Fever. The statement that "patient Jones has a temperature," has always annoyed us, since even a stone in the forest has a temperature. What was meant was that the patient has a fever, which is to say that his or her temperature is elevated above normal. Normal temperature includes the recognition that each of us has a daily rhythm of body temperatures. This normal rhythm peaks about 6 P.M. each

day, with an increase of as much as half a degree Celsius over the basal level. This is normal temperature far short of the bone-aching, hectic, sheet-sweating expression of the physiology of a body temperature of 104°F or 42°C.

The causes of fever are legion, but the mechanisms are well described (Table 5–3). Any substance capable of causing fever is generally called a **pyrogen.** There are bacterial pyrogens and chemical agents, such as etiocholanolone, a steroid, that also raise the body temperature. There are endogenous pyrogens derived from leukocytes of the polymorphonuclear class as well as from macrophages and monocytes. It now seems that cells of the reticuloendothelial system are able to synthesize this low-molecular-weight protein (15,000 MW) soon after they are so stimulated, usually by phagocytosis of bac-

Table 5–3.   Proposed Mechanism of Fever Production

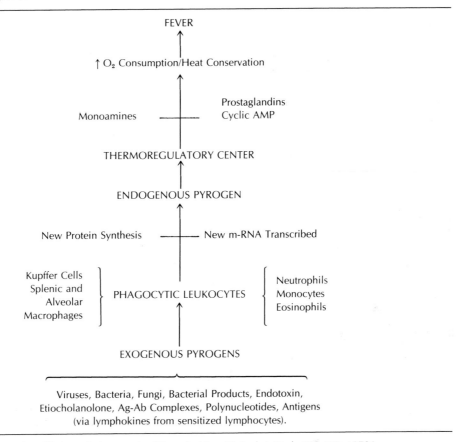

(From Dinarello, C.A., and Wolff, S.M.: Pathogenesis of Fever in Man. N. Engl. J. Med., *298*:607, 1978.)

teria. In elegant studies, Bodel has shown that cells including the monocyte, macrophages, Kupffer cells, and granulocytes, when isolated, contain no pyrogen, but that after stimulation, they produce pyrogen for many hours or for several days. Pyrogens, whether they are exogenous or endogenous to the host, act on the neurons of the thermoregulatory center of the anterior hypothalamus. The signals that adjust this thermostat increase the metabolic rate, oxygen consumption, and the respiratory rate, and cause involuntary muscle contractions (shivering) to take place in order to generate the rise in temperature called for by the pyrogen.

It is of some interest that the pyrogens that have been characterized to date are all small molecules and are capable of acting in dilutions that are impossible to measure with any accuracy. There is evidence now that prosta-

glandins may be mediators of fever; drugs such as aspirin, a classic treatment for fever, suppress prostaglandin synthesis. The effect of these drugs in reducing fever is directly proportional to their ability to block the synthesis of prostaglandins.

In theory, the role of fever is to increase the rate of metabolic reactions, and in this sense we must assume that fever has had some survival value. The thesis is that the host is better able to manage higher temperatures than the bacterium or parasite. In the 1920's, sweat boxes were used (the preantibiotic era) in an attempt to treat patients with syphilis; the rationale being that the delicate spirochete would succumb to the higher temperatures, whereas the human could tolerate the heat.

It is of some consequence that temperatures of over 105°F may irreversibly denature proteins, and that fevers of 107°F and over are frequently fatal. It is desirable to bring down the higher temperatures by any means, for example, baths, ice, water, and drugs such as aspirin.

Leukocytosis. An increase in the number of circulating white blood cells in the peripheral blood has been referred to earlier as an example of systemic response to injury. Whether the injury is myocardial infarction or bacterial pneumonia, the presence of injury is often revealed to the clinician by the increase (normal 5,000 to 7,000 white blood cells/mm^3) in numbers up to 30,000/mm^3. The spectrum of change includes a departure from the normal pattern of white blood cells to one in which polymorphonuclear leukocytes generally circulate in great excess, and in which even immature forms (band or stab nuclei) are seen on the examination of the smear of the peripheral blood.

Results of Inflammation

The effective inflammatory response meets the challenge of injury with the varied panoply we have sketched. Microcirculatory, cellular, humoral, and systemic reactions are like an ancient Roman army meeting the foreign enemy's spearmen and gladiators. The net result is to isolate, wall off, starve out, or annihilate the invader, if indeed it is injury due to a biologic agent, and to prepare the way for the next sequence of events, the repair of the damage (healing). In general terms, the inflammatory response has modified the vascular supply to the injured area and has alerted the host by a variety of signals to send troops continuously to the beleaguered zone, to initiate the machinery for antibody synthesis, and to arm the host for faster metabolic activity. The localization of the injury by slowing the flow in and out of the inflamed area, the presence of a scaffolding (fibrin) on which the active cellular defenders can climb, hand over hand, and can engage in combat with the bacterial invaders, and the general alarm reaction initiated through the release of adrenal hormones all take place in an effective sequence unless the host is debilitated, or unless aspects of the response are inhibited by drugs such as are used to treat cancer or to suppress the inflammatory response. In brief,

the results are an effective containment of the injury.

Complications of Inflammation

However, there are other sides to the inflammatory process, particularly when it is elicited by a bacterial or infectious agent, and we shall consider them under the general heading of complications of inflammation.

Let us consider the prototype of a bacterial attack introduced through a puncture wound of the skin, where the original inflammatory response is not successful in containing and destroying the implanted microorganisms. When the inflammatory sequence is successful, there is no spread or evolution of the injury. This spread may take one of 3 common routes. The first and most threatening is the entry of the bacteria by lymphatic, venous, or other route into the blood stream. If the numbers of bacteria are sufficient and virulent, we call this septicemia, and its effect is to escalate the warfare from a small affair to a systemic and life-threatening episode. Norman Bethune, the Canadian missionary surgeon who was a hero of modern China for his battlefield efforts during the Revolution, died from septicemia following his accidental inoculation when he cut himself while operating in an infected area. The diffusion of bacteria into the natural culture media of the blood, where there are few means by which the host is able to contain and to wall off the bacteria, and to facilitate phagocytosis, used to be invariably fatal, as the old term "blood poisoning" implied. However, with the development of antibiotic and drug sensitivity assays, the outcome is not necessarily fatal today. One result of the embolization of bacteria, represented by septicemia, is the potential for seeding bacterial colonies to grow in an infinite number of anatomic sites, in addition to the site of entry. Widespread abscesses may form in many organs of the body. This outcome of uncontrolled infection is due to an ineffective inflammatory response.

The most common evolution of inflammation in response to bacterial injury is the development of an abscess. An abscess may be defined as a cavity in a tissue. It contains pus. The importance of an abscess is not that it exists, but that in order to exist it has had to make a place for itself in a vital organ, and by so doing has inevitably destroyed some of the tissue of that organ. It is one thing to have an abscess in one segment of one lobe of one lung, and quite another to have an abscess in the speech center of the brain. The evolution of the abscess is the story of inflammation, but its physiologic consequence may be to destroy irretrievably some functioning tissue. The history of an abscess begins when the bacterial invaders gain a foothold in a particular tissue and the defensive reaction walls off the bacteria and builds a boundary of fibrin and cells around the margin. At the same time, a large number of phagocytes, attracted by the prey, sally into the area where tissue is dying and where bacteria are multiplying. Subsequently, the limited life span of the polymorphonuclear leukocytes reduces them and the ingested bacteria to a yellowish liquid without life, but rich in enzymatic debris. This is pus. The eventual fate of the liquid-filled cavity is to rupture, usually to the surface if the abscess is in the skin, a most common site. Abscesses deep in vital organs such as the liver may rupture through the surface of the organ into the appropriate body cavity, in that case the peritoneum, and spread the infection (peritonitis), or they may become enclosed again in some larger space, for example, between the liver and the diaphragm. In lung abscess, inflammation may frequently extend to the pleural surface and may involve the pleural space. Pus in the pleural space is commonly referred to as an empyema.

When an abscess lies deep in the tissues and eventually finds its way to rupture and drain the necrotic, purulent material, it creates a track leading from the abscess to the surface that is called a **sinus**. Should the abscess join 2 mucosal surfaces (bowel to bowel), or an internal organ and the skin, this connection is often referred to as a **fistula**, or abnormal communication between 2 compartments.

Because the rich enzymatic content and the presence of fibrin in acute inflammation are not easily resolved, the effect of inflammation on otherwise normal organs is to create a fabric of new contacts or adhesions among surfaces that had been smooth, shiny, and nor-

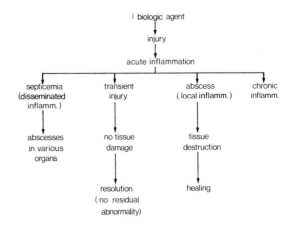

Fig. 5–11. This scheme outlines some possible outcomes of acute inflammation.

mally lubricated. This phenomenon allows spatial adjustments to take place as necessary within cavities such as the peritoneum. These fibrinous adhesions, as they are called, are testimony to the fire within. The adhesions may bind the surface of the lung to the chest wall, the epicardial surface of the heart to the pericardium, or the surfaces of the small or large bowel to one another. One result of this new, unplanned contact is to predispose a patient to obstruction in the gastrointestinal tract. The most common cause of intestinal obstruction is the formation of adhesions, the result of earlier inflammation, usually the simple reaction to surgical intervention. The more common outcomes of inflammation are shown in Figure 5–11.

Anergy. Finally, we should note that in some cases the expected does not happen. In the very old, very young, and very sick, inflammation does not occur in a normal way. The failure to mobilize the defensive reactions has been termed anergy. In so many instances it is the presence of pain, fever, and leukoyctosis that signifies the presence of injury. The diagnosis of appendicitis is easier since we have come to understand the pattern. The diagnosis of meningitis is usually made more obvious because of the inflammation that involves nerve roots. Can you imagine the diagnostic dilemma when, in a case of appendicitis, there is no pain in the right lower quadrant, no fever, no leukocytosis, and the patient becomes progressively sicker?

Or the situation where coma supervenes without the telltale sign of a stiff neck in meningitis? In these situations, the appropriate therapy is not given because the diagnosis is obscured by the absence of the usual pattern of inflammation. Thus inflammation is more than a biologic phenomenon. In the practice of medicine it often presents the clue to the correct diagnosis.

HEALING OR REPAIR

Speaking teleologically, the aim of the efforts in response to injury is to restore the organism to its original state, if possible, and the steps toward this goal can be arbitrarily separated. However, it is difficult to state categorically at any one moment where inflammation ends and where healing begins. Nonetheless, there are features of each process that are particular to inflammation or to healing. For example, the presence of large numbers of polymorphonuclear leukocytes is characteristic of acute inflammation, and the presence of abundant, if not exuberant, fibroblasts and new collagen is typical of scar formation, a particularly important part of healing.

For the purpose of this chapter, it is well to remember that we are discussing generalities about biologic phenomena that are derived from many different specific examples. For instance, healing in the skin is different from healing in the cornea, which has no blood vessels. Healing in the heart is different, because it is constantly working, from healing in a skeletal muscle that has been splinted. Healing in the liver is different from healing of the femur. In these instances, healing may be different because the nature of the injuries may vary. Mechanical trauma, a one-time occasion, may initiate a series of responses that appear different, with a beginning, a middle, and an end, from the healing that takes place in the face of chronic irritation or metabolic injury, as in nutritional cirrhosis.

With these provisos, we shall consider an arbitrary division of the process from injury to restoration of normal function, and then we shall discuss specific examples of healing in different tissues.

An arbitrary list of steps, starting with injury, could be stated as follows: 1. **Injury.** This can be of many kinds, from thermal burns and surgical incisions to infections and ischemic necrosis. Important considerations are the size, extent, and degree of local hemorrhage, and the kind of tissue damage. Obviously a small puncture with a sterile needle invokes a different type of healing from a fracture of a long bone with massive hemorrhage.

2. **Inflammation.** The vascular, cellular, and systemic responses already discussed are an important preparation for restitution of normal structure and function.

3. **Debridement.** Although the removal of dead, dying, injured, or foreign material from an injury could just as easily be considered part of inflammation, it is an essential part of healing. In the presence of foreign bodies (splinters, glass, bacteria), the process of healing is aborted and inflammation persists, invariably distorting the restoration to normal. This debridement is effected most conventionally by enzymatic means. However, it is one of the achievements of medicine that the intervention of the physician, who removes the nonviable materials, actually accelerates the repair process. In older times, maggots were sometimes used to debride complicated wounds, and, more recently, purified enzymes (streptokinase) have occasionally been used for that purpose.

4. **Repair.** The ingrowth of new capillaries, the migration of fibroblasts, the elaboration of collagen, ground substance, and elastic fibers, and the recovery of areas where the epithelium has been lost are all unequivocal steps in healing. When a group of epithelial cells of the skin or intestinal mucosa have been killed by whatever means, the neighboring cells perceive in some way this loss of integrity of the membranous barrier and begin to migrate over the basement membrane in efforts to resurface the lost area (Fig. 5–12A,B,C). This migration can be seen within minutes of injury, and within hours there is an increase in mitosis in the adjacent cells, which begin to multiply in order to replace the lost cells. The signal for this re-epithelization is believed to be the loss of the cell-to-cell attachments typical of all epithelia.

A

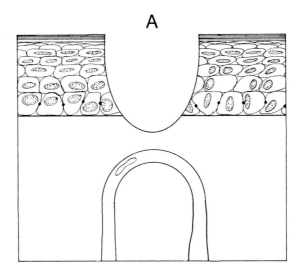

B   C

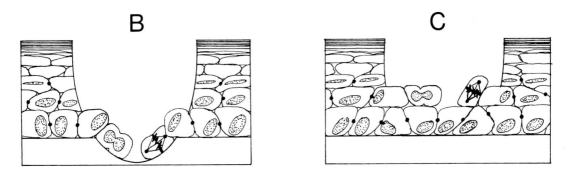

Fig. 5–12.   These drawings show: *A,* the injury of the epithelium; *B,* the mitosis and migration of the germinal cells; and *C,* the continuing attempt to repair the epithelial lesion.

5. **Remodeling.** The final phase in repair is the remodeling of the newly manufactured tissue in response to the demands of normal use. Typically, a new scar on the skin of the arm or the hand is first as smooth as glass, but with use and time it develops wrinkles and calluses just like the old skin. However, it may not develop the freckles or the hairs that were once there, since the regeneration may not include all the elements of the original tissue. Nowhere is remodeling so elegantly seen as in the final healed result of a fractured long bone in a young person.

For an illustration of healing, we shall take a simple skin wound, in which the incision has sundered the epithelium and the subcutaneous tissue down to the underlying muscle

(Fig. 5–13). It is the typical kitchen knife accident, treated at home with a small adhesive bandage and soon forgotten as healing takes place over the ensuing 4 or 5 days. The wound kills a few hundred thousand cells of the epidermis, splits the basement membrane, and ruptures small and large blood vessels in its path. These blood vessels bleed briskly into the defect between the severed edges; the coagulation cascade is initiated by the liberation of tissue thromboplastins from the damaged cells. At this point, some response by the person whose finger is cut may modify the entire subsequent course. Washing and exploring the wound may hemolyze red blood cells and may renew the bleeding; putting the cut finger into the mouth may introduce

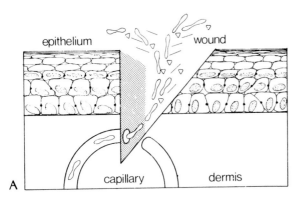

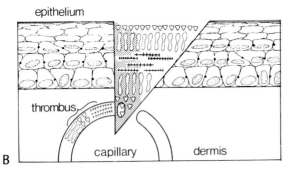

Fig. 5–13. This drawing suggests the changes that take place with time in the restoration or healing of a wound. At the top (A), a fresh injury with red blood cells, fibrin, and platelets indicated, the fibrinogen as the single lines, the platelets as the triangles. At the bottom (B) an organized clot has formed.

mixed bacterial flora, but it may also have cleansing value; and compression of the wound may enhance and facilitate the clotting mechanisms. Tincture of iodine or strong oxidizing agents may impair healing because, although they may kill some bacteria, they also kill the very cells that lie at the margins of the wound and thereby destroy the front wave that can heal the incision.

Next is the initiation of the inflammatory response by the kinins and the peptides liberated from the damaged tissue. Simultaneously, the epithelial cells that have lost their neighboring contacts begin to move to find a similar cell (loss of contact inhibition). This movement causes a flow of epithelial cells toward the free or cut margin. The attenuation of the covering sheet of cells is met later by new cells arising from mitosis in the germinal epithelium of the epidermis. If the cut mar-

gins are brought together by an adhesive bandage, suture, or pressure, as in Figure 5–14, then the migrating epithelial cells may meet their counterparts and join in a single sheet within a day or so. This renewal of epithelium and approximation of the underlying tissue is called **healing by first intention.**

In the deeper layer of the skin wound, fat cells have been ruptured, elastic fibers severed, nerves rendered, and the fabric of the interstitial tissue altered by the cataclysm of microcosmic catastrophe. Bringing together the severed edges staunches the blood flow, accelerates coagulation, and apposes the tissues. The inflammatory process is soon in progress, and there are attempts to realign the vascular network. New capillaries form from

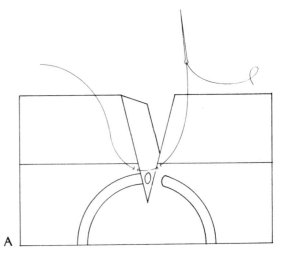

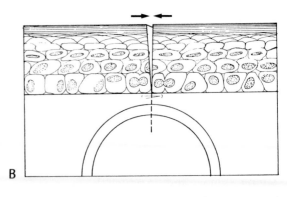

Fig. 5–14. A and B, This figure illustrates the importance of apposition in a fresh injury, showing the approximation of the wound edges.

the neighboring ones. Fibroblasts differentiate from paravascular cells or are transformed from existing quiescent fibrocytes. Soon the cytoplasmic machinery prepares collagen in soluble or monomeric (unpolymerized) form to be delivered into the interstitial space, where the collagen will mature, polymerize (aggregate to form macromolecules), and form fibrils of indeterminate length but of great tensile strength. The sequence of events during healing is shown in Figure 5–15, which illustrates the time course of the deposition of extracellular materials and its relationship to the tensile strength of the wound.

The rate at which the repair by newly formed collagen, a "magic weave" repair, takes place is of real consequence to the restoration of normal function of a tissue. Not until the restoration of the mechanical integrity of

the tissue has occurred is it safe to remove the surgeon's sutures, or to apply physical stress to the recent incision line. For example, the simple stress of a cough may initiate the breakdown of the gossamer-like fabric of fibrin and cells of a two-day-old wound. The patient in whom wound dehiscence (rupture) most commonly occurs after an operation is the person with chronic lung disease who coughs constantly. Other important causes of failure of normal healing are malnutrition, vitamin deficiency, absence of essential elements such as zinc, and the presence of infection. A marginally successful blood supply or atherosclerosis also predispose a person to inadequate healing and wound dehiscence.

A second pattern of healing is best illustrated when the injured edges are not brought together within a short time (hours), and where the edges are left separated, either exposed to the air or separated by a large clot or by necrotic tissue (Fig. 5–16). The defect created by the injury may be deep or superficial, small or extensive, but the distances to repair in cellular terms are vast. The process of repair must proceed from the base of the wound and must attempt to fill in the defect from the bottom. This pattern of healing is called second intention, and is much slower than healing by first intention. Because of its very nature, this slower pattern of healing often leads to a palpable or visible defect years later in the form of scar tissue. The process consists in man of budding capillary loops growing slowly into the crusted, overlying area (scab), which is composed of serum proteins and clot. The appearance of the capillary loops, with their accompanying perivascular

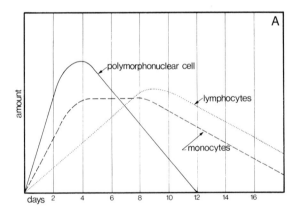

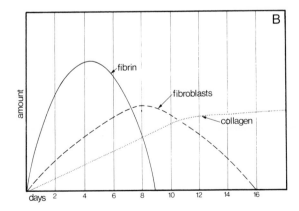

Fig. 5–15. *A,* This graph shows the sequential changes of polymorphs, lymphocytes, and monocytes in comparative numbers. *B,* This shows, at the same time, changes in the presence of fibrin, fibroblasts, and collagen.

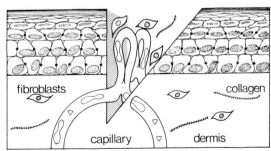

Fig. 5–16. This drawing illustrates granulation tissue. The capillary buds and the presence of perivascular cells are shown in the drawing.

cells and fibroblasts, is red and friable, bleeding at the slightest provocation, and has a granular appearance. It has been called a variety of names such as granulation tissue and "proud flesh." Scar tissue such as is formed in a defect caused by a burn or an extensive loss of epithelium may conform to the original shape and size of the damage; however, in general, scar tissue has the tendency to contract as it gets older. Marked deformities and shortening in the area may result (contractures), leading to a loss of function. The Hiroshima maidens had to undergo many plastic reconstructive procedures because of the contractures on the exposed areas of their skin. Another outcome of scar formation may be the exuberant overgrowth of the new connective tissue that results in a protuberance above the old surface plane. This raised, healed area, seen frequently in surgical wounds, is called a keloid. After many months or years, it may subside to match the surrounding tissue elevations as remodeling takes place. The wonder of it is that healing takes place at all, not that there are occasional excesses in response.

We have discussed healing in the skin and have described what happens in a system that is largely two-dimensional. Healing occurs, of course, in many organs besides the skin. After an infarct, the heart cannot regenerate new muscle, and although the remaining fibers compensate by increasing in size (hypertrophy), the necrotic area is replaced in 6 weeks by firm, white connective tissue that has no contractile capacity. Some organs, such as the kidney, may respond to injury by replacement with new tubules, so that a scar does not appear. However, in other instances where the damage is considerable or continuous, there may be scar tissue present as testimony to the previous injury. The most successful of the many appearances of healing is the replacement of damaged tissue by identical but new tissue. Unfortunately, this cannot take place in many tissues of man, where the important cells have lost their power to undergo mitosis (for example, neurons in the brain, heart muscle cells), but in other organs (the liver and epithelium of the gastrointestinal tract, for example), repair can be effected by simple replacement. The many factors that

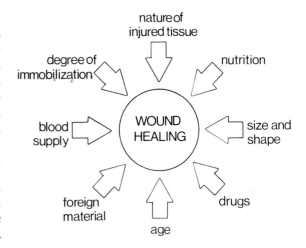

Fig. 5–17. This illustrates the many different factors that may modify wound healing.

come to bear on the healing process are shown diagrammatically in Figure 5–17.

Principles of Treatment. In the treatment of any disease, the doctor may adopt one or both of 2 methods: he may assist the healing powers of Nature, and/or he may directly attack the cause of the illness. Rest of the inflamed part is one of the most important of all therapeutic measures. Activity may act as an additional irritant, and may disperse the bacteria through the tissues and increase the area of inflammation. It tends to break down the barrier that the leukocytes try to build around the bacteria. Thus the inflamed finger is splinted, the inflamed arm is placed in a sling, the inflamed eye is shaded so that it cannot be used, and purgatives are avoided as if they were poison in the treatment of the inflamed bowel.

A second principle is drainage. The quickest way to get an abscess to heal is to open it and to drain the pus. This procedure not only allows the infecting bacteria to escape, but it also relieves the tension in the inflamed area, and thus encourages the further flow of healing substances from the blood vessels, in addition to relieving the pain. However, if pus has not yet formed and if a barrier of leukocytes has been built around the bacteria, the knife may do more harm than good, for it may open fresh channels for the spread of the infection. Drainage is essential in infections of enclosed spaces such as the pleural and peritoneal cavities.

Heat, in the form of fomentations or poultices, is one of the oldest methods of treating inflammation. The warmth sends messages up the sensory nerves of the part to the spinal cord; these messages pass down the nerves to the blood vessels and cause the latter to dilate, so that additional blood is brought to the part, thus adding to the supply of leukocytes and antitoxins. Cold, in the form of an ice-bag or cold compresses, relieves the pain by causing the vessels to contract thus diminishing the swelling of tissues that is responsible for pain. Cold seems to be particularly effective in treating athletic injuries and local trauma.

A direct attack on the invading bacteria by antibiotics has come to occupy so dominant a place in the treatment of inflammation due to infection that we sometimes lose sight of the healing powers that used to be our only hope, powers that proved to be sufficient in most cases.

Finally, we have anti-inflammatory agents such as acetylsalicylic acid, butazolidine, and cortisone, each of which has its place in the management of acute and chronic inflammation (Fig. 5–18). However, the aids to the heal-

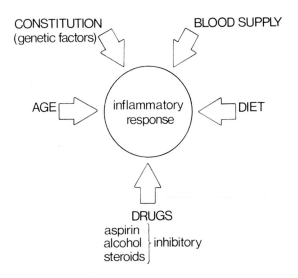

Fig. 5–18. This scheme illustrates factors that can alter the inflammatory response.

ing process reviewed earlier far outweigh the value of individual drugs.

In conclusion, we should recognize that whereas inflammation and healing have been represented here as beneficial biologic responses (Table 5–4), in each instance there are examples in which the deleterious effects of

Table 5–4.　Chronologic Sequence of Events in Wound Healing

DAYS AFTER WOUNDING	CELLULAR ACTIVITY	VASCULAR CHANGES	DEPOSITION OF INTERCELLULAR SUBSTANCES
2	Phagocytosis of blood, tissue debris, etc. Proliferation and mobilization of histiocytes and fibroblasts	Dilation of marginal capillaries and arterioles	Edema with perivascular metachromatic material
4	Multiplication of acid mucopolysaccharide-producing fibroblasts Bipolar fibroblasts with fine argyrophilic prolongations	Proliferation of capillary buds with neoformation of abundant capillaries	Increasing edema with more generalized deposition of acid mucopolysaccharides Appearance of free amino acids such as glycine and proline
6	Transformation of all fibroblasts into bipolar cells in active fibrogenesis, arranged perpendicular to capillaries	Maximum of capillary proliferation reached	Begins the disappearance of edema and acid mucopolysaccharides Appearance of fine argyrophilic fibrils with tendency to arrange perpendicular to capillaries
8	Fibroblasts decrease in size and number, their prolongations are less abundant and appear continuous with intercellular fibers	Number and caliber of blood vessels decrease	Fusion of argyrophilic fibers which become thick acidophilic collagen bundles
	Most fibroblasts appear as fibrocytes	Few and narrow capillaries	Abundant collagen

(From Perez-Tamayo, R.: *Mechanisms of Disease.* Philadelphia and London, W. B. Saunders, 1961.)

the process may outweigh the benefits. Chronic inflammation, as in rheumatoid arthritis, can destroy joints and permanently cripple; the formation of adhesions and scar tissue can obstruct vital pathways, as in mitral stenosis, or in the case of hydrocephalus following meningitis. We must therefore recognize these processes for what they are—responses to stimuli that depend on many factors for their final result.

SYNOPSIS

Inflammation and healing are a continuum.

Vascular and cellular phases of inflammation can be separated arbitrarily.

Systemic responses to inflammation are leukocytosis and fever.

Acute, subacute, chronic, and granulomatous inflammations differ in cellular and temporal terms.

Physical, chemical, bacterial, and immunologic injuries all lead to inflammation.

The advantages and disadvantages of inflammation are opposite sides of the same coin.

Factors that enhance healing include rest, adequate nutrition, a good blood supply, normal protein metabolism, and adequate stores of vitamins and trace metals.

Terms

Phagocytosis	*Lymphocyte*	*Septicemia*
Chemotaxis	*Plasma cell*	*Ulcer*
Polymorphonuclear leukocytes	*Granuloma*	*Fibroblast*
Pyrogen	*Giant cell*	*Granulation tissue*
Macrophage		

FURTHER READING

Adams, D.O.: The granulomatous inflammatory response. A review. Am. J. Pathol., *84*:164, 1976.

Atkins, E., and Bodel, P.: Clinical fever: its history, manifestations and pathogenesis. Fed. Proc., *38*:57, 1979.

Bendtzen, K.: Biological properties of lymphokines. Allergy, *33*:105, 1978.

Bucher, N.L.R.: Experimental aspects of hepatic regeneration. N. Engl. J. Med., *277*:686, 1967.

Dannenberg, A.M., Jr.: The antiinflammatory effects of glucocorticosteroids: a brief review of the literature. Inflammation, *3*:329, 1979.

Dinarello, C.A., and Wolff, S.M.: Pathogenesis of fever in man. N. Engl. J. Med., *298*:607, 1978.

Dubos, R.J.: The microenvironment of inflammation. Lancet, *269*:1, 1955.

Dunphy, J.E.: The fibroblast—a ubiquitous ally for the surgeon. N. Engl. J. Med., *268*:1367, 1963.

Fine, R.: Inhibition of alveolar macrophage chemotaxis by ethanol and prostaglandin E_1. Am. Rev. Respir. Dis., *117*:273, 1978.

Goodwin, J.S., and Webb, D.R.: Regulation of the immune response by prostaglandins. Clin. Immunol. Immunopathol., *15*:106, 1980.

Greenbey, A.G., et al.: Wound dehiscence. Arch. Surg., *114*:143, 1979.

Henkin, R.I.: Zinc in wound healing. N. Engl. J. Med., *291*:675, 1974.

Majno, G.: *The Healing Hand: Man and Wound in the Ancient World.* Cambridge, Harvard University Press, 1974.

Movat, H.Z. (Ed.): *Inflammation, Immunity and Hypersensitivity.* New York, Harper & Row, 1971.

Newhouse, M., Sanchis, J., and Bienenstock, J.: Lung defense mechanisms. N. Engl. J. Med., *295*:990, 1976.

Quie, P.G., and Cates, K.L.: Chemical manifestations of disorders of neutrophil chemotaxis. In *Leukocyte Chemotaxis.* Edited by J. I. Gallin and P. G. Quie. New York, Raven Press, 1978.

Stossel, T.P.: Phagocytosis. N. Engl. J. Med., *290*:717, 1974.

Zweifach, B.W., Grant, L., and McCluskey, R.T. (Eds.): *The Inflammatory Process.* New York and London, Academic Press, 1965.

The Immune System and Its Disorders

6

The development of immunity, in the broadest sense, is a process by which the body learns from experience of past infections to deal more efficiently with subsequent ones.—MACFARLANE BURNET.

Early in the course of evolution, animals learned to protect themselves against external enemies by developing armor, spines, or poison. Some enemies gained access to the interior of the body and adopted the life of a parasite. They were recognized by the wandering cells we have described in Chapter 5 (macrophages), and attempts to evict the newcomers were not always successful. An acceptance or **tolerance** of the newcomer was often acquired by the host after it had remained for some time. This tolerance demanded some adaptation to the foreign agent, which frequently secreted substances or was acknowledged to be different from the host by virtue of different biochemical markers on its surface. Perhaps the visitor was successfully repulsed after a lengthy battle. We now know that if the host is visited again by the same unwanted guest, the cellular and humoral mechanisms are able to recognize the intruder because of the previous visitation, and react more vigorously to reject him, we say, because of their previous **sensitization**.

Classically, immunity takes 2 forms: the cellular response, in which lymphocytes and their relatives are concerned with a direct confrontation, and the humoral response, characterized by antibodies that circulate in the serum after having been produced by a cell somewhere in the body following the original sensitization. However, the immunologic mechanisms are not so simple, because every cell and every host has genetically determined markers on all its cells from the time of its creation. These substances are the hallmark of our individuality. Blood group determinants A, B, and O; the Rh factors; and transplantation antigens are all examples of these inherited differences among persons.

The capacity to develop antibodies to any antigen is related both to the presence of lymphocytes in the blood and to the presence of lymphoid tissue somewhere in the body. This unique defensive system permits the host to mobilize a cytologic army (lymphocytes) against invaders, and to spread the serologic equivalent of gas warfare (antibody production). However, this complicated defensive apparatus can sometimes backfire, as when the wind blows poison gas back over the troops who launched it. The immunologic defense system can be turned on tissues of the host itself. The concept of **autoimmunity** is described later in this chapter.

We shall outline first the normal function of the immune system: the cells involved and the types of antibody and immunologic reactions. We shall then discuss 2 general disorders of this system: first, when it is deficient, and second, when it is overreactive. Finally, we shall consider immunity as it relates to transplantation and to autoimmune disease.

CELLS OF THE IMMUNE RESPONSE

There are 2 populations of cells that function directly in the immune response. First is the lymphocyte, a cell capable of detecting foreign cells or material. There are 2 general kinds of lymphocytes: "B cells," derived from the bone marrow, and "T cells," derived from the thymus (Fig. 6–1). Both types of lymphocytes originate from stem cells in the bone marrow; some stem cells later migrate to the thymus, where they develop into mature T cells. Finally, T cells migrate to various lymphoid tissues around the body. Several lymphoid elements affect the differentiation of B cells.

"B cells" were originally so called because in birds these lymphocytes arise in the bursa of Fabricius, a lymphoid organ lying in the avian rump (Fig. 6–2). Human B lympho-

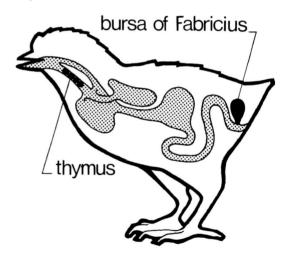

Fig. 6–2. The bursa of Fabricius, site of B cell differentiation in the chicken. (Adapted from David, J.R.: Cellular immunity and hypersensitivity. In *Immunology*. Edited by B. A. Thomas. Scope Monograph Series. Kalamazoo, Michigan, Upjohn Co., 1975.)

cytes were therefore also regarded as bursadependent; however, no bursa equivalent has been convincingly identified in man. In human beings, B cells develop first in fetal liver, then in spleen, then in adult bone marrow.

B cells, whose secretory products help protect us against bacteria, also retain immunoglobulins or antibodies attached to their surface membranes. When these antibodies come into contact with an antigen (foreign particle or cell), the antibody on the cell surface interacts with the antigen, and the B cell differentiates into a plasma cell. Plasma cells then actively produce and secrete antibodies specific for the antigen that originally stimulated the differentiation of the original B cell. Antibodies circulate in the blood, and for this reason the B cell antibody response is often called the **humoral** component of the immune response.

T cells do not have soluble antibody on their surfaces; nevertheless, they react specifically with antigen, then they proliferate. Finally, they participate in a series of reactions leading to the destruction of the antigen. Because the types of reaction mediated by T cells can be experimentally transferred to recipient subjects by white blood cells, and *not* by serum, the T cell system is referred to as the **cellular** component of the immune response,

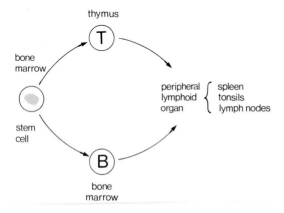

Fig. 6–1. Differentiation of lymphocytes. Cells of the immune system begin as multipotential (stem) cells in the bone marrow. They may differentiate into several types of blood cells and lymphocytes (see Fig. 5–9). The two types of lymphocytes mature in different locations as described in the text, then migrate to lymph nodes throughout the body.

or "cell-mediated immunity." Among the most important functions of the T cells are protection of the host against tumors, intracellular bacteria, viruses, parasites, and the rejection of transplants. T cells also appear to influence B cells in some way (Fig. 6–3).

If all the lymphocytic cells in the circulation are assessed by various techniques to determine whether they are either B or T cells, the total number is always short of 100%. The few lymphocytes that are neither one nor the other are termed "null cells," and it is not yet clear whether they represent cells that have lost their surface determinants or cells that have not yet gained an identity.

The second general type of cells important in the immune response belong to the reticuloendothelial (RE) system. These cells are nonspecific "scavengers" of foreign or antigenic material; they ingest material that is recognized by the lymphocytes as being foreign. RE cells form a diverse group, but all are phagocytic. They are found in many tissues of the body, but mainly in the spleen, liver, lymph nodes, and bone marrow. The most important cells we shall consider are the monocytes and their tissue counterparts, the macrophages.

Macrophages in the simplest sense have been recognized for 100 years as the cellular

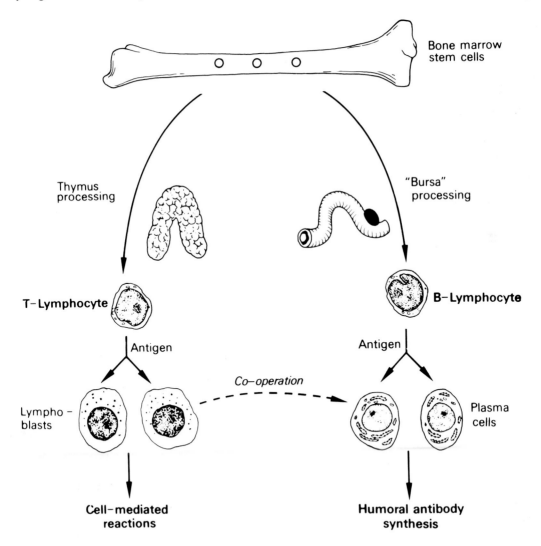

Fig. 6–3. This figure illustrates the processing of lymphocytes. Proliferation and transformation to cells of the lymphoblast and plasma cell series occurs following antigenic stimulation. Cooperation between T and B cells can take the form either of help or of suppression. (From Roitt, I.: *Essential Immunology*. Oxford, Blackwell Scientific Publications, 1977.)

crows of our hematopoietic system; they always appear where there is dead or dying material to be scavenged. They are found in the lung after pneumonia has run its course, and they carry away the cellular debris to regional lymph nodes. Some macrophages are permanent residents of the lung (alveolar macrophages), and some are domiciled in the liver (Kupffer cells). Now there is evidence that they also affect the early stages of infection, particularly with organisms such as the tubercle bacillus in which humoral immunity is not effective, by both ingesting and transporting such bacteria to regional lymph nodes, where cellular immune mechanisms are alerted to the danger, and where specific reactivity is initiated (Fig. 6–4).

Interaction between macrophages and lymphocytes may form the initial step of the immune response (Fig. 6–5). We believe that the macrophage picks up material and carries it to the lymph nodes, where the material, if antigenic, stimulates the lymphocytes to differentiate (and to produce antibody in the case of B cells). The lymphocytes and antibody seek the antigen in the tissues, from which the T cells secrete substances that attract monocytes from the blood and cause them to differentiate into macrophages. These substances also attract other

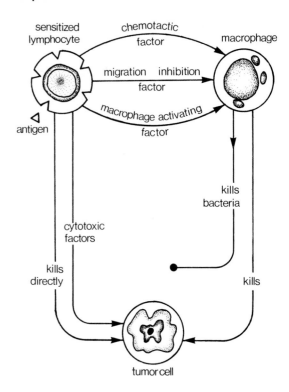

Fig. 6–5. This figure shows a more detailed outline of the macrophage-lymphocyte interaction in the tissue. Chemotactic factors, secreted by T cells, attract macrophages to the area, and migration inhibition factors prevent them from leaving. (From David, J.R.: Cellular immunity and hypersensitivity. In *Immunology*. Edited by B. A. Thomas. Scope Monograph Series. Kalamazoo, Michigan, Upjohn Co., 1975.)

macrophages to the area and prevent them from leaving. While still in the tissue, the lymphocytes then indicate to the macrophages what material is to undergo phagocytosis. This process is referred to as **macrophage activation**. The phenomena of macrophage-lymphocyte interaction and of macrophage activation are new insights into the complex nature of the defense mechanisms that are taken for granted when they work normally. Moreover, defects or alterations in these activities provide new explanations for the susceptibility of some persons to infections. Tables 6–1 and 6–2 list some mechanisms that activate and depress macrophages.

Although macrophages do not determine the specificity of the immune response, they are important in identifying and initiating the immune response.

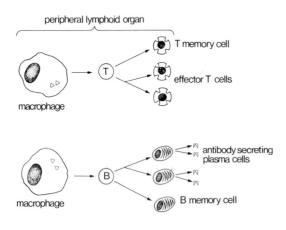

Fig. 6–4. A schematic representation of macrophage and lymphocyte interaction. The macrophage finds antigenic material in the tissue and brings it to the lymph node. The antigen stimulates T and B cells to differentiate into effector T cells and plasma cells, capable of responding specifically to that antigen. It is thought that at some stage in this differentiation memory cells are formed which remain in the lymph node and await the next exposure to the same antigen.

Table 6–1. Macrophage Activators

1. Specific fixed cellular antibodies
2. Antigen-antibody complexes and other humoral factors
3. Glass or plastic surfaces
4. Phagocytosed particulate material (carbon, etc.)
5. Microbial products (cell wall, etc.)
6. Interferon inducers
7. Lymphokines

Table 6–2. Macrophage Suppressors

1. Specific antimacrophage serum
2. Irradiation
3. Silica, Thorotrast
4. Corticosteroids
5. Antimetabolites and anti-inflammatory agents
6. Certain viruses, fungi, protozoa
7. Reticuloendothelial system blockade

ANTIGENS

Before we dive deeper into the turbulent waters of the immune response, let us discuss what we are responding to immunologically. An **antigen** is a substance that, when introduced into the body, provokes an immune response to which an antibody reacts specifically. This antigen could be a bacterium or another biologic agent, a toxin, a protein, or almost any other kind of macromolecule. In cellular or viral antigens, the antigen which combines with antibody is not the whole cell or virus but some protein or molecule on the surface (or possibly inside).

Antigens are usually foreign to the host. Occasionally, the immune system loses part of its ability to distinguish between self and nonself, so that a tissue or a substance belonging to the host is perceived by the lymphocytes as antigen, and is subsequently attacked. The result is so-called "autoimmune" disease.

There are small, simple substances (molecular weight of less than 1,000) that do not evoke an immune response by themselves, but that can do so if complexed with larger carrier molecules. In this bound form these substances behave as antigens and react with antibodies, once the latter are formed. Such small substances are called **haptens**. The carrier molecules are frequently host proteins such as albumin.

ANTIBODIES

In the simplest sense, the term antibody means exactly that: a substance that has been raised in the self as an antagonistic (protective) response to some nonself material (antigen). Antibodies have the unique ability to distinguish among almost identical antigens, much as a cylinder lock distinguishes among nearly identical keys. Antibodies were recognized in theory long before they were identified, and it was not until the era of modern physical chemistry that antibody activity was shown by electrophoresis to reside in the globulin fractions of human serum.

The term antibody currently designates a member of the family of serum proteins often referred to as **immunoglobulins**. (Recently, immunoglobulins have also been found in alpha-2, beta, and delta globulins). Serum has been shown to contain at least 5 different immunoglobulins, which are designated by their abbreviations IgG, IgM, IgA, IgD, and IgE (Table 6–3). All these different classes of proteins are approximately the same size (molecular weight 160,000), except for IgM, which is much larger (molecular weight 900,000) (Table 6–4). Each class is made up of similar parts of chains of amino acids (heavy and light chains), but each antibody molecule may be different by virtue of the specific nature of its amino acid sequence and three-dimensional arrangement. Of the 5 types of gamma globulin, IgG represents the largest proportion (80%) in the normal serum. This antibody is directed against common infectious agents such as viruses, bacteria, and toxins. IgG is the only type of immunoglobulin capable of crossing the placental barrier and therefore capable of protecting the fetus during the maturation of its immune system.

IgM, the largest molecule (Fig. 6–6), constitutes between 5 and 10% of the circulating antibody, and is important to the primary immune response. This large molecule may have as many as 10 antibody reaction sites.

IgA globulins differ in that they are found in secretions such as tears, saliva, and mucus of the respiratory tract. Therefore, we think of

Table 6–3. Biologic Properties of Major Immunoglobulin Classes in the Human

	IgG	IgA	IgM	IgD	IgE
Major characteristics	Most abundant Ig of internal body fluids particularly extra-vascular where it combats microorganisms and their toxins	Major Ig in sero-mucous secretions where it defends external body surfaces	Very effective agglutinator; produced early in immune response —effective first line defense vs. bacteremia	Present on lymphocyte surface	Raised in parasitic infections. Responsible for symptoms of atopic allergy
Complement fixation					
Classical	+ +	–	+ + +	–	–
Alternative	–	+	–	–	–
Cross placenta	+	–	–	–	–
Fix to mast cells (in homologous skin) and basophils	–	–	–	–	+
Cytophilic binding to macrophages and polymorphs	+	–	–	–	–

(From Roitt, I.: *Essential Immunology.* 3rd Ed., Oxford, Blackwell Scientific Publications, 1977.)

Table 6–4. Physical Properties of Major Human Immunoglobulin Classes

	IgG	IgA	IgM	IgD	IgE
WHO Designation	IgG	IgA	IgM	IgD	IgE
Sedimentation coefficient	7S	7S, 9S, 11S*	19S	7S	8S
Molecular weight	150,000	160,000 and polymers	900,000	185,000	200,000
Number of basic 4-peptide units	1	1, 2*	5	1	1
Heavy chains	γ	α	μ	δ	ϵ
Light chains $\kappa + \lambda$	$\kappa + \lambda$	$\kappa + \lambda$	$\kappa + \lambda$	$\kappa + \lambda$	$\kappa + \lambda$
Molecular formula†	$\gamma_2\kappa_2, \gamma_2\lambda_2$	$(\alpha_2\kappa_2)_{1-3}$ $(\alpha_2\lambda_2)_{1-3}$ $(\alpha_2\kappa_2)_2 S^*$ $(\alpha_2\lambda_2)_2 S^*$	$(\mu_2\kappa_2)_5$ $(\mu_2\lambda_2)_5$	$\delta_2\kappa_2(\delta_2\lambda_2?)$	$\epsilon_2\kappa_2, \epsilon_2\lambda_2$
Valency for antigen binding	2	2, (? polymers)	5(10)	?	2
Concentration range in normal serum	8–16 mg/ml	1.4–4 mg/ml	0.5–2 mg/ml	0–0.4 mg/ml	17–450 ng/ml‡
% total immunoglobulin	80	13	6	1	0.002
Carbohydrate content, %	3	8	12	13	12

*Dimer in external secretions carries secretory component—S.
†IgA polymers and IgM contain J chain.
‡ng = 10^{-9} g.
(From Roitt, I.: *Essential Immunology.* 3rd Ed., Oxford, Blackwell Scientific Publications, 1977.)

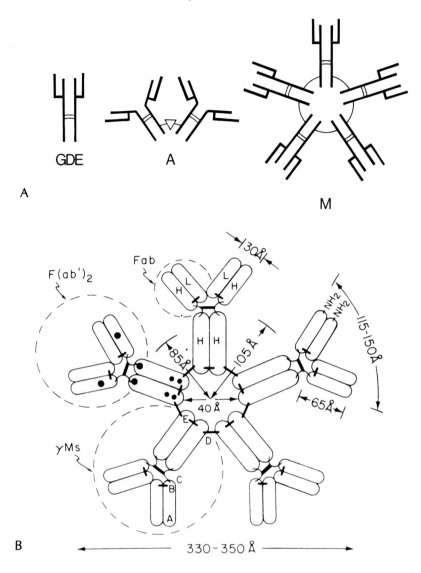

Fig. 6–6. *A,* This figure shows schematic representations of the 5 types of antibody molecules. The unit of light and heavy chains constitutes the molecules of IgG, IgD, and IgE shown at the left. IgA is shown schematically in the center, and IgM, the largest molecule, is at the right. The pieces of the molecule IgM are represented in the diagram *B,* and the dimensions are shown in the scale at the bottom.

them as antibodies that help to protect the mucosal barriers, which are exposed and susceptible to attack by bacteria. IgA globulins represent about 5 to 10% of the normal total antibody in the host. There are IgA molecules in the serum as well as in the secretions, and these molecules may not be identical.

IgE is concerned with acute allergic responses such as asthma, hay fever, and anaphylaxis, and aid in protection against parasites. IgD is found as a surface marker on B cells, usually in association with IgM. Its function is unclear.

Antibody Synthesis

It seems that for an antibody to appear in the serum in response to an infection such as an acute streptococcal sore throat, it is necessary for several cellular reactions to take place: recognition, transfer, synthesis, and secretion of antibody in significant amounts requires time, perhaps as much as 2 or 3 weeks.

A step-by-step sequence in simplified terms involves recognition of antigen by a macrophage, transportation or migration by the macrophage containing the antigen to the lymph node, transfer of antigenic information to lymphocytes and there, once the plans are drawn, specifications made, the factory goes to work and proliferation of antibody-forming cells (plasma cells) occurs. As Fagraeus showed in 1949, the appearance in the serum of immunoglobulin is closely correlated with the appearance in the lymphoid tissue of plump, rich RNA-containing cells, which have been referred to as plasmablasts.

In these cells, the first sites of antibody production are in the granular reticulum around the nucleus (the perinuclear cisternae). Soon the plasma cell has developed a rich, rough reticulum, whose cisternae are filled with newly synthesized antibody, which is then secreted from the cell surface where it finds its way to the serum. At this time we believe that each plasma cell is capable of synthesizing only a single type of immunoglobulin at a time.

None of this takes place in man during the days immediately after birth, and the predominant immunologic protection that a newborn has is the passively acquired antibody transferred from the mother while the child is in utero (IgG can cross the placenta). Immunologic competence matures slowly and IgA begins to be synthesized at about 3 weeks of age, IgG at 6 weeks. During these first weeks the lymphoid tissue of the newborn is developing. It is important to remember that at the other extreme of life (after 60), lymphoid tissue atrophies, and elderly people frequently become immunologically unresponsive (anergic). In the

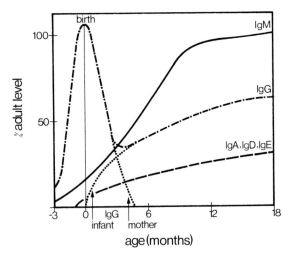

Fig. 6–7. The development of serum immunoglobulin levels in human beings. This diagram illustrates the time course of development of different immunoglobulins up to the age of 18 months. (From Roitt, I.: *Essential Immunology.* Oxford, Blackwell Scientific Publications, 1977.)

newborn, the thymus gland is a large and well-developed organ whose function was unsuspected as recently as 25 years ago. Today, we know that the thymus plays an important role in populating the rest of the body with lymphocytes, which are responsive to antigenic stimulation and are capable of being cytotoxic (T lymphocytes), that is, ca-

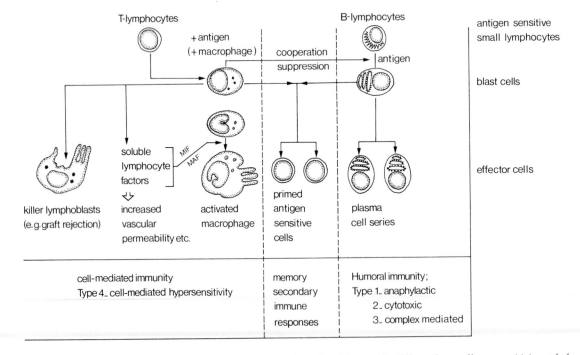

Fig. 6–8. This diagram illustrates the interrelationships of B and T cell activity, and the different forms of hypersensitivity and of immunity associated with each type of lymphocyte. (Adapted from Roitt, I.: *Essential Immunology.* Oxford, Blackwell Scientific Publications, 1977.)

pable of killing other cells. Experiments in animals have shown that the removal of the thymus from the newborn will arrest the development of immunologic responses, and will lead to infections that prematurely overwhelm and kill the animal. Removal of the thymus will also deprive the animal of the ability to reject transplantation.

Precisely how cells make antibodies is not clear, but various theories have attempted to explain the exquisite matching of antibody to antigen. The specificity has been likened to the matching of keys to locks, and it is easy to accept that once a key has been made that fits a particular lock, it is easy to make many more keys on the same pattern. Unfortunately, it seems clear that antigens do not act as templates. It seems that a cell is able to produce an antibody of only one specificity, but it may switch from one type of molecule to another, e.g., from antidiphtheria IgM to antidiphtheria IgG.

In any case, the production of newly synthesized antibody follows the same general rules as outlined in Chapter 1 for protein synthesis. Ribosomal synthesis of antibody is achieved by attached ribosomes, but the original stimulus and the cytoplasmic steps that determine the conformation of the protein are not clear. It is of interest that the synthesis of different classes of antibodies occurs at different rates (Fig. 6–7), as well as in different amounts and at different times, depending on whether it is a primary exposure to an antigen or a secondary or anamnestic response (see p. 151). The synthesis of antibody is also under genetic control, so that there may be some immunologic truth to the folktales that certain families are healthier than others.

Without controls over the persistence of antibody synthesis we would be drowning in antibody, similar to the plight of the sorcerer's apprentice, who could not turn off the torrents of water. Antigen concentration must have a regulatory ef-

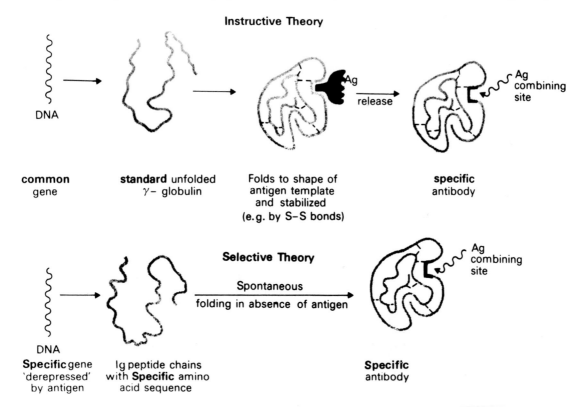

Instructive Theory

common gene   **standard** unfolded γ– globulin   Folds to shape of antigen template and stabilized (e.g. by S–S bonds)   **specific** antibody

Selective Theory

Spontaneous folding in absence of antigen

Specific gene 'derepressed' by antigen   Ig peptide chains with **Specific** amino acid sequence   **Specific** antibody

Fig. 6–9. Comparison of instructive and selective theories. According to the instructive theory, the antigen (Ag) acts as a template around which a standard unfolded antibody chain can be molded. The antibody then stabilizes in this configuration and forms an antigen-specific combining site. This is analogous to instructing a tailor to make a suit to fit our proportions.

The selective theory contends that the genes contain all the information required for the synthesis of specific antibodies, including the antigen combining site. Presence of the antigen "switches on" the gene, which mobilizes production of antibody specific for that antigen.

Current evidence supports the selective theory of antibody production. Antibody molecules can be unfolded experimentally by ribonuclease or by a reduction of the disulfide bonds. They can be refolded in the absence of antigen, and they can recover their antigen-specific properties spontaneously. This means that the information held in the primary amino acid sequence is sufficient to allow the correct antigen-specific bonding site to be formed by spontaneous folding. (From Roitt, I.: *Essential Immunology.* Oxford, Blackwell Scientific Publications, 1977.)

fect on the continued production of antibody, but it is not clear how this is perceived by B cells. T cells have also been shown to regulate antibody production, both as helpers and as suppressors. These interrelationships are schematically illustrated in Fig. 6–8.

The theories of antibody synthesis may be reduced to: the selection of antibody-producing cells and the instruction of antibody-producing cells (Fig. 6–9). Roitt has illustrated these opposing alternatives by drawing a parallel with the selection of a suit from an infinite number on a rack, with differing neck, shoulder, and arm lengths, as compared with ordering from the tailor a suit cut precisely to a person's measurements.

In the 1940's, it became clear that antibodies arose in lymphatic tissues; simple experiments demonstrated that an antigen injected into a foot stimulated the regional lymph nodes to change their cell population, and that antibody could be found in the lymphatic vessels draining the particular nodes following a suitable interval of time. Today, when lymph nodes are enlarged and swollen (e.g., around the elbow or in the axilla of the arm that has an abscess of the hand), one should recognize that, in addition to serving as a filter, the nodes are actively producing antibody.

For a moment it may be useful to sketch the anatomy of the lymph node (Fig. 6–10) and to illustrate the traffic flow through the different areas that can be recognized (Fig. 6–11). The

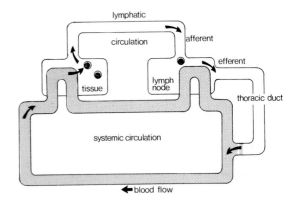

Fig. 6–11. Traffic and recirculation of lymphocytes. Blood-borne lymphocytes enter the tissues and lymph nodes and leave through the draining lymphatics. The efferent lymphatics finally emerging from the last node in each chain join to form the thoracic duct, which returns the lymphocytes to the blood stream where it empties into the left subclavian vein. (Adapted from Roitt, I.: *Essential Immunology*. Oxford, Blackwell Scientific Publications, 1977.)

respective areas of the lymph node that are populated by B and T cells are illustrated.

The lymph nodes therefore form a network of watch towers, replete with a garrison of warriors who form a secondary line of defense against such foreign agents as bacteria, much as the watch towers of Roman days stretched across northern England to defend against the Vikings.

ANTIBODY-ANTIGEN REACTIONS

The interaction of antibody with antigen follows physical chemical rules. The amount of precipitate or of complex varies with the proportions of antigen and antibody. *In vivo* this may affect the nature of the body's reactions.

When antibody and antigen interact, they form what is known as an **immune complex**, a large and complicated molecule or mass of molecules that seems to be composed of more than just the antigen and antibody (complement, for example). This material then triggers or initiates several mechanisms: agglutination, opsonization and complement fixation are 3 such mechanisms. Agglutination refers to the clumping of bacteria in masses. Antibody appears to link antigen molecules on the surface of neighboring cells. This pro-

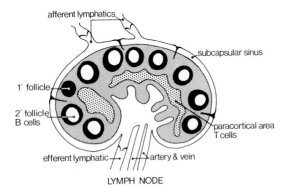

Fig. 6–10. A diagrammatic representation of a human lymph node. A primary follicle contains an aggregation of B cells that has not yet been stimulated by antigen. After antigenic challenge, these form secondary follicles containing pale-staining germinal centers of large, proliferating lymphoid cells and macrophages. T cells reside in the paracortical areas. (Adapted from Roitt, I.: *Essential Immunology*. Oxford, Blackwell Scientific Publications, 1977.)

cess can be interpreted as an aid to confine or to limit the spread of infection. Opsonization is the name given to the process of coating the bacteria with antibody. This process enables the polymorphonuclear leukocytes to ingest bacteria more easily. Opsonization and agglutination occur when the antigenic stimulus is cellular, or attached to a cell. When the antigen is an unattached macromolecule, the antigen-antibody combination becomes a massive macromolecular complex also easily phagocytized.

When antigen and antibody interact and combine in the body, a series of reactions involving serum proteins is triggered. These particular proteins are collectively called **complement** (Fig. 6–12). There are 9 separate proteins in complement (C1–C9), which react sequentially in the following manner: The immune complex (Ab-Ag) interacts with the first component of complement (C1), converting C1 into an active enzyme. C1 then acts on 2 other serum complement components. This action produces more active enzymes and some biologically active byproducts. Each new enzyme formed activates another member of the sequence, resulting finally in the production of cytotoxic complex that is able to punch holes in cell membranes. The cell to which the immune complex is attached is unable to maintain its internal environment and collapses as does a balloon that lands on a thistle (Fig. 6–13).

Various by-products of these immunologic reactions are part of the inflammatory response. Some molecules are chemotactic and attract polymorphonuclear leukocytes and monocytes. Some cause histamine to be released from mast cells in the tissue; histamine then increases vascular permeability, which brings more cells and more antibody to the site. Other molecules make the surface of the antigenic cell stick to a phagocytic cell, which greatly increases the likelihood of the destruction of the antigenic cell.

Immune complexes can also be useful in diagnosis. If a patient is suffering from an infection by an unknown biologic agent, tests

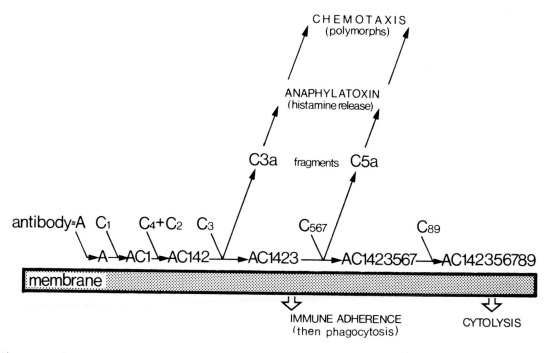

Fig. 6–12. The sequence of complement activation. This sequence of biochemical interactions is much like a cascade. The immune complex activates C1, creating AC1, which activates C_4 and C_2, creating another active complex AC142. This activates C_3 yielding more active enzymes and AC1423, which goes on to activate C567, and so on. The active fragments are important in the defense process; chemotactic substances attract phagocytic polymorphonuclear leukocytes, and histamine increases vascular permeability, allowing blood cells to flood into the area. (Adapted from Roitt, I.: *Essential Immunology.* Oxford, Blackwell Scientific Publications, 1977.)

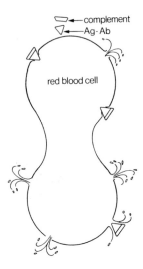

Fig. 6–13. This figure shows a red blood cell being lysed by antigen-antibody complexes.

can be performed on his serum to determine what antibodies are present. For example, if the infection is suspected to be 1 of 4 possible agents, the serum may be mixed with each of the 4 suspect antigens and then observed to see which provokes immune complex formation, visualized as a precipitate. The antigen that forms the complex must be specific for the patient's antibody. We conclude that this antigen is the likely cause of the infection. This is the principle that lies behind several new diagnostic tests.

Radioactively labeled tumor antibody may also be used to find tumors too small to be seen with the naked eye that carry antigens on their cell surfaces.

IMMUNITY

The beneficial and usual consequence of the immune response is called **immunity**. The immune host is resistant to particular diseases or poisons. Immunity comes about when the host is exposed to an antigen and, as a result of this exposure, acquires the capacity to recognize, react with, and neutralize the antigen the next time it is encountered. Anyone who has ever had diphtheria, even a mild, barely noticeable case, is immune for life. On every subsequent occasion that this person is exposed to diphtheria, immunologic memory mobilizes a response so

fast that the toxin is neutralized before it produces the disease.

This accelerated immune response on second infection is called an **anamnestic response** (Greek *anamnesis,* memory). It occurs in about half the time it took to mobilize the first or primary response (Fig. 6–14). Lymphoid tissue contains greater numbers of plasma cells this time, and more cells produce more antibody. This process probably results from the presence of "memory" cells that developed at the time of initial exposure.

The anamnestic response will occur at any time during a person's lifetime when there is exposure to antigen. However, the response does diminish slightly as time from the initial exposure passes. In vaccinations this diminished response can be overcome by giving repeated doses of antigen, known as "boosters," to reawaken waning immunity (Fig. 6–15).

Anergy is the opposite of the anamnestic response. The immune response may be either retarded or ineffective in elderly, debilitated, malnourished, and seriously ill patients, in persons with overwhelming infections or cancer, or for reasons we do not understand. In these instances, the immune mechanism seems paralyzed and unable to respond to the presence of normal antigen, much less to reply with a rapid and effective

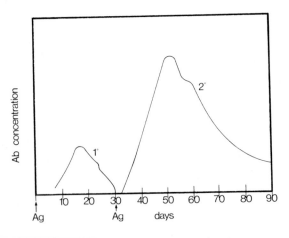

Fig. 6–14. The primary versus the secondary immune response. The secondary response is greater and more immediate because of the presence of memory cells formed during first exposure. (Adapted from Weiser, R.S., Myrvik, Q.N., and Pearsall, N.N.: *Fundamentals of Immunology.* Philadelphia, Lea & Febiger, 1969.)

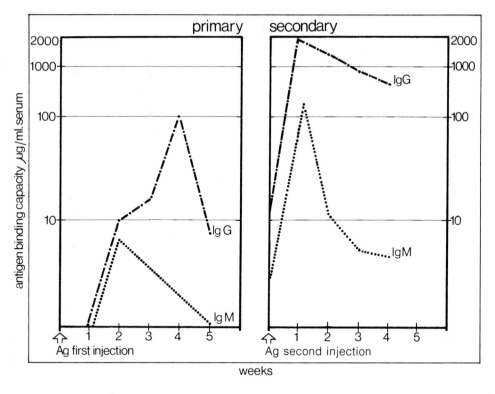

Fig. 6–15. The synthesis of antibodies in the mouse during primary and secondary responses to bovine serum albumin. The IgM response to a secondary challenge is not much greater than it was during first exposure. The secondary response is largely an IgG response produced by "memory" B cells. A secondary response elicited by a "booster" injection will literally "boost" immunity to a high level, as shown. (Adapted from Roitt, I.: *Essential Immunology.* Oxford, Blackwell Scientific Publications, 1977.)

amount of antibody. The ineffective immune state (anergy) has become the focus of recent interest, and is used currently to define how ill a patient is. It has become evident that both acute and chronic illness may render someone anergic, and that this anergy can be reversed by supportive measures such as hyperalimentation and successful management of shock.

Immunity can be either active or passive. Active immunity refers to the process of antibody formation in response to an antigen. This process can be induced naturally, by infection by the pathogenic organism, or artificially, by vaccination by either injection or ingestion of a particular antigen that has been rendered harmless but retains its antigenic properties. This process stimulates antibody production and hence produces active immunity without causing the disease. For example, bacteria and viruses may be killed in such a way that their antigenic components remain intact. The process of rendering

someone resistant or immune (e.g., through vaccination) is called immunization.

Passive immunity means that the infected host does not form his own antibody, but is given injections of antibody from another (immune) person or animal. This procedure is useful in emergencies. However, it is only a temporary measure. The person who receives such passive antibody has no immunologic memory of the infection, and copes no better with a second infection of the same organism. In addition, in cases of passive immunity, antibody is soon metabolized and excreted by the host; actively immune hosts continually replace lost antibody. Passive immunity is also acquired naturally, before birth. Maternal antibodies are transferred across the placenta to the fetus. Thus there are 4 ways of acquiring immunity: (1) **by being exposed to infection** (active, natural); (2) **by inoculation of dead or harmless organisms** (active, artificial); (3) **by transfer of antibodies from**

mother to fetus (passive, natural); and (4) **by transfer of antibodies from a previously immunized person or animal** (passive, artificial).

TOLERANCE

Another phenomenon, **tolerance**, should be discussed briefly. In the era of transplantation, it is interesting to observe that some persons, twins, for example, accept potentially foreign antigens, whereas others of different genetic backgrounds reject tissues because of activation of cellular and humoral immunologic mechanisms. In the pattern of Huxley's *Brave New World*, when it was discovered that a person exposed to foreign tissue during the first few weeks of life retains this tolerance to the foreign tissue into adult life, the thought of vaccinating infants in anticipation of future organ transplantations was discussed. It has since become evident

that tolerance may be acquired at both ends of the range of antigenic stimulation. That is, both small and large doses of antigen may make a host accept a foreign material (Fig. 6–16). The differences between unresponsiveness or tolerance and anergy are still unclear and may be merely semantic.

Anergic states occur in congenital immunologic deficiencies, or they may be acquired in a variety of conditions later in life. Congenital immunologic deficiencies can involve B cells, T cells, or both, depending on the disease. Such a disorder usually becomes apparent within the first 6 or 8 months of life.

Agammaglobulinemia is the condition in which B cells are either absent or are remarkably few in number. The infant makes little immunoglobulin of his own. However, he usually appears to be healthy for the first 5 or 6 months after birth because he is protected by maternal immunoglobulin (transferred through the placenta or in milk). Disease be-

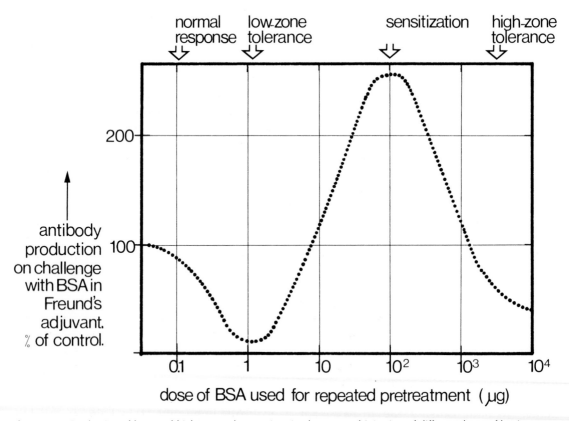

Fig. 6–16. Production of low- and high-zone tolerance in mice by repeated injection of different doses of bovine serum albumin (BSA). Tolerance was then tested by inoculating the animals with BSA in a highly antigenic form in adjuvant. Pretreatment with either a small or a large dose of BSA elicits little antibody response or tolerance. (From Roitt, I.: *Essential Immunology.* Oxford, Blackwell Scientific Publications, 1977.)

comes evident as the maternal immunoglobulin disappears; the infant suffers from repeated infections, usually resulting in early death. This condition is generally familial and sex-linked, being confined to males. The T cell system is unaffected in this disease.

T cell deficiencies result from hypoplasia of the thymus. Infants with this disorder have little thymus tissue and few, if any, T cells. Thus these children are vulnerable to viral and fungal infections as well as to some bacterial infections. B cells and serum immunoglobulins may be relatively unaffected, but because some types of T cells help B cells to produce antibody to some antigens, a defect in T cells may manifest itself as a defect in B cells as well. Diseases involving combined B and T cell deficiencies have been reported.

B and T cells are not the only elements of the immune response that can be deficient. Any disorders in the complement or reticuloendothelial systems impair the host's ability to respond appropriately. However, because these disorders are not immunologic, they are not considered here.

Congenital immune deficiencies are rare compared with the acquired types of immune disorder.

Suppression of immune and inflammatory reactions occurs in several situations. The most common instance is a person who takes corticosteroids in substantial amounts. Severe injury, debilitating disease, and infections with virus or massive tuberculosis can also cause the anergic response, in injury and disease, by methods that are poorly understood, and, in the use of corticosteroids, by interfering presumably with the lymphocytes directly. Anergy also occurs in patients who have neoplastic diseases, particularly Hodgkin's disease. Conversely, it has been hypothesized that these debilitating neoplastic diseases emerge because of a failing immune system. Finally, anergy occurs sometimes in old age for reasons that are not clear.

HYPERSENSITIVITY

The opposite side of the coin to anergy or tolerance can be thought of as hypersensitivity. This section discusses diseases caused by the immune response: diseases in which the immune system produces tissue damage and disordered function rather than immunity. In these diseases, immune complex formation and complement activation ultimately destroy the host's tissue.

The terms used to describe this type of phenomenon are confusing and misleading. Therefore, before describing the diseases themselves, we shall examine the terminology.

The first term used to refer to disease of this nature was the word "allergy," which originally meant an "altered state of reactivity." In recent years, however, the word "allergy" has become a nonspecific term that can be applied equally to ragweed, to eggs, or to mothers-in-law. Efforts to find a more precise description of immune phenomena produced the term "hypersensitivity."

The notion of a hypersensitivity reaction or of a state of hypersensitivity has even passed into the jargon of the layman and is used casually to mean hypercritical. However, in biology and in the context of this chapter and book, the term refers to an altered state of reactivity. Thus all who have been immunized may be potentially hyperreactive should they encounter the appropriate antigen. The term best applies to those cases in which an untoward or destructive rather than a simple neutralizing or defensive reaction occurs. There are instances of this extraordinary inflammatory reaction in which edema and even death take place following exposure to an agent to which the person is allergic or **hypersensitive**.

Hypersensitivity can best be thought of as an increase in sensitivity to a particular antigen, or as an abnormal overreaction by an oversensitive immune system. Persons who experience such a reaction, be it to pollen, to metal, or to penicillin, may be considered to be more sensitive to that antigen than the rest of the human population, which does not normally react to that antigen. Hence, the former may be referred to as "hypersensitive individuals." In fact, they are really only "sensitive" to the antigen, whereas the rest of the population is "nonsensitive."

Familiar examples may help to express this idea. Ten per cent of the North American population experiences hay fever; these persons are then described as hypersensitive to plant pollen, relative to the remaining 90% who produce no reaction to pollen. Most persons react to bee venom with pain, redness, and swelling, but a few are truly hypersensitive and respond with a systemic, life-threatening reaction, and may die as a result of a bee sting.

In all attempts to define hypersensitivity, one thing must remain clear, that is, that in all hypersensitivity diseases, antigens, when introduced to the body, evoke immune processes that damage the host (Table 6–5). These processes involve the same basic pathways that lead to immunity on other occasions: antibody formation, immune complex formation, and complement activation, for example. When immunity is the result of the immune response, the invading antigen is neutralized, and on second exposure the defense is so successful that there is no evidence of disease. In the hypersensitivity state, second

Table 6–5. Atopic Conditions

CONDITION	COMMONLY ASSOCIATED ALLERGENS
Allergic rhinitis	Inhalants (spores, pollens, animal dander)
Extrinsic asthma	Mold spores
Atopic conjunctivitis	Inhalants (spores, pollens, animal dander)
Atopic dermatitis	Various food allergies Drug hypersensitivities: especially penicillins, sulfonamides, streptomycin Local anesthetics Heavy metals Reactive chemicals
Urticaria-angioedema	Insect bites Food allergies
Gastrointestinal allergy	Food allergies (cereals, milk, eggs, shellfish, fruit) Drug hypersensitivities
Serum sickness syndrome Anaphylaxis	Drugs, especially penicillin Heterologous antisera Vaccines Iodinated radiographic material

(Adapted from Bach, M.K.: Reagin allergy. In *Immunology*. Edited by B.A. Thomas. (Scope Monograph Series.) Kalamazoo, Michigan, Upjohn Co., 1975.)

exposure leads to self-destructive reactions that can be catastrophic, such as the anaphylactic reaction to a bee sting.

All allergic or hypersensitivity reactions have been divided into 4 groups, 3 mediated by humoral antibody, and 1 mediated by T cells (see Table 6–6). Most of these reactions have features that are found in "normal" immune responses; it is only when there is exuberant, unregulated control of some features that one can observe "hypersensitive" reactions leading to damage of the host's tissues.

Type I—Anaphylaxis

Everyone knows a person who, on a spring day, has a fit of sneezing and weeping even with wheezes, or someone who visits a house in which a family of cats has made its home for many years on the only available sofa, where the visitor sits, trying to make conversation as his eyes run and he itches furiously. This allergic reaction to contact with pollen or dander is mediated by IgE or reaginic antibody. On first exposure, IgE antibody is formed; it binds to mast cells or tissue basophils, cells that contain granules of histamine and other vasoactive amines in the cytoplasm (Table 6–7). On subsequent exposure to the same antigen, the binding of antigen to antibody causes degranulation of the mast cells and basophils, which results in a marked vasomotor, vascular and axonal response characteristic of inflammation (Fig. 6–17). The substances released cause smooth muscle contraction and stimulate the nerve endings, in addition to increasing capillary permeability. This response leads to wheals, flare, and itching. The reaction occurs locally in some instances and systemically in others, for reasons that are not well understood.

Local anaphylactic-type reactions are seen in some persons who have an inherited tendency (idiosyncrasy or atopy) to overreact to normal environmental antigens. Ninety per cent of the population do not react to the presence of these substances. Such persons tend to form IgE in response to dust, cat fur, and plant pollen, for example. The common reaction site is the mucous membranes of the

Table 6–6.   4 Types of Hypersensitivity Reactions

	ANAPHYLACTIC (TYPE 1)	CYTOTOXIC (TYPE 2)	COMPLEX-MEDIATED (TYPE 3)	CELL-MEDIATED (TYPE 4)
Antibody-mediating reaction	IgE, mast cell binding	IgG or IgM	IgG	Receptor on T-lymphocyte
Antigen	Usually exogenous	Cell surface	Extracellular	Extracellular or cell-surface
Response to intradermal antigen:				
maximum reaction appearance	30 min Wheal and flare	— —	3 to 8 hrs Erythema and edema	24 to 48 hrs Erythema and induration
histology	Degranulated mast cells, edema, eosinophils	—	Acute inflammatory reaction; predominant polymorphs	Perivascular inflammation: polymorphs migrate out leaving predominantly mononuclear cells
Damaging agent	Biochemical mediators from IgE-sensitized cells produce tissue response	Complement may or may not be involved	Complement and polymorphs produce tissue damage	Lymphokines released from antigen-sensitized lymphocyte, reactions produce tissue damage
Transfer sensitivity to normal subject	←——————————— Serum antibody ———————————→			Lymphoid cells, transfer factor
Examples	Atopic allergy, e.g., hay fever	Hemolytic disease of newborn (Rh)	Serum sickness; complex glomerulonephritis	Tuberculin skin reaction; contact dermatitis

Table 6–7.   Pharmacologic Mediators of Anaphylaxis

	HISTAMINE	SEROTONIN	SLOW REACTIVE SUBSTANCE A	EOSINOPHIL CHEMOTACTIC FACTOR
Structure	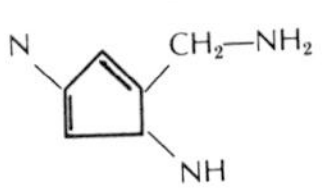 (chemical structure shown)	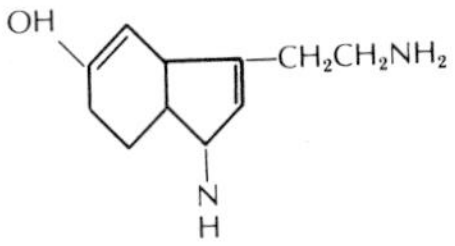 (chemical structure shown)	Unknown	Unknown
Molecular Weight	97	146	Around 600	Below 1,000
Origin	Mast cell granule	Mast cell granule	?	Mast cell granule
Action	Vasodilator	Vasodilator	Slow acting vasodilator, smooth muscle contraction	Chemotactic for eosinophils

(Adapted from Bach, M.K.: In *Immunology*. Edited by B.A. Thomas. (Scope Monograph Series.) Kalamazoo, Michigan, Upjohn Co., 1975.)

1st exposure

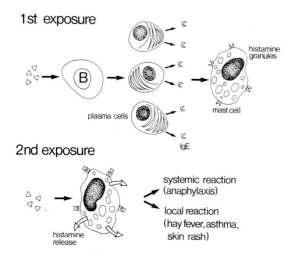

2nd exposure

Fig. 6–17. This figure illustrates the Type I hypersensitivity reaction. On first exposure to antigen, B cells proliferate and differentiate into plasma cells that produce antibody. The antibody attaches to the surface of mast cells and basophils. On second exposure the antigen combines with the antibody, which triggers degranulation of the attached cells.

nasal sinus. There histamine and the other amines cause local edema and other inflammatory responses.

Hay fever is one of the best-known examples of local Type I reaction. The attacks are strictly seasonal, occurring in spring, summer, or autumn, depending on whether the patient is hypersensitive to the spring pollens of trees, summer pollens of grasses, or fall plants such as ragweed. Symptoms of itching, congestion of the eyes, violent paroxysms of sneezing, and a profuse watery discharge from the nose (called rhinorrhea) are typical. The particular protein responsible can usually be identified by means of skin tests, i.e., scratching the arm and rubbing in the suspected protein; if an inflamed area or wheal is produced, the patient is hypersensitive to that protein. When the protein is identified, the patient may be desensitized against it by means of repeated small injections of the protein before the onset of the hay fever season. The aim of desensitization is to produce excess antibody in the person's blood, so that the antigen will be destroyed before it reaches the tissues. (It is in the tissues that the allergic reaction is triggered.) This procedure may render the sensitive person partially or totally insensitive.

Far more serious is systemic anaphylaxis, usually referred to simply as anaphylaxis (Greek *ana* [to reverse] and *phylaxis* [to guard]). The term describes the situation in which the expected or anticipated immunity does not follow exposure to a small dose of toxin, but instead an extraordinary susceptibility to small doses of antigen results.

The mechanisms involved in this reaction are basically the same as those of the local reaction: IgE is formed, attaches to mast cells and basophils. However, in this case, the site of the reaction is not limited to the nose; it occurs all over the body. The substances released by IgE-antigen complexes cause a massive generalized change in capillary permeability, leading to hypotension and shock. In different mammals there are different responses, but in man there frequently is smooth muscle contraction, particularly in the bronchial tree, which causes respiratory distress or asthma-like symptoms. Edema of the larynx may threaten to obstruct the airways and sometimes requires an immediate tracheostomy.

Anaphylaxis is often life-threatening, but if it is treated immediately with adrenalin and antihistamines, and if the airways are kept open, the patient will usually survive. Immediate treatment is crucial, as the reaction could follow an intravenous or intramuscular injection of a drug in about 15 minutes. In North America, death due to anaphylaxis shock following a bee sting, or to exposure to a drug such as penicillin, may occur in as many as 4,000 people annually.

The foregoing are 2 kinds of Type I or anaphylactic sensitivity: atopic reactions usually limited to the mucous membranes of the upper respiratory tract, but sometimes also involving the skin and systemic reactions (anaphylaxis).

Type II—Cytotoxic

The second general type of allergic reaction is an antibody-dependent cytotoxic reaction, in which an antigen, when introduced to the body, binds to either red blood cells, leukocytes, or platelets. Alternatively, blood cells from another person may be transfused into someone, and, as you know, these cells already have antigens on their surface. Antibody against these cells is formed, which subsequently complexes with antigen, complement is fixed, and the blood cells with immune complexes on their surfaces are lysed. The effect of this phenomenon depends on the type of cell being destroyed as well as on the severity of the allergic reaction. If the antibody is located on red cells, red cells will be destroyed, leading to hemolysis, jaundice, and anemia. If leukocytes are involved, the result may be an increased susceptibility to infection, whereas the result of antiplatelet antibodies will be thrombocytopenia and hemorrhagic manifestations (Fig. 6–18).

Cytotoxic reactions have been seen occasionally with penicillin therapy. The drug becomes attached to the red-cell membrane. Antibodies are formed that complex with the drug, complement is activated, and the red cell is destroyed.

The same principle is involved when a patient is given a transfusion of mismatched blood (this is not a hypersensitivity reaction; the immune system is merely acting normally to destroy foreign material). In a mismatched transfusion, the donated blood cells are recognized as foreign; they have antigens on the cell's surface against which the host has antibodies. For example, a person with Type A blood has A antigens and anti-B antibodies. If he is transfused with Type B blood, the anti-B antibodies will complex with B antigens on the surface of the donor's blood cells and will cause hemolysis of the donor's cells. A large amount of blood breakdown products will soon accumulate in the body and result in jaundice or even in the accumulation of red blood cell casts in renal tubules, which can lead to acute renal shutdown.

Symptoms of such a transfusion reaction are restlessness, anxiety, flushing, chest or lumbar pain, tachypnea (rapid breathing), tachycardia (rapid heart rate), and nausea. These symptoms may be shortly followed by shock and renal failure.

There are other instances of this same type of reaction: Rh incompatibility (Fig. 6–19), autoimmune hemolytic anemia, and Goodpasture's syndrome, to mention some.

Type III—Complex-Mediated Hypersensitivity

Immune complexes can produce disease when they are deposited in the walls of blood vessels. The immune complex (antigen-antibody) activates complement and attracts neutrophils in the normal manner. The reactions that follow destroy the cells in the immediate vicinity, in this case the endothelial cells of the vessel wall.

There are both systemic and local versions of this process. The local reaction occurs principally in the presence of antibody excess, the systemic reaction generally with antigen excess.

Maurice Arthus showed that rabbits that had been hyperimmunized and had developed high levels of precipitating antibody reacted violently to the **intradermal** injection of soluble antigen. This resulted in a large, red, swollen reaction that reached the maximum size about 6 hours after the injection. Histology of this area shows an intense infiltration with polymorphonuclear leukocytes. Special studies show antigen, antibody, and complement all within this lesion, which often is accompanied by thrombosis and necrosis of the vessel walls (Fig. 6–20). This whole process can be blocked by remov-

exposure to antigen

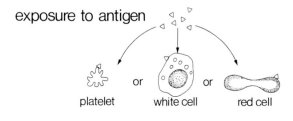

platelet   white cell   red cell

antibody formation

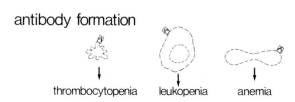

thrombocytopenia   leukopenia   anemia

Fig. 6–18. The cytotoxic reaction. In the Type II reaction only 1 exposure to the antigen is necessary. The antigen attaches itself to the surface of a circulating blood cell, then when antibody is formed and complexes with the antigen, complement is activated and the host cells are destroyed. Which type of disease results depends on the particular blood cells that are destroyed.

pregnancy 1

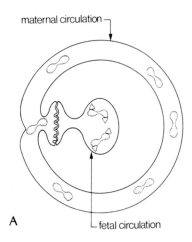

maternal circulation

fetal circulation

A

immediately after birth of first baby

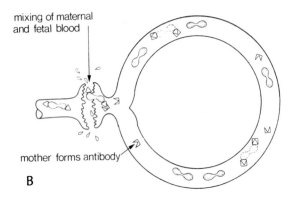

mixing of maternal
and fetal blood

mother forms antibody

B

births 2,3,4, etc.

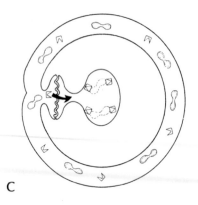

C

Fig. 6–19. *A,* An illustration of a Type II or cytotoxic immune reaction involving Rh antigens. In this disease, the mother is Rh negative (i.e., has no Rh antigen), and the father is Rh positive (i.e., his red blood cells have Rh antigen on the surface). The fetus has inherited the Rh antigen from his father. Normally maternal and fetal blood do not mix; rather the placenta allows capillaries from both systems to come into close contact so that nutrients, oxygen and fetal wastes can pass across the capillary walls from one circulation to the other. Therefore, the fetal Rh antigen is contained within the fetal circulation. *B,* At birth, mixing of maternal and fetal blood may occur as the placenta breaks away. Should the Rh antigen enter the maternal system in this way, the mother will recognize the Rh antigen as foreign and will form anti-Rh-antibody, which will destroy any fetal red blood cells in her system. Her first child is safe, since he or she has already been born, because the full-blown maternal immune response does not occur until 2 weeks after childbirth. *C,* However, if her next child is also Rh positive, there will be problems. The mother will still have some anti-Rh-antibody in circulation, which she may continue to produce at a low rate. This antibody is small enough to cross through the placental capillary system and into the fetal circulation, where it will destroy fetal red blood cells. Thus the second child will be anemic at birth. The plight of the third child will be worse, because the maternal response increases every time. The fourth child may die *in utero.*

The treatment for this condition is simple. The mother and her baby are blood-typed when the baby is born. If Rh incompatibility is found, then the mother is given a dose of anti-Rh-antigens. This removes the Rh antigen from her system before she mobilizes her own immune response. A few weeks later, the donated Rh antibody is also cleared from the system. When the next child is conceived, the mother's immune system has no recollection of an Rh antigen, since she has never produced it herself.

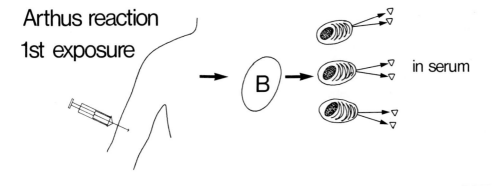

Arthus reaction
1st exposure

B

in serum

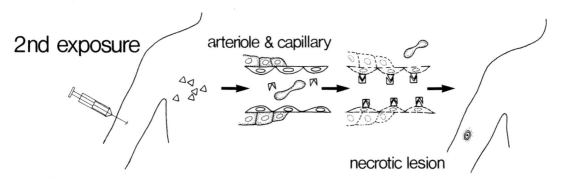

2nd exposure

arteriole & capillary

necrotic lesion

Fig. 6–20. This diagram illustrates an Arthus reaction. Antibodies are formed when a small amount of antigen is introduced into the body. The antibodies attach themselves to the capillary endothelium at the spot where the antigen was injected. The next exposure to antigen produces immune complexes that lead to the destruction of endothelial cells by the host's own immunologic defense.

ing complement or polymorphonuclear leukocytes from the serum of the experimental animal before the injection of the challenging antigen.

Similar types of reaction may be initiated by the inhalation of antigen, as in the case of poultry breeders who are sensitized by years of exposure. When challenged by the dust raised during cleaning of the chicken coop, an acute attack of wheezing and respiratory embarrassment can take place. This has been reproduced many times in experimental animals and is also the explanation for Farmer's lung, an attack occurring after a farmer is exposed to the spores and antigens from moldy hay.

A local sensitivity may also occur in the skin when a foreign protein is injected subcutaneously many times during 1 or 2 weeks. At first

there is no reaction, as in the case of most vaccinations or of a dose of insulin, but there are many instances in which the injection of vaccines or antibiotics may bring about extensive necrosis and gangrene. This reaction can be avoided if a skin test with a dilute amount of the substance is done first.

The local reaction, which begins within an hour of the injection and reaches a peak by 12 to 24 hours, is characterized by destruction of the capillary, arteriolar, and venular walls with hemorrhage, fibrinoid necrosis, and thrombosis. We believe that the cause of this lesion is the precipitation of antigen-antibody and of complement in the vessel walls. On first exposure to the antigen, antibody is formed and is deposited along the capillary wall in the area of injection. The next injection of antigen leads to antibody-antigen complexes, and to complement fixation. The antigen/antibody/complement complex is chemotactic to polymorphonuclear leukocytes and brings many of these cells to the site where the liberation of their enzymes increases the further destruction. To aggravate the situation further, the immune complexes are able to trigger the coagulation factors that lead to the observed thrombosis.

Serum Sickness. No previous exposure is necessary for this reaction, which occurs only in the presence of antigen excess. The symptoms appear about 10 days to 2 weeks after passive immunization with horse serum (e.g., horse tetanus antitoxin). Antigens in the horse serum evoke antibody synthesis, which leads to the formation of immune complexes (Fig. 6–21). These complexes circulate throughout the body and are deposited at various points in the blood vessels of the skin, joints, and kidneys. Complement is activated at these sites, neutrophils arrive, and tissue destruction commences as in the previous example. (Substances other than horse serum have been known to cause this disease, e.g., penicillin.)

Type IV—Cell-Mediated Reactions (Tuberculin Hypersensitivity)

The first 3 types of toxic immune reactions discussed are mediated by **soluble** antibody. The fourth type is mediated by the T lymphocytes and involves essentially the same mechanisms as the protective response of T cells. This reaction takes at least 12 hours to develop. It does not occur in persons without a thymus, and it is characterized by the presence of macrophages and lymphocytes rather than of polymorphonuclear leukocytes (because of the cellular response, the reaction is frequently referred to as "delayed hypersensitivity").

Poison ivy, contact dermatitis, eczema, and the tuberculin reaction are all examples of this type of allergy. Testing with patches containing the allergen usually defines the specific material to which one is sensitive because of the reddening, weeping, blisters, and hyperplasia of the epidermis that result after topical exposure (Fig. 6–22).

Many persons are hypersensitive to such foods as oysters, fish, strawberries, pork, cereals, eggs, and milk. In these persons, a

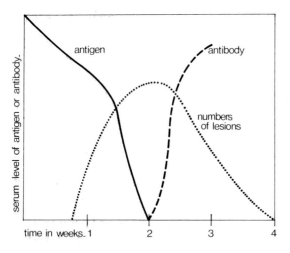

Fig. 6–21. This diagram illustrates the immune response to radioactively labeled antigen in immune AgAb complex disease. Circulating AgAb complexes can be measured about a week after injection of antigen. With the appearance of these immune complexes, the clinical and histologic manifestations of the disease develop.

When the number of immune complexes decreases, lesions begin to heal. This evidence, along with demonstration of the complexes in the lesions themselves, implicates immune complexes as a cause of Arthus reactions and of serum sickness. (Adapted from Sell, S.: Immunopathology (hypersensitivity diseases). In *Pathology*, 7th Ed. Edited by W. A. D. Anderson and J. M. Kissane. St. Louis, C. V. Mosby, 1977.)

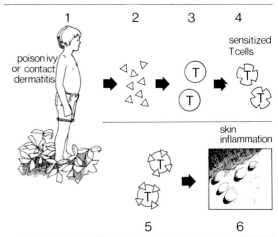

Fig. 6–22. This diagram illustrates cell-mediated hypersensitivity. Contact with poison ivy allows the antigen to enter the skin where it evokes a T-cell response. T cells are sensitized by the antigen, and then interact with it to cause dermatitis.

small amount of the food in question may produce an immediate attack of vomiting and diarrhea accompanied by collapse, of urticaria and other skin eruptions, or of asthma. The fault lies in the person, not in the food, clearly illustrating that "what is one man's meat is another man's poison." The search for the article at fault may tax the detective powers of the physician to the utmost. It may be found by means of skin tests, or even more reliably by elimination of one article after another from the diet. It should be realized, however, that food allergy is rare in the adult.

Hypersensitivity to plant poisons is a common affliction. Such plants as poison ivy, poison oak, and the genus *Primula* (primrose family) may set up a severe inflammation of the skin (*dermatitis venenata*) when the sensitive person touches the leaves. Even the smoke of burning poison ivy can bring about the same result. It often happens that florists develop hypersensitivity only after they have been handling plants of the genus *Primula* for many years, a fact that suggests induced rather than natural hypersensitivity.

Studies have shown that the cell-mediated delayed type reactions depend on the intact thymus. Lymphocytes that arise in the paracortical area of the lymph node are responsible for this type of reaction, whereas the humoral immunity depends on the integrity of the germinal follicle of lymph nodes and on the presence of structures analogous to the bursa of Fabricius in man.

Few classification schemes neatly contain every existing piece of biologic data, and the attempt to classify immunologic reactions presented here is no exception. Many clinical examples of hypersensitivity cannot be easily fitted into any one of these classes. For example, hypersensitivity to insulin among diabetics does not readily fit into a single category.

Allergic reactions to insulin form one of the most complicated examples of medicine. Without insulin, the patient is severely diabetic and incapacitated; with insulin, he or she may uncommonly have a local or even a systemic allergic reaction. Fortunately, the art of the allergist has ways to resolve the dilemma. Since the allergy is most often due to contaminants of the insulin injection, several

steps can be taken. The first is to use purer preparations of insulin to avoid the noninsulin impurity. There are several degrees of purity, depending on the preparative methods. A second step is to use antihistamines locally, and a third step in the management of this reaction is to desensitize the patient by lowering the dose of insulin to about 20% of the present dose and only gradually increasing it. Anaphylactic or systemic reactions to insulin, as to any foreign substance, are fortunately rare, but the local reactions are bothersome enough.

TRANSPLANTATION

The replacement of a failed organ (kidney, liver, heart) by a donated new organ has become a medical fact despite technical and immunologic barriers to its success. Each of us is so special that we normally recognize and reject the tissues of another person when they are introduced into our body. We refuse to accept the foreign tissue and usually produce antibodies against it. An inflammatory reaction rejects the transplant.

Many early insights resulted from P. B. Medawar's work arising from his interest in skin grafts of burned patients. He showed that whereas the first graft might be tolerated for a few weeks, a second graft was rejected in a much shorter time. Of course, this did not happen with grafts of the patient's own skin (autograft), but grafts from other species (xenografts) were always rejected, as well as grafts from other human beings.

The graft survives better if the donor and recipient are related. One study of renal transplants illustrated this fact by showing that 60% of kidneys donated by siblings, 50% of those donated by parents, and 30% of cadaver kidneys remained functional after 5 years.

A failed skin graft illustrates the rejection process. First the graft becomes vascularized as part of normal healing. Then it becomes heavily infiltrated with lymphocytes, macrophages, and plasma cells, so that within a week it becomes dark, hard, and thick. After 2 weeks the blood flow through the graft stops suddenly, resulting in thrombosis and necro-

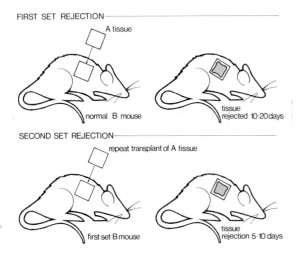

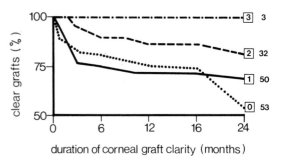

duration of corneal graft clarity (months)

Fig. 6–24. This figure shows the influence of HLA (human leukocyte antigens) matching on duration of corneal graft success. The boxed numbers represent the numbers of HLA antigens shared by both donor and recipient. The numbers of patients studied are shown in unenclosed numerals to the right of the boxes. When a corneal graft is rejected, it becomes cloudy. The grafts where HLA antigens are in common are most successful, whereas those grafts in which no HLA matching exists, or where only one HLA antigen is shared, show a different failure rate than those where 2 or more HLA antigens are shared. (From Morris, P.J., Batchelor, J.R., and Festenstein, H.: Matching for HLA in transplantation. Br. Med. Bull., 34:259, 1978.)

Fig. 6–23. Skin graft rejection. When skin from A mouse is grafted onto B mouse, B rejects the tissue within 10 to 20 days. The next time skin is grafted from A to B, rejection occurs in half the time, which shows that memory of the first contact has been retained. (Adapted from Barrett, J.T.: *Basic Immunology and Its Medical Application.* St. Louis, C. V. Mosby, 1976.)

sis. Finally it is shed as a dark, dry scab (Fig. 6–23).

Examination of rejected grafts shows many lymphocytes and macrophages as well as thrombosis of the blood vessels in a full-thickness graft. The vascular lining (endothelium) of a successful graft is usually derived from the host's blood vessels. The grafts that are rejected early frequently fail because of thrombosis and occlusion of their blood vessels, particularly if the graft is a kidney.

If a second graft from the same donor is placed on the same recipient at a later date, the graft will be rejected in only a few days, as opposed to 3 weeks. It will not even become vascularized. This is known as "second set" rejection, and seems to be mediated by humoral antibody, whereas the first set is mediated by T cells. Fortunately for clinical transplantation, not all grafts are rejected, and some are rejected less vigorously than others. The vigor with which a graft is rejected depends on the histocompatibility of the donor and the recipient (Fig. 6–24). This term refers to the degree of similarity of donor and recipient antigens, or to the literal compatibility of donor and recipient tissue.

There appear to be 2 antigen systems that

play major roles in histocompatibility. The first is the ABO blood group system. Donor-recipient pairs must be matched for blood type in accordance with the usual rules for blood transfusions (i.e., Type A recipients require Type A donors). The second group of antigens is called human leukocyte antigens (HLA antigens), which, as the name suggests, are present on white blood cells, but are also present on all nucleated cells to various degrees. Each person inherits 4 HLA antigen types from each parent, and so has a total of 8 HLA types. For obvious genetic reasons, there is a greater probability that siblings will carry the same antigens and therefore will have more compatible tissue. Thus the degree of histocompatibility is determined by the number of HLA antigens that the donor and recipient share (as well as by ABO blood type). This degree, in turn, is reflected in the strength of the immune rejection response produced by the recipient. The link between a person's HLA type and his ability to elicit a specific pattern of antibody response correlates with the fact that the genes responsible for the 2 functions are closely situated on the same chromosome.

The presence of varying frequencies of HLA antigen types has recently been linked with many diseases. It has been observed that persons suffering from certain diseases have the same particular HLA combinations. Thus the HLA system appears to serve as a genetic marker, an indication that someone may be susceptible to a certain disease. This idea has been discussed in Chapter 3, and we shall return to it later in our discussion of genetics.

Much tissue transplantation between different persons is considered to be of questionable value because of the problem of rejection. However, in certain instances, transplantation has proved to be invaluable. Autogenous transplants in man are of course most desirable, and these are used in skin grafts. Heterologous transplants have also proved to be of great use, particularly in cases of bone, fascia, nerves, blood vessels, and the cornea of the eye. In these instances, we are using not the cells, but the **intercellular substance** of the transplant. Even though antibodies may destroy the cells, the intercellular substance acts as a scaffold on which the cells of the host are able to build a new structure. This is particularly well illustrated in arterial transplants, which provide a temporary skeleton on which a new vessel can be constructed.

IMMUNE SUPPRESSION

It is sometimes desirable to suppress the immune response. This is done after transplantations, in the hope that the recipient will accept the graft, and in instances where disease is produced by immune mechanisms (see autoimmune disease). The immune response can be suppressed by radiation, chemotherapy, and the use of corticosteroids. Radiation and chemotherapy destroy the lymphocyte population by interfering with cell replication, which prevents formation of specifically sensitized T cells and antibody. Corticosteroids suppress the inflammatory response in general.

The risk when immunosuppressive agents are used is that ordinary bacteria and fungi, which are normally successfully handled by the body, may cause infection. Such infections are referred to as **opportunistic**, since they have seized the chance to gain access to the weakened host.

AUTOIMMUNE DISORDERS

The idea of being allergic to oneself seems strange, and yet the idea that the body may react to certain of its own tissues in an adverse way has been clearly demonstrated. However, the problem related to the concept of autoimmune disease is that we are not sure whether the so-called autoantigen has been previously damaged by some injury that has changed its structure from self to "slightly nonself." Autoimmune diseases may be defined as diseases **that result from antibodies or immune cells produced by the host that react with some of that host's own antigens**. The antigens may be in the serum or in the cells of a particular tissue, such as the thyroid gland. To be scientific about the concept, criteria to establish that a particular disease is of autoimmune etiology have been proposed:

Criteria for Autoimmune Disease

1. The antigen in question should be present in the affected tissues, and the lesions should show round cells and immunoglobulin in the affected tissue.
2. Antibodies that react with these antigens should be present in all cases of this disease.
3. The disease can be passively transferred to normal persons or to animals with cells or serum of the affected host.
4. The disease should have the appearance typical of allergic disorders and should respond to anti-inflammatory drugs such as corticosteroids.

Some examples of autoimmune diseases are given in Tables 6–8 and 6–9.

To summarize, we have outlined the features of the immune system and have discussed some disorders that are clearly of allergic rather than of infectious or other etiology. Currently, the pendulum has swung far in the direction of explaining many additional diseases of the reticuloendothelial system, the endocrine glands, the bowel, the liver, and central nervous system, as all being disorders of the immune system. In some instances, there are good grounds for this designation (Hashimoto's disease), whereas in others, the evidence is scanty (Crohn's disease). For those who are hearing about disease for the

Table 6–8. Spectrum of Autoimmune Disease

ORGAN-SPECIFIC ← ————————————————————————————— → NONORGAN-SPECIFIC

Hashimoto's thyroiditis	Goodpasture's syndrome	Autoimmune hemolytic anemia	Primary biliary cirrhosis	Systemic lupus erythematosus (SLE)
Primary myxedema	Myasthenia gravis	Idiopathic thrombocytopenic purpura	Active chronic hepatitis HB_s-ve	Discoid LE
Thyrotoxicosis	Juvenile diabetes	Idiopathic leukopenia	Cryptogenic cirrhosis (some cases)	Dermatomyositis
Pernicious anemia	Pemphigus vulgaris			Scleroderma
Autoimmune atrophic gastritis	Pemphigoid		Ulcerative colitis	Rheumatoid arthritis
Addison's disease	Sympathetic ophthalmia		Sjögren's syndrome	
Premature menopause (few cases)	Phacogenic uveitis			
Male infertility (few cases)	(?? Multiple sclerosis ??)			

(Goodpasture's syndrome, Myasthenia gravis, Juvenile diabetes are bracketed together.)

(From Roitt, I.: *Essential Immunology*. 3rd Ed., Oxford, Blackwell Scientific Publications, 1977.)

Table 6–9. Some Autoimmune Diseases

DISEASE	ANTIGEN	LESION
Autoimmune hemolytic anemia	Red blood cells	Erythrocyte destruction
Hashimoto's thyroiditis	Thyroglobin	Infiltration of thyroid by lymphocytes and plasma cells, destruction of follicular cells and germinal cells
Pernicious anemia	Intrinsic factor	Blocking antibody prevents binding of vitamin B_{12} to intrinsic factor. B_{12} is necessary for red blood cell maturation (see Chap. 3)
Systemic lupus erythematosus	DNA, nucleoprotein, blood clotting factors, IgG	Systemic disease. Widespread lesions of connective tissue in skin, kidney glomeruli, joints, serous membranes, and blood vessels
Myasthenia gravis	Skeletal and heart muscle acetylcholine receptor	Blocks neuromuscular transmission leading to muscle weakness
Rheumatoid arthritis	IgG	Local Arthus reaction in synovial tissues and fluid leading eventually to joint destruction

first time, listen with a critical ear to the claims that a particular disease of uncertain cause is of an immunologic etiology. The most important message of this chapter is that not all inflammation is caused by physical, chemical, or biologic (in the sense of bacterial, viral, or protozoal, for example) injury, but rather that the interaction of antigen and antibody can serve as a potent agent for tissue destruction.

SYNOPSIS

Response to antigen depends on macrophages, which are nonspecific, and immunocytes, which react specifically with an antigen.

Immunocompetent cells are of 2 types: B cells, which secrete antibody, and T cells. Passive transfer of maternal immunity to fetus occurs *in utero* and lasts for a short time after birth.

Antigen and antibody combine to form immune complex. This triggers several mechanisms, one of which is complement fixation.

After a single exposure to an antigen, the host recognizes and destroys it faster the next time. This is the anamnestic response.

Hypersensitivity refers to the altered state of reactivity that is destructive rather than defensive.

Systemic anaphylaxis is a massive allergic response that involves widespread change in capillary permeability that leads to shock and respiratory distress.

A cytotoxic allergic reaction causes destruction of cells in the blood or tissue.

Immune complex disease involves thrombosis and necrosis of small blood vessel walls either locally or systemically.

Cell-mediated hypersensitivity is a delayed allergic reaction in which T cells interact with antigen to cause inflammatory lesions in the skin.

Terms

Immunity	*Lymphatic tissue*	*Atopy*
Sensitization	*Immune complex*	*Cytotoxic*
Tolerance	*Complement*	*Delayed hypersensitivity*
Autoimmunity	*Anamnestic response*	*Transplantation*
T cells	*Active/passive immunization*	*Rejection*
B cells	*Anergy*	*Immunosuppression*
Antigen	*Hypersensitivity*	*Arthus reaction*
Antibody	*Anaphylaxis*	

FURTHER READING

Austen, W.G.: Heart transplantation after ten years. N. Engl. J. Med., *298*:682, 1978.

Beer, A.E., and Billingham, R.E.: Transplantation in nature. Perspect. Biol. Med., *22*:155, 1979.

Bowman, J.M., and Chown, B.: Prevention of Rh immunization after massive Rh-positive transfusion. Can. Med. Assoc. J., *99*:385, 1968.

Burnet, F.M.: Autoimmune disease. I. Modern immunologic concepts. II. Pathology of the immune response. Br. Med. J., *2*:645, 729, 1959.

Good, R.A., and Yunis, E.: Association of autoimmunity, immunodeficiency and aging in man, rabbits and mice. Fed. Proc., *33*:2040, 1974.

Guttmann, R.D.: Renal transplantation. N. Engl. J. Med., *301*:975, 1038, 1979.

James, L.P., Jr., and Austen, K.F.: Fatal systemic anaphylaxis in man. N. Engl. J. Med., *270*:597, 1964.

Mayer, M.M.: Complement, Past and Present. (The Harvey Lectures, Series 72.) New York, Academic Press, 1978.

Patterson, R., Zeiss, C.R., and Kelly, J.K.: Classification of hypersensitivity reactions. N. Engl. J. Med., *295*:277, 1976.

Roitt, I.: *Essential Immunology*, 3rd Ed. Oxford, Blackwell Scientific Publications, 1977.

Russell, P.S., and Winn, H.J.: Transplantation. N. Engl. J. Med., *282*:786, 1970.

Schwartz, R.S.: Another look at immunologic surveillance. N. Engl. J. Med., *293*:181, 1975.

Bacterial Infections

7

The bacterium is nothing, the soil is everything—Pasteur

One bacterium gives rise to hundreds of millions in the course of 24 hours, provided the conditions are suitable, i.e., food, moisture, and temperature. This enormous increase is possible under laboratory conditions because reproduction is not a complicated process; 1 bacterium simply divides into 2. Bacteria are so small they cannot be seen with the naked eye, but only with the oil immersion lens of the light microscope. When stained with chemical dyes they can be seen to vary in size and shape, and have been divided into 3 groups: **cocci**, which are round, **bacilli**, which are rod-shaped, and **spirilla**, which are, as the name implies, spiral.

Typically, pneumonia is caused by a coccus, tuberculosis by a bacillus, and syphilis by a spirillum. Diplococci grow in pairs, staphylococci in clusters like grapes, streptococci in long or short chains. Bacteria are named according to the disease they produce, but new and more complex nomenclatures have replaced the old. What was once called *Bacillus tuberculosis* is now known as *Mycobacterium tuberculosis; Bacillus typhosus* is now called *Salmonella typhi*. New names have been attributed to the cultural requirements of the organisms, or to the appearances of the organisms in culture media. Fortunately, some bacteria (staphylococci, streptococci) have escaped this renaming process. For our purposes, we shall use the common and important names.

When a microorganism invades tissues or a host, 1 of 3 things may happen: 1. The bacterial invader may die, which is most likely. 2. The microorganism may survive without giving rise to disease, but may cause an immune reaction in the host, which short-circuits subsequent infections. 3. Exceptionally, the microorganism survives, multiplies, and produces clinically apparent disease that may prove fatal not only to the host, but often, necessarily, to the microorganism.

Although bacteria may be the living form responsible for many of man's afflictions, these small organisms are also responsible for many good things in our lives. Bacteria derive their sustenance from already dead materials, whether plant or animal. Their role is to return the complex elements of living forms to a simpler, elemental nature. Thus the floor of the forest, littered with leaves, is rendered to humus by millions of bacteria. Other bacteria play more specific roles, such as those that are able to capture nitrogen in its gaseous form and affix it in an organic form, from which it can be converted eventually into protein. We use different terms to define the different roles of bacteria. Bacteria that live on dead materials are called saprophytes, whereas those that live on living material are known as parasites.

Physicians tend to be preoccupied with disease-producing (pathogenic) bacteria and are apt to forget that most bacteria are harmless, if not beneficial. We can go so far as to say that without bacteria life would long ago have ceased on this planet, for they keep the building blocks of metabolism in circulation. Bacteria prepare the substrate for plants, which in turn are eaten by animals. Without bacteria, the nitrogen cycle would come to a full stop and the existence of all higher forms of life would be impossible. It used to be thought that life in animals and in man was impossible without the presence of bacteria, particularly those in the bowel. We now know this is not true because various forms of life (birds and mammals) have been raised in germ-free environments. It is interesting, in the light of the previous chapter, to remark on

Table 7–1. Predominant Microbial Species Found in Various Human Anatomic Regions

REGION	MICROORGANISM	% INCIDENCE
Skin	Staphylococcus epidermidis	85 to 100
	Staphylococcus aureus	5 to 25
	Propionibacterium acnes	45 to 100
Nose and nasopharynx	Staphylococcus epidermidis	90
	Staphylococcus aureus	20 to 85
	Hemophilus influenzae	12
Mouth and tooth surfaces	Staphylococcus epidermidis	75 to 100
	Staphylococcus aureus	Common
	Streptococcus mitis and other alpha-hemolytic streptococci	100
	Lactobacillus	95
	Actinomyces israeli	Common
	Hemophilus influenzae	25 to 100
	Bacteroides fragilis	Common
	Fusobacterium nucleatum	15 to 90
	Candida albicans	6 to 50
	Borrelia vincentii	Common
Ileum	Distal portion may have small numbers of Enterobacteriaceae and anaerobic gram-negative bacteria	
Large intestine	Gram-negative bacilli:	100
	Bacteroides fragilis	
	Fusobacterium nucleatum	
	Gram-positive bacilli:	20 to 60
	Lactobacillus	25 to 35
	Clostridium perfringens	
	Enterococcus (group D streptococcus)	100
	Escherichia coli	100
	Klebsiella spp.	40 to 80
	Enterobacteriaceae	40 to 80
	Proteus spp.	5 to 55
	Candida albicans	15 to 30
Vagina and uterine cervix	Bacteroides spp.	60 to 80
	Clostridium spp.	15 to 30
	Staphylococcus epidermidis	35 to 80
	Candida albicans	30 to 50
	Trichomonas vaginalis	10 to 25

(Adapted from Pelczar, M., Jr., et al.: *Microbiology*, 4th Ed. New York, McGraw-Hill, 1977.)

what happens to animals brought from a germ-free to a normal environment. All guinea pigs die of overwhelming infection within 48 hours; 50% of mice also die, but rats and chickens show no ill effects.

Many regions of the body are normally inhabited by bacteria (see Table 7–1). Occasionally, when a host's defenses are weakened, or when these bacteria leave their natural habitat and migrate to another part of the body, where they are less welcome, disease develops. These bacteria are called opportunistic microorganisms, because they cause trouble only when the opportunity arises. Table 7–2 shows the types of opportunistic and other infections known to occur when host resistance is compromised.

Outside the body it is easy enough to kill bacteria by means of agents that are capable of denaturing their protein, or of interfering with their metabolism. It is much more difficult to do so in the living body because substances, such as carbolic acid, that kill the bacteria are injurious to body cells. Specific treatment that attacks bacteria without injuring body cells has developed only in the last 40 years. Modern antibiotics such as penicillin and streptomycin have been prepared from fungi in the soil and can kill bacteria *in vitro* with startling rapidity. In the living body they may not do this directly, but they prevent bacteria from multiplying, thus giving the defenses of the body time to mobilize

and attack the invaders. We speak of **bacterio-static** agents and of other antibiotics that are **bacteriocidal.** It is true, in addition, that antibiotics that kill unwanted bacteria may also kill those useful inhabitants of the intestine. Bacterial overgrowth by more pathogenic organisms may lead to greater complications.

The effects of bacteria are achieved principally by enzymes directly secreted into the immediate bacterial environment. Bacterial enzymes break down complex food materials—whether protein, carbohydrate, or fat—into amino acids or peptides and short chains of carbon and acetic acid. These substances can be assimilated and used by the bacteria. The enzymatic activity in the intestine results in the decomposition of the organic material that has been ingested. As we have said, decomposition returns to the soil those elements that can be used in the next cycle of growth. Intestinal bacteria have been called nature's fertilizer factory. Bacteria serve also outside the body to purify sewage and to make it inoffensive, as in a compost heap. Many essential vitamins such as the B complex are formed by the bacteria in the large intestine of man, and are then used by him.

The activity of bacteria is manifest in various ways. Fermentation of carbohydrates results in the production of gas and acid, which are used by the professional microbiologist to identify certain bacteria, and by the industrialist in the manufacture of alcohol, vinegar,

Table 7–2.   Infections in the Compromised Host

	MAJOR DEFECTS	ETIOLOGIC AGENTS	INFECTIONS
Burns	Tissue necrosis, loss of epithelial barrier, lymphocytopenia	*Streptococcus pyogenes* *Staphylococcus aureus* *Pseudomonas*	Cellulitis Bacteremia Pneumonia
Diabetes	Reduced vascular supply, decreased leukocyte chemotaxis	*Staphylococcus aureus* *Candida* Enteric bacilli *Mycobacterium tuberculosis*	Cellulitis Urinary tract infection Bacteremia
Thermolytic disease	Reduced monocyte-macrophage function	*Salmonella* *Streptococcus pneumoniae*	Bacteremia Pneumonia Osteomyelitis Meningitis
Cystic fibrosis	Bronchial obstruction by hyperviscous mucus	*Staphylococcus aureus* *Pseudomonas*	Bronchitis Pneumonia

(From Thorn, G.W., et al. (Eds.): *Harrison's Principles of Internal Medicine,* 8th Ed. New York, McGraw-Hill, 1977.)

cheese, and many good things. Pasteur was first drawn to the study of bacteria by his work on the fermentation of wine. The breakdown of proteins (proteolysis) into simpler substances, some of which smell foul, is achieved by the enzymes of anaerobic bacteria. The decomposition of dead tissue is an example of proteolysis. Toxin production varies from bacteria to bacteria. Comparatively few bacteria produce exotoxins, that is, poisons excreted by the living bacteria. Diphtheria bacillus and the clostridia group of spore-bearing, gram-positive bacilli are examples. The organisms of tetanus, gas gangrene, and botulism, 3 members of the clostridia group, illustrate the variation in action and types of exotoxin. Tetanus bacilli grow under anaerobic conditions (without air) in dead tissue, and there produce an exotoxin that causes no local inflammatory reaction, but rather passes along the course of the peripheral nerves to the central nervous system. There it causes catastrophic clinical results, but still without apparent tissue damage. The organisms of gas gangrene, on the other hand, produce profound and widespread local damage in wounds by means of their enzymes. Finally, the bacilli of botulism do not need to live in the tissues of the host, but

proliferate in insufficiently sterilized canned goods. There they elaborate one of the most deadly poisons known, which kills swiftly when ingested. When an exotoxin is treated with formaldehyde, it no longer causes disease when injected, but confers immunity. Such a modified toxin is called a **toxoid**. Toxoids are used more particularly for protection against diphtheria and tetanus. Practically all bacteria contain endotoxins, which are liberated when the bacteria die and disintegrate. Examples are the gram-negative intestinal bacilli.

Spread of Infection. Different pathogenic or disease-producing bacteria have different portals of entry to the body. Some may be introduced through the skin, but most enter through natural passages. Some prefer the respiratory passages, others the alimentary or the genitourinary tracts. Some are discharged from the body in feces and urine, others by the mouth, nose, respiratory tract, saliva, and even the blood by means of insect bites. Knowledge and appreciation of these routes are necessary if the spread of infection is to be prevented. When an infection is transmitted intentionally through a series of laboratory animals, the **virulence** is likely to be increased, probably because the bacteria adapt

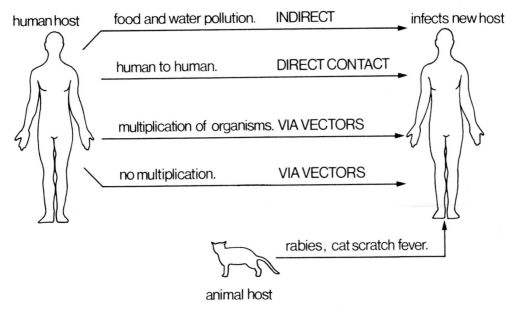

Fig. 7–1. Transmission of pathogenic microorganisms from person to person occurs in a variety of ways, ranging from direct contact, to fomites, and by intermediate vectors. Animals may also transmit pathogens to humans. (From Pelczar, M., Jr., et al.: *Microbiology.* 4th Ed. New York, McGraw-Hill, 1977.)

themselves to their environment. The same thing is seen in human epidemics, in which virulence increases until a peak is reached, followed by a decline, perhaps because only the resistant members of the community remain to be infected. There are 4 principal methods of spread: (1) physical contact, (2) air, (3) food and water, and (4) insects or other vectors (Fig. 7–1).

PHYSICAL CONTACT. The contact may be direct, the infecting bacteria not surviving outside the body; the classic example is venereal disease. The contact may also be indirect, through **fomites,** that is to say, clothing, utensils, and other possessions of the patient, the bacteria surviving for some time outside the body.

AIRBORNE INFECTION. Bacterial and viral infections of the respiratory tract are transmitted through the air by dust or droplets. Dust infection comes from bacteria in dried sputum that become attached to dust particles; this is

particularly true of tuberculosis. Droplet infection is the basis of epidemics of upper respiratory disease. It is estimated that 20,000 droplets containing possible pathogens may be expelled by one sneeze, and that droplets 1 mm in diameter may pass over a distance of 15 feet. Were it not for natural and acquired defenses we might all be ill.

FOOD-BORNE INFECTION. This constitutes an important public health problem (Fig. 7–2). The possibility of infection by food or water must be considered in every major epidemic of intestinal disease. Epidemics of typhoid, dysentery, and cholera are due to infection of food or water.

INSECT-BORNE INFECTION. Insects are important conveyors of infection, not only bacterial, but also viral and protozoal. Thus plague is spread from the rat to man by the rat-flea, typhus by lice, and yellow fever virus and the malaria parasite by mosquitoes. It is obvious how necessary is a knowledge of the spread of

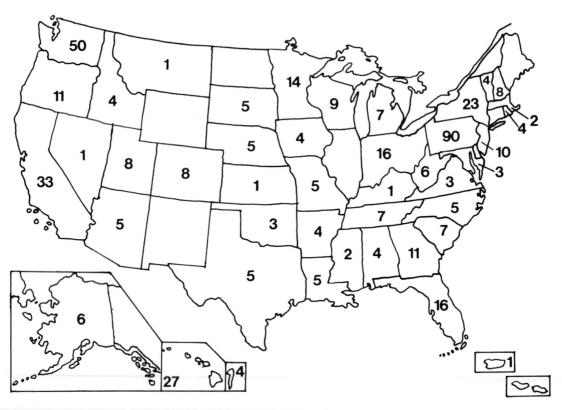

Fig. 7–2. This map shows the reported food-borne and water-borne disease outbreaks in 1974. (Insets illustrate, left to right, Alaska, Hawaii, Guam, Puerto Rico, and Virgin Islands.) These outbreaks affected 15,489 persons in 44 States, Puerto Rico, the District of Columbia, and Guam. The numbers are the numbers of such outbreaks in each state. (Adapted from Center for Disease Control: Foodborne and waterborne disease outbreaks, annual summary, 1974. Atlanta, United States Public Health Service, 1976.)

infection by insects if some of the great scourges of the tropics are to be controlled.

Diagnostic Methods. It might be thought that it would be a simple matter to determine the bacterial agent causing a given disease. In some cases this is easy, but in others it may be extremely difficult. Robert Koch established the criteria necessary to justify the assumption of an etiologic relationship in 1881. These 4 criteria have long been known as **Koch's postulates.**

Koch's Postulates

1. The suspected organism must always be present in the lesion.
2. It must be grown in pure culture on laboratory media.
3. It must cause the same disease when injected into a susceptible animal.
4. It must be recovered from the experimental animal.

The most notable of the many contributions that Koch made to bacteriology was his demonstration of the true cause of tuberculosis, for in the space of a year he: demonstrated the tubercle bacillus in the lesions by special staining, grew the bacilli on a medium that he invented, reproduced the disease by injecting the culture into suitable laboratory animals, and recovered tubercle bacilli from these animals. Such conclusive proof of the bacteriologic cause of disease is not always possible, but it serves as a model for outlining the causal relationships in any disease. Thus Koch outlined a philosophically sound basis for establishing the etiology of any disease.

Special stains and cultural characteristics are of value in recognizing and classifying certain bacteria. The aniline dye, methylene blue, will stain most bacteria satisfactorily, but 2 special methods are invaluable. The first of these is **Gram's stain**, in which the film is stained with gentian violet followed by iodine, and then decolorized with alcohol and counterstained. Bacteria that resist the decolorization and so remain stained blue are said to be **gram-positive**; those that are decolorized by the alcohol, but are shown up by a counterstain of a different color, are said to be **gram-negative**. This method is indispensable in routine laboratory work, for it separates bacteria, both cocci and bacilli, into 2 great groups. The second method is **acid-fast staining**. The term "fast" is taken from a German word meaning resistant. Bacilli that resist decoloration with acid after being stained red with hot carbol fuchsin are said to be

acid-fast. The reader will appreciate that acid-fast corresponds to gram-positive; in the former, acid is used as the decolorizing agent, in the latter, alcohol. The only important members of the acid-fast group are the bacilli of tuberculosis and of leprosy. There are many other special stains, but these 2 are mentioned because we refer frequently to acid-fast bacilli and to gram-positive and gram-negative organisms in the course of this chapter.

Cultural characteristics are also important in determining the nature of an infection. The 4 requirements for successful culture are food, temperature, moisture, and oxygen. Food is represented by the culture medium. Some media suit some types of bacteria; other media, such as those containing hemoglobin, are better for other types. Moisture is essential, because water is as vital to bacteria as to all other forms of life. It is for this reason that a swab of infective material must never be allowed to dry out in its passage from the bedside to the laboratory by being left lying around. The temperature best suited for pathogenic bacteria is usually that of the body to which they are accustomed, so that the incubator in which the media are placed is kept at 37°C (98.4°F). Oxygen, represented by air, is required for growth by most bacteria; they are said to be aerobic. Some can live with or without air. An important group are peculiar enough to demand absence of air for continued growth; they are therefore called anaerobic bacteria or anaerobes, and the laboratory technique must be regulated accordingly. To this group belong the spore-bearing bacilli that live in soil that has been fertilized by manure, and infect wounds contaminated with such soil, the most important being the bacillus of tetanus and the bacilli that cause gas gangrene.

In summary of the diagnostic aspects of bacterial infections, we may say that an immediate laboratory diagnosis of the nature of the infective agent has become of prime importance, so that appropriate antibiotic therapy may be started at the earliest possible moment. The first step is gram-staining of the smears, which allows a preliminary classification before the final culture and sensitivity tests become available. An exact bacteriologic diagnosis is far more necessary than formerly because microorganisms respond so differently to different chemotherapeutic agents.

Host Reactions to Bacteria. Different bacterial pathogens produce widely differing lesions. Some are focal, others diffuse; some evoke acute inflammatory response, others are granulomatous, and so on. A general idea of the types of the infecting agent may be gathered from a consideration of the character and histologic appearance of the lesions (Table 7–3), but absolute certainty can only come from such bacteriologic techniques as staining the organisms in smears or tissue, growing them in culture, reproducing the disease in an animal, or demonstrating the presence of antibodies by appropriate serologic methods.

Suppurative lesions are produced in most cases by one or another of the pus-forming (pyogenic) cocci. When the suppuration remains localized, the lesion forms an abscess, with necrosis of tissue and collections of polymorphonuclear leukocytes. Diffuse suppuration spreading through the interstitial tissue without abscess formation (cellulitis) is more likely to be caused by hemolytic streptococci. **Granulomatous inflammation** is characterized by a reaction composed of both

Table 7–3. The Syndrome Approach to Infection

TYPE OF INFECTION	COMMON ETIOLOGIC AGENT
Skin and subcutaneous tissue	*Staphylococcus aureus*
Sinusitis	*Streptococcus pneumoniae* *Staphylococcus aureus*
Pneumonitis	*Streptococcus pneumoniae, Mycoplasma pneumoniae Mycobacterium tuberculosis*
Bacterial endocarditis	*Streptococcus viridans Staphylococcus aureus*
Gastroenteritis	*Salmonella, Shigella* Enteric viruses
Peritonitis, cholangitis, intra-abdominal abscess	*Escherichia coli,* enterococcus *Bacteroides,* anaerobic streptococcus
Urinary infection	*Escherichia coli, Klebsiella*-Enterobacter *Proteus,* enterococcus
Meninges	*Streptococcus pneumoniae Hemophilus influenzae Neisseria meningitidis* Various viruses

(Adapted from Thorn, G.W., et al. (Eds.): *Harrison's Principles of Internal Medicine,* 8th Ed. New York, McGraw-Hill, 1977.)

round cells and giant cells. The classic example is, of course, tuberculosis.

Changing Picture of Infection. Under normal conditions, life in the bacterial world is a constant competition for survival. If the local environment becomes unfavorable, the power to mutate or to bring latent enzyme systems into play becomes apparent. Modern conditions, particularly the widespread and often unnecessary use of antibiotics, have greatly exaggerated this tendency. In the Toronto General Hospital, resistant strains of *Staphylococcus aureus* rose from 6% in 1947 to 60% 4 years later. We were faced with a situation in which our hospitals were filled with carriers of antibiotic-resistant strains of staphylococci ("hospital staph"). These strains were present in the nose and throat of both patients and staff, and the distance between the nose of a surgeon and a surgical wound is very short. The incidence of penicillin-resistant staphylococci was much higher in hospital inpatients than in outpatients, and it was still lower in the general population.

A chemotherapeutic agent can displace the normal harmless flora of the throat, which is soon replaced by intestinal bacteria, also harmless in their proper habitat. In the new environment, however, they may cause serious local infections and may even invade the blood stream. It is indeed a paradox that the more an antibiotic is used (or abused) in a hospital community, the less valuable it becomes. As we have already seen so frequently, what is potent for good can be powerful for evil, and the wonder drugs may become harbingers of death (Table 7–4).

We must not suppose that this changing picture of bacterial infection is a new thing. The incidence, character, and severity of microbial diseases change from one generation to another, probably owing to changing environmental conditions, to the development of immunity in the population, or to the introduction of prophylactic measures, such as vaccination against smallpox and toxoid inoculation against diphtheria. In such cases we may turn for an explanation to the natural tendency to mutation in the rapidly recurring generations of bacteria. *The Andromeda Strain*, Michael Crichton's science fiction novel, is

Table 7–4. Infections in Compromised Host: Iatrogenic

	MAJOR DEFECTS	ETIOLOGIC AGENTS	INFECTIONS
Glucocorticosteroids	Decreased cellular immunity Decreased chemotaxis	*Staphylococcus aureus* Enteric bacilli Some viruses *Candida*	Cellulitis Bacteremia Pneumonia
Cytotoxic drugs	Neutropenia Monocytopenia Lymphopenia	Enteric bacilli *Candida* *Pseudomonas*	Bacteremia
Antibiotics	Colonization by resistant bacteria	*Staphylococcus aureus* *Pseudomonas* *Serratia*	Superinfections
Prosthetic devices	Foreign body	*Staphylococcus aureus* Enteric bacilli *Candida*	Abscesses Bacteremia

(From Thorn, G.W., et al. (Eds.): *Harrison's Principles of Internal Medicine,* 8th Ed. New York, McGraw-Hill, 1977.)

based on this premise. Leprosy practically disappeared in England during the sixteenth century. Long before the modern era of chemotherapy, syphilis had changed its character profoundly, and the mortality rate from tuberculosis had fallen steadily since 1945. It would appear that the changing picture of infection, although partly man-made, is also partly natural. We must admit, however, that the majority of fatal infections used to be produced by streptococci, staphylococci, and tubercle bacilli, originating in apparently healthy persons outside a hospital. Now the commonest culprits are gram-negative bacilli, staphylococci, viruses, and fungi.

Lest the picture presented in the foregoing paragraph be too depressing, we may recall that of the children born in London between 1762 and 1771, two-thirds died before the age of 5 years. This was in the century called the Age of Reason. There was certainly no danger of an exploding population. At the same period and in the same country, Queen Anne had 12 pregnancies, but not 1 child survived. Improved living conditions and, in particular, improved sanitation altered this picture significantly. (Until the mid-nineteenth century the water supply to the city of Vienna ran though the municipal cemetery, which allowed the dead to infect the living.) Modern antibacterial therapy has also contributed greatly to human survival.

STAPHYLOCOCCAL INFECTIONS

The staphylococcus is a gram-positive organism that grows in small clusters like a bunch of grapes. There are 2 principal forms, *Staphylococcus aureus* (golden) and *Staphylococcus albus* (white), depending on the color of the colonies on solid media. The white form is always present on the skin and is usually, though by no means always, harmless. It is usually the cause of the stitch abscesses of the skin that sometimes follow a surgical operation.

The staphylococcus is a pyogenic organism, a pus-producer, and is a common cause of acute inflammation. It enters the body through cracks in the skin, often as a result of local irritation. The mere pricking of a pimple may start the infection. In contrast to streptococci, the staphylococcus usually produces inflammation that remains localized. Some staphylococci produce an enzyme, coagulase, which causes a marked formation of fibrin from the fibrinogen of the plasma. The coagulase-positive organisms are more dangerous, because the film of fibrin protects them from the action of antibodies and antibiotics. The presence of this enzyme is a reliable criterion of virulence. It must be admitted that the fibrin tends to limit the spread by blocking paths of dissemination. Some strains of staphylococci produce a "spreading factor," hyaluronidase, which markedly increases the permeability of the tissues. Certain strains can form an extremely powerful exotoxin in culture.

We must always remember that staphylococci are normal inhabitants of the body. They have been called the jackals of the microbial parasitic world, usually unable to mount an attack against the healthy body, but ready to invade the tissues when resistance is lowered by other disease states.

The chief lesions may be external or internal. External lesions occur in the following places: (1) **Skin pimples** are staphylococcal infections in the surface layer of the skin; **boils** are in the deeper layer; and a **carbuncle** is a large collection of pus in the subcutaneous tissue that communicates with the surface by several openings. **Infected wounds and stitch abscesses** are caused by staphylococci. (2) Boils on the upper lip and nose are of especial importance, as the infection is apt to pass back along the facial vein (which has no valves) into the cavernous venous sinus in the base of the skull, with a resulting **thrombophlebitis**, a condition of grave danger. (3)

On the eyelid staphylococci may cause a **stye**. Internal lesions take the form of abscesses principally in the bones (osteomyelitis) and kidneys. Some persons are subject to repeated staphylococcal infections, particularly boils, and recurrent infections suggest that there may be some lack of normal defense mechanisms. Certain strains of staphylococci produce a toxin that is a common cause of food poisoning. A classic case of this disease is illustrated in Figure 7–3.

STREPTOCOCCAL INFECTIONS

The streptococcus is a gram-positive organism identical in appearance with the staphylococcus except that it grows in chains of varying length instead of in clusters. It is more difficult to grow than the staphylococ-

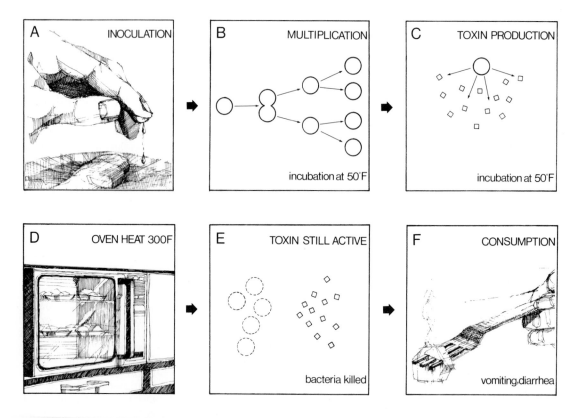

Fig. 7–3. An outbreak of staphylococcus food poisoning on an international jet flight. *A,* A cook preparing ham and omelet breakfasts for an international flight has blisters on 2 fingers that are infected with staphylococci. The cook handles at least 205 portions of ham, which are kept at room temperature for 6 hours during preparation of the food trays. *B* and *C,* The contaminated food trays are stored overnight at 50°. Staphylococci multiply at temperatures over 40°, and as they multiply they produce a toxin that is a common cause of food poisoning. *D* and *E,* The food trays are loaded onto the plane. In 6 to 7 hours, they are heated in 300° ovens for 15 minutes, treatment that cannot inactivate the toxin. *F,* The passengers are served. From 2 to 6 hours later, those who ate the contaminated food begin to experience staph food-poisoning symptoms: nausea, vomiting, cramps, and diarrhea.

cus, and flourishes best on media enriched with blood (blood agar).

Streptococci can be divided into 2 groups, depending on the reaction on blood agar. In the first group, **hemolytic streptococci**, the bacteria cause hemolysis or breaking down of blood in the medium, so that colonies are surrounded by a colorless halo. In the second group, the bacteria produce a green color on the blood agar. This group is called *Streptococcus viridans*. The hemolytic group causes more acute and virulent infections than the viridans group. Nevertheless, *Streptococcus viridans* is an important cause of disease. It gives rise to focal or limited infection in the tonsils, at the roots of teeth, in the sinuses of the nose and face, and in the valves of the heart, where it causes bacterial endocarditis, a condition that used to be uniformly fatal.

The habitat or natural home of the streptococcus is the mucous membrane of the respiratory and intestinal tracts. It is found less often on the skin. It tends to produce spreading inflammation that extends widely throughout the tissues in comparison with the circumscribed lesions caused by the staphylococcus. This power of infiltration seems to depend largely on the power to produce fibrinolysin and hyaluronidase. **Fibrinolysin** prevents the formation of fibrin and tends to dissolve any that has formed, thus eliminating the fibrin barrier to the spread of infection. **Hyaluronidase** is the enzyme that digests hyaluronic acid, the mucopolysaccharide of the ground substance that forms a natural obstacle in the interstitial compartment.

Some of the most widespread infections, such as septicemia and peritonitis, are caused by streptococci. It is the commonest cause of puerperal sepsis, the frequently fatal infection that used to follow childbirth. Most cases of septic throat, tonsillitis, and ear infection are due to streptococci.

Streptococcal infections may start in 2 different ways: (1) Cocci already present on the mucous membrane may invade the underlying tissue owing to some lowering of resistance. It is in this way that tonsillitis, streptococcal pneumonia, and appendicitis may be produced. (2) Virulent streptococci may be introduced from outside the body through the skin or mucous membrane. It is in this way that a surgeon's hand may be infected while operating on a septic case, or that the uterus may be infected owing to lack of care during or after delivery.

Two manifestations of streptococcal infection are of so special a character that they merit separate descriptions; they are erysipelas and scarlet fever. Two others, namely rheumatic fever and glomerulonephritis, are sequelae not caused by the *Streptococcus pyogenes* directly, but representing an immunologic response. The first 3 will be described here, and the last will be discussed in connection with diseases of the kidney.

Erysipelas. This is an acute, spreading inflammation of the lymphatics of the skin caused by hemolytic streptococci with marked rash-producing power. The usual site is the face or scalp, the bacteria probably entering from the nose. The inflamed skin is of a bright red color and curiously firm. Like other streptococcal and staphylococcal infections, erysipelas is accompanied by fever and leukocytosis.

Scarlet Fever. This is an acute streptococcal fever characterized by a high temperature, sore throat, and a widespread rash, often followed by complications in the ear, kidneys, and lymph nodes of the neck. The throat is always actively inflamed, and this is probably the starting point of the infection, which may spread along the eustachian tube (the communication between the throat and the ear) and cause acute inflammation of the ear. The lymph nodes of the neck are swollen and sometimes abscesses are formed in them. The tongue shows a rash similar to that of the skin, so that it has a strawberry appearance.

The symptoms are caused by the erythrogenic toxin of the streptococcus. When this toxin is injected into the skin, and a red area appears in the course of a few hours, the patient has no natural antitoxin in his blood, i.e., he is susceptible to scarlet fever. In early childhood nearly everyone shows a positive reaction, but with increasing years the number of persons susceptible steadily decreases, since most persons are exposed to infection too slight in degree to cause the disease, but sufficient to stimulate the formation of antibody. These infections are called **subclinical**, and are the most frequent type of infection, especially in polio, tuberculosis, and infectious hepatitis.

Rheumatic Fever. This acute inflammation principally affects the joints and the heart, and is accompanied by sore throat. It may be regarded as a complication of infection with group A hemolytic streptococci, usually located in the throat or tonsils. These bacteria are not found in the organs attacked by rheumatic fever, such as the joints and the heart. Because high antibody titer to a surface antigen of streptococcus (ASO) can be shown in the serum, we believe that **these organs have become hypersensitive or allergic to the streptococci or its product**. It is not clear why the heart and serous membranes of the joints or blood vessels in the brain are the targets of injury, and it is even more mysterious why the heart valves (mitral and aortic) should become scarred 20 years after the acute episode.

We cannot explain why only a few persons show the rheumatic response to streptococcal infection, and why 75% of the cases occur in children, or at least before the age of 20 years. There appear to be several unknown factors. The incidence of rheumatic fever parallels in a striking manner the incidence of hemolytic streptococci in the throat. Both are common in cold, damp climates, but rare in many parts of the tropics.

The most striking and obvious **clinical feature** in rheumatic fever is acute inflammation of the **joints**, which become tender; the slightest movement of the joint produces excruciating pain. The inflammation is not a suppurative one; there is little destruction of tissue, and when the infection subsides the joints return to their normal condition. The acute joint symptoms such as swelling and pain are greatly relieved by the use of anti-inflammatory salicylates, which are practically a specific remedy for this infection.

The same is not true, however, of the **heart**. During the acute illness there may be no evidence of any cardiac lesion, but months or years later symptoms of these lesions may make their appearance. Both the heart valves and the heart muscle are attacked, but the lesions need not be described here in detail, as they will be considered in connection with diseases of the heart. The characteristic microscopic lesion is the Aschoff body, marked by fibrinoid necrosis and collections of large chronic inflammatory cells. It is evident that the heart lesions of rheumatic fever are much more serious than the joint lesions, although it is the latter that first claim the attention of the patient and the doctor. For this reason, an important element in the treatment of rheumatic fever is bed rest, so that the affected heart may have every chance of recovering to the greatest extent possible. Moreover, in some persons, particularly in children, the inflammation in the joints may be so slight that the disease is not diagnosed as rheumatic fever, yet the heart may be seriously affected. Patients with rheumatic heart disease may therefore give a history of repeated sore throats, but not of the acute joint pains. For all this the truth of the saying becomes apparent that "**rheumatic fever licks the joints, but bites the heart.**"

Treatment of rheumatic fever consists of a combination of skilled nursing and drug therapy. During an attack of acute rheumatic fever, damage may occur to the heart valves and to the heart muscle, and may progress unrecognized at first. During the period in which any activity of the rheumatic process is suspected, the patient should be kept at rest in bed until the signs of the acute stage are past. This may require many weeks or months. The use of salicylates, and of cortisone, during this acute phase relieves the symptoms and may prevent some of the progress of the disease. Fortunately, with early treatment of streptococcal sore throats, acute rheumatic fever and its long-term complications, mitral and aortic valve disease, are becoming rare.

PNEUMOCOCCAL INFECTIONS

The pneumococcus is a gram-positive diplococcus surrounded by a polysaccharide capsule. It is a pyogenic organism, with a marked ability to excite the formation of fibrin. The chief lesion produced is lobar pneumonia, in which pulmonary alveoli are filled with an exudate composed mainly of polymorphonuclear leukocytes and fibrin. Other lesions caused by pneumococci are endocarditis, pericarditis, peritonitis in children, meningitis, and middle-ear infections.

LEGIONNAIRE'S DISEASE

Another pneumonia of current interest came into prominence during the summer of 1976 when many persons who were attending a convention of the American Legion in

Philadelphia were stricken by a serious and frequently fatal (15%) respiratory illness. Epidemiologic work since the outbreak has identified the organism responsible, a previously unidentified gram-negative bacillus that can be propagated in embryonated egg yolk sacs, and has been designated *Legionella pneumophila*.

This organism seems to thrive in warm, moist places; the current and previous outbreaks occurred between June and November in the northern hemisphere, and have been traced to cooling towers or evaporative condensers, or to exposure to cleaning such equipment. Although there are different types of *Legionella pneumophila*, the availability of serologic diagnostic methods has made it possible to diagnose other epidemics of respiratory illness retrospectively. An epidemic of a two- to five-day acute febrile illness in Pontiac, Michigan, of 144 people who worked, paradoxically, in a county health department building, was shown to be due to this organism. Two other similar outbreaks, one in St. Elizabeth's Hospital, Washington, D.C., and another in Spain, were both so identified.

Clinical Pattern. The disease has an incubation period of 2 to 10 days and appears with malaise, headache, and muscular aches and pains, without previous upper respiratory tract illness. A nonproductive cough, with chest pain and sometimes vomiting, diarrhea, and delirium are often present. Patients have ranged in age from 10 to 84 years, with a median age of 55 years. Males seem to outnumber females 3:1. Chest films show patchy, multilobar involvement with consolidation, and pleural effusions are frequent. Fortunately, erythromycin seems to be effective in treating the disease. In this sophisticated age, it is a wonder that a disease caused by a hitherto unknown bacterium has been discovered.

MENINGOCOCCAL INFECTION

We now turn to the gram-negative neisseria. The 2 members of the group that concern us are *Neisseria meningitidis* and *Neisseria gonorrhoeae*. They resemble each other morphologically as closely as the proverbial 2 peas. In addition to being gram-negative, they are bean-shaped diplococci with the convex surfaces opposed. Both the meningococcus and the gonococcus are found in large numbers within the polymorphonuclear leukocytes of pus, an environment in which, unfortunately, they seem to flourish.

The **meningococcus** is a normal inhabitant (commensal) of the nasopharynx, and in times of epidemic 90% of persons in a crowded army camp may be carriers. It does not grow readily on culture media. The meningococcus is sensitive to sulfonamides and a wide range of antibiotics, and it is pleasant to learn that, unlike the case of the staphylococcus, acquired resistance is unknown. The bacteriologic diagnosis of meningococcal meningitis is made by examining the **cerebrospinal fluid**, obtained by lumbar puncture, for the tell-tale gram-negative intracellular diplococci. The cerebrospinal fluid bathes the central nervous system and therefore shares any inflammation of the superficial layers. The disease used to be frequently fatal, but modern antibiotic therapy has entirely altered the prognosis. The lesions and clinical features of meningococcal meningitis are described in the chapter on the nervous system.

GONOCOCCAL INFECTION

In physical appearance and staining characters, the gonococcus is identical to the meningococcus. It is harder to grow in culture than the meningococcus. When allowed to dry, it dies immediately when removed from the body. The gonococcus is a complete parasite living on a human host; it does not live in the body as a harmless commensal. With these facts in mind it is surprising that the gonococcus manages to hold its place in the natural world, but that it does succeed is only too evident.

Gonococcal infection is a venereal disease, transmitted through sexual intercourse. The initial site of infection is the mucous membrane of the anterior urethra in men, and the urethra, vaginal glands, and cervix in women. Once the gonococcus reaches the male or female genital tract, it makes itself at home. The initial process is an acute suppuration developing in a few days after infection, with a copious discharge of pus loaded with intracellular gonococci. If prompt and effective treatment is given, the discharge disappears like magic and the infection clears up.

The untreated case is a different matter. The inflammation becomes chronic, spreads upward, and is followed by fibrosis. This leads to stricture of the urethra and stenosis of the vas deferens in men, causing sterility, whereas in women the fallopian tubes are closed and converted into bags of pus, with sterility again a frequent result.

The treatment of gonorrhea is an important public health problem. When the sulfonamides were first introduced, the gonococcus proved to be so susceptible that it seemed as if the disease might be completely eliminated, especially since the organism is unable to live outside the body. Soon, however, most strains became resistant. Penicillin took the place of the sulfonamides with complete success, but again the sad story of resistant strains was repeated. Then came streptomycin, but the gonococci proved as resourceful as ever. Yet they had once again

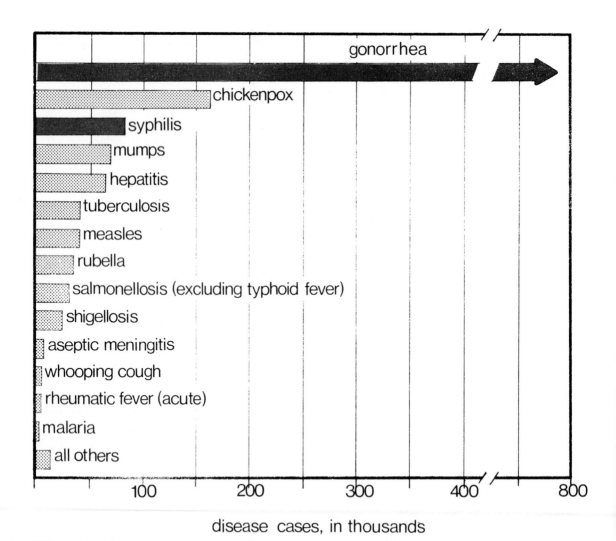

Fig. 7–4. The striking importance, in numbers of cases, of sexually transmitted diseases as compared with other communicable diseases is illustrated in this chart published by the United States Public Health Service. About 800,000 cases of gonococcal infections were reported in 1973 in the United States. (From United States Public Health Service.)

become sensitive to the sulfonamides. And so the battle of attack and defense continues with varying fortunes (Fig. 7–4).

DIPHTHERIA

The diphtheria or Klebs-Löffler bacillus (*Corynebacterium diphtheriae*) is a thin gram-positive bacillus, often slightly curved. It stains irregularly with methylene blue, some parts appearing dark while others remain light; for this reason the bacilli may have a granular appearance. There is apt to be pleomorphism, i.e., variation in structure, and some of the bacilli may have an expanded end, giving an Indian-club appearance. The bacilli are easily stained and easily grown in culture within 24 hours. Löffler's blood serum (solid) is the standard medium for this purpose. Under the microscope the bacilli present an arrangement that suggests a box of split matches.

Unlike many of the other pathogenic bacteria, the diphtheria bacillus does not invade the tissues of the patient. It remains on the surface of the mucous membrane of the throat and produces a powerful exotoxin, which kills the cells with which it comes in contact. It also excites a plentiful production of fibrin. The dead or necrosed cells are not shed off, but are bound together by the threads of fibrin to form a tough, leathery layer known as the false or **pseudo membrane**, so called because it is not a natural or true membrane of the body (Fig. 7–5). The name diphtheria is from the Greek meaning leather. Sometimes the nose and, rarely, the ear, conjunctiva, and even wounds may be affected. In each of these instances a diphtheritic (false) membrane is formed, which is swarming with bacilli. The incubation period is from 2 to 7 days.

The danger to the patient is twofold: (1) he may die of suffocation owing to the false membrane's obstructing the air-passages, especially the glottis; (2) the toxin may be absorbed into the blood and cause damage to either the heart or the peripheral nerves.

Infection may be spread directly from person to person, or indirectly by infected articles such as cups, handkerchiefs, and even books. Direct infection may be from a patient,

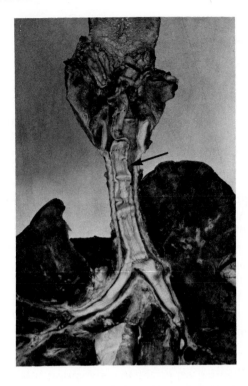

Fig. 7–5. This photograph shows the membrane (at arrow) lining the trachea and bronchus in a case of diphtheria. This membrane is composed of fibrin and polymorphonuclear leukocytes and is sufficiently large to obstruct the airways. Today, immunization against diphtheria makes such a lesion exceedingly rare. (McGill University, Department of Pathology Museum.)

but often it is from a healthy carrier, i.e., a person carrying diphtheria bacilli in the throat, but not suffering from the disease; often, indeed, he has never had a previous clinical attack, but has established a complete immunity, presumably from a subclinical infection.

Immunity against diphtheria may be natural or artificial. About 85% of nursing babies have natural immunity which comes from the mother. This immunity disappears after 8 months. Most children are therefore susceptible, and 80% of the deaths used to occur in children under 5 years of age. Susceptible children can be immunized by means of diphtheria **toxoid**. This diphtheria toxin has been rendered harmless by the addition of formalin. The immunity is of variable duration, but usually lasts for several years. These procedures are of value both for persons who have been exposed to infection and for children during an outbreak of diphtheria.

WHOOPING COUGH

Also known as **pertussis**, this disease is caused by a minute gram-negative bacillus, which is found in great masses entangled in the cilia of the bronchial mucosa. It is known as *Hemophilus pertussis* because it belongs to the group of hemophilic bacilli, so named since they require hemoglobin for growth in the culture medium.

This disease has largely disappeared in North America today owing to the universal practice of immunization with **DPT** or diphtheria, pertussis, and tetanus vaccine.

As with diphtheria, it is children who are in danger. About 33% of the cases and 90% of the deaths occur in children under 3 years of age.

The disease used to come in periodic epidemics, especially in early spring and late summer.

TUBERCULOSIS

This disease is a chronic, destructive inflammation caused by *Mycobacterium tuberculosis*, and is one of the most widespread of all diseases. It is particularly prevalent among peoples who live under crowded conditions in which droplet infection is facilitated, and in people who are debilitated through malnutrition or other causes. However, it is seen frequently in all ages, sexes, and all economic groups. The lesions may be small and self-limited, and the presence of the infection may only be demonstrable by means of laboratory tests, but it is there nonetheless. It is evident that the natural defensive power of the body against tuberculous infection is sufficiently great to hold it in check in the majority of instances of exposure. This defense may be broken down on the one hand by an infection such as influenza, which undermines the health, by overwork, by poor hygienic conditions, or by insufficient food, and on the other hand by a fresh, overwhelming dose of tubercle bacilli. The long-continued use of cortisone, as prescribed for rheumatoid arthritis, may not only disguise the symptoms, but may also depress resistance and activate the disease.

The **tubercle bacillus** is a thin, curved rod with a waxy coat that does not grow on ordinary culture media. It can be stained in a specific way, being colored red by carbol fuchsin and retaining the color after treatment by acid, which removes the color from other bacteria (acid-fast). Another example of an acid-fast organism is the bacillus of leprosy. On account of its waxy sheath the tubercle bacillus is an exceptionally hardy germ. It may live outside the body for months.

Immediate diagnosis is made by direct microscopic examination of the infected material (e.g., sputum, urine) rather than by culture, as is done with most bacteria, because the bacilli do not grow readily on culture media and several weeks may need to elapse before the colonies can be seen. Inoculation of a susceptible animal such as a guinea pig is of great value, but again several weeks must pass before the animal develops evidence of the disease.

There are 2 forms of tubercle bacilli, the human and the bovine, the latter causing disease in cows as well as in man. The organisms are identical under the microscope, but can be differentiated by special culture methods and by the inoculation of animals.

Tuberculosis used to head the list of the killing diseases, so that Osler called it the "Captain of the Men of Death." During the nineteenth century, man slew on the battlefield 19 million persons, but during the same period the tubercle bacillus slew 34 million. The disease is steadily becoming less common as well as less dangerous, and in most communities tuberculosis sanatoriums are closed for lack of patients. These facts must not breed a spirit of false complacency, for it is estimated that at the present time there are 30 million infected persons in the United States, and that 2 million of them will develop active tuberculosis in their lifetime. It used to kill the young adult; now it is often seen in the aged. The reduction in the tuberculosis rate is due to the following factors: (1) improved social living conditions with better nutrition, fresh air, and sunlight; (2) education in hygiene, so that people lead more healthful lives as regards exercise and fresh air; (3) segregation of the sick in sanatoriums and destruction of tuberculous sputum; (4) earlier seeking of medical advice; (5) improved methods of treatment; (6) improved case finding by population surveys, chest roentgenograms; and (7) vaccination of high-risk populations, such as nurses and medical students, with Bacille-Calmette-Guerin vaccine (BCG).

Routes of Infection. In trying to prevent a disease, it is essential to know the route of infection. In the case of tuberculosis, infection may occur in a number of ways.

1. By Inhalation. The most likely source of infection from man is the sputum of a patient with active tuberculosis of the lungs. The bacilli may be inhaled from sputum that has dried and has been changed into dust. The bacilli are soon killed by sunlight, but may survive a long time in the dark. When a patient with pulmonary tuberculosis coughs, he infects the air in the immediate neighborhood with millions of tubercle bacilli contained in tiny drops of moisture. It has been estimated that a moderately advanced case may expel from 2 to 4 billion bacilli in 24 hours. These figures give some idea of the infectivity of such a patient. Inhalation of sputum is probably the most important method of infection in the adult, for the "dose" of bacilli will be much larger than in the case of inhaled dust, and a large dose has much to do with breaking down the resistance of the exposed person. It is evident how vitally important it is to instruct the patient with pulmonary tuberculosis how to behave so that he will not be a source of danger to those with whom he comes in contact. Attention to certain rules of hygiene, which are also rules of polite behavior, such as coughing into a handkerchief and never expectorating on the floor, remove some of the danger from living in close contact with a patient suffering from active tuberculosis. The technique of prevention, however, must be as unremitting and relentless as the similar technique in an operating room. Bacilli may also be inhaled from the mouth into the lungs in minute droplets of fluid. It is probable that many children become infected through the introduction of bacilli into the mouth by contaminated hands followed by inhalation into the lungs. The danger to a child crawling about the floor on which tuberculous sputum has been expectorated is self-evident. The principal methods of infection are then by inhalation (e.g., dust, droplet) or ingestion.

2. By Swallowing. Children may readily acquire tuberculosis by drinking infected cow's milk. Here the bacillus is of the bovine type, and the lesions are naturally abdominal, either in the bowel or in the abdominal lymph nodes. However, the nodes in the neck may also be infected by bacilli passing through the tonsils. The amount of infection with the bovine tubercle bacillus in a community depends on the strictness of the milk inspection. The importance of the rigid sanitary control of milk supplies to children is obvious.

3. Through the Skin. Although this method is rare, it is important to the laboratory technician and the nurse, because the disease may be acquired through the handling of infected material. A warty lesion develops on the hand, and the infection may spread up the arm to the lymph nodes in the axilla.

Pathogenesis. The tubercle bacillus may invade the blood stream. The infection may spread in 3 ways: (1) **Through the tissues**. In the organ infected, unless the defense forces gain mastery, the disease gradually spreads until the greater part of that organ is destroyed. (2) **By the lymphatics**. The bacilli tend to spread from the site of infection along the lymphatic vessels to the lymph nodes that drain the part, where they set up tuberculous disease. Thus the nodes in the neck are infected from the tonsil, the nodes in the chest from the lung, the abdominal nodes from the bowel. (3) **By the blood stream**. A tuberculous lesion may perforate the wall of a vessel and discharge millions of bacilli into the blood stream. These are arrested in every organ in the body, where they cause the formation of numberless minute lesions the size of a pin's head; these are called miliary tubercles and the condition is known as generalized miliary tuberculosis. In addition to this massive infection, occasional bacilli may enter the blood stream and set up a single tuberculous focus in one organ such as kidney or bone, causing collapse.

Lesions. Tuberculosis is a chronic inflammation. The characteristic cell of the inflammatory exudate is the macrophage, which becomes changed in character so that it has a swollen pale body and indefinite outlines. These characteristics are due to the fact that the fatty envelope of the bacillus is dissolved and taken up by the cells, which in their new form are called **epithelioid cells** (epithelial-like) and are the most characteristic single feature of the tuberculous reaction (see Chap. 5). The bacilli are surrounded by a mass of these cells, which are actively phagocytic. Sometimes a number of epithelioid cells fuse together to form a large **giant cell**, with as many nuclei as there are cells in its formation. Further out there is a zone of

lymphocytes, also called small round cells. There is none of the dilation of blood vessels nor exudation of serum that is so characteristic of acute inflammation, and for this reason the heat and redness of acute inflammation are also absent.

The collection of inflammatory cells around the clump of tubercle bacilli forms a little mass that becomes visible to the naked eye and is called a **tubercle** or **miliary tubercle** (Latin *milium*, a millet seed). This is the standard lesion of tuberculosis, and is found in whichever organ the disease occurs, be it lung, kidney, or brain. Indeed, it is the tubercle that originally gave the disease its name. As the bacilli spread throughout the organ, large numbers of tubercles are formed, and these grow ever larger, fuse together, and thus come to form extensive tuberculous areas.

Meanwhile a further change takes place in the center of the tubercle. The cells are killed by the bacilli, undergo necrosis, and finally lose all vestige of structure and fuse together to form a cheesy mass, which is called caseous (cheesy) material, the process being known as **caseation**. In the course of time the caseous material may become liquefied, so that a cavity or cavities are formed in the organ, or the material may calcify.

Any organ of the body may be involved by tuberculosis. It is exceptional, however, for more than 1 or 2 organs to be attacked at the same time, except in miliary tuberculosis. Although a bone such as the femur must necessarily be infected from the blood stream, it is nevertheless unusual for other bones to be involved in the same case. It is difficult to give a satisfactory explanation for this behavior.

The lungs and pleura are most frequently attacked, and pulmonary disease accounts for 85 to 90% of all deaths from tuberculosis. Lymph nodes come next, most often those in the hilum of the lung, less frequently the abdominal nodes. Tuberculosis of the larynx is a serious form, secondary to pulmonary tuberculosis. The intestine may be the seat of tuberculous ulcers, due in children to the drinking of infected milk, in adults to the swallowing of tuberculous sputum. The bacilli may spread from these ulcers to the peritoneum and may cause tuberculous peritonitis. Tuberculosis of the kidney is not uncommon. It tends to spread down to the bladder, and in men it may infect the prostate and the testes (see Fig. 20–25). In women, the fallopian tubes are often infected, a condition known as tuberculous salpingitis. The bones and joints are often involved, especially in children; in the spine the condition is called Pott's disease. Tuberculous meningitis is the most fatal form, although antibiotic therapy has now greatly changed the former gloomy picture. Other organs may also be attacked, but the aforementioned are the most common.

The microscopic picture in tuberculosis is characteristic and readily recognized, but it must be borne in mind that a histologic diagnosis of the disease has its limitations.

Possible Outcome. Tuberculosis is a fight in which the forces of attack and defense, of destruction and conservation, are usually evenly balanced. **The outcome depends on 2 main factors: the resistance of the tissues and the size of dose of the bacilli.** If the resistance is good and the dose small, there is a proliferation of fibrous tissue around the tubercle that limits the spread of the infection and eventually invades the tubercle and converts it into a mass of scar tissue known as a healed tubercle. This process of encapsulation and scarring is seen particularly well in the lung, and may occur even when the tuberculous area is of considerable size. Tuberculous scars are commonly found at the apex of the lung, and these scars often contain calcium, which is deposited in the caseous material as healing occurs, and which can be detected in the roentgenogram. Healing of the tuberculous lesion is by far the most common outcome.

When the dose of bacilli is larger, or the resistance of the patient is lowered, the disease tends to progress slowly, but fibrous tissue is continually forming, so that the destruction of tissue is gradual, and the process may be halted after it has lasted for a long time. Halting, however, is not synonymous with recovery, and unless the patient pays strict attention to the rules of hygiene, the process may light up again, with recurrence of the severe symptoms. The patient is, metaphorically, sitting on a barrel of gunpowder, and he must not forget that fact.

Finally, the infection may be overwhelming and resistance may be at a minimum. In these cases there is almost pure destruction with practically no attempt at limitation; the disease rages like a fire throughout the lung, huge cavities are formed, and the patient dies in the course of a few weeks or months. These are the cases that used to be popularly and justifiably known as galloping consumption. The fatal outcome of pulmonary tuberculosis was often due to rupture of the lesion into a vein or artery and hemorrhage into the lung. The tragic heroine, Camille, of A. Dumas, died in such a way, and many Victorian tragediennes faded away with pulmonary tuberculosis.

Though particular mention has been made of the lung, because it is the organ most commonly attacked by tuberculosis, it will be understood that the same variations of the disease may occur in any organ with the same caseation cavity formation, fibrosis, calcification, and so on. When we think about these varied possibilities, it becomes obvious that nothing could be more different from the story in, say, infection by the pyogenic cocci, thus illustrating the difference between an acute and a chronic type of infection.

Many years ago, Osler illustrated the possible outcome in tuberculosis by reference to the parable of the sower. "Some seeds fell by the wayside, and the fowls of the air came and destroyed them;" these are the bacilli that are scattered broadcast from an infectious case, but few are inhaled by other persons, and the majority of these bacilli die. "Some fell on stony places;" these bacilli fail to grow in immune persons, or form only small lesions that wither away "because they have no root." "Some fell among thorns;" these seeds grow, but the protecting forces serve to choke them. "But others fell on good ground and sprang up and bore fruit a hundredfold;" these are the cases in which the dose is overwhelming and resistance is at a minimum.

Treatment and Prevention. The **treatment** of tuberculosis, whether of the lung or elsewhere, has been revolutionized by modern chemotherapy. The bacilli easily acquire resistance to the individual drugs, but combinations of the drugs are remarkably effective.

Prevention rather than treatment is of course the ideal method of controlling a disease that used to be such a scourge. Nothing could be done before Koch first showed that tuberculosis was a bacterial disease and therefore infective. There are 2 sources of infection: the human patient with pulmonary tuberculosis and infected cow's milk (bovine infection). The latter, which used to be of special importance in children, can be combated by the testing of dairy cows with tuberculin, by pasteurization of milk, and by other public health measures. Spread of infection from the patient can be prevented by careful disposal of the sputum and by education in the dangers of unguarded coughing and spitting. Tubercle bacilli can live outside the body as long as they have food and moisture and are protected from direct sunlight. Under these conditions they may survive for months. Gauze used for the collection of sputum can be burned. If the patient does not go to a sanatorium, the other members of the household should undergo a periodic check-up by the tuberculin test and roentgenographic examination for the development of infection.

With such an insidious disease as pulmonary tuberculosis it is not possible to be certain that all danger of infection has been eliminated. Now we have a method of immunizing those most likely to be exposed to infection, such as children, nurses, and hospital employees, by inoculation with **BCG**. This is short for the **Bacille-Calmette-Guerin** vaccine, which is a bovine strain of tubercle bacillus rendered avirulent by prolonged culture on special media. The bacilli, which are living, have lost all power of producing disease, but when injected, they still have an immunizing power against infection with a virulent strain. It is a remarkable fact that the method was introduced as long ago as 1922 by the French bacteriologist Calmette as a means of protecting infants born into tuberculous families, but the method did not gain general favor by reason of the fear of injecting a live culture. This fear has proved to be groundless. The reader will recognize that the principle is similar to that of the oral (Sabin) vaccine for protection against poliomyelitis and that it is related to toxoid immunization against diphtheria. The drug Isoniazid has also proved of great value in protecting persons who live in household contact with an open case of tuberculosis.

LEPROSY

This disease was significant in medieval Europe, until the Black Death killed so many infected persons that leprosy almost disappeared. At that time, "leprosy" was used to describe a number of different infections that affected the skin in conspicuous and horrible ways. The disease as we know it today is caused by a rod-shaped bacillus, *Mycobac-terium leprae*, first identified in 1873 by a Norwegian doctor, Armauer Hansen. Like its relative, the *Mycobacterium tuberculosis*, *Mycobacterium leprae* is acid-fast. It has never been cultivated *in vitro*, and only recently has it been possible to grow it on animal tissue.

At present there are probably 10 to 20 million people with leprosy in the world, many of them living in tropical countries where the disease is more common. In the United States, 419 cases were reported between 1971 and 1973, mostly in California, Texas, and Hawaii.

Leprosy is classified into 3 types: lepromatous, tuberculoid, and borderline. Lepromatous leprosy involves extensive skin lesions, nasal symptoms (stuffiness) and, in males, infiltration and scarring of the testes, which leads to sterility. In addition, there is some neurologic involvement. Tuberculoid leprosy is characterized by fewer skin lesions and by pronounced nerve involvement, leading to muscle atrophy, crippling, and blindness when the facial nerve is involved. Borderline leprosy is a combination of the other 2 types.

Effective chemotherapy is available, and many of the deformities of the advanced disease can be prevented by proper attention.

SYPHILIS

Like tuberculosis, syphilis is a chronic inflammatory disease of long duration, but it differs in that it is a venereal disease. It is acquired by contact with a syphilitic lesion in a patient suffering from the disease, usually during sexual intercourse, so that the first lesions to appear are on the genital organs. Sometimes, however, the primary lesion may appear on the fingers as in the case of a doctor examining a syphilitic patient, or on the lips from kissing an infected area.

Bacteriology. Although syphilis has been the subject of study for hundreds of years, our modern knowledge of the disease is based on 3 great discoveries made in the course of 5 years at the beginning of the twentieth century, for its cause was discovered in 1905 by Schaudinn, an invaluable test for its presence was introduced by Wassermann in 1906, and a specific treatment in the form of arsenic (606) was given to the world by Ehrlich in 1910.

The **cause** of syphilis is a delicate spiral-shaped organism, *Treponema pallidum*, formerly called *Spirochaeta pallida*. It cannot be grown on any of the ordinary culture media nor stained by ordinary staining methods. It is best demonstrated by the dark-field method, in which a special attachment to the microscope enables the organisms to be seen as bright white threads against a dark background. The early lesions, both on the genital organs and in the mouth, contain enormous numbers of treponemata (still commonly referred to as spirochetes), so that these lesions are highly infectious. The spirochete resembles the gonococcus in its inability to survive outside the body.

Immunology. A patient suffering from syphilis is immune to reinfection. This immunity, which becomes established as soon as the primary lesion develops, is associated with the appearance of 2 distinct antibodies in the serum, namely syphilitic reagin and treponema-immobilizing antibody. Reagin is a substance normally present in the plasma in small amount associated with gamma globulin (IgE). It reacts as does antibody with certain extracts of normal tissues. In syphilis, reagin is greatly increased in amount, as a result of the interaction of the treponema with tissue, and this substance forms the basis of the complement fixation (Wassermann) and the precipitin (Kahn) reactions. The **complement fixation test** is a method for demonstrating a pathologic increase of reagin, using an antigen-like lipid substance present in bovine heart muscle and other tissues. There are now various modifications of the Wassermann such as the Kolmer, Kline, and Eagle, but they are often still referred to as the Wassermann reaction (WR). The technique, by means of which "fixation" of complement is recognized to have taken place, is outlined in the previous chapter. It will be seen that the Wassermann is in no sense a specific test for syphilis, because a syphilitic antigen is not used but, fortunately, it works in practice. The **Kahn** and the **VDRL (Venereal Disease Research Laboratory) precipitation** or **flocculation tests** are also nonspecific, depending on the production of a precipitate by the interaction of an increased amount of reagin (antibody) with a tissue antigen containing lipid. Precipitation tests are more sensitive in treated cases, so that the VDRL test may be positive when the WR has become negative.

The **treponema-immobilization (TPI) test**, unlike the complement fixation and precipitation methods, is a specific test for a true syphilitic antibody. Living spirochetes from the testis of a rabbit are immobilized and finally killed by serum from a patient with syphilis as shown by dark-field microscopy.

Finally it must be emphasized that in all laboratory tests for syphilis the results of a wrong report are so far-reaching and disastrous that the most meticulous care is needed not only in the performance of the test, but also in the collection and labeling of the sample of blood.

Natural History of the Disease. Syphilis seems to have lost much of its virulence since it was first introduced into Europe by the sailors of Christopher Columbus returning from the New World. At that time it swept through Italy like a pestilence, so that it came to be called *lues* (a plague), the name by which it is still known at the present day. This is another example of the natural changing picture of disease. Until recently, however, syphilis was one of the most common and important diseases in the world. It has now fallen from this high estate because of treatment with penicillin, and the late manifestations, particularly those due to involvement of the central nervous system, are rapidly becoming a thing of the past. At the same time it must not be thought that syphilis is no longer to be feared, because the current social revolution has been accompanied by a dramatic increase in all venereal diseases.

What may be called the natural history of the disease is peculiar and highly interesting, and can be divided into 3 stages known as primary, secondary, and tertiary. For 3 or 4 weeks after infection, the person feels well and shows no evidence of the disease. Then a lesion known as the primary sore or chancre appears at the site of infection. It takes the form of a curiously hard nodule, quite painless, which may become ulcerated, enormous numbers of spirochetes being discharged from the raw surface. The lesion consists of masses of chronic inflammatory cells, with no sign of acute inflammation. In the course of a few weeks it heals and may or may not leave a tell-tale scar. The regional lymph nodes, i.e., those that drain the part, are enlarged and hard in the primary stage. Usually these are the nodes in the groin, but if the primary lesion is on the lip the nodes below the jaw will be involved. At the end of the primary stage, the patient appears to have recovered, but the reaction to a serologic test on the blood has now become positive, and shows that, although the patient seems to be so well, he is really suffering from active syphilis.

The secondary lesions appear after 2 or 3 months, and are due to the spirochetes's having been carried far and wide throughout the body by the blood stream from the primary lesion. The skin, mucous membranes, and lymph nodes are principally affected. A variety of **skin rashes** may appear, which may easily be mistaken for some other skin disease. White patches develop on the mucous membrane lining the mouth, tongue, and tonsils; they are called **mucous patches**, and as they discharge countless spirochetes they are highly infective. The **lymph nodes** all over the body become slightly enlarged. All of these secondary lesions finally disappear without leaving any trace, and the patient again appears to be well, although results of serologic tests are still positive.

In about one-quarter of all untreated cases late complications (tertiary lesions) occur. The tertiary lesions appear after an interval of many years, with something of the inevitability of a Greek tragedy.

Tertiary syphilis may involve the central nervous system, the spinal cord, or the cardiovascular system. In addition, there used to be a further complication in which the loss of proprioception due to dorsal column disease resulted in a knee or ankle joint that became generally unusable. Today, fortunately, tertiary syphilis is extremely rare.

The diffuse lesions are of 3 types: (1) **cardiovascular,** (2) **central nervous system,** and (3) **spinal cord lesions.** They are essentially destructive, and even if they do heal they leave the organ damaged and badly scarred. Syphilis frequently attacks the arteries; in the brain, the small arteries become thickened and narrowed so that thrombosis is apt to develop; in the main arteries such as the aorta, the wall becomes so weakened that the diseased part of the vessel dilates and forms a bulging known as an **aneurysm.** The most serious of all the tertiary lesions are those in the nervous system, which may develop many years after the original infection. The spinal cord may be involved by tabes dorsalis, also known as locomotor ataxia, or the chief lesions may be in the brain causing general paresis, also known as general paralysis of the insane. We do not know why only about one-quarter of those affected with primary syphilis go on to develop any of the tertiary complications.

An investigation of the natural history of syphilis was conducted by the United States Public Health Service in Macon County, Alabama, from 1932 to 1972. When published, this study, called the Tuskegee study, received much criticism because the subjects of the experiment were intentionally not given any treatment for their disease, and were not informed of this fact. Today, this appears to us to be unethical conduct. Although we cannot completely excuse actions of the experimenters on philosophic grounds, this study needs to be viewed in its proper historical context. When the study was begun in 1930, the only pertinent literature on syphilis suggested that the disease ran a benign course, and that the available treatment was of questionable effectiveness. Under these circumstances, a study on natural history seemed desirable. In 1943, penicillin was recognized to be an efficient treatment in the early stages of syphilis. However, use of this treatment in the later stages of the disease was not fully accepted until a decade later, by which time such treatment would have had little therapeutic effect on the subjects of the study. Finally, we must remember that informed consent is a recent idea, and that the United States Public Health Service did not adopt it as policy until 1966. (Readers interested in a detailed account of this case should read Benedek's article, listed at the end of this chapter.) Experimentation with human life is a complex ethical issue, but we should be careful not to use modern ethical standards to judge events that occurred in a different intellectual climate. (Can past experimentations with human life be justified in all circumstances simply by explaining the intellectual climate under which the experiment took place?)

Congenital Syphilis

A child infected with syphilis, which may be congenital, from the mother before birth does not necessarily show signs of the disease at birth. Indeed, with regard to congenital syphilis, there are 3 possibilities: (1) The child may be born dead, usually showing well-marked evidence of syphilis. The disease used to be an important cause of stillbirth. (2) The child may be born alive with external evidence of syphilis. The skin shows inflammatory patches on the buttocks, the spleen is enlarged, and the mucous membrane of the nose is ulcerated with subsequent destruction of the bridge of the nose (saddle nose of congenital syphilis). (3) The child may appear healthy at birth, but lesions appear later. These lesions are on the whole similar to those of acquired syphilis, but in addition the teeth may be small and peg-shaped, and the cornea of the eye may become hazy and opaque.

COLIFORM BACTERIA

The intestine is the natural home of myriads of gram-negative, motile bacilli, most of which are not only harmless, but serve a useful purpose, such as synthesizing vitamin K and members of the B complex, so that we must beware of banishing them too completely by overenthusiastic antibiotic therapy. In addition to the harmless organisms, such as the **Coliform** group, that cause disease when implanted in tissue with diminished resistance, others, such as the **Salmonella** (typhoid) and **Shigella** (dysentery) groups, are pathogens, which invade the intestine in contaminated food and water, and set up inflammation in the wall of the bowel.

These various gram-negative bacilli are indistinguishable from one another morphologically, but the coliform organisms are lactose-fermenters, producing acid and gas from this sugar, whereas the majority of the pathogens are not, a simple means of laboratory differentiation.

Escherichia coli. This gram-negative, motile bacillus, is generally a harmless inhabitant of the bowel, but it is a common cause of acute and chronic inflammation elsewhere, especially when supported by other organisms. It can cause acute inflammation in the appendix and gallbladder, as well as in the pelvis of the kidney and the urinary bladder in cases of obstruction to the outflow of urine. Its toxins (endotoxin) are an important cause of shock. It is in children, in the aged, and in surgical cases that infection with *E. coli* is most to be feared.

Proteus and Pseudomonas. These 2 groups of motile gram-negative intestinal bacilli have come to assume increased importance because of their extreme resistance to antibiotics, so that they tend to supplant other bacteria when such therapy is long-continued. The proteus group ferments carbohydrates; the pseudomonas group does not, but produces a distinctive blue-green pigment (*Bacillus pyocyaneus*). Both groups only become dangerous invaders when general resistance is lowered or when local tissues are damaged. The urinary tract is most frequently involved. Pseudomonas infections are now common in burns.

TYPHOID FEVER

The gram-negative, motile bacillus that causes typhoid fever belongs to the salmonella group, and its official name is *Salmonella typhosa*, but we shall refer to it as the typhoid bacillus. The salmonella group differs from *E. coli* in that it comprises non-lactose-fermenters, and although powerful pathogens, they are nonpyogenic in action, and indeed suppress the polymorphonuclear leukocytes, which are the hallmark of suppuration. The motility of the organisms is due to the presence of numerous flagella.

The infection is spread from some person with typhoid bacilli in his digestive tract. This person may be a patient suffering from the disease, or he may be a **carrier**. A carrier is one who has had an attack of the disease, sometimes so mild that it fails to be diagnosed, but who continues to harbor the bacilli after recovery. Commonly, the bacilli live in the gallbladder of the carrier, from which they pass into the intestine and are excreted in the feces. A carrier is only dangerous to others if he is a food-handler (e.g., a cook or a dairy farmer), or if the infection can be transmitted from the carrier's excreta to food or water, as in the case of troops on active service or of contamination of wells from cesspools in the country. The patient suffering from an attack of typhoid fever is an active source of infection, but knowledge and care on the part of those nursing him should prevent spread of the infection to others.

The infecting agent has to be swallowed to produce the disease, and the bacilli may be conveyed by infected water, milk, or food, or by direct contagion. Epidemics can usually be traced to either water or milk infection. Water infection is generally due to fecal contamination. Food and milk infection may be caused by the contaminated fingers of a nurse who has been looking after a typhoid patient, by a cook or dairy farmer (usually a carrier), or by flies. A most famous example of the danger of a cook's being a carrier is that of Typhoid Mary, a cook in New York, who was responsible for at least 50 cases of typhoid fever, many of whom died, before she was finally tracked down. Oysters grown in shallow water at the mouths of infected streams occasionally have been responsible for outbreaks. Apart from water- and milk-borne epidemics, the important causes of infections are the fouling of food by fingers and by the feet of fecal-feeding flies.

Typhoid fever used to be a common disease. Now it has vanished from our cities. In 1910 there were 4,637 deaths from typhoid in 78 United States cities with a total population of 22 million; in 1936 there were only 342 deaths from this disease in 78 cities with a population of 36 million, and the majority of these cases were infected in the country. This is a triumph of sanitation in the prevention of disease.

Lesions. In typhoid, lesions are in the lymphoid tissue of the intestine, the spleen, the abdominal lymph nodes, and the bone marrow. The intestinal lesions are most marked at the lower end of the small intestine. Here the lymphoid tissue is collected into small masses in the deeper part of the mucous membrane that are called Peyer's patches. The bacilli, which have been swallowed, lodge in these masses and cause an inflammatory reaction with accompanying swelling of the patches. By the end of a week, the mucous membrane covering the patches is shed and the underlying lymphoid tissue becomes necrotic, disintegrates, and is lost, so that many ulcers of varying depths are formed. As a rule, the ulcers heal by the end of the third week, but 1 or more of the ulcers may extend deeply, just as in the case of a gastric ulcer, until finally perforation may occur into the abdominal cavity. The gallbladder is always infected, although the lesions may be negligible. The bacilli live in the bile and pass down into the bowel. Most of the bacilli in the stools come from the gallbladder, not from the ulcers in the bowel. The bacilli in the typhoid carrier come from the gallbladder. The bacilli are carried by lymphatics to the abdominal lymph nodes, and these are markedly enlarged. The organisms also enter the blood stream, by which they are conveyed to all parts of the body. The spleen is considerably enlarged, so that it often can be felt by the physician. Microscopic examination of the bone marrow shows the presence of masses of the characteristic mononuclear inflammatory cells (typhoid cells) that are found in all the lesions.

Symptoms. These are partly general, partly intestinal, and partly related to the blood and blood-forming organs.

The general symptoms are fever, headache, malaise, lethargy, and a clouding of the mind, which gives the name to the disease (Greek *typhos,* a cloud). The **fever** usually lasts about 3 weeks, but sometimes considerably longer. The temperature chart is characteristic; the temperature rises gradually for a week, remains elevated (103° to 105°F) for a week, and gradually returns to normal during the third week. There is none of the sudden rise and fall (crisis) so characteristic of lobar pneumonia. About the end of the first week small red patches appear on the abdominal wall; these are known as **rose spots.** Bronchitis and nosebleeds are early symptoms. The center of the tongue is heavily furred. The fever, headache, and lethargy are due to the toxins of the bacilli in the blood stream. The rose spots are caused by clumps of bacilli lodging in the capillaries of the skin.

The intestinal symptoms are abdominal discomfort, and constipation or diarrhea. With diarrhea, the feces may have an appearance described by the unpleasantly vivid term "pea-soup stools." **Hemorrhage** from the bowel may take place owing to an ulcer's having opened into a blood vessel. The hemorrhage may be severe and may prove fatal. It usually occurs late in the disease, at about the third week, and is accompanied by a sudden drop in the temperature. An even more serious complication is **perforation** of the bowel, owing to the penetration by an ulcer of the entire thickness of the intestinal wall. Perforation also usually occurs in the third week. The intestinal contents are poured into the abdominal cavity, and may cause a fatal peritonitis unless an immediate operation is performed. As the patient may have a deep ulcer and yet be only slightly ill, it follows that every case of typhoid fever must be treated with the greatest care. The recognition of the symptoms of perforation is the nurse's duty, and it is no exaggeration to say that the patient's life is literally in the nurse's hands. Perforation causes a sudden, sharp, intense abdominal pain different from any the patient may have experienced hitherto, but it only lasts a few seconds, and is quickly followed by a feeling of complete relief. This remarkable relief causes the ignorant observer to fall into grave error, but to the instructed mind it is a clear indication of the intense gravity of the situation. The subsequent peritonitis produces a very few symptoms, because of the dulled condition of the patient's mind.

Diagnosis. The 4 most valuable laboratory tests are: (1) blood culture, (2) the Widal agglutination test, (3) the demonstration of the bacilli in the feces, and (4) the leukocyte count. **Blood culture** is positive at the beginning of the disease (the period of bacteremia) and during the first week. The **Widal test** indicates whether antidotes against typhoid bacilli in broth culture are present in the blood. A few drops of blood are taken from the finger or the ear and allowed to clot; a drop of the serum is then added to a drop of a broth culture of typhoid bacilli and examined under the microscope. If the result is positive, the bacilli are seen to become agglutinated into small clumps; if negative, they remain separate. The test has a great reputation, but in many cases of typhoid it does not give a positive reaction until late in the disease, by which time the diagnosis is self-evident. After recovery, the agglutinins persist for months and sometimes for years, and the test is frequently negative in carriers. **Bacilli in the stools** are most numerous in the third week, and they are found even more readily in carriers. Culture of the bile obtained by duodenal drainage is one of the best methods of detecting a carrier. The **leukocyte count** shows leukopenia from the beginning of the illness. In the first week blood culture, in the second the agglutination test, and in the third week culture of the stool may be expected to yield positive findings.

A clinical picture resembling typhoid fever but milder in type may be caused by other members of the salmonella group, more particularly *Salmonella paratyphi* A and B. Paratyphoid A infection is more common in Asia; paratyphoid B, usually due to dairy products, occurs in Britain and North America. The vaccine used for protection against typhoid is known as TAB; this label indicates that it contains all 3 types of organisms. Other more common types of the salmonella bacteria cause gastroenteritis (*Sal-*

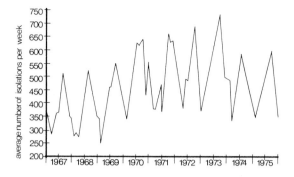

Fig. 7–6. This graph shows the reported human isolations of salmonellas in the United States from 1967 to 1975. The most commonly isolated varieties of salmonella in this period did not include the typhoid bacillus, but are pathogenic and usually cause mild gastroenteritis. The incidence of the isolations shows a consistent seasonal pattern with the greatest number reported between July and November. (From Center for Disease Control: Morbid. Mortal. Weekly Rep. 25, 1976.)

monella enteritidis), particularly in children under the age of 5 years. The incidence pattern of these and other salmonella diseases is seasonal (Fig. 7–6).

FOOD POISONING

This term denotes acute gastroenteritis (with the exception of botulism) caused by bacterial contamination of food or drink. The condition is a toxemia rather than a bacterial invasion. There are 2 distinct forms of different origin, but with a similar clinical picture: (1) the **infection type**, in which bacteria in the contaminated food multiply and produce their toxins in the bowel, and (2) the **toxin type,** in which toxins are produced in the food before ingestion. Both forms are marked by violent vomiting and diarrhea accompanied by severe prostration. The symptoms usually begin 6 to 12 hours after the infected food has been eaten, being naturally earlier in the toxin type, and perhaps delayed for 24 hours in the infection type.

The infection type is usually caused by one of the Salmonella group (although not by the typhoid bacillus itself), sometimes by one of the Shigella (dysentery) group. The food (animals or game birds) usually has stood for 2 or 3 days, but it does not smell nor does it look bad. The outbreak is likely to involve all the members of a family or the guests at a large

social gathering or picnic where there is a common food supply, probably imperfectly cooked or shielded from infection. In the toxin type, the poison is formed in the food before it is eaten, so that the onset is early, sometimes within an hour. Typically, the food may be pastry or cream sauce. The bacteriology is obscure. It is known that some strains of *Staphylococcus aureus* and some *Proteus* strains can produce a powerful enterotoxin in decomposing meat. The different problem of botulism must be mentioned here, although it is discussed in relation to the anaerobic spore-bearing clostridia. The spores of *Clostridia botulinum* can survive boiling for hours and, if they develop in canned goods, they produce one of the most powerful poisons known. (One gram of the toxin can kill 33 million mice!) The symptoms are due to the action of the toxin on autonomic nerve endings.

YERSINIA

Human illness caused by *Yersinia enterocolitica* was first described in New York State in 1933. It has since been reported in Northern Europe, in Japan, and in Canada. In 1976, an outbreak of yersiniosis in New York was found to be due to contaminated chocolate milk that children were drinking at school. The predominant symptoms were acute abdominal pain and fever.

BACILLARY DYSENTERY

Dysentery is an acute colitis characterized by **diarrhea.** Two entirely different diseases are known by this name as the result of ancient usage; they are bacillary dysentery and amebic dysentery, only the first of which will be considered here. The bacillus belongs to the **Shigella group,** of which there are several types, only a few being pathogenic. These gram-negative bacilli differ from the coliform and typhoid organisms in 2 respects: (1) they are nonmotile, and (2) they damage the bowel not by invading it at first, but by secreting a powerful **exotoxin** that produces necrosis of patches of the wall of the colon and lower part of the ileum, followed by ulceration.

Infection is acquired through the ingestion of contaminated food and water, just as in the case of typhoid. The infection may come from a patient suffering from the disease or from a carrier. Like amebic dysentery, the disease is prevalent in the tropics, but it also may occur in a temperate zone, especially when persons are crowded together under poor hygienic conditions. In the past it has been a great destroyer of armies in the field. It is prevalent in large mental hospitals, and it is an important cause of acute diarrhea associated with the passage of pus and blood in children, especially in hot weather.

CHOLERA

Asiatic cholera, like leprosy, is a disease that I trust the reader will never encounter, but he ought to know something about it. It is caused by a motile, gram-negative bacillus shaped like a comma, and therefore easily distinguished from the ordinary gram-negative bacilli seen in the stools. It is called *Vibrio cholerae*, and the disease is known as Asiatic cholera because the lower basin of the Ganges is the area where the disease is endemic and from which fearful epidemics spread across the world before it was known that infection was due to drinking water polluted by fecal discharge. The vibrios release a powerful endotoxin, which causes intense dilatation of the capillaries along the length of the small and large intestine. Huge quantities of watery fluid pour into the lumen from the dilated capillaries, and the result is a **dehydration** so profound that it kills the patient in 75% of untreated cases. The vibrios proliferate in the watery fluid as in a culture, so that the "rice-water stools" are intensely infective and can contaminate wells, streams, and other sources of drinking water. Before this was known, 50,000 persons died of cholera in England in 1831. Treatment consists in restoring fluid and electrolytes to the blood at the earliest possible moment. Prophylactic inoculation is of value, but ensuring a pure water supply is infinitely more important. Today, treatment by replacement of fluid and electrolyte loss by mouth saves thousands of lives annually.

PLAGUE

This disease is caused by the pest bacillus (*Yersinia pestis*), a small, gram-negative, extremely virulent organism. There is no more terrifying chapter in the story of disease than that of plague. The great plagues of the Middle Ages were worse than any wars. The Black Death came the nearest to exterminating the human race, for it killed 25 million people in Europe at a time when the population of that continent was very small (Fig. 7–7). Zinsser, in his delightfully written *Rats, Lice and History*, refers to plague and typhus as "those two calamities sharing with human ferocity the greatest responsibility of wholesale sorrow, suffering, and death throughout the ages."

The bacillus usually enters the body through the skin by means of the bite of a flea, which carries the infection from the rat to man. Indeed, plague is primarily a disease of rats. A human epidemic is accompanied or preceded by a rat epidemic. When a rat dies, the infected fleas leave it and go in search of a new and preferably human victim. A patient with plague is not infective unless fleas carry the infection from him to others.

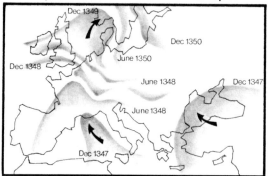

Spread of Black Death in Europe.

Fig. 7–7. This figure illustrates the spread of the plague, or Black Death, as it was called, through Europe in the mid-fourteenth century. The disease was brought to Europe from the East, probably by Mongol armies and commercial caravans, who began to travel vast distances after the founding of the Mongol Empire by Genghis Khan (1162 to 1227). (Adapted from Carpentier, E.: Autour de la peste noire: famines et épidémies dans l'histoire du XIVe siècle. Annales—Economies, Sociétés, Civilisations, 6:1062, 1962.)

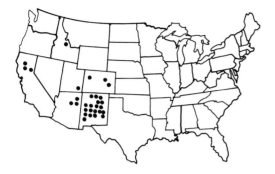

Fig. 7–8. This map shows the incidence and distribution of plague in the United States from 1965 to 1970. Each dot represents one case. (From Gilbert, E.F., and Huntington, R.W.: *An Introduction to Pathology.* New York, Oxford University Press, 1978.)

There is no inflammation at the site of the flea bite, but the nearest lymph nodes become swollen and acutely inflamed, forming masses called buboes. It is these masses that give the disease its name of bubonic plague. The bacilli then invade the blood stream and are found in enormous numbers in the internal organs. The patient dies of overwhelming septicemia before there is time for marked lesions to develop. The mortality is extremely high, and the patient may be dead in less than 24 hours.

Sometimes an epidemic takes a pneumonic form, in which the infection is spread by droplets of sputum. Pneumonic plague is one of the most deadly and rapidly fatal of all infections.

The control of plague consists in exterminating rats and in preventing them from leaving a ship that comes from a country in which plague is prevalent. This is done by placing large discs on the ship's cables, which prevent the rats from running down the ropes. The problem of the flea is met with insecticides. This dreaded disease has not been entirely wiped out, and a few cases are occasionally reported in the United States (Fig. 7–8).

TULAREMIA

This plague-like disease affects animals principally, but it may spread from them to man. It is caused by another organism, *Fran-*

cisella tularensis. Ground squirrels and jack rabbits are the animals most often affected. The name comes from Tulare County in California, where an epidemic of the disease killed many ground squirrels. Infection is carried from animals to man (1) by biting fleas, (2) by ticks, and (3) most often by contact with skins of infected rabbits. It is seen, therefore, in farmers, hunters, butchers, housewives, and others who are likely to skin rabbits. In man the disease is fortunately not nearly so fatal as in animals.

The bacteria enter through cuts and cracks in the skin, and an ulcer develops at the site of infection. In this respect the disease differs from plague. The regional lymph nodes are swollen and tender, as in plague. There is prolonged fever and prostration. Recovery is the rule, but convalescence may take some months. In fatal cases, areas of necrosis are found in the internal organs.

UNDULANT FEVER

This disease is caused by a small organism midway in form between a coccus and a bacillus. For this reason it is called neither, but is given the name of its discoverer, Sir David Bruce, and is known as brucella. Infection with brucella (**brucellosis**) is essentially an animal disease, attacking particularly cattle and goats. The germs infecting these 2 kinds of animals are of slightly different strains, although indistinguishable under the microscope. That infecting goats is known as *Brucella melitensis*, because it was first discovered by Bruce in the goats on the island of Malta. The strain infecting cattle is called *Brucella abortus*, because it produces contagious abortion in these animals. Infection in swine is caused by *Brucella suis*. Man acquires the infection by drinking cows' milk or goats' milk. Brucellosis is said to be the most common illness conveyed to human beings from animals. In North America, the only infecting agent that need be considered is *Brucella abortus*.

The disease is extraordinarily prevalent in cattle. In some parts of the eastern states, 90% of the herds are infected. Fortunately, the abortus infection is not so pathogenic for man as the melitensis form. Most of the persons who drink infected cows' milk show no sign of the disease, though they may have agglutinins in the blood, indicating that they have been infected. However, the disease undoubtedly used to be much more common than is usually thought. Its importance lies in the possibility of confusion with such long-continued fevers as typhoid, miliary tuberculosis, and subacute bacterial endocarditis. These are all serious diseases, whereas in undulant fever the mortality rate is less than 2% (Fig. 7–9).

The disease begins insidiously with an evening rise of temperature, and the patient may be ill for some time without knowing that he has any fever. The fever may come in waves, hence the name undulant fever, although this feature is often absent. Its most striking characteristic is its remarkable persistence; 3 months is an average duration, but it may last for years. Persistent weakness, muscle pains, joint pains, and marked perspiration with a sweet sickly odor to the sweat are some of the common features and may easily pass unrecognized. The patient may feel extraordinarily miserable, and a doctor remarked on recovering from the disease: "If the cows felt as miserable as I did, I do not blame them for aborting." Strange to say, there are no characteristic lesions, merely those of any septicemia.

The most reliable means of diagnosis is the test for agglutinins in the blood against *Brucella abortus*, a test identical to the Widal test for typhoid. Agglutination in a dilution of over 1 in 300 indicates active disease; agglutination in a dilution of 1 to 80, in the absence of clinical symptoms, indicates latent infection. The most satisfactory antibiotic treatment is with tetracycline, which seems to be specific for undulant fever and prevents relapses.

ANTHRAX

The anthrax bacillus is a large, square-ended, gram-positive bacillus, which forms spores outside the body. The spores are resistant to chemical disinfectants and also to heat. They may remain alive in the soil for many years, and when they finally enter the body again, they develop into bacilli. This is a fact of profound importance. The organisms grow readily in culture. They are aerobic, in marked contrast to the anaerobic spore-bearers to be considered.

Anthrax is a disease of animals, principally cattle and sheep. It is prevalent in European animals, but is much less common in North America, so that in this country the human disease is correspondingly uncommon. Cattle and sheep are usually infected by feeding on pasture contaminated by spores from other victims of the disease, a fact originally discovered by Pasteur. It is indeed remarkable that more than 100 years ago, the father of bacteriology immunized sheep against anthrax by means of a vaccine consisting of the bacilli attenuated by culture at a raised temperature.

Man is infected from animal material, not from other persons, usually from the hides of cattle or from the wool of sheep. The skin is the common site of infection, but the disease may be acquired by those using infected shaving brushes, or working with the hides of diseased cattle. The spores may be inhaled into the lungs, usually in the process of the "carding" of wool; the pulmonary form is known as "woolsorters' disease."

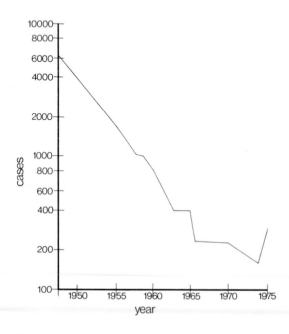

Fig. 7–9. Human brucellosis, United States, 1947 to 1975. (From Center for Disease Control: Morbid. Mortal. Weekly Rep., *25*, 1976.)

The skin lesion is called a malignant pustule and is easily recognized. A pimple appears on the surface of the hand, forearm, or face, which develops into a boil and then a pustule containing blood-stained fluid swarming with anthrax bacilli. The surface turns black, and then presents a highly characteristic appearance. If it is recognized and promptly excised, recovery follows. If not, the blood stream is invaded, the bacilli multiply with frightful rapidity, filling the capillaries of all the organs, and death soon results. A specific antiserum gives good results when used in conjunction with early excision of the lesion. The pulmonary form is almost always fatal. Penicillin and tetracycline have been used with beneficial results in anthrax infections in recent years.

ANAEROBIC SPORE-BEARERS

All the bacteria considered so far are able to live and multiply in air, or rather in oxygen. They are aerobes. We now come to a group that cannot do so, and in particular the genus *Clostridium*, composed of many members that live in the soil, where they take part in the process of putrefaction, so that they are readily ingested in vegetables and establish themselves in the colon. Being strict anaerobes, they are unable to multiply in living tissue which is supplied with oxygen, confining themselves to dead tissue in which they can manufacture lethal toxins. All the clostridia are large gram-positive bacilli that produce spores that can survive in dry earth for years and are extremely resistant to heat and antiseptics. The 3 important pathogens of the group are: (1) *Clostridium perfringens*, causing gas gangrene, (2) *Clostridium tetani*, causing tetanus, and (3) *Clostridium botulinum*, causing botulism.

Gas Gangrene

The common cause of gas gangrene is *Clostridium perfringens,* although other members of the clostridia group are sometimes responsible. This anaerobic bacillus, discovered by the great American pathologist William Welch in 1891, is sometimes referred to as *Clostridium welchii*. It occurs in the intestinal tract of men and animals, where it does no harm, but wounds may become infected either by soil containing animal manure or by contaminated clothing. It is in war wounds that *Clostridium perfringens* infection is of the greatest importance. The bacillus is short, plump, gram-positive, produces spores, and is surrounded by a capsule that gives it a characteristic appearance.

Unlike ordinary disease-producing bacteria, it does not invade living tissue, but grows only in dead or injured tissue in which there is a sufficiently low supply of oxygen to meet its requirements. It is therefore a saprophyte. It flourishes in muscles that have been torn up by bullets or by fragments of shrapnel, have been deprived of their blood supply, and are thus anaerobic.

The chief characteristic of *Clostridium perfringens* is that it produces gas from the muscle sugars, so that it is commonly called the "gas bacillus," and the disease itself is known as gas gangrene. The gas is the result of fermentation, which may be defined as the splitting of a complex organic compound (in this case, muscle sugar) into simpler elements. The gas spreads along the muscle sheaths, separating these from the muscles, and bubbles of foul-smelling gas and blood-stained fluid can be pressed up and down the length of the muscle. This fluid is highly toxic, so that it kills the muscle fibers, which are then invaded by the bacteria. The process is one of putrefaction or breaking down of muscle, and is marked by a terrible odor. A toxin is also produced, which poisons the patient. Against this toxin an antitoxin has been prepared.

The most important part of the **treatment** of gas gangrene is to reduce the likelihood of anaerobic environment for the organisms by adequate surgical treatment to remove dead tissue and blood clots. The use of antiserums and large doses of penicillin have also been effective in controlling this type of infection in wounds.

Tetanus

Clostridium tetani, the tetanus bacillus, is a slender anaerobic organism with a spore at one end, giving it a characteristic, drumstick-like appearance. It lives in the intestine of horses and occurs in about 15% of horses' feces, so that it is found in soil that has been fertilized with manure.

This bacillus causes a dangerous wound infection, which results when infected soil or the dirt of streets gains entrance to a wound. The spores can live in dust for long periods. Another source of infection in surgical wounds used to be catgut, which is prepared from the intestine of the horse, not the cat. If this is imperfectly sterilized, the spores may persist, and later cause infection in the wound.

The organism remains localized in the wound and does not invade the tissues. In this respect it is the exact opposite to the clostridia causing gas gangrene. As it is anaerobic, it grows best when other bacteria are present that kill the tissue so that the supply of oxygen diminishes.

The tetanus bacillus is dangerous because it produces one of the most powerful toxins known, far more virulent than the most deadly snake venom. The toxin gradually passes along the nerves from the wound to the spinal cord. There it becomes anchored to the motor nerve cells, which it stimulates, so that the muscles become rigid and the patient is thrown into terrible convulsions. The jaw muscles are involved early by stiffness, and the mouth cannot be opened. Hence the common name of the disease is lockjaw.

The incubation period, i.e., the time between infection and the first appearance of symptoms, is considerable, for the toxin travels along the nerves slowly. The average time is 7 to 10 days. In wounds of the face it is shorter, as there is less distance for the toxin to travel. In other cases it may be several weeks. This long incubation period is fortunate, because it makes preventive inoculation possible. When the possibility of tetanus is suspected, and this should be the case in all street accidents or contaminated wounds, a prophylactic injection of tetanus antitoxin is given. This neutralizes the toxin before it has time to reach the nerve cells in the spinal cord. After that it is usually too late to do much good, as the toxin is firmly anchored to the nerve cells. In wartime, every wounded soldier received a dose of antitetanus serum on the chance that the wound might have become infected with tetanus.

Botulism

Clostridium botulinum is essentially a soil bacterium, but it is also found in the intestine of domestic animals. This anaerobic bacillus is entirely different in its action from anything so far considered. We are not concerned with the organism itself, for it does not grow in the human body. However, it does grow in spoiled sausage (Latin *botulus*, a sausage), preserved meat, canned vegetables, and ripe olives. Its spores are resistant, and if the temperature employed in home canning is insufficient, the bacilli will produce a potent toxin which, if taken even in tiny amounts, may cause death. The condition is called botulism. The toxin does not produce any inflammation in the stomach or intestine, but is absorbed and acts on the brain, producing eye disturbances such as double vision and squint, and finally coma and death. The symptoms are apt to be mistaken for those of encephalitis, so that the correct diagnosis of food poisoning may be missed. Prevention is the best treatment, and this means proper attention to detail in home canning.

SYNOPSIS

Bacteria as a biologic form are utilitarian, and higher organisms depend on them.
Bacterial infections may be local or systemic diseases.
Bacterial endotoxins and enzymes are causes of injury.
Antibodies to bacterial antigens are aids to diagnosis.
Hypersensitivity to bacterial antigens is a cause of tissue injury.
Koch's postulates are a paradigm for the germ theory of disease.
Tuberculosis is a model of infectious disease in which tissue destruction, immunity, and hypersensitivity all exist.

The carrier state, as in typhoid fever, is an important complication of infectious disease.

Spores of bacteria represent an important factor in the spread of disease.

Terms

Bacteriostatic	*Staphylococci*	*Cholera*
Bacteriocidal	*Streptococci*	*Plague*
Virulence	*Scarlet fever*	*Tetanus*
Fomites	*Pneumococcus*	*Incubation period*
Vectors	*Diphtheria*	*Spores*
Gram stain	*Tuberculosis*	

FURTHER READING

Bates, J.H.: The changing scene in tuberculosis. N. Engl. J. Med., *297*:610, 1977.

Benedek, T.G.: The "Tuskegee Study" of syphilis: analysis of moral versus methodologic aspects. J. Chronic Dis., *31*:35, 1978.

Black, R.E., et al.: Epidemic yersinia enterocolitica infection due to contaminated chocolate milk. N. Engl. J. Med., *298*:76, 1978.

Blake, P.A., et al.: Cholera—a possible endemic focus in the United States. N. Engl. J. Med., *302*:305, 1980.

Burnet, F.M.: *Natural History of Infectious Disease,* 2nd Ed. Cambridge, Cambridge University Press, 1953.

Crichton, M.: *The Andromeda Strain.* New York, Knopf, 1969.

Dondero, T.J., et al.: An outbreak of legionnaires' disease associated with a contaminated air conditioning cooling tower. N. Engl. J. Med., *302*:365, 1980.

Dubos, R.J.: Historical evolution of infectious diseases. Can. Med. Assoc. J., *79*:445, 1958.

Jesson, O., et al.: Changing staphylococci and staphylococcal infections. N. Engl. J. Med., *281*:627, 1969.

Fekety, F.R., Jr., et al.: Bacteria, viruses and mycoplasma in acute pneumonia in adults. Am. Rev. Respir. Dis., *104*:499, 1971.

Fraser, D.W.: Legionnaires' disease: four summers' harvest. Am. J. Med., *68*:1, 1980.

Gilbaugh, J.H., and Fuchs, P.C.: The gonococcus and the toilet seat. N. Engl. J. Med., *301*:91, 1979.

Hammerschlag, M.R.: Chlamydial pneumonia in infants. N. Engl. J. Med., *298*:1083, 1978.

Mackowiak, P.A.: Microbial synergism in human infections. N. Engl. J. Med., *298*:21, 1978.

Pelczar, M., Jr., et al.: *Microbiology,* 4th Ed. New York, McGraw-Hill, 1977.

Salton, M.R., and Tomasz, A.: Mode of action of antibiotics on microbial walls and membranes. Ann. N.Y. Acad. Sci., *235*, 1974.

Sanford, J.P.: Legionnaires' disease—the first thousand days. N. Engl. J. Med., *300*:654, 1979.

Taylor-Robinson, T., and McCormack, W.M.: The genital mycoplasmas. N. Engl. J. Med., *302*:1003, 1980.

Wilson, G.S., and Miles, A.: *Topley and Wilson's Principles of Bacteriology, Virology and Immunity,* 6th Ed. London, Edward Arnold, 1975.

Zinsser, H.: *Rats, Lice and History.* Boston, Little, Brown, 1935.

Viruses and Other Intracellular Parasites

8

Repetition is the only form of permanence that nature can achieve—SANTAYANA

We come now to viruses, a class of small but powerful life forms. Viruses have some, but not all, of the capabilities of most living things, and depend on a phase of intracellular growth. They cannot multiply without a living cell for a host and thus are obliged to infect living things as diverse as bacteria, plants, and human beings. Viruses are as varied in their structure and as different in their biologic impact as this universality suggests. The role of viruses as disease-causing agents is well known, but animal viruses have also been invaluable tools to experimental biologists in unraveling the basic mechanisms of nucleic acid and protein synthesis and membrane assembly. Viruses can be studied *in vitro* in cell culture. Their streamlined life cycle has revealed key functions of molecular biology in all living forms. They have been a ready source of mutants, whose pathogenic effects aid in understanding normal function, and they represent a relatively pure source of biologic material for biochemi-

cal analysis. From such viruses we have been able to learn much about the biology of nucleic acids and about viral infections in general.

The history of virology and viral diseases is remarkable. More than 100 years ago, Pasteur showed that disease could be produced by agents too small to be seen with the microscope, so minute that they are not held back by the finest filter. They refuse to grow on culture media. These unknown agents were called viruses. It is amazing to learn that he was able to immunize persons suspected of being exposed to a viral infection, namely rabies. Equally remarkable was Jenner's success in 1796, when he immunized persons against smallpox, which we now know to be a viral disease. The first virus to be actually demonstrated was in a plant disease, tobacco mosaic. The first demonstration of an animal viral disease in 1898 was foot-and-mouth disease of cattle. In 1901 came the proof of the first viral disease in man, namely yellow fever. But it is in the last 25 years that the most startling progress has been made. This advance has largely been due to the discovery that viruses can be grown outside the body in tissue culture. This was done first in the yolk sac of a hen's egg (the living embryo) and more recently in a tissue culture of the epithelial cells of monkey kidney. For this work, Enders and his associates were awarded the Nobel prize. The virus not only grows luxuriantly in these epithelial cells, but is also present in large quantities in the supernatant fluid. The tissue culture technique is also used for the development of vaccines, especially for poliomyelitis. Not so long ago the public had never heard of viruses, but now everyone diagnoses his or her own complaints as being due to a virus.

VIRAL STRUCTURE AND FUNCTION

The general anatomy of a virus is a nucleic acid core within a well-structured protein coat, which may or may not be surrounded by a lipid envelope. The nucleic acid may be RNA or DNA; it directs the replication of many new viral genomes, and codes for various viral proteins. Some of these proteins are the structural components of the virion; some are enzymes that facilitate the replication and growth of the virus in the cell. The host provides the energy, the substrates, and the synthetic machinery for viral growth (Fig. 8–1). A virus is an elegant, elementary, extraordinary parasite.

The nature of the virus-host relationship varies enormously, ranging from relatively benign coexistence, similar to a stowaway on a ship, to massive destructive takeover, as a hijacker redirects the flight destination and purpose, and ultimately destroys the plane to achieve his personal goals. A virus may enter a cell and neither change its cellular structure nor disturb its function. This phenomenon is seen in some enteroviruses (cultured from the stools of infected persons who therefore act as carriers), the Coxsackie viruses, for example. At the other extreme we have the explosive effects of the yellow fever virus on the liver cells, and the poliomyelitis virus on the anterior horn (motor) cells of the spinal cord. There is thus a world of difference between viral infection and viral disease. In viral infection, which is much more common than viral disease, the virus may sojourn indefinitely in the comfortable surroundings of the cell. It may simply be a boarder, as in some cases where viral genes remain in the cell but are not expressed. At some later time, this genome may become active and its effects may become apparent. Alternatively, the sojourning virus particle may become one of the family, and multiplication of the virus proceeds without damage to the cell. Various circumstances such as age, stress, or nutritional or hormonal imbalance may upset the harmony and may convert the latent virus into a virulent one. Bacterial infection may also spark this conversion, one of the best examples being the well-known relation between herpes simplex ("cold sore") and pneumococcal infection. In viral disease, the normal functions of the cell may be rapidly shut off, as the virus directs cell machinery to manufacture virus particles. The cell may be blown to pieces by the explosive proliferation of the virus, but evidence of cellular degeneration, known as the cytopathic effect of the virus, is much more common.

Viruses pose an interesting evolutionary dilemma. The rules of natural selection and survival of the fittest apply to viruses as well as to the rest of the biologic world. Any genetic change that increases the efficiency of viral proliferation enhances the ability of that virus strain to survive. However, more efficient proliferation may result in rapid elimination of the host. Viruses need their hosts in order to grow; destroying the host during infection is obviously counterproductive. This parasitic need leads to a modulation or tempering of virulence in wild virus populations so that virus and host may coexist. Therefore, many viral infections are productive but inapparent. Our concept of viruses as agents of disease comes from those cases where the effects of infection are apparent or perhaps even fatal.

The viral life cycle involves several stages. A virus must find susceptible cells. These may be restricted to a single species of animal, or to a particular type of tissue. Susceptibility is usually determined by the presence of appropriate receptors on the cell membrane. This is an example of the

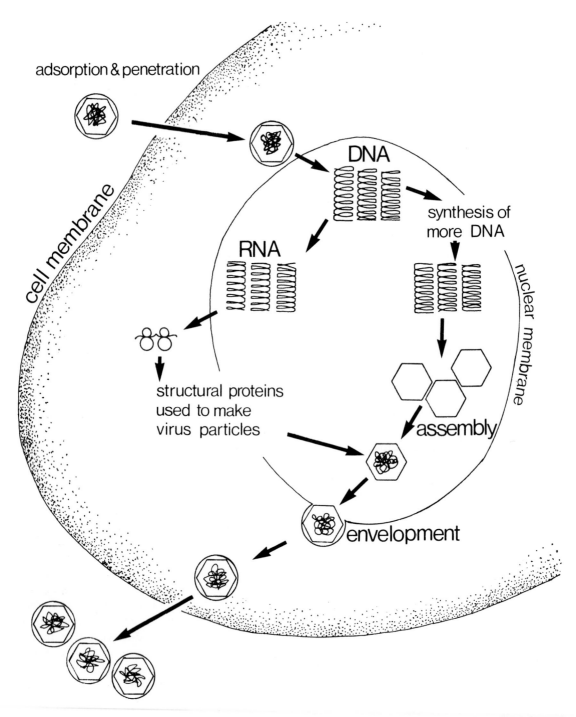

adsorption & penetration

cell membrane

DNA

synthesis of
more DNA

RNA

nuclear membrane

structural proteins
used to make
virus particles

assembly

envelopment

Fig. 8–1. This diagram shows the various steps in the entry, development, assembly, and formation of viral particles. The virus shown in the upper left with its coat must gain access to the nucleic acids of the cell, where new synthesis of viral particles takes place. Subsequently, assembly of the viral particles occurs. The cell is usually destroyed in the process. (Adapted from Dales, S.: The uptake and development of vaccinia virus in strain L cells followed with labeled viral deoxyribonucleic acid. J. Cell Biol., *18*:51, 1963.)

fine-tuned coevolution of a virus and its host. A virus binds to the receptors of the cell and penetrates the cell (by fusion to the membrane, or phagocytosis), where it is uncoated and initiates the cycle of nucleic acid transcription and translation. The result is the synthesis of viral proteins and the replication of new viral genomes. The nature of these processes, along with virion structure, is the basis of contemporary viral classification. DNA viruses have a DNA genome, as do their hosts. The replication of DNA from DNA, and the transcription of DNA to RNA to protein is thus similar to normal cell function. Host enzymes may be employed for these functions. Viruses may use all the existing cell machinery, or they may bring about their own modifications. The more complex the virus (the greater the number of its components and the functional proteins it encodes), the more "independence" it has in its intracellular cycle. By supplying variant polymerases, viruses can grow in nondividing cells, in the cytoplasm rather than in the nucleus, or they can shift the net effect of synthesis to viral functions and away from those of the host.

RNA viruses are the only living forms to have RNA alone as their genomic information. Since cells do not normally copy RNA from RNA, viruses must bring along their own such enzymes. RNA viruses may be single-stranded or double-stranded, although most are single-stranded. Their genome may be a single linear strand, or it may be segmented. Single-stranded RNA is classified as follows: "+ RNA" functions directly as mRNA (messenger RNA), that is, it is translated into proteins. "− RNA" must first be copied, and the complementary "+ RNA" serves as the mRNA. In + strand viruses, the RNA of the virus may serve directly as a message. Replication is accomplished by synthesizing a complementary − RNA, and then by making many new + virion RNA's from this template. In − strand viruses, complementary + RNA must be made first, for use as mRNA and as the template for virion − RNA synthesis.

Once the replication and protein synthetic pathways have been accomplished (with or without an accompanying cessation of host functions), the new virions must be assembled and released. In some cases, viruses accumulate and cell lysis causes their dispersion. In other cases, the new virions assemble at the cell membrane, bud out, and finally pinch off without disrupting the cell. Released viruses are then "inert" particles until they encounter new host cells and begin the cycle again.

In addition to lysis, other adverse effects are exerted by viruses. They may cause fusion of cells into syncytia or giant cells. Viruses are also capable of converting cells to a neoplastic state, changing the growth pattern of cells dramatically, so that they become unrecognizable and are malignant for the host.

As well as the lethal cellular effects of viral infection, many symptoms of disease are related to the host's reaction to viral growth. Viral infections often cause fever, which accompanies many common symptoms. Viruses and virally infected cells are also often highly antigenic and mobilize the immune system. Reactions of virus and circulating antibodies are often responsible for the rashes associated with viral disease. Inflammation and tissue damage result from mobilized cellular immunity; the release of previously inaccessible cellular components is responsible for the damage associated with viral infections involving the central nervous system. In these cases it is the host-virus interaction, rather than the virus by itself, which causes the damage. Finally, following viral infections, persons are more susceptible to bacterial infections for reasons that are not always clear; this susceptibility is responsible for many fatalities in viral-associated diseases. For example, the influenza virus kills the epithelium cells lining the respiratory tract. This epithelium is a primary barrier against bacterial invaders, and, once destroyed, a bacterial pneumonia may easily invade and overcome an elderly or weakened person.

IMMUNITY AND RESISTANCE

The immune response of the host is often part of the evolution of disease in viral infections; it is also often part of the controls that limit viral disease. Viruses elicit circulating antibodies (IgG and IgM) and evoke localized antibodies present in body secretions (IgA). These antibodies may either curtail the viral infection or prevent its spread to secondary targets. It is often during the secondary spread of infection that the most serious complications of viral infection arise.

The immune response to viruses is the key to the success of vaccination. Vaccination is the process by which the host is rendered immune to a pathologic organism without suffering through the disease itself. As Pasteur and Jenner discovered, there are 2 ways of producing immunity without producing disease. One is to use a dead form of the virus, the other is to use a live nonpathogenic form that has the same antigenic properties as the virulent form. In the first type, the virus is killed in such a way (e.g., by heat) that it can no longer replicate, but its antigenicity is preserved. The dead virus stimulates production of antibodies without causing disease. The antibodies circulate in the blood stream, but other defenses such as those in the tissue rather than in the blood can only be stimulated by live viral infection. Thus vaccination with dead virus may not provide adequate protection. The other method of vaccination involves using an attenuated, live virus that has the same antigens as the pathogenic virus, but that causes no disease. We owe this method to the English physician, Jenner, at that time a country practitioner, who observed that milkmaids who had had cowpox were immune to smallpox. He then used the living virus of cowpox (vaccinia), which causes a mild disease, to prevent smallpox infection. (The word vaccination is derived from this experience, Latin *vacca* meaning cow.) Today, viruses can be attenuated by repeated replications in a laboratory culture, where, deprived of normal host conditions, they lose their virulence. (However, the smallpox vaccine is still derived from cows with cowpox.) When attenuated virus is used in vaccination, normal infection is mimicked and tissue antibodies are produced as well as circulating antibodies. The disadvantages of this method are several: usually there are more disease-like symptoms after live vaccination, and occasionally there are other contaminants in live vaccine preparations. Sometimes the attenuated virus changes or loses its potency. Inapparent but concurrent infections in the host may interfere with the replication of the attenuated virus, therefore, with the appearance of the desired immunity. Finally, a live virus will be released from persons so vaccinated. This may present a danger to nonimmune persons in their environment, especially if more virulent viruses (as sometimes happens) arise during the course of the infection. It is important to realize that each new infection in a new host provides the virus with the opportunity for mutation. Three different things may happen as virus is passed from host to host: the virus may stay the same, or it may become either more or less virulent.

There has been tremendous debate over the relative merits and dangers of the 2 types of vaccine: dead or live attenuated virus. The controversy surrounding the use of the Sabin polio vaccine (attenuated), or the Salk vaccine (dead) provides the best example.

An irony of the great improvements wrought by vaccination should be mentioned here. In nature, frequent inapparent infections with endemic viruses often provide immunity that moderates the effects of a more virulent strain. This is caused by the inapparent infection limitation of the number of susceptible hosts in the population, thereby limiting the chances of mutation. Vaccination campaigns can, and, ideally, do completely eliminate nonimmune hosts and destroy the virus. At this point, the public temptation and sometimes the general practice is to stop vaccination. This has now happened with the smallpox virus; travelers are no longer required to have vaccination certificates. The next generation may be exposed to an epidemic.

Some viral diseases do not lend themselves well to vaccination. These are diseases that result from many viral serotypes. The term serotypes refers to the different antigenic properties that members of a virus species may possess. For example, there are 3 serotypes of poliovirus identical in all respects except for the surface markers (proteins) that serve as antigenic stimuli to the host immune system. Vaccination with 1 polio serotype provides no protection against the other 2, hence poliomyelitis vaccines contain all 3 types. The host who has formed all 3 antibody types for polio, is immune to the disease. Poliomyelitis does not present a big vaccination problem. However, in the case of influenza, or of the "common cold," the number of serotypes is much greater, and it is impractical to protect against the large number of strains occurring in the wild. Similarly, natural immunity from an infection does not protect against later bouts with different serotypes. Hence we all contract many colds, but only 1 case of measles.

Since viruses must have a host, they have had to evolve along with host defenses such as immunity. Some viruses, such as influenza, have established mechanisms for frequent change, so that immunity as a result of prior infection does not block their infection. Other viruses can survive only in large populations, where the introduction of new preimmune hosts is frequent enough to provide for the maintenance of the virus. The childhood diseases of mumps and measles fit this pattern. Other viruses persist in the host and are reactivated years later. Still others are maintained in an animal reservoir, in which breeding is sufficiently rapid that there are always new hosts, although each infection may kill or may induce lifelong immunity.

In addition to the host's immune response, there is another general, antiviral defense mechanism. Cells that have been infected with virus produce and secrete a glycoprotein capable of inhibiting or interfering with the growth of many viruses, the stimulus for this probably being viral nucleic acid. This protein has been named **interferon**, and it seems to have many of the properties of a viral antibiotic. Interferon spreads to other cells in which it creates an antiviral state that renders those cells unable to support viral replication. The antiviral state may also be produced in the original infected cell and may modify the ongoing infection cycle. This defense mechanism is different from the immune system.

Immune antibodies are specific, differing for each disease, but interferon is constant, no matter what the infecting virus. Antibodies only begin to make their appearance relatively late in the disease, whereas interferon is found in large quantities often during early stages of infection (Fig. 8–2).

Some viruses are potent inducers of interferon; others are not. Infections in which viral transcription and translation are rapid are inefficient in inducing interferon (for example, poliomyelitis). Paradoxically, some viruses that are poor inducers of interferon have been shown to be sensitive to its action; these viruses represent likely targets for interferon therapy.

TRANSMISSION

The usual routes of transmission of viral infections are through the respiratory or gastrointestinal tracts. Unhygienic conditions and crowded environments are key factors in viral spread and control. Viruses may also spread by direct skin contact, as in animal or insect bites. **Arboviruses** (*ar*thropod-*bo*rne) are transmitted by insect vectors. The insect is not a passive carrier; arboviruses are capable of productive growth in insects although no disease is present. Insects then transmit the viruses to a plentiful reservoir of animal hosts, where disease results. Arboviruses are not endemic to human populations, but rather they become significant after migrations into new environments. These infections are among the most virulent and lethal of human diseases, yellow fever, for example.

Viruses have been classified historically by the tissue they infect, by their size or shape, and more recently by their nucleic acid and enzymatic characteristics. Table 8–1 outlines a contemporary catalog of viruses (Fig. 8–3).

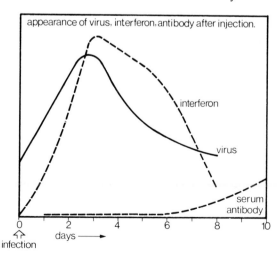

Fig. 8–2. This graph show the temporal sequence between the appearance of virus, the appearance of interferon, and the appearance of serum antibodies following infection. (Adapted from Roitt, I.: *Essential Immunology.* Oxford, Blackwell Scientific Publications, 1977.)

RNA VIRUSES

These are viruses whose genome is composed of RNA. We shall consider first the smallest and simplest of the RNA viruses.

Picornaviruses. These viruses (Italian *pico*, small, and −rna) fall into 2 general subdivisions: enteroviruses (polio-, Coxsackie, echo-) and rhinoviruses.

Table 8–1. Major Groups of Viruses Infecting Human Beings

GENERIC NAME, NUCLEIC ACID, AND PROTOTYPE VIRUS	SIZE, NM	ETHER-SENSITIVE	ENVELOPE	SYMMETRY

Picornavirus (RNA):
    Coxsackie viruses A and B; echo, entero-, rhino-,
    and polioviruses
	17 to 30	No	No	Cubic

Reovirus (RNA)	74	No	No	Cubic

Arbovirus (RNA):
    Group A (equine encephalitis, Semliki Forest)
    Group B (Japanese B, Russian tick-borne, yellow
    fever, dengue)
    Group C (Morituba, Oriboca)
    Ungrouped (Rift Valley, Colorado tick fever,
    sandfly)
	20 to 100	Yes	?	

Myxovirus and paramyxovirus (RNA):
    Influenzas A, B and C: parainfluenza, mumps,
    rubeola; respiratory syncytial
	80 to 200	Yes	Yes	Helical

Rhabdovirus: rabies (RNA)	65 to 180	Yes	Yes	

Arenavirus (RNA):
    Togavirus: rubella (most arbovirus of groups A
    and B)
	50	Yes	Yes	

Papovavirus (DNA): "Warts" simian virus 40	45 to 55	No	No	Cubic
Adenovirus (DNA)	65 to 85	No	No	Cubic

Herpesvirus (DNA):
    Herpes simplex, monkey B, varicella-herpes zos-
    ter, cytomegalovirus, Epstein-Barr
	120 to 180	Yes	Yes	Cubic

Poxvirus (DNA): Variola, vaccinia, molluscum contagiosum	150 to 300	Yes or no	Yes	Cubic
Human hepatitis (nucleic acid unclassified): Infectious hepatitis, serum hepatitis				

(Adapted from Thorn, G.W., et al. (Eds.): *Harrison's Principles of Internal Medicine.* 8th Ed. New York, McGraw-Hill, 1977.)

They are nonenveloped viruses that have within their icosahedral shells a single + strand RNA genome of 2.7×10^6 daltons, which serves as the mRNA for 1 long polypeptide, which is subsequently cleaved to the mature proteins. In addition to 4 structural proteins, 1 of the additional proteins is the poliovirus replicase. Replication of the RNA through a double-stranded intermediate supplies a pool of virion RNA. Replication, translation, and assembly of the virus occur in the cytoplasm. Shutdown of host RNA and protein synthesis is rapid and dramatic. Newly assembled virions are released by lysis of the infected cell.

ENTEROVIRUSES. These are unusually acid- and bile-resistant. In light of their transmission by ingestion and their intestinal site for multiplication, this resistance is teleologically understandable. They can be grown in tissue culture with striking cytocidal effects.

Poliovirus comes in 3 serotypes that are infectious only for primate cells. Interestingly, most poliovirus infections are inapparent. Of those that are clinical, many cause a mild disease with headache, nausea, and fever. A few cases progress to aseptic meningitis, with pains in the back and neck, ending in rapid and complete recovery. In approximately 15% of the cases, the poliovirus causes flaccid paralysis, frequently with loss of anterior horn cells and the consequent loss of muscle innervation, which may be prolonged and often is irreversible.

After ingestion of the virus, there is a one-

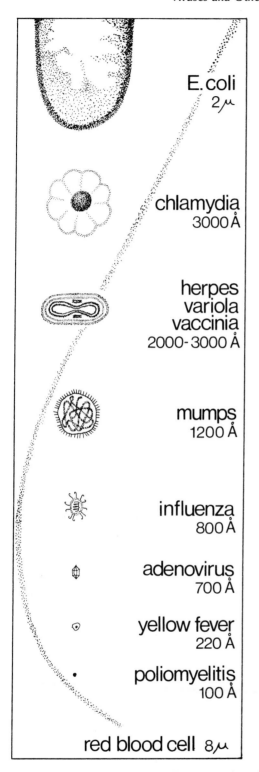

E. coli
2μ

chlamydia
3000 Å

herpes
variola
vaccinia
2000-3000 Å

mumps
1200 Å

influenza
800 Å

adenovirus
700 Å

yellow fever
220 Å

poliomyelitis
100 Å

red blood cell 8μ

Fig. 8–3. This illustration shows the relative sizes of a red blood cell, half of which is shown in a silhouette the length of the figure, and a bacterium (E. coli), which is shown in the upper part of the field. Chlamydia, herpes, mumps, and the smaller viruses are also indicated. (Adapted from Pelczar, M., Jr., et al.: *Microbiology.* 4th Ed., New York, McGraw-Hill, 1977.)

to two-week incubation period with viral multiplication in the lymphoid tissues of the pharynx and gut. This period may be followed by viremia and distribution of the virus to secondary target organs. Poliovirus replicates preferentially at this stage in the anterior horn cells of the spinal cord and causes the characteristic paralysis. (Greek *polios* (gray) refers to the gray matter of the spinal cord.)

Antibody to poliovirus is serotype-specific—thus the importance of having all 3 types in the vaccine. Antibody is produced locally in the intestine during infection, and prevents reinfection with the same serotype. If generalized viremia does occur, there must be preexisting circulating antibodies to halt the paralytic path. In rarer cases, the virus may travel along nerve fibers to the brain, causing bulbar paralysis.

Environmental factors that increase the likelihood of paralysis have been discussed and described, such as pregnancy, fatigue, and tonsillectomy. Early in the twentieth century, with poorer sanitation, poliovirus was endemic. Most people suffered inapparent or mild infections at a young age. As hygiene improved, this widespread (herd) immunity changed. People were more likely to be exposed later in childhood, when the chances of serious complications are higher. There were also significant numbers of susceptible nonimmune persons, and the virus usually spread in an epidemic fashion when it appeared. Poliomyelitis has been brought dramatically to a near halt with the advent of the Salk (dead) and Sabin (live) vaccines. In 1952, just before the Salk vaccine became generally available in the United States, there were 3,145 deaths and 21,269 cases of paralysis, whereas in 1969 there were only 19 cases of paralytic polio and not a single death.

Coxsackie viruses have a similar life cycle and are responsible for many illnesses. These include febrile abdominal illnesses, rashes, upper respiratory tract infections, meningitis, and myocardiopathy. Recent findings also implicate a Coxsackie virus in the etiology of juvenile-onset diabetes mellitus. There are far too many serotypes to make vaccines a sensible or practical possibility.

Echoviruses cause similar symptoms and signs, including rashes and meningitis.

RHINOVIRUSES. Although they are more acid-labile, these viruses are similar to the enteroviruses. They have a clear preference for growth *in vitro* at 33°C rather than at 37°C. This preference is consistent with their localization in the nasal passages, which are cooler than the core body temperature. Rhinoviruses are the causative agents of many of our "common colds." Experimental work has shown that nasal entry is the most efficient mode of infection, and that virus shedding starts as soon as 24 hours after entry and can continue for weeks. Edema of mucous membranes, fluid exudation, increased secretory activity of submucosal glands, and coughing are at their peak 2 to 3 days after infection. This continues for about a week. The virus titer is highest in nasal secretions rather than in saliva. Sneezes are contagious. Antibodies are stimulated by rhinovirus infection; whether clinical improvement is a function of antibody intervention or of interferon induction is debatable.

Togaviruses. These viruses are composed of an RNA genome inside a capsid, which in turn is enveloped (hence Latin *toga*, cloak). The togaviruses are also single-stranded, + RNA viruses with a genome of 4×10^6 daltons. The term togavirus refers to the morphology of the virus, whereas the term arbovirus refers to the mode of transmission (*arthropod-bo*rne). Thus a virus could have a coat and still be spread by insects.

Togaviruses multiply in the cytoplasm and replicate much as do picornaviruses. Host protein synthesis shuts off rapidly; RNA synthesis stops late in infection. The togaviruses are enveloped in a membrane. During their assembly, viral cores line up at the cell membrane under patches in which viral glycoproteins have become embedded. The virions then bud off, surrounded by a lipid and glycoprotein envelope. This budding leaves the cell intact. Although the togaviruses have a one-piece genome, they translate their proteins from more than 1 mRNA derived from the virion genome. This is a first step toward genetic complexity, and probably allows more evolutionary or adaptive flexibility than the simple system employed by picornaviruses. With 2 messages, the timing and relative quantities of protein synthesis can differ.

Many togaviruses are arboviruses (indicating their transmission by an insect vector to a reservoir of animal hosts). The animal population supplies new susceptible hosts through breeding; the high virus titers in the animal blood during the viremic phase provide a rich source for viral passage by the blood-sucking ticks and mosquitoes. The virus grows abundantly within the insects but without killing the cells. *In vitro*, arboviruses have been shown to infect insect and vertebrate cell cultures, which demonstrates variability with respect to the host environment. The ability of the same virus to replicate effectively in insects and in a variety of birds and mammals was one of the first supports for the universality of the genetic code.

YELLOW FEVER. Arbovirus infections have been of broad economic and political significance to man. The real interest, indeed romance, of yellow fever is not so much the virus that causes it as the means by which the virus is transmitted. Until 1900, it was believed that the disease was due to unsanitary conditions, that the infection was probably conveyed from the sick to the healthy by intestinal discharges. In that year, the American Yellow Fever Commission under Walter Reed determined to put to the test the theory that a mosquito might carry the infection, as had already been shown to be the case in malaria. At that time no animal was known to be susceptible to the disease, so human volunteers had to be used. These persons allowed themselves to be bitten by mosquitoes that had already fed on yellow fever patients. One member of the Commission, Dr. Carroll, developed yellow fever and nearly died; a second, Dr. Lazear, became even more desperately ill and finally did die.

The centuries-old problem of yellow fever had at last been solved. The disease was transmitted by a mosquito, the female *Stegomyia* (different variety from the *Anopheles* that carries malaria). If the *Stegomyia* could be destroyed, the scourge of the tropics could be eradicated. How this was done by General Gorgas cannot be related here, but success was complete. The control of yellow fever opened up South and Central America, made Rio de Janeiro habitable, and made the Panama Canal possible.

These arthropod-borne viruses are injected into the capillaries of the host with saliva when the insect bites. The viruses multiply in the vascular endothelium and the reticular cells of lymph ·nodes, liver, and spleen. This phase is characterized by viremia, and may represent the full course of the disease. Togaviruses are potent stimulators of interferon. Progress of the infection may cause arthralgia and rashes. In the case of yellow fever, the virus attacks the capillaries and kills the capillary cells, causing hemorrhaging, particularly in the liver and the kidneys. The most characteristic lesions are in the liver, which shows areas of necrosis, inclusion bodies, and rupture of the biliary passages with escape of bile into the blood. The chief symptoms are fever, vomiting, diarrhea, and intense jaundice, so that the skin turns yellow. In epidemics there is a mortality rate of 80%. It is therefore little wonder that the disease was dreaded by Europeans. Other arboviruses cause encephalitis that results in paralysis, coma, and death. Because of the extensive viremia accompanying these viral diseases, survivors have a lifelong, type-specific immunity. There is now an effective yellow fever vaccine that employs a lab-attenuated strain.

RUBELLA. Also known as German measles virus, this is a non-arthropod-borne togavirus that causes human disease. The virus is transmitted by inhalation, after which it multiplies in the upper respiratory tract and passes into the blood stream by means of the cervical lymph nodes. It causes a trivial rash, which involves the face and is probably due to localized antigen-antibody reactions. There is 1 serotype, and immunity is long-lasting.

The importance of rubella is that it affects the fetus of pregnant women in the first trimester. It exerts teratogenic effects on the fetus such as blindness, deafness, heart defects, and retardation. The mechanism is unknown, but it is likely that infected fetal cells survive but divide too slowly or abnormally. The virus spreads through contiguous cells of the fetus. This renders maternal antibody inefficient in halting the infection. Thus organs derived from infected cells are often improperly developed. Clearly, exposure to rubella virus of pregnant, nonimmune women may have serious consequences.

Rhabdoviruses. These viruses are similar to the togaviruses in that they are enveloped. The most famous is the rabies virus.

The rhabdoviruses are bullet-shaped, enveloped viruses with a 4×10^6 dalton genome consisting of a single piece of $-$ strand RNA. Viral proteins include a nucleocapsid protein, a surface glycoprotein, a matrix protein, and putative polymerase proteins. The glycoprotein spikes of the virus have hemagglutinating activity. The proteins are translated from multiple messages (each coding for 1 protein) derived from the single genomic RNA, and thus can vary in the timing and level of their synthesis. In some cases host functions are shut off completely; in other instances infected cells continue to produce virus persistently. The virus enters cells by membrane fusion or phagocytosis. Newly produced virions leave the cell by budding. Frequently, characteristic acidophilic inclusions known as Negri bodies appear in the cytoplasm of the ganglion cells at the base of the brain. These are ribonucleoprotein complexes that persist in the cells but are not released and not infective.

RABIES VIRUS. This rhabdovirus infects most warm-blooded animals. Bats are thought to be asymptomatic carriers. Their urine, which they spray when flying, contains the virus, and even the air of densely populated bat caves may be dangerous to breathe. In other hosts, the disease is violent and usually fatal. A characteristic behavior of rabid animals is the frenzied biting of other animals. Since the virus is present in saliva, it is spread effectively.

Symptomatic rabies occurs in roughly one-half of exposed cases; the incubation time, usually 1 to 3 months, may range from 1 week to 1 year. The disease begins with general malaise and hyperesthesia in the wound. The principal symptoms, whether in animal or in man, are terrific cerebral excitement and rage, spasm of the muscles of the pharynx, especially at the sight of water, so that the patient is unable to drink, and generalized convulsions. It is one of the most terrible of all diseases, and when symptoms have developed, is almost always fatal. The virus does not spread from the wound by means of the blood stream, but rather along the neurons. Amputation of the infected area can halt the disease. The lesions are entirely microscopic, for the brain appears normal to the naked eye. Microscopically, there is degeneration of the nerve cells and collars of inflammatory cells around the small vessels, but the pathognomonic feature is the presence of Negri bodies. When a dog suspected of rabies has bitten a person, it must be killed and its brain examined for Negri bodies. After exposure to the disease, persons are usually given immune serum, followed by rabies vaccine. This procedure is generally effective because of the long incubation period of the disease. It is remarkable that the modern treatment of rabies was introduced by Pasteur, who knew nothing of filterable viruses. He found that the spinal cord of rabbits infected with the disease was rich in the infective agent, as shown by the results of animal inoculation. He also found that he could lower the virulence by drying the spinal cord; the longer the drying, the lower the virulence. Pasteur then used the material of low virulence as a vaccine, with which he repeatedly inoculated the person bitten by the rabid animal. By this means the patient built up resistance to the virus, so that by the time it reached the spinal cord some 2 months later, he had become immune. If the Pasteur treatment was commenced immediately after the bite, there was complete prevention in every case. Surely this was a stroke of pure genius in the earliest days of microbiology! And Pasteur was a chemist, not a doctor of medicine! Control of rabid animals, vaccination of dogs, and effective treatment protocols have greatly reduced the frequency of symptomatic rabies.

Paramyxoviruses. These viruses include the causative agents of mumps, measles, and some respiratory diseases.

They are enveloped viruses with a genome of one − strand of RNA 7×10^6 daltons in size. They can be grown in culture without extensive cell destruction. Cytologic characteristics are acidophilic inclusions and the frequent fusion of infected cells to form giant syncytia (multinucleate masses of protoplasm produced by the merging of cells). Viruses multiply in the cytoplasm, using a viral transcriptase, and are released by budding through the cell membrane. Proteins are translated from multiple messages, and precursor proteins are cleaved during maturation. These processing steps probably involve host functions and are often essential in producing fully infectious virions. Proteins include nucleocapsid, matrix, and glycoprotein; glycoprotein spikes most often have hemagglutinating activities, and sometimes hemolysin potentiation as well. There is no dramatic shutdown of host cell functions. Paramyxoviruses associated with human disease are parainfluenza viruses 1 to 4, mumps, measles, and respiratory syncytial virus (RSV).

PARAINFLUENZA VIRUSES. Infecting the epithelia of the upper respiratory tract, symptomatic after a two- to six-day incubation period, these viruses may cause fever, pharyngitis, and bronchitis. In infants, lower respiratory tract involvement is common; one of the best-known complications is croup, an acute laryngotracheobronchitis caused primarily by parainfluenza 1. These viruses replicate locally in the respiratory epithelium and are highly contagious. Reinfection with similar serotypes is common, since the relevant antibody is tissue IgA, which is neither abundant nor long-lived. Even in the presence of circulating antibody, the disease progresses unchecked.

In adults, RSV causes upper respiratory infections that are indistinguishable from colds. In infants, it can cause serious lower respiratory tract infections, in which secondary bacterial infection is the rule. These infections reach epidemic proportions annually in urban centers. *In vitro*, RSV can be grown in primate cultures, in which it causes huge syncytia. The paramyxoviruses may spread by fusing cells rather than by freely circulating, and so may escape the effects of the antibody response.

MUMPS VIRUS. This produces characteristic inclusions and syncytia in culture. Its glycoproteins possess hemagglutinin, hemolysin, and neuraminidase activity. One-half of mumps infections are inapparent. There is a sixteen- to eighteen-day incubation period. The virus multiplies in the upper respiratory tract and lymph nodes, and 3 to 5 days of viremia follow, which may bring the virus to characteristic target organs. The virus has a proclivity for glands. The most common symptom by far is swelling of the parotid (salivary) gland(s). In postpubescent males, orchitis with or without resultant sterility is frequent. Meningitis follows in roughly 10% of the cases. Infection stimulates interferon and antibody production. Antibodies to the hemagglutinin antigen are thought to be the most long-lived and relevant to immunity. There is now an effective mumps vaccine.

MEASLES VIRUS. This virus can be grown in culture and also produces striking syncytia and cytoplasmic inclusions. Inapparent infections are rare. After inhalation, the virus multiplies in the epithelia of the upper respiratory tract, where it may spread to lymph nodes and lymphocytes. In 9 to 12 days, antibody levels rise in the blood and the rash appears, commencing with Koplik's spots (red ulcerations inside the cheek). The rash is probably due to an antigen-antibody reaction. Recovery is usually rapid and complete. There is now an effective attenuated vaccine.

In a few cases, encephalomyelitis may develop as a result of delayed hypersensitivity, when lymphocytes infiltrate infected neural tissue, sometimes causing demyelinization. Even more rarely, a slow neurologic disease, SSPE (subacute sclerosing panencephalitis) is found in older children with a previous history of measles. SSPE patients have high levels of antibodies to most measles antigens, and tissue of the central nervous system contains a measles-like virus. The role of persistent measles virus in causing this disease is being investigated.

Multiple sclerosis (MS) is another disease in which measles virus is implicated. The epidemiology of this demyelinating disease suggests that a precipitating event could be a measles infection in late adolescence. Another possible explanation is outlined in the chapter on the central nervous system. Many MS patients have elevated levels of antimeasles antibody in their serum and cerebral spinal fluid. Viruses that seem to persist by slow growth, avoiding immune eradication by spreading through fusing cells rather than through the bloodstream, appear to be of newfound biologic importance.

Orthomyxoviruses. This class includes **influenza viruses,** types A and B.

These are enveloped viruses with roughly 550 glycoprotein spikes per virion. Their glycoproteins have hemagglutinin and neuraminidase activities. The A and B types are distinguished by the nucleoprotein antigen; with these types, strains are characterized by glycoprotein antigenic variations. The genome of the virus occurs as 9 distinct pieces of − strand RNA, totaling 5×10^6 daltons, each of which is transcribed to mRNA for translation. This segmented genome not only allows for multiple messages that permit translational control, but also for high levels of recombination among the different influenza genes. This recombination is probably responsible for the extensive antigenic changes that influenza virus undergoes rapidly.

After inhalation, influenza virus establishes an upper respiratory infection with a one- to two-day incubation period. The first phase is characterized by constitutional symptoms of fever, chills, and aches. A more obvious respiratory infection follows, with cough, coryza, and rhinorrhea. High titers of virus are released in nasal secretions.

To establish infection, influenza virus must bypass any local IgA present from previous influenza infections. In addition, there are glycoprotein inhibitors of viral attachment in the nasal mucus that are attacked by the viral neuraminidase. This interaction causes the runny fluid exudate of influenza respiratory disease. Although influenza virus can be grown *in vitro* in cell cultures with no cytopathic effects, the result of *in vivo* infection is necrosis and shedding of the respiratory epithelium. This epithelium is the first line of defense against bacterial infection, which occurs with great ease when the infected epithelium is destroyed and the raw surface of the trachea and respiratory tree is subject to invasion and attack by normal bacterial inhabitants of the upper airways. A secondary or superinfection results in pneumonia, which is the cause of high fatality rates in influenza epidemics.

Because the main obstacle to the establishment of influenza is a relatively small amount of tissue IgA, any antigenic changes that allow the virus to bypass this line of defense are strongly selected. Changes in the viral hemagglutinin (an antigenic marker) are the primary mode of antigenic drift, by which a new, slightly different strain of influenza appears and is more successful in establishing infection and in spreading among a population. This occurs every few years. At intervals of roughly 10 to 15 years, a dramatically different strain appears, a so-called antigenic shift. We believe this results from the recombination of a human influenza virus with a virus from a different species of animal host, perhaps by an exchange of 1 of the 8 genomic pieces. This new strain can find a large pool of susceptible hosts, and it causes the great influenza epidemics that have been disastrous in recent medical history. Serologic studies of persons of all ages have allowed the sketching of a profile of influenza antigenic drift and shift for the last hundred years.

Arenaviruses. These round or oval enveloped viruses are characterized by electron-dense internal granules. Their genome appears as 2 pieces of single-stranded RNA; the virions package host RNA species as well.

LASSA FEVER VIRUS. This virus is transmitted by respiratory or alimentary route. It replicates in local lymph nodes, and invades reticuloendothelial tissue, inhibiting the effects of immune-related cells. Capillary damage is usual. Antibody buildup may stem the disease. The febrile stage can last from 1 to 3 weeks. Thirty to 66% of hospitalized cases are fatal. This rare disease is seen primarily in Africa, but laboratory cases have been reported recently. Most known arenavirus infections are thought to originate from contact with infected rodents, the natural reservoir. The viruses tend to be localized in distinct geographic areas. Interestingly, pathologic arenaviruses of man can at times induce persistent infections with no discernible effect on the host.

Retroviruses. These are a unique class of enveloped viruses. Their genome consists of 2 identical + strand RNA's of 3×10^6 daltons each. When infection takes place, RNA is transcribed to DNA by the viral reverse transcriptase. The DNA is made double-stranded and then integrates permanently into the host genome. From this integrated copy, virion RNA and viral messages may be transcribed, proteins may be synthesized, and virions may be assembled at the cell membrane. The viruses are nonlytic and may be expressed indefinitely. Many of these viruses have been shown to be natural causes of cancer in a range of animal species. In some cases, these viruses are inherited as cellular genes by all members of an animal population. Presumably, germ line cells were infected early in evolutionary history and the virus was maintained in the genome. These endogenous viruses may be either fully expressed or latent. Although no human retroviruses have yet been found, their importance in animal disease makes them worth mention here.

DNA VIRUSES

Since these viruses have a DNA genome, as does the host, life-cycle pathways of replication and transcription can rely to a greater extent on the normal cellular enzymatic machinery. Some simple DNA viruses use only host enzymes. With increasing complexity, DNA viruses bring in their own polymerases. These viruses are bigger and more complicated than RNA viruses, and they can replicate in a greater variety of cell locations. Some stimulate resting cells to grow, others replicate independently of the host genome. Perhaps because of this potential for control of DNA replication and growth in cells, almost all DNA viruses have been shown to have an oncogenic potential in animals. As we shall discuss, there is a growing evidence for the viral origin of some human cancers. The importance of latent and persistent infections with DNA viruses will also become apparent.

Viral Hepatitis, Types A and B. Both infectious and serum hepatitis are now known to be viral in origin, and have been reclassified as viral hepatitis types A and B. They are caused by hepatitis A virus (HAV) and hepatitis B virus (HBV), respectively. Molecular studies are incomplete, but the HBV virion, the Dane particle, has been partially characterized. This spherical particle has an envelope bearing the HB_s antigen, a core carrying the HB_c antigen, and a partially double-stranded, circular DNA genome that is approximately 2×10^6 daltons in size (Fig. 8–4). The host range of these viruses is limited to primates; no appropriate tissue culture system has been found despite 40 years of continued effort.

Epidemiologic studies have been more complete regarding HBV infection, which is widespread and often inapparent. Among healthy blood donors in the United States and Western Europe, 3 to 15% show immunologic evidence of previous infection, and .1% are chronically infected with HBV. Roughly 1 to 5% of HBV infections are clinically severe, and may present long-term complications.

HAV is generally transmitted by the fecal-oral route, although contaminated water systems and food supplies have also been incriminated. Type A hepatitis epidemics have occurred. There is a month-long incubation period, during which the virus replicates in nonhepatic sites. Viral excretion begins after roughly 3 weeks. In the postincubation phase, viral excretion declines, anti-HAV IgM titers rise, and jaundice become noticeable. Damage to the liver may result from the immune response. The onset of type A hepatitis is usually abrupt and febrile, with malaise, fatigue, nausea and abdominal discomfort. Pooled human immune serum is an effective

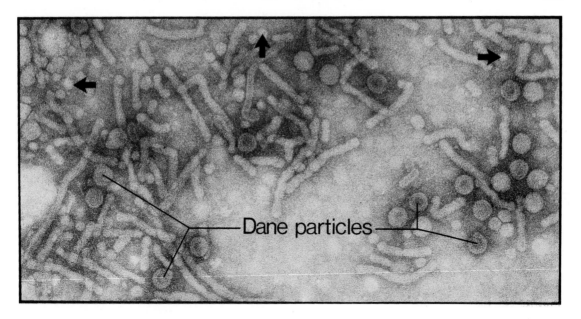

Fig. 8–4. This electron micrograph shows the Dane particle and HB antigen particles (arrows) in a negatively stained preparation. × 155,000 (Courtesy of Dr. S. N. Huang, Pathology Institute, McGill University.)

treatment for preventing or attenuating infection in exposed or potentially exposed persons.

HBV is most often transmitted by blood transfusions, contact with inadequately cleansed medical instruments contaminated with blood, and by dirty needles used either in tattooing or by drug users. The primary site of replication is unknown, but evidence of the virus in the liver does not appear until some weeks after infection. The immune response complicates the characteristic hepatic damage. Antigenemia is typical. Type B disease is more insidious and less febrile in its onset, but it tends to be more prolonged than type A infections. Passive immunization with immune serum globulin is an accepted treatment of probable contacts.

Papovaviruses. With their double-stranded, closed circular genome of 5×10^6 daltons, these viruses are enclosed in an icosahedral virion. Although papovaviruses have been of great value to molecular virologists in studying gene expression and oncogenic transformation, they are mentioned only briefly here. A subgroup of these viruses is implicated in a progressive neurologic disease. Another papovavirus, human wart virus, causes benign overgrowths of the epidermis.

Adenoviruses. These large viruses have a 23×10^6 dalton double-stranded genome. The adeno-

viruses are a cause of upper respiratory disease. The genome is often found in a circular conformation with the ends linked by a terminal protein; this shape facilitates infection. The nonenveloped particle is icosahedral, and the capsid contains at least 14 proteins. Virions are relatively stable and suited to survival outside the host. Susceptible cells are thought to have 10^4 receptors per cell. After entry, multiple mRNA's are synthesized in the nucleus, copying different regions along both strands of the DNA at different times. Significant RNA processing is involved in the temporal control of the viral protein synthesis. Shortly after infection, host DNA synthesis is stimulated, perhaps to ready the cell for virus replication. Later in infection, host DNA, RNA, and protein synthesis are inhibited. Viral DNA is replicated in the nucleus, using the cellular polymerase; levels of adenovirus DNA reach that of total uninfected cell DNA. Particles are assembled in the nucleus, where they form characteristic crystalline arrays. They are released on disruption of the infected cell.

There are at least 31 serotypes of human **adenoviruses.** These are endemic, and only some 50% of childhood infections cause symptomatic disease. The common adenovirus disease is an acute respiratory infection with the pharynx as the site of viral multiplication, and an incubation period of 5 to 7 days. The frequent recovery of adenovirus from tonsils of patients who do not have an adenovirus-like disease suggests frequent inapparent and chronic infections. Virus shedding usually outlasts the duration of the disease. Transmission is usually through respiration or by the fecal-oral route. Adenovirus accounts for about 5% of viral respiratory disease. There are a few examples of more serious adenovirus complaints, one of which, ARD (acute respiratory disease), is a disabling respiratory ailment prevalent among new military recruits. Adenoviruses have also been shown to have oncogenic potential in animals.

Herpesviruses. The *herpes simplex virus* is one of the most widely distributed viruses in the general population. The reason is that after the initial attack, the virus continues to live and to multiply in the cells in a latent stage. The herpesviruses are large, with a double-stranded linear DNA genome of 100×10^6 daltons and an unusually high guanine and cytosine content. The DNA is associated with proteins in a barbell formation, and is surrounded by a protein capsid, outside of which is a lipid envelope. The virions are acid-labile. Their DNA codes for at least 49 proteins, 33 or more of which are virion components. There are 162 capsomers in the icosahedral capsid. The lipid envelope is thought to be derived largely from the nuclear envelope. DNA replication occurs in the nucleus and may employ the host polymerase. The herpesvirus genome is known to code for some enzymes involved in DNA synthesis; their role remains unclear. After mRNA transcription and cytoplasmic protein synthesis, the proteins are returned to the nucleus where virion assembly occurs. The envelope is acquired during the process of budding out. Host protein synthesis is shut down; host RNA synthesis is reduced by 75%. The particular strains of herpesviruses will be discussed in the context of their various diseases.

HERPES SIMPLEX, 1 AND 2. These 2 related viruses cause primary infections during childhood that are usually inapparent. Although they can each establish infection anywhere on the body, type 1 is usually transmitted orally and causes infections of the upper body, primarily of the mouth, and type 2 is transmitted genitally and causes infections of the lower body. When apparent, symptoms appear after about a week, appearing as sores that result from lytic viral replication. Complications are more serious when babies are infected during birth with vaginal HSV-2. Another serious site of herpes infection is the conjunctiva of the eye; severe infections can cause blindness. Luckily, this infection is responsive to topical application of antiviral agents that interfere with DNA metabolism.

The real significance of herpes simplex virus (HSV) is not in its primary infection, but in its persistence in a latent state following infection. Fever, radiation, sunlight, and other stresses can activate herpes. The most common presentation of HSV-1 reactivation is the "cold sore," or "fever blister" on the lip. Experimental evidence suggests that the virus remains in a latent state in the sensory nerve ganglia, and travels in times of stress to the epidermis, where it can replicate freely. Circulating anti-HSV antibodies do not halt this reactivation. The evolutionary advantage of such persistent infections for the virus is obvious; the prevalence of anti-HSV antibodies in primitive societies suggests an early origin and widespread prevalence of these viruses.

There has been much attention focused on the possible role of HSV-2 in uterine cervical cancer. HSV-2 does infect cervical tissue, and there is a greater frequency of anti-HSV-2 antibodies in women with cervical cancer than in the general population. HSV-2 and cervical cancer are both rare in women with little or no sexual activity. Both HSV-2 and cervical cancer correlate epidemiologically with early onset of coitus and multiple sexual partners. Although the evidence is not complete, it seems likely that there is a sexually transmissible agent involved in cervical cancer. Herpesviruses do have oncogenic potential *in vitro* and in laboratory animals.

HERPES ZOSTER VARICELLOSUS. In primary infection, this herpesvirus is responsible for **chickenpox** (varicella). The virus is thought to enter through the oropharynx, the upper respiratory tract, conjunctiva, or perhaps through the skin. The virus replicates by spreading through contiguous cells. Infected cells display ballooning and develop intranuclear inclusions. Virus circulates in the blood and lymph, stimulating an immune response. After a week, the immune response is overpowered, viremia increases, and systemic symptoms of fever and malaise appear. There are successive crops of skin vesicles, red macules with a centrally placed vesicle of clear fluid ("dewdrop"). Different stages of macule, pustule, and scab can be seen simultaneously; the lesions occur centripetally, primarily on the trunk. Virus is present in these lesions for less than 1 week. The disease is normally mild, and immunity to exogenous infection is lifelong. There is only 1 known serotype. Widespread disease and fatal pneumonia can arise in immune-compromised children and also in adults, in whom accompanying pneumonia is common.

After varicella infection, the virus is thought to persist in dorsal root or cranial nerve ganglia. Various stresses may cause a reactivation of the virus, causing it to travel down a sensory nerve with accompanying pain. Blisters develop on the area supplied by the nerve; the lesions are unilateral and terminate abruptly at the midline. This is **zoster** ("girdle") or **shingles,** an illness plaguing .3% to .5% of the population per year. More than one-half of those affected are over 50 years of age. The virus in the zoster lesions is identical to that in chickenpox; one may contract chickenpox from a person who has zoster lesions. This again underlines the selective advantages of such reactivatable latent infections.

CYTOMEGALOVIRUS. This herpesvirus is primarily associated with chronic or latent infections of the salivary gland, most of which are inapparent. Occasionally, hepatitis or pneumonitis occurs. Frequently the infection is activated in persons undergoing immunosuppressive therapy, inducing an interstitial pneumonia. Transplacental infection can be fatal to the fetus, or it may leave a child mentally retarded.

EPSTEIN-BARR VIRUS. The agent of **infectious mononucleosis,** this is a ubiquitous virus that causes many inapparent infections, especially when contact occurs in childhood. Transmission can be respiratory or through the mouth, frequently through the salivary exchange of kissing. In 4 to 7 days, malaise and lethargy appear, accompanied by pharyngitis and enlargement of cervical and axillary lymph nodes. Fever and chills may occur, and the spleen may become enlarged. The disease usually runs its course in 1 to 2 weeks, but prolonged discomfort can occur. When the Epstein-Barr virus (EBV) enters the host's mouth, it probably first replicates in the epithelia of the mouth and throat. The virus is spread through the blood and lymph and infects B lymphocytes. Various changes in the lymphocyte population occur, with a characteristic appearance of atypical T lymphocytes. Some but not all infected B cells are killed. Recently, the profile of the immune response

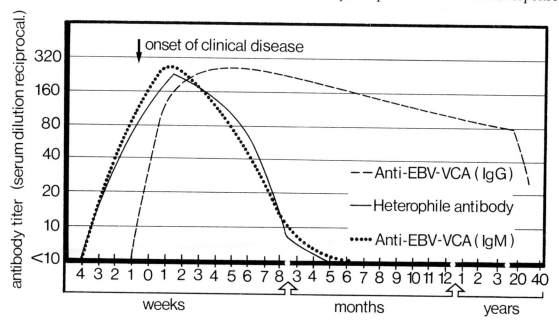

Fig. 8–5. The relative antibody titers during the evolution of infectious mononucleosis is shown in the accompanying graphs. The onset of clinical disease appears within one week of infection. The life-long immunity to anti-EB virus is shown in the top line. (From Schleupner, C.J., and Overall, J.C., Jr.: Infectious mononucleosis and Epstein-Barr virus. I. Epidemiology, pathogenesis, immune response. Postgrad. Med., 65:83, 1979.)

has been studied. IgM and then IgG antibodies to the virus capsid antigen (VCA) first appear, followed by transient IgG antibodies to D, a diffuse viral antigen found in nuclei and cytoplasm of infected cells. Finally, lifelong antibodies appear to Epstein-Barr nuclear antigen, which is virally induced. Heterophil antibodies arise and are diagnostic for the disease (Fig. 8–5).

EBV is not a simple lytic virus. The virus can induce either lytic or abortive infections. In cell cultures, EBV can establish latent infections of 2 types. The herpesvirus DNA has been found in 2 forms: as independent circles, and as segments integrated into the host chromosome. When latent cultures are derepressed, 2 types of particles are obtained, those with full lytic capabilities and non-lytic transforming particles. The latter can transform (immortalize) B cells *in vitro*. EBV-transformed cells all express the EBNA antigen, and it appears that transformation reflects the presence of integrated herpes DNA. Although B cells from EBV⁻ persons die after a short period in culture, B cells from EBV⁺ persons are transformed and grow indefinitely in culture.

It is likely that EBV persists in a latent form in B cells of infected persons, and that the disease is lytic and is a self-limiting leukemia kept in check by the immune system. Carriers may continue to shed virus, again underlining the selective advantage of a virus that is able to establish a persistent infection. Finally, EBV has been shown to be oncogenic in laboratory primates.

EBV is intimately associated with 2 human cancers, Burkitt's lymphoma and nasopharyngeal carcinoma. **Burkitt's lymphoma** affects 1 in 10,000 children per year, primarily aged 6 to 8 years, in the warm, wet lowlands of Africa. It is a rapidly growing lymphoma of the neck and jaw. EBV is endemic in the locale of incidence, and infection usually occurs early in childhood. Patients with Burkitt's lymphoma (BL) have roughly tenfold higher titers of anti-EBV antibodies than the normal African child. Ninety-eight per cent of monoclonal BL tissue contains EBV DNA, whereas it is not found in other lymphomas. The clinical prognosis of the disease correlates with anti-EBV antibody profiles (Fig. 8–6). When therapy results in a decrease in the anti-R antibody (an early EBV antigen) titer,

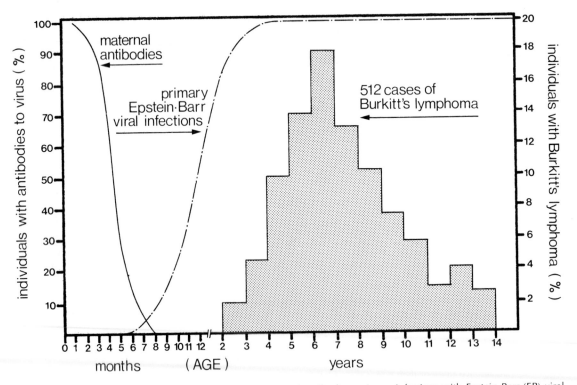

Fig. 8–6. This graph shows the relationships among maternal antibodies, primary infections with Epstein-Barr (EB) viral infections, and 512 cases of Burkitt's lymphoma. The Burkitt's lymphoma cases were preceded by infections with EB virus. (From Henle, W., Henle, G., and Lennette, E.T.: The Epstein-Barr virus. Sci. Am., *241*:48, 1979.)

recovery is likely; persistence or increase in the anti-R titer after therapy usually implies a fatal recurrence. It is unlikely that all the monoclonal tumors would arise in the small number of EBV-infected lymphocytes by chance. It seems probable that EBV infection or transformation is necessary but not sufficient for the onset of BL. Since the area of BL prevalence is coincident with that of malaria, the possibility of malaria as a cofactor has been suggested. Malaria is thought to weaken the immune response and to enhance lymphocyte proliferation. The seasonal variation in BL onset implies that the cofactor is environmental. It is also true that BL tissue has a chromosomal translocation involving segments of chromosomes 8 and 14; similar rearrangements have been observed in other lymphomas.

Nasopharyngeal carcinoma occurs in several limited geographic locales and racial groups. Genetic factors and chemical carcinogens have been suggested as etiologic agents. All biopsies have revealed EBV DNA in the carcinoma tissue. Patients have high titers of anti-EBV antibodies, especially to the D antigen; uniquely, IgA is frequently present in these cases. Patterns of antibodies to VCA and D antigens parallel tumor enlargement and regression after treatment, and also foreshadow tumor reappearance. Although causation has not been proven, experimental and epidemiologic data point to EBV, and perhaps to other herpesviruses, as human tumor viruses.

Poxviruses. This is the largest, most complex group of DNA viruses. The only true poxvirus we consider here is the causative agent of smallpox. Under older systems of classification, a number of important diseases were categorized as "poxes." The name is derived from the vesicopustular skin eruptions that characterize these diseases. In the Middle Ages, when diseases began to be named, there were 4 types of pox, or pocks. These were known as the Great Pox (syphilis), the Small Pox (variola), Cow Pox (vaccinia), and Chicken Pox (herpes zoster varicellosus), so-called because the chicken typified something gentle and mild. Syphilis, of course, is not caused by a virus. The herpes simplex virus is one of the most widely distributed viruses in

the general population. The reason for this is that after the initial attack, the virus continues to live and multiply in the cells in the latent stage.

These are at least 20 proteins in the brick-shaped virion, within which is a 100×10^6 dalton double-stranded genome. After absorption onto specific receptors, the virus undergoes sequential uncoating steps, the last of which requires early mRNA synthesis and translation. The virus codes for several enzymes involved in DNA metabolism. Uniquely, these DNA viruses multiply in the cytoplasm, in characteristic factories known as Guarnieri bodies. There are early and late phases of mRNA and protein synthesis. Several thousand virions are released from the disintegrating cells as rapidly as 5 hours after infection.

The most significant poxvirus for our discussion is variola, the etiologic agent of **smallpox**. This was one of the most virulent of infectious diseases. All races of men were susceptible, and no one from childhood to old age was exempt. Actual contact, direct or indirect, with a patient was not necessary for transmission. It swept through the country with the speed of a prairie fire. (Other virus diseases, such as influenza, may travel with the same terrifying speed.) Small wonder, then, that in bygone years nearly everyone, high or low, rich or poor, bore the marks of "the pox" on his or her face. The picture in seventeenth-century England is drawn thus by the vivid pen of Macaulay: "The smallpox was always present, filling the churchyards with corpses, tormenting with constant fears all whom it had not stricken, leaving on those whose lives it spared the hideous traces of its power, turning the babe into a changeling at which the mother shuddered, and making the eyes and cheeks of a betrothed maiden objects of horror to the lover." Now almost no doctor living in countries where this book is likely to be read has ever seen a case of smallpox (Fig. 8-7).

The virus enters through the respiratory route, multiplying for 1 to 2 weeks in the lymph nodes and lungs. Cell lysis is typical. Two days of febrile viremia follow. During this circulatory phase, virus localizes in the skin and grows in nodules. These are most frequent on the extremities; this may occur because the high temperature inhibits viral growth, and the extremities remain cooler

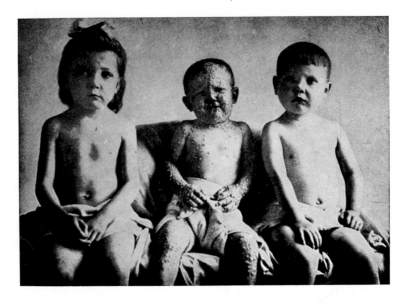

Fig. 8–7. The value of vaccination. Three of a family exposed to smallpox; the child in the middle unvaccinated, the others vaccinated one year before (Schamberg and Kolmer.)

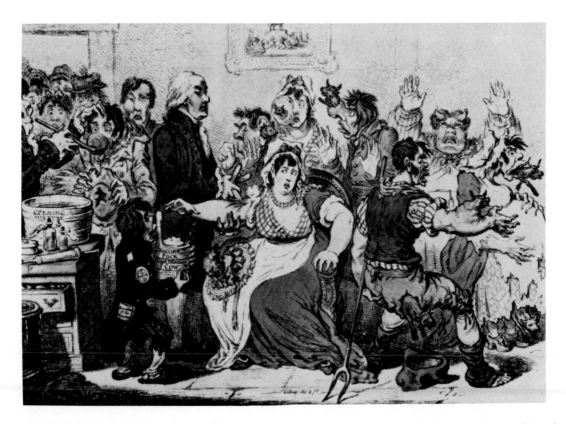

Fig. 8–8. This caricature by Gillray (1802) illustrates the ridicule to which Jenner's discovery of vaccination was subjected. (From a print in the Wellcome Institute for the History of Medicine.)

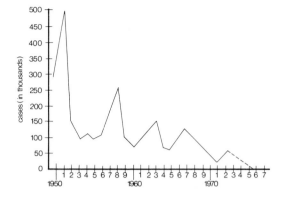

Fig. 8–9. The graph shows the decreasing incidence (worldwide) of smallpox during the last 2 decades. (From World Health, Jan.–Feb., 1968.)

than the trunk. At first these nodules are solid papules, but in a few days they become converted to pustules that may cover the face and the entire body. There is swelling and "ballooning" of the epithelial cells, which goes on to liquefaction of the cells, often followed by superinfection due to streptococcal infection. In chickenpox there is also swelling of the epithelial cells, but superinfection with streptococci is uncommon. The epithelial cells adjoining the lesions contain characteristic cytoplasmic Guarnieri bodies. Scabs are formed over the pustules. As the scabs dry they are cast off and changed into dust, each particle of the dust being covered with the virus. From this description it will be seen how important the problem of nursing is, especially in a community that has not been adequately vaccinated. As the pustules heal, scars of varying depth are left in the skin. Thus the dangers of smallpox are twofold: (1) death, and (2) disfigurement.

Smallpox has always been in the foreground of vaccine research. It was first found that the related cowpox virus would induce only a mild disease in human beings but would stimulate lasting immunity to the more severe smallpox virus (Fig. 8–8). Today, massive vaccination campaigns have eliminated smallpox as a threat in most areas of the world (Fig. 8–9).

UNCONVENTIONAL VIRUSES

There is a class of unconventional viruses that are responsible for slow neurologic dis-

eases. These viruses are by definition filterable, but they are thermostable and ultraviolet-insensitive. No nucleic acid assignment has been made. No apparent immune response or inflammatory lesions accompany their infections. They induce slow degenerative diseases known as subacute spongiform virus encephalopathies.

Kuru is one such disease found only among a single ethnic group in New Guinea. The virus is present in diseased brain tissue and can be passed to primates. It appears that the virus was spread by contact with and ingestion of infected brain tissue. Cannibalism as a mourning tribute was prevalent from 1920 until 1950; with its cessation, the disease is on the decline. Apparently, the virus slowly accumulates in the central nervous system and gradually destroys tissue. Eventually neurologic symptoms appear, with tremors progressing to motor incapacity and death.

Creutzfeldt-Jakob disease is caused by a similar virus that produces analogous disease on inoculation into primates. The symptoms are diffuse mental disorientation proceeding to dementia, mutism, rigidity, and death. This rare disease appears worldwide and is transmissible.

CHLAMYDIAL INFECTIONS

Another group of diseases (trachoma, lymphogranuloma venereum, psittacosis) was thought until recently to be caused by agents included as viruses, although the agents showed some peculiar features, and had been separated as the largest viruses known. They have been called Bedsonia, Miyagawanella, Prowazekia, and a confusing array of other names.

These agents were considered to be unusual because they were sensitive to some antibiotics, but similar to other viruses, they required living cells for replication. We now know that these agents differ from viruses in that they have 2 nucleic acids, yet they differ from bacteria in that they have a limited metabolic capability. They are nonmotile spheroids, 0.3-1.0 μ in diameter, with a discrete cell wall analogous to those of gram-negative bacteria. They can be stained by Giemsa stain, and can multiply within cells by binary fission without undergoing the eclipse phase typical of viral multiplication, in which phase the particles are dispersed in the nucleoplasm or cytoplasm of the host cell and cannot be visualized.

Chlamydiae are medically important because they are causative agents of several diseases that are endemic, and because the agent may reside within the host for long periods of time before causing clinically apparent disease. People who have left trachoma-endemic areas without evidence of active disease for decades may develop acute eye infection in their 60's or 70's; this disease is the most common worldwide cause of blindness. These same organisms cause genital infections such as urethritis and cervicitis. Currently chlamydia is believed to be the commonest cause of urethritis, other than gonorrhea. The importance of these infections is that they usually are transmitted to the consort, and may ultimately threaten the health of the newborn.

Trachoma

The chlamydial organism causes 3 types of conjunctivitis: infections in the newborn, adult inclusion conjunctivitis, and trachoma.

During passage through the birth canal, newborn children may acquire infection of the conjunctiva that appears as a mucopurulent discharge, is generally considered to be benign and self-limited, and responds to antibiotic therapy. This disease is estimated to occur about twice per 1,000 live births, but recent estimates suggest this may be a gross underestimation. Other complications in the newborn are otitis and pneumonitis.

In the adult, acute conjunctivitis often occurs, and significant numbers of cases have been traced to chlamydial infections usually acquired from exposure to or discharge from the genital tract. It is likely that many of the cases of so-called "swimming pool conjunctivitis" are due to chlamydial infections.

The chronic form of conjunctivitis, seen most commonly in North Africa, sub-Sahara Africa, the Middle East, and Southeast Asia, is the leading preventable cause of blindness in the world. The term trachoma was coined by a Sicilian physician in 69 A.D., but the dis-

ease has been described as early as 1500 B.C. in the Ebers papyrus. It was widespread in early times, as now, and afflicted both Cicero and Horace. It was introduced to Europe by returning crusaders and by Napoleon's troops coming from Egypt. The disease is still a problem in the United States where it exists in Indian reservations of the southwest. It has been found to be a disease of families, with the agent passing from child to child, sparing none under 2 years of age. The inflammation advances by superinfection with bacteria that causes scarring of the lids, so that the eyelashes turn inward to abrade the cornea constantly, leaving a scar through which no light can penetrate to the retina.

Reiter's Syndrome

This disease complex with an eponym for its designation is the simultaneous occurrence of conjunctivitis, arthritis, mucocutaneous lesions, and urethritis not caused by gonorrhea. Reiter's syndrome occurs principally in men between the ages of 20 and 40, and may either occur acutely or wax and wane. We used to believe the causal agent was the gonococcus, but cultures were negative and subsequent studies have incriminated chlamydia as the offending agent. This entity is considered more completely in the section where HLA antigens are discussed because of the unusually high association with HLA W-27 markers.

Psittacosis

The final disease caused by these agents is the acute febrile illness in which fever, headaches, muscle aches, and dry cough with interstitial pneumonia can be identified. This acute illness has been reported in pigeon breeders, people who have pet budgies, finches, or parrots, chicken or turkey farmers, poultry processors, and pet store personnel, or in children. Since we now know that the organism (serologically different from the other chlamydia) can be passed from birds to man, this is called a zoonosis, a disease harbored by an animal vector and transmitted on occasion to the human being. It responds to tetracyclines, and the problem is to make the correct diagnosis.

RICKETTSIAE

These organisms are small bacteria and perhaps should be included in that chapter, but for decades they have been considered a biologic form intermediate between bacteria and viruses, so we shall discuss them here, although the concept is no longer acceptable. Rickettsiae have a gram-negative-bacteria-like cell wall, prokaryotic DNA with a genome approximately equivalent to Neisseria, and a complement of ribosomes. They often have a microcapsule or slime layer and are capable of substantially independent metabolic activity, but they are only known to grow within cells. For this reason specifically, we include them here.

All rickettsiae are transmitted by arthropod vectors. They were first observed in 1909 by H. T. Ricketts in the blood of patients with Rocky Mountain spotted fever, and in the tick that carried the disease. The next year, Ricketts found similar organisms in the intestine of lice that had fed on a patient with typhus. It is appropriate that these organisms should be named after Ricketts, since he died of infection with these agents during his studies.

Typhus Fever

This acute infectious fever that used to be one of the great scourges of man is caused by *Rickettsiae prowazekii*, and it may be noted that Prowazek also died of the disease. The infection is carried by the louse. Until this apparently simple discovery was made, we were powerless to control this plague or to explain the historic association of typhus epidemics with wars, famines, and wretchedness. However, the discovery of the vector of typhus left unsolved the problem of the smouldering embers of the infection in interepidemic periods, for the human louse soon dies of intestinal hemorrhage when infected with typhus. The secret reservoir of infection was found to be the domestic rat, transmission from animal to animal being through the agency of the rat flea. If the rat dies and the rat flea is hard put to find a new

host, he may bite man. The louse now has its chance, and if the victim is lousy and lives in a lousy community, the result is an epidemic. The patient may survive, but the poor louse is doomed. Any reader who may wish to know more about the fascinating story of typhus in war and history should turn to Zinsser's delightful and entertaining, *Rats, Lice and History*.

The onset of the disease is acute, with high fever, great weakness and prostration, a hemorrhagic rash, and mental apathy passing into stupor. The characteristic microscopic lesion is a swelling of the vascular endothelium throughout the body, including the skin and the central nervous system, the cytoplasm of the cells being crowded with rickettsiae. This is accompanied by thrombosis and hemorrhage that account for the symptoms. Curiously enough, in the louse the organisms are confined to the epithelial cells lining the gut, so that the excreta are swarming with rickettsiae which, when deposited on the skin, may enter through scratches and abrasions. Bacot, one of the leading workers in this field, died of typhus although he never was bitten.

We feel that we should apologize for devoting so much space to a disease that we sincerely hope the reader will never encounter, but we have been carried away by the fascination of the subject.

Other Rickettsial Diseases

Five other diseases are known to be caused by rickettsiae. These will merely be mentioned. (1) Tsutsugamushi fever is a typhus-like infection, also known as **scrub typhus**. It is endemic in Japan, Malasia, and the East Indies, and the infection is transmitted by the bite of the infected larva of certain mites that live in rotting vegetation and tall grass, hence the name scrub typhus. (2) **Rocky Mountain spotted fever** bears a remarkable resemblance to typhus fever in regard to symptoms, lesions, and bacteriology. It used to be thought that the disease was confined to the Rocky Mountain region of the United States, but it is now known that the infection may be acquired over a considerable part of the United States and in southern Canada (Fig. 8–10). The disease is conveyed by a wood tick. As in

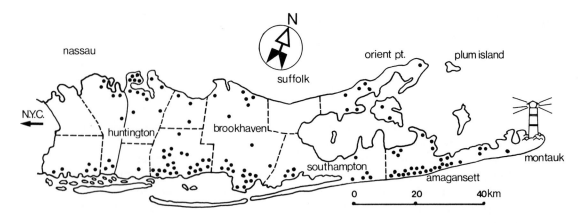

Fig. 8–10. This map of Long Island in New York State shows the distribution of cases of Rocky Mountain spotted fever in 1978. This disease is transmitted by the wood tick. Note the distribution at the seashore. (From Benach, J.L., et al.: Changing patterns in the incidence of Rocky Mountain spotted fever on Long Island (1971-1976). Am. J. Epidemiol., *106*:380, 1977.)

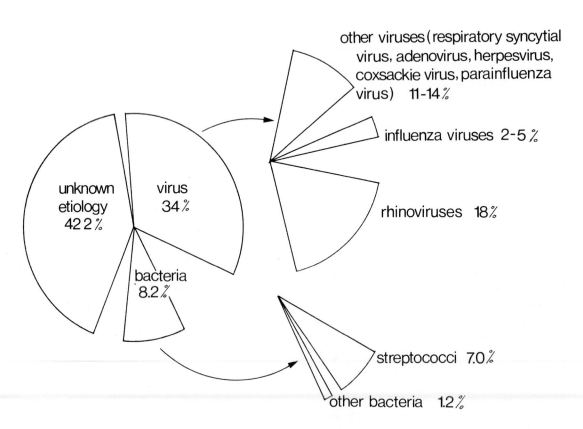

Fig. 8–11. This diagram shows the relative importance of different viruses and bacteria in causing respiratory tract infections. (After *Patterns of Diseases*, Morris Plains, N. J., Parke, Davis and Company, 1961.)

the case of typhus, laboratory workers may acquire the disease without being bitten by the tick. (3) **Trench fever** is so-called because it was the commonest of all the diseases affecting the troops in France during the trench warfare period of World War I. Infection was carried by the body louse. The mortality was so low that nothing is known of the lesions in man. (4) **Rickettsial pox** is a new rickettsial disease recognized in New York in 1946. The name is due to an eruption not unlike that of chickenpox. Infection is caused by the bite of a tick. The prognosis is uniformly favorable. (5) **Q fever** is a rickettsial disease that derives its name from having been first described in Queensland, Australia. The infection is carried by rodents and is spread by ticks. The remarkable feature of the disease, which is

widespread throughout the world, is the absence of any relation between the lesions, which take the form of pneumonic patches in the lungs, and the clinical picture, which is that of a typhoid-like state with a complete absence of respiratory symptoms. The mortality rate is low.

To conclude, it is important to keep some perspective in understanding the place of viruses as agents that cause disease in general. The accompanying diagram (Fig. 8–11) shows the proportions of respiratory tract infections caused by different viruses and bacteria. Of the unknown causes, one could estimate that half at least may be caused by viruses, leading to a grand total of 50% of all respiratory tract ailments, one of man's most common afflictions, being of viral etiology.

SYNOPSIS

Viruses are obligate intracellular parasites.

Viruses do not reproduce by dividing, but by directing the synthesis and export of a large number of like progeny.

Viruses can be classified by size, tissue specificity, and nucleic acid content.

Viruses may lyse cells, or they may alter their morphology or growth patterns.

Many viral infections are inapparent.

Viruses have been shown to be among the causes of cancer in animals.

Viral infections stimulate an immune response. In addition to curbing infection, the immune response can cause severe complications.

Viruses can exist in latent forms.

Viruses may be spread by droplet, blood, sewage, and insect vectors.

Terms

Arbovirus	*Interferon*	*Syncytia*
Cytopathic effect	*Latent virus*	*Viremia*
Eclipse	*Lysis*	*Virulent*
Inclusion bodies	*Persistent virus*	*Virion*

FURTHER READING

Baron, S.: The interferon system. A. S. M. News, *45*:358, 1979.

Evans, A.S. (Ed.): *Viral Infections of Humans: Epidemiology and Control.* New York, Plenum Medical Book Co., 1976.

Fenner, F., et al.: *The Biology of Animal Viruses.* New York, Academic Press, 1974.

Fenner, F., and White, D.O.: *Medical Virology.* New York, Academic Press, 1970.

Foege, W.H.: Should the smallpox virus be allowed to survive? N. Engl. J. Med., *300*:670, 1979.

Henle, W., Henle, G., and Lennette, E.T.: The Epstein-Barr virus. Sci. Am., *241*:48, 1979.

Kilbourne, E.D.: *Molecular Epidemiology—Influenza as Archetype.* (Harvey Lectures, Series 73.) New York, Academic Press, 1979.

Leclair, J.M., et al.: Airborne transmission of chickenpox in a hospital. N. Engl. J. Med., *302*:450, 1980.

Schachter, J.: Chlamydial infections. N. Engl. J. Med., *298*:428, 1978.

Fungal Infections

9

Infectious disease is merely a disagreeable instance of a widely prevalent tendency of all living creatures to save themselves the bother of building the things they require. —ZINSSER

Fungi represent another type of organism than bacteria; unlike plants, they lack pigments necessary to manufacture their own food and therefore depend on other forms of life. Fungi may assume different appearances during their life cycle, and can exist as microscopic forms (yeast), or in large colonies (mushrooms). Historically, many diseases of medical importance caused by fungi (histoplasmosis, coccidioidomycosis), have been mistaken for those caused by protozoa, and other diseases once classified as fungal are now considered to be bacterial (nocardia, actinomycosis). Regardless of how they are classified, fungi are assuming greater importance than ever, because we now successfully treat most bacterial diseases and keep people safe longer from the traditional infectious agents by various techniques.

Fungi are omnipresent in the air, so that they are apt to contaminate culture media, to grow as molds on food, and to be generally troublesome. Fortunately, few are pathogenic. For growth they require a high humidity, warmth, and a free supply of oxygen. Any gardener trying to grow roses and prevent "black spot" knows this. The warmth and humidity of the tropics are particularly favorable for their multiplication, so it is natural that fungal diseases should be much commoner in tropical countries and in the south-ern United States. Some reproduce only by budding, but others bud with failure to separate, giving rise to long branching filaments known as hyphae, which form masses called mycelia. A fungus causing an infection can be grown on culture media or demonstrated in the tissue, preferably with special stains such as PAS (periodic acid-Schiff) and silver methenamine.

The subject of fungal infections, known as the mycoses or mycotic diseases, is acquiring a new importance by reason of the use and abuse of multiple antibiotics. These wipe out the harmless bacteria with which the fungi are accustomed to live and that restrain fungal growth. With elimination of the bacteria, the fungi occupy the field, to multiply without restraint, and to assume the role of pathogens. Damage to the tissues is not caused by toxins, but is the result of allergic necrosis due to sensitization to the proteins of the fungi. Skin tests for hypersensitivity to these foreign antigens are of great value in many instances. Fungi are more resistant than bacteria to drying and to the action of antibiotics, which, after all, are derived primarily from fungi. With modern medical treatment involving many people in chemotherapy for cancer, immunosuppressive therapy for transplantation, and antibiotic therapy for common bacterial infections, we see greatly increased numbers of hospital patients who succumb to fungal diseases such as candidiasis, aspergillous infections, and mucormycoses. Because these fungi normally cannot infect a human being but are successful in the debilitated or immunologically deprived patient, such fungal diseases are called opportunistic infections. The fungi that cause superficial infections spread from animals to man, whereas those that cause systemic infections seem to come from the soil, vegetation, and bird droppings. Only a few of the pathogenic fungi will be considered in this text.

HISTOPLASMOSIS

This disease has an extraordinary history. The causal organism, named at that time *Histoplasma capsulatum*, was first demonstrated in 3 fatal cases in the Panama Canal Zone in 1906, and was believed from its appearance to

be a protozoon animal parasite. The disease was believed to be confined to the tropics and to be uniformly fatal. Some 30 years later, the organism was cultured and shown to be a fungus, not a protozoon. This discovery proved to be the breakthrough, for the culture of the fungus was used as the antigen for a histoplasmin skin sensitivity reaction, to be followed shortly by a complement fixation test. These procedures proved to be revolutionary, for they showed that infection with the fungus was prevalent in the northeastern and central part of the United States, the central Mississippi Valley in particular, and that in much lesser degree it was worldwide in distribution (Fig. 9–1). From the skin tests it soon became apparent that there were 2 different forms of the disease: 1 mild, localized, and common; the other severe, disseminated, rare, and nearly always fatal. In endemic areas, histoplasmin tests show that up to 75% of the population may be infected by the fun-

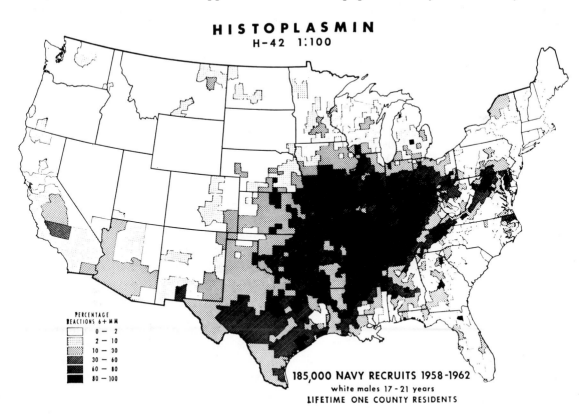

HISTOPLASMIN
H-42 1:100

PERCENTAGE
REACTIONS 6+ M M
0 – 2
2 – 10
10 – 30
30 – 60
60 – 80
80 – 100

185,000 NAVY RECRUITS 1958-1962
white males 17 - 21 years
LIFETIME ONE COUNTY RESIDENTS

Fig. 9–1. This map of the United States shows the histoplasmin positive skin tests for 185,000 navy recruits between 1958 and 1962, illustrating their lifetime residence. The Mississippi River valley is the location of most of the fungal infections caused by this organism. (From Comstock, G.W.: In *Maxcy-Rosenau Preventive Medicine and Public Health,* 10th Ed. Edited by P. E. Sartwell. New York, Appleton-Century-Crofts, 1973.)

gus without any clinical evidence of disease. The infection does not appear to be transmitted directly from person to person, but to be inhaled in the dust from the soil, where the fungus can be demonstrated. Many domestic animals are susceptible to infection, and several epidemics have been associated with contamination of the soil by animal excreta, especially that of pigeons and chickens.

Typically the epidemic will be a small group of persons involved in demolition or in cleaning out old silos or chicken coops, who become ill after an incubation of 1 to 2 weeks. Attack rates may reach 100% and cough, fever, and prostration are the typical symptoms in the illness, which lasts 1 to 3 weeks. This mild form is a benign inhalation infection of the lungs. At least 95% of cases are asymptomatic. It is startling to find roentgenographic evidence of extensive infiltration in the lungs with no symptoms or physical signs. The lymph nodes at the hilus of the lung are nearly always enlarged. A few patients have cough, fever, and loss of strength (Table 9–1).

The rare progressive form is an entirely different story, with a nearly always fatal finish. Acute disseminated histoplasmosis is generally the result of a heavy infection with the

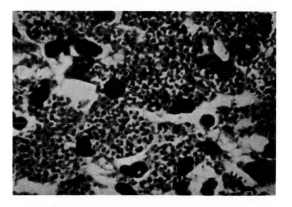

Fig. 9–2. Cells of the lymph node packed with *Histoplasma capsulatum.* (From a section by Dr. W. A. D. Anderson. In Boyd, W.: *Textbook of Pathology* Philadelphia, Lea & Febiger.)

fungus or of poor resistance in young children and debilitated elderly persons. Tubercle-like nodules and necrotic foci are found in the lungs, liver, spleen, and kidneys, together with ulcerating lesions of the mouth, larynx, and intestine in many cases. Microscopically the reticuloendothelial cells are crowded with the organisms, which bear a remarkable resemblance to the protozoa causing leishmaniasis (Fig. 9–2).

COCCIDIOIDOMYCOSIS

Approximately 100,000 new cases of coccidioidomycosis occur per year in the United States, with about 70 deaths. It is said to be as common as chickenpox in some areas, and the medical interest lies both in the morbidity it causes and in the rarer, but often fatal, fulminant case. The disease is commonly called San Joaquin Valley fever and came into prominence during the early days of World War II when large numbers of recruits were stationed in that area, and later prisoners of war as well. These military men often became symptomatic, with a first diagnosis being made of pulmonary tuberculosis. Skin testing 25 years ago showed the distribution of positive reactors (Fig. 9–3).

The causative agent is a dimorphic fungus (Fig. 9–4) that grows naturally and on media as a mold, but in man or in laboratory animals it may appear as spherules that contain endospores. The endemic region for the organ-

Table 9–1.   Clinical Characteristics of Infected and Reinfected Persons in an Outbreak of Histoplasmosis at an Arkansas Courthouse in July, 1975

SYMPTOM	FREQUENCY IN 50 SEROLOGICALLY CONFIRMED CASES (%)
Fever	100*
Chills	76
Weight loss	44†
Cough	72
Headache	72
Myalgia	78
Chest pain	74
Arthritis	26
Mouth ulcerations (size unknown)	12
Erythema nodosum (red swelling on legs)	18

*Average 39.1°C (102.6°F)
†1.8 kg to 5.6 kg
(From Dean, A.G., et al.: An outbreak of histoplasmosis at an Arkansas courthouse, with five cases of probable reinfection. Am. J. Epidemiol., *108*:36, 1978.)

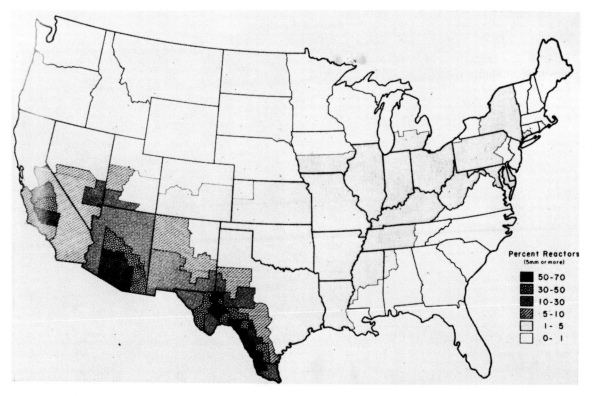

Fig. 9–3. This map of the United States shows the location of reactors to skin testing for coccidioidomycosis. (From Comstock, G.W. In *Maxcy-Rosenau Preventive Medicine and Public Health*, 10th Ed. Edited by P. E. Sartwell. New York, Appleton-Century-Crofts, 1973.)

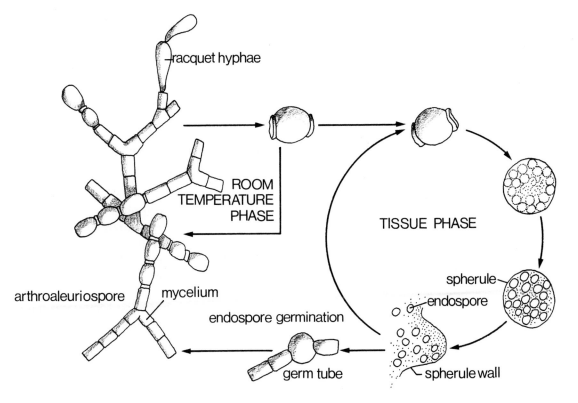

Fig. 9–4. This drawing illustrates the appearance of the fungus coccidioidomycosis. The hyphae of the fungus are shown on the left. An intermediate form between the hyphae and the microspheres appears at the top (between the arrows). The tissue phase (endospores) is shown on the right. (From Drutz, D.J., and Catanzaro, A.: Coccidioidomycosis. Am. Rev. Respir. Dis., *117*:559, 1978.)

Table 9–2. Frequency of Symptoms in 27 Archeology Students with Laboratory-Confirmed Coccidioidomycosis

SYMPTOM	FREQUENCY (%)
Cough	89
Fever	82
Headache	74
Chest pain	70
Chills	67
Shortness of breath	63
Malaise	59
Myalgia	52
Rash	52
Night sweats	44
Phlegm	30
Erythema nodosum	15
Meningismus	15
Weight loss	11

(From Drutz, D.J., and Catanzaro, A.: "Coccidioidomycosis. Part II." Am. Rev. Respir. Dis., *117*:727, 1978.)

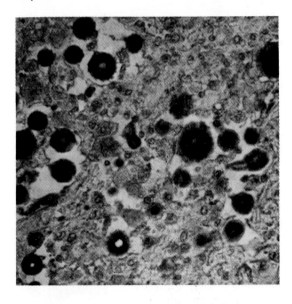

Fig. 9–5. *Cryptococcus neoformans* shown in Alcian blue stain. The thick capsules of the organisms have been preserved by mounting in glycerin jelly. (Kindness of Dr. R. W. Mowry. In Boyd, W.: *Pathology for the Physician.*)

ism is the southwest, where the fungi survive in rodents' burrows and in the sandy soil. The fungus infects swine, cattle, and sheep, but they, like man, are largely resistant to infection. It has been reported in dogs, in horses, and even in tigers.

The disease is acquired by inhalation of the spores, therefore the dustier, drier, and richer the soil is with the agent, the better the chance for exposure.

The clinical symptoms are outlined in Table 9–2.

CRYPTOCOCCOSIS (TORULOSIS)

A subacute or chronic infection caused by *Cryptococcus neoformans* (*Torula histolytica*), cryptococcosis or torulosis may involve the lungs, skin, and other parts, but it has a special predilection for the meninges and brain, so that it is always dangerous (Fig. 9–5). In the lungs, the smaller lesions are easily mistaken for tubercles, but sometimes they are as large as an orange. The infection favors tissue weakened by reason of infancy, before resistance has had time to be established, of old age, of chronic debilitating illness, or of the displacement of the normal friendly bacterial inhabitants by antibiotics, and the balance is tilted still more decisively from health to disease.

BLASTOMYCOSIS

This is a chronic granuloma caused by a yeast-like fungus known as *Blastomyces*. The organisms are spherical, 2 or 3 times the diameter of a red blood cell, and show 2 characteristic features: (1) a clear double contour, and (2) budding yeast-like cells. The disease and the fungus that causes it occur in different forms in different parts of the world. Thus there is North American, South American, and European blastomycosis. The last is better named cryptococcosis, described in the foregoing section.

The North American form may be cutaneous or systemic. In the cutaneous (the common) variety, skin papules, which later ulcerate, develop especially on the face, the back of the hand, and the front of the leg. The disease spreads over the surface, so that a large area may be involved. In the systemic and naturally much more dangerous variety, infection spreads by the blood stream throughout the body, setting up nodules and abscesses usually in the lungs, but any organ may be involved.

South American blastomycosis, a chronic granulomatous disease of the skin, viscera, and lymph nodes that is most common in

Brazil, is caused by a much larger fungus with numerous buds. The most characteristic feature is enlargement of the lymph nodes, particularly those of the neck, present in practically every case.

CANDIDIASIS

Candida, a saprophytic, dimorphic fungus, is commonly present on mucous membranes (oral cavity, genitalia), and in the gastrointestinal tract of man. Normally, the organism does not cause disease, but it has become increasingly a serious threat to life when there is prolonged therapy with antibiotics, corticosteroids, or immunosuppressive drugs, or in the presence of uremia, leukemia, hyperalimentation, or intravenous catheters.

The organism normally thrives in conditions of moisture and will appear as white patches involving the vagina, axillary folds, or mouth. When these patches occur in the mouth, they are known as thrush, and consist of growing mycelia, branching mycelial filaments with budding yeast-like cells that have thin walls. Normally, the infection is limited to the surface epithelia, but more cases of fungemia (blood stream infection) are being reported, often similar to and difficult to distinguish from endocarditis caused by other organisms.

Antibodies are made to the fungus and, in suspected cases, a serum agglutinating antibody titer can be done. It is also helpful to examine the buffy coat to see if the yeast-like organisms can be stained within the white blood cells. Tissue diagnosis by histologic examination is often diagnostic. Amphotericin B is the modern drug of choice, but its administration carries risks and it is wise to be certain of the diagnosis before beginning therapy.

MUCORMYCOSIS (PHYCOMYCOSIS)

This is another example of a disease caused by aerobic saprophytic fungi that are normally not pathogenic for man, but reside in soil and decaying matter. Again, in the debilitated host, someone with another illness such as diabetes mellitus, uremia, acidosis, burns, or cancer, or who has been receiving steroids,

radiotherapy, chemotherapy, or antibiotics, these fungi may grow, prosper, and cause disease.

The organism normally grows as hyphae with a wide angle of branching, and typically invades and obstructs blood vessels leading to thrombosis and infarction, particularly in the lung in man. The organisms may involve branches of the retinal or cerebral vessels, sometimes arising in a sinus infection, or they may penetrate the gastrointestinal tract and compromise the circulation to the liver. These organisms may also cause weakening of the arterial wall, leading to the particular type of aneurysm called mycotic.

Diagnosis can be established by staining the suspected tissue, or by growing the organism from the sputum or blood. Mucormycosis is to be suspected in all instances in which the patient's defenses are compromised. It is best regarded as a complication of other disease, a true example of opportunistic infection.

DERMATOMYCOSES

This in common language is ringworm, which suggests that all dermatomycoses have the same etiology, and implies that the treatment may be the same. The dermatomycoses resemble each other in that areas of redness occur in patches on the skin of the head, groin, between the fingers and toes, or in the axilla, but the specific fungi are different. Because they are highly contagious, they are often difficult to treat in crowded conditions, or in those areas where facilities for personal hygiene are not available. These infections are communicated by means of contaminated clothing and structures such as the floors of rooms. Although not dangerous, dermatomycoses are notoriously difficult to treat. The following are some common forms.

Ringworm of the Scalp. This disease is also known as tinea (not to be confused with taenia or tapeworm). For some reason it affects only children. It is contagious, and in schools and institutions it may assume epidemic proportions. The fungus, known as *Trichophyton* (Greek *thrix*, hair and *phyton*, plant) invades and lives in the hair and in the roots of the hair; this explains why it attacks the scalp, why it produces bald patches, and why it is so difficult to eradicate.

Ringworm of the Groin. The causal fungus invades the epidermis, and is therefore known as an *Epidermophyton*, and frequently occurs in schools and among young athletes.

Interdigital Ringworm. This form occurs between the fingers and toes, and has become common because of the increased use of gymnasiums, locker rooms, showers, swimming pools, and the like. The frequency of the disease has in places been enormous. The association of the disease with various sports is the reason for its common name, "athlete's foot." The fungus usually responsible is *Epidermophyton.*

To put fungal infections in some perspective, of 1,251 cases seen in hospital between 1972 and 1974, 102 were candidal, 44 were aspergillous, 9 were mucormycoid, and the remainder were minor dermatomycoid infections.

SYNOPSIS

Biologic factors in fungal growth limit its infectivity.

Opportunistic infections are the most serious fungal threat to human life.

Superficial fungal infections are common, deep infections are rare.

Terms

Mycelia	*Hyphae*	*Epidermophyton*
Yeast	*Mycoses*	

FURTHER READING

Conant, N.F., et al.: *Manual of Clinical Mycology,* 2nd Ed. Philadelphia and London, W. B. Saunders, 1954.

Dean, A.G., et al.: An outbreak of histoplasmosis in an Arkansas courthouse with five cases of probable reinfection. Am. J. Epidemiol., *108*:36, 1978.

Drutz, D.J., and Catanzaro, A.: Coccidioidomycosis. Am. Rev. Respir. Dis., *117*:559, 1978.

Flynn, N.M., et al.: An unusual outbreak of windborne coccidioidomycosis. N. Engl. J. Med., *301*:358, 1979.

Goldstein, E., and Hoeprich, P.D.: Problems in the diagnosis and treatment of systemic candidiasis. J. Infect. Dis., *125*:190, 1972.

Medoff, G., and Kobazaski, G.S.: Pulmonary mucormycosis. N. Engl. J. Med., *286*:86, 1972.

Rubenstein, E., et al.: Fungal endocarditis. Medicine, *54*:331, 1975.

Animal Parasites

10

Nature is a labyrinth in which the very haste you move with will make you lose your way. —BACON

An animal parasite is a member of the animal kingdom that has acquired the power of living in the body of another animal. The parasite may or may not produce disease in the host. Here we are concerned only with the human host and with pathogenic (disease-producing) parasites. Most parasites have developed a remarkable habit; they spend a part of their life cycle in 1 host (man) and another part of the cycle in another host (an animal). The second host may be of any size, from a cow to a mosquito, but each parasite has its own particular animal host; the cow and the mosquito are not interchangeable. Moreover, the second host is a necessity, not a luxury; unless it can be found, that particular parasite will die. It is evident that knowledge of this dependence places a powerful weapon in the hands of persons involved in the prevention of parasitic diseases. Finally, the second host may be responsible for conveying the disease to man, as in the case of the mosquito and malaria.

One of the most remarkable features of a parasite's life cycle is that the eggs produced in the body of an animal or man do not develop in the same animal. They may develop into larvae in the soil, but usually they must be ingested by another host and develop there. The **definitive host** is the host of the adult parasite (sexual cycle), and the **intermediate host** is the host of the embryo (asex-

ual cycle). Man is the definitive host of the common tapeworms, but the intermediate host of the malaria parasite.

We can agree that animal parasites have evolved a remarkable and perilous method of completing their life cycles, for unless the appropriate intermediate host comes along, the family of the parasite is doomed, as the eggs cannot develop in the definitive host. To meet this hazard, parasites have learned to produce eggs in numbers that in some instances are astronomic. The fish tapeworm of man lays several million eggs daily and lives for several years, whereas the stomach worm of the sheep lays an egg every 10 to 20 seconds. The problem of reproduction has been simplified in some tapeworms by the male's being dispensed with entirely!

Before discussing various animal parasites, we might look at the question of parasitism from the point of view of the parasite. When an animal decides to adopt this way of life, it must be prepared to make certain sacrifices. The host provides the parasite with all the comforts of life, so that organs of locomotion and those of special sense required for hunting prey or avoiding enemies disappear. The parasite does not necessarily damage the host; they may live in harmony for many years. Indeed the successful parasite does not jeopardize the survival of the host, because in so doing it jeopardizes its own survival.

However, the pathogenic parasites must occupy our attention. These occur commonly even in temperate climates, and, when tropical parasites are included, we meet some of the most important diseases of mankind. Only a few of the more serious will be considered here. Disease-producing parasites belong to 2 great groups: protozoa, or unicellular organisms, and worms, which fall under the category of metazoa. The worms are divided into roundworms, tapeworms, and flukes.

PROTOZOA

Amebiasis. This condition is commonly the cause of dysentery, an inflammation of the colon. The danger of dysentery, apart from the inconvenience, is dehydration, electrolyte loss, and loss of blood in the acute stages. With more chronic disease, perforation, peritonitis, and abscesses may occur. The clinical pattern of infections other than dysentery depends on the organs involved. Apart from the bowel, liver abscess is most common, and spread from there to the lungs may also occur. Symptoms of these infections are nonspecific and heralded by fever and malaise. To make the diagnosis, one must

suspect the presence of such abscesses, which may be identified today by technetium-sulfur colloid liver scans, or by gallium citrate studies. Ultrasound studies may also reveal a hollow cavity with internal echoes (Fig. 10–1), but, of course, none of these techniques identify the causal organism, only the presence of a lesion. In order to make the diagnosis, it is necessary to identify the ameba with the microscope.

The ameba is a single, large cell, recognized by its motility in a fresh specimen of feces. It often contains ingested red blood cells. In chronic cases of amebiasis, such as are seen in temperate climates, the ameba becomes globular and is converted into a cyst with a thick, outer capsular layer. The cysts are the infective form of the parasite, for the active form is killed by the gastric juice as it passes through the stomach. Multiplication in this simplest of all animals is by direct division; there is no sexual stage.

Infection is usually the result of fecal contamination of water supply or food. The chief danger is from a carrier rather than from a patient suffering from the active form of the disease. Two reasons for this are: In the first place, the danger from the patient is obvious,

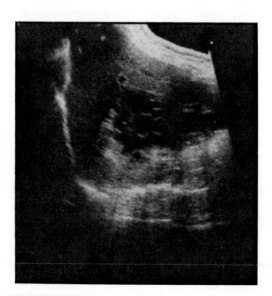
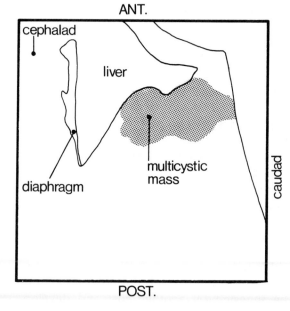

Fig. 10–1.   *A,* This ultrasound scan of the liver shows a multiloculated cystic mass in the inferior portion of the liver. The dense white line at the top indicates the position of the diaphragm. *B,* The drawing illustrates the position of the multicystic mass, which is typical of an echinococcal cyst.

and precautions can be taken to prevent the spread of the infection, whereas the carrier is unsuspected. The second reason is that the parasites discharged from the carrier in the form of cysts are much more resistant to the action of the gastric juice than are those from the patient with the active disease. For this reason, the amebas are able to pass through the stomach and to reach the large bowel, where they set up fresh lesions of the disease.

Recently, another amebic infection in man has been identified in which free-living aquatic amebas are able to infect man and to cause meningitis, most frequently from swimming areas.

The diagnosis is made by finding the amebas in the stools, but in order that they may be recognized, they must be living and moving. On being passed from the body, they soon lose their power of movement, especially when they are chilled. A specimen of stool (a tiny amount is required) should be placed in a warm receptacle, which is then wrapped so as to prevent chilling, and immediately dispatched to the laboratory, where it should be delivered directly to the pathologist, and not merely laid down on a table, where it may be overlooked for some time. Unless these precautions are taken, it will be impossible to detect the amebas.

Malaria. This disease is caused by a minute unicellular parasite, known as a plasmodium. Part of the life cycle is spent in man and part in the anopheles mosquito. Destruction of this type of mosquito will be followed by the disappearance of malaria. The disease is the most widespread serious malady affecting the human race, although necessarily confined to those parts of the world infested by the anopheles mosquito. Greece, a land of heroes, fell in a few centuries to be a land of slaves, largely because of malaria. The disease still constitutes the greatest public health problem in the world. In certain tropical regions, everyone is infected with malaria from early infancy until death. Such persons never know for a single day the feeling of perfect health. Malaria is responsible, either directly or indirectly, by weakening resistance, for about 2 million deaths every year in India alone, and it is estimated that about 100 million suffer annually from the disease in that country.

When an infected mosquito bites man, it injects the parasites into the blood stream. Each parasite enters a red blood corpuscle and multiplies inside it until it destroys the corpuscle, which then bursts and liberates the new parasites into the blood. These attack new red corpuscles, multiply inside them and destroy them. It is obvious that in this way billions of parasites may be produced, and billions of red blood corpuscles may be destroyed, so that the patient will develop a profound anemia. The time taken by the parasites to multiply in the blood cells is always the same, so that the billions of blood cells all burst at the same time and liberate the new parasites into the blood stream at the same time. This massive discharge of parasites into the blood produces sudden high fever and an attack of shivering known as a rigor. The temperature rapidly falls, and may remain normal until the next batch of parasites is liberated. One form of parasite completes this part of its life cycle every 48 hours, and so the fever and chills occur every other day; as this is every third day (counting the day of the attack), this form of the disease is known as tertian malaria. In another form, the life cycle occupies 72 hours; the attack of fever occurs on the fourth day (counting the day of the attack), so that the disease is known as quartan malaria.

The human part of the life cycle is asexual, i.e., 2 sexes are not necessary for reproduction. However, this asexuality can continue for a certain time only. Unless rejuvenation of the parasite occurs by sexual reproduction, for which the mosquito is necessary, the parasite will die. Sexual forms, male and female, are present in human blood, but they are unable to unite. Their chance comes when the mosquito bites a malarial patient and sucks his or her blood into her stomach (it is only the female of the species that does the biting). The male and female forms now unite, and the fruit of the union is a fresh brood of rejuvenated parasites, which make their way to the mosquito's proboscis and wait to enter the blood of the next person the insect happens to bite. Thus the mosquito not only carries on the life cycle of a parasite, but conveys it from person to person. The complete life cycle of the parasite is illustrated in Fig. 10–2.

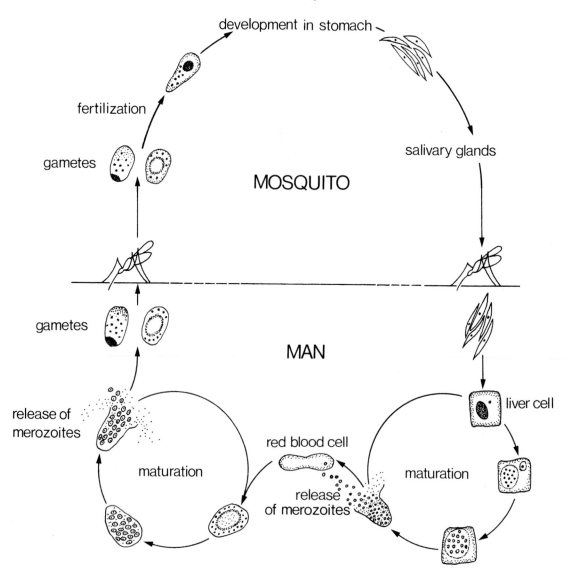

Fig. 10–2. This diagram shows the life cycle of the malaria parasite. The sexual forms are taken up by the mosquito where they develop and are subsequently reinfected into man, where the infectious agent is liberated from the liver. It then inhabits the red blood cell, where it develops again.

The diagnosis of malaria is suggested by the chills and regular repeated attacks of fever, but it can only be made with certainty by finding the parasites in the red cells in a smear of the patient's blood. The best time to make the blood examination is just before the onset of a chill. The spleen is large, and in acute cases it is soft, but in chronic cases it becomes hard.

The control of malaria in the districts of the world in which it is common has been aided by intensive campaigns against the mosquito by measures such as drainage of marshes and the treatment of stagnant water with oil or DDT to kill the larvae of the mosquito. It is of interest to recall the original meaning of the word malaria. It means bad air (Italian *malo*, bad, and *aria*, air) and is a reminder of the days when the disease was thought to be transmitted by the miasmic vapors of marshes. It was the mosquitoes, not the miasmas, that lived in the marshes.

Many drugs are used in the treatment of a patient with malaria, and these have been improved greatly during recent years. The common drugs in use are quinine, chloroquine, pentaquine, mepacrine, and pamaquine. An important advance has been the introduction of mepacrine and chloroquine as means of suppression of the disease during times of exposure in malarial countries.

The drugs are effective in treating malaria because they kill the immature forms of the protozoa by interfering with the oxidation of glucose and lactate and by inhibiting oxygen consumption. The difficulty in treating any disease is to find an agent that is toxic to the parasite but harmless to the host, and in cases where the parasite has a complex life cycle, it is fortunate if any drug can be found to be effective for more than 1 stage of the parasite's cycle.

Sleeping Sickness. Trypanosomes are spindle-shaped protozoan parasites characterized by a macronucleus in the center, a micronucleus at 1 end, an undulating membrane, and a flagellum (Fig. 10–3). Sexual development occurs in an invertebrate host, the tsetse fly, which transmits the infection from 1 person to another. Asexual reproduction occurs in the blood of the intermediate host, namely man and many wild animals. There are many varieties of trypanosomes and many tsetse flies. Trypanosomiasis is confined to tropical Africa, since this region is the habitat of the tsetse fly.

Human trypanosomiasis, or African sleeping sickness, is caused by *Trypanosoma gambiense* (called after the Gambia river, in which district the fever is prevalent), and is carried by the tsetse fly, *Glossina palpalis*. The trypanosomes live in the blood, causing fever, weakness, emaciation, and enlargement of the cervical and other lymph nodes. It is only later that they invade the central ner-

vous system and cause true sleeping sickness with its characteristic lethargy and coma. Trypanosomes are easily demonstrated in the blood during attacks of fever and in the cerebrospinal fluid when symptoms of sleeping sickness have developed.

Toxoplasmosis. The protozoan *Toxoplasma gondii* is found throughout the world in many species of warm-blooded animals; members of the cat family appear to be the definitive host. The 3 forms of toxoplasma, the trophozoite, cyst, and oocyst, are variously responsible for the acute infection and the latent infection, but the oocyst exists only in the cat family (Fig. 10–4). When formed in cat intestine, the oocyst is excreted in the feces and matures in 1 to 21 days, after which it is infectious. This suggests that kitty litter boxes and human infants do not make a good match.

Toxoplasma is widespread in distribution, and results in lymphadenopathy in man. It causes congenitally acquired infection that is often characterized by cerebral calcifications and chorioretinitis in newborns (3,000 cases per year in the United States). In addition, toxoplasma often causes fatal encephalitis in the immunologically compromised host.

The disease is best diagnosed by serologic tests for specific toxoplasma antibodies. The trophozoite may be identified with Giemsa stains in tissues, and isolation by injection into mice is a useful procedure. A case can be made for serodiagnosis in all women before pregnancy, since acquisition of toxoplasma

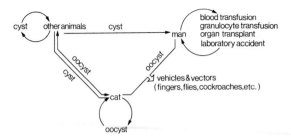

Fig. 10–4. This diagram illustrates the life cycle of the toxoplasma organism. The cat is a preferential host. The organism may be excreted in the feces of the cat and infest other animals, such as mice. The cyst in man may be transferred from man to man by blood transfusion, laboratory accident, or organ transplant. (From Krick, J.A., and Remington, J.S.: Toxoplasmosis in the adult—an overview. N. Engl. J. Med., *298*:550, 1978.)

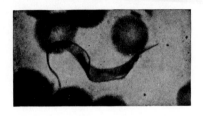

Fig. 10–3. Trypanosoma gambiense. × 1500.

by the pregnant patient is a grave risk to the fetus. However, such testing is not yet routine in the United States.

An epidemic of toxoplasmosis occurred in patrons of a riding stable in Atlanta in 1976. Thirty-seven became ill with toxoplasmosis. The source was traced to 2 cats and 2 kittens; the instance of disease was highest in the riders who came daily to the stable and spent most of their time at the end of the stable where cat feces were most abundant.

Leishmaniasis, or kala-azar, is simply referred to in passing as another worldwide protozoal disease.

NEMATODES OR ROUNDWORMS

Metazoal parasites are 2 cell layers thick and are unfortunately more complex structurally than protozoa; they include the worms, so far as this chapter is concerned, and we shall consider these parasites as follows: (1) nematodes or roundworms, (2) cestodes or tapeworms, and (3) trematodes or flukes. Such parasites can infest any compartment of the body and can navigate through the host during different parts of their life cycle. They have an awesome potential for travel through the intestinal tract across the gut barrier into the bloodstream to rest in the liver, or to migrate into the lung. From there, the egg or worm may be swallowed, or it may enter and obstruct the lymphatics, there to cause elephantiasis, or it may find its way into the eye or brain. Eosinophilia in the peripheral blood is often present. This is always suggestive of a helminth (parasitic worm) infection, being part of an allergic reaction to the foreign protein of the worm. In the case of the nematodes, which form the largest group, with a few exceptions, no intermediate host is required for completion of the life cycle.

Hookworm disease (ankylostomiasis). This is one of the most prevalent diseases; it has been estimated that there are some 100,000,000 cases in the world. It is a disease of warm and tropical climates and used to be prevalent in the southern part of the United States. The worm, which is less than 3 cm in length, occurs in large numbers in the duodenum and jejunum. The mouth is armed with 4 teeth or hooklets that attach it to the wall of the duodenum and that give the worm its name (Greek *ankylos,* hooked, and *stoma,* mouth). The method by which the hookworm reaches the duodenum is one of the romances of medicine. The young embryo worm lives in warm, moist ground, bores through the skin of a person's bare feet, enters a vein, and is carried by the blood to the lung, where it is arrested. Here the worm escapes into the bronchi and starts to climb up the trachea. When it reaches the upper end, it descends the esophagus, passes through the stomach, and reaches the end of its long journey in the duodenum. Large numbers of hookworms arrive here and fasten themselves to the wall of the bowel. In time they produce marked anemia with profound lassitude and weakness. This is not remarkable, seeing that hundreds, sometimes thousands, of the little worms have been found hanging onto the wall of the intestine, sucking blood as a baby would suck milk (Fig. 10–5). No intermediate host is required for the development of the hookworm. As many as 10,000,000 eggs may be laid at one time. If these are deposited in warm, moist soil, they develop into active embryos, which await a passerby with bare feet, so that they may penetrate the skin and start on their odyssey to the duodenum, where they complete their life cycle.

Roundworm disease (ascariasis). This worm resembles the earthworm in size and shape,

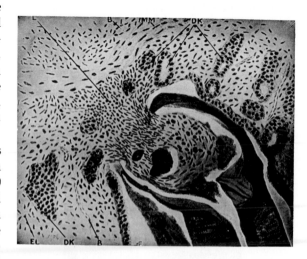

Fig. 10–5. This histologic section shows the method of attachment of the hookworm to the wall of the human intestine.

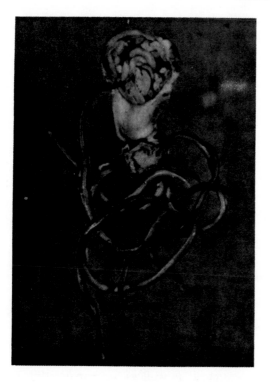

Fig. 10–6. This photograph shows the Ascaris lumbricoides in the appendix. (Kindness of Dr. C. H. Lupton, Jr.; Boyd, W.: *Textbook of Pathology.* Philadelphia, Lea & Febiger.)

and is a common inhabitant of the intestine, especially in children (Fig. 10–6). Infection is due to swallowing the eggs of the worm on uncooked vegetables.

This sounds simple, but the reality is far from simple. The capacity of the uterus has been estimated at about 27,000,000 eggs and the daily output for each female at 200,000, quite a difference from the human female. Indeed the ascaris seems to be bent on an "exploding population." But when the developing eggs hatch into larvae in the intestine, they are not content to develop there without following the strange example of the hookworm. So they penetrate the wall of the bowel, are carried to the heart and then the lungs, where they are filtered out, and pass up the trachea and down the esophagus into the intestine! With this voyage of discovery behind them, they are content to develop peacefully into adult worms. We can wonder how on earth such a method of development could have been evolved, but we are left without an answer.

Pinworm or threadworm disease (enterobiasis). Enterobius vermicularis is a common parasite in the intestine of children. The worms are only 8 mm long, and, when passed in the stools, they resemble a moving piece of white thread. They cause marked irritation and itching of the skin around the anus. Infection is due to swallowing contaminated vegetables and fruits. Masses of pinworms may be found in the vermiform appendix, but they are not responsible for acute appendicitis, as was once believed. An easy diagnostic procedure is to apply transparent adhesive (Scotch) tape to the perineal area of the person who has the irritation and itching. Pinworms may be readily identified when they stick to the tape, although they are not easily seen in the skin.

Trichinosis. Every parasitic worm seems to take pride in developing a special way of life, and trichinella, or trichina as it used to be called, is no exception. The disease trichinosis is caused by a tiny roundworm that passes its complete life cycle in the body of a single animal. However, unless the host is eaten by another animal, the embryos die, surely a curious arrangement to have been evolved by a worm, but apparently a satisfactory one. Owing to improvement in meat inspection and changes in the handling and distribution of meat, trichinosis has become comparatively rare. Larvae in pork may be rendered noninfective by heating to 55°C (131°F) or by freezing at −15°C (5°F) for about 3 weeks.

The parasite infects a variety of animals, in particular the rat, the bear, the pig, and man. The pig becomes infected by eating the rat, and man becomes infected by eating the pig, but the life cycle comes to an end with man, because he is not eaten. Epidemics occur, particularly in Germany, from eating imperfectly cooked pork in sausages. The embryos ingested in the infected pork develop in the intestine into tiny adult male and female worms, only 1 to 3 mm long. The resulting ova develop into embryos, which are discharged into the blood, are carried to all parts of the body, and invade various organs. However, the embryos can only develop in the voluntary muscles and die out elsewhere (Fig. 10–7). Every muscle in the body may be infected, but full development of the embryo

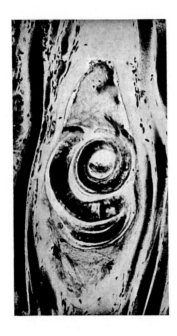

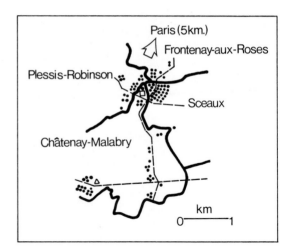

Fig. 10-8. This map of villages near Paris shows the outbreak of trichinosis at the dots. Source of this outbreak is believed to have been infected horse meat. (From Bourée, P., et al.: Outbreak of trichinosis near Paris. Br. Med. J., 1:1047, 1979.)

Fig. 10-7. This section shows the appearance of Trichinella spiralis in human muscle. × 75. (Boyd, W.: *Textbook of Pathology.* Philadelphia, Lea & Febiger.)

into an adult worm is not possible unless the parasite finds itself in the digestive canal of another animal. In man the embryos cause myositis, an acute inflammation of the muscles, which become hard, swollen, and often painful. Fever is a common symptom, and there is a marked and characteristic eosinophilia, of great diagnostic value. Diagnosis is made immunologically or by skin test, and only rarely today by biopsy.

The clinical pattern of trichinosis is fever (65%), headache (61%), muscle aches (59%), and periorbital edema (57%). An increased eosinophil count (97%) is the signal that alerts the clinician to the suspicion of trichinosis. Elevated muscle enzymes confirm this diagnosis and are present in 93% of patients. These figures are taken from an outbreak of trichinosis in the suburbs of Paris in January, 1976 (Fig. 10-8). The epidemic was presumed to be traced to horsemeat, although no horses were examined.

Filariasis. In this infection by a nematode worm, the adult worm lives in the lymphatics while the larvae travel in the blood. It is a disease of tropical countries, because the culex mosquito is necessary for completion of the life cycle as well as for transmitting the infection.

The life history and habits of the filaria are remarkable even for an animal parasite. The adult worm, only 0.5 to 1 cm in length and extremely thin, lives in the lymphatics, especially in those of the groin and pelvis. The male and female live together, and the ova develop in the uterus of the female into active larvae, known as microfilariae, which are eellike bodies so thin that they pass through the smallest capillaries. They are therefore found in the blood (Fig. 10-9), but only at night, because it is at night that the culex makes its appearance, sucks the blood of the patient, and thus allows completion of the life cycle of the parasite. This beautiful piece of timing is made possible by a daily cyclical parturition by the females and by the rapid death of the microfilariae. Before midday, the turgid females are crammed with microfilariae, but after 2 P.M. the uterus is empty until the next day, for the larvae are in the blood awaiting the mosquito at sundown. The larvae do the patient no harm, and this nocturnal periodicity may go on for years. When the mosquito bites an infected person, the larvae pass with the blood into the insect's stomach. They penetrate the stomach wall and lodge in the thoracic muscles. Here they develop into

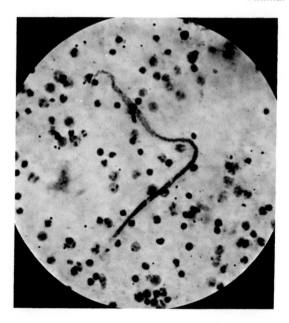

Fig. 10–9. This microscopic view shows a microfilaria in blood. × 300.

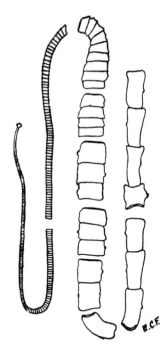

Fig. 10–10. This drawing shows the appearance of a tapeworm. Its head is in the small segment on the left. (From Faust: *Human Helminthology.* Philadelphia, Lea & Febiger.)

young worms, which make their way to the base of the proboscis and await injection into man, where sexual development may be attained and reproduction takes place.

Although the larvae in the blood do no harm, the adult worms are apt to produce lymphatic obstruction, especially as they are present in masses. Elephantiasis may develop as a result of obstruction of the lymphatics. This is a condition in which the tissues become enormously thickened and indurated, the legs resemble those of a young elephant (hence the name), and the scrotum is huge. The diagnosis of filariasis is made by demonstrating the larvae in the blood at night, but it is elephantiasis caused by the adult worms that constitutes the real disease.

CESTODES OR TAPEWORMS

We now pass to a different type of worm. Tapeworms are of various kinds, but they all spend part of their life cycle in man and part in another animal. A tapeworm gets its name from its shape, for it is long and narrow, like a piece of tape (Fig. 10–10). The head is small and the body long. There are 4 tapeworms of importance in human pathology. Three of these pass the sexual or adult stage in man and

the asexual or cystic stage in an animal, hence the name cestode. The fourth passes the adult stage in an animal (dog) and the cystic stage in man. The easiest way to remember the names of tapeworms is by the name of the animal that acts as the second host. All of these worms are known by the generic term, taenia.

Beef tapeworm (Taenia saginata, Taenia mediocanellata). This common tapeworm of the United States and Canada may be 10 meters long, but its head is only 2 mm in diameter. It lives in the intestine, and the body of the female is crowded with eggs that are discharged in the stools. If these eggs are swallowed by cattle, they are carried to the muscles, where they pass through a second phase of the life cycle and develop into cysts. If the beef from an infected cow is eaten imperfectly cooked, human infection will result, and the cystic parasite will grow into the full-length adult in the intestine. The diagnosis is made by examining the stools for fragments of the worm (segments) that become broken off and discharged.

Pork tapeworm (Taenia solium). This worm is similar to the beef tapeworm, but it is smaller, only 3 meters long. The second host is the pig, and human infection results from eating infected pork that contains the tiny cysts.

Fish tapeworm (Diphyllobothrium latum). This very long worm passes the cystic stage in some of the larger freshwater fish, such as pike and perch. There is no danger in eating these fish provided they have been properly cooked, and the same is true of the beef and pork. Infestation used to be found chiefly among the fish-eating peoples in the Scandinavian countries, Russia, and parts of Asia, but more recently it has been imported into the United States and Canada, and is now indigenous in the districts around the Great Lakes and Lake Winnipeg. The eggs are discharged from the ripe segments at the rate of 1,000,000 a day, but the segments are empty and shriveled when shed, in this respect differing from the other 2 tapeworms. It follows that in stool examinations the presence of ripe segments indicates the beef or the pork tapeworm; the presence of eggs indicates the fish tapeworm.

Dog tapeworm (Echinococcus granulosus). This disease is commonly called hydatid disease and is caused by 1 of 2 species (*Echinococcus granulosus,* or *E. multilocularis*) of tapeworm that live in the intestines of dogs and wolves. This worm is entirely different from the other 3 in the following respects: (1) It is small, 8 mm long. (2) It is the cystic stage that is passed in man; the adult stage occurs in the dog. (3) The cysts often cause serious symptoms in man and may prove fatal. Human infection is usually due to ingestion of unboiled vegetables soiled by the excreta of dogs. The dogs are infected by eating the flesh of infected sheep. The disease in man, which is most prevalent in Australia, South America, and other great sheep-raising countries where infected dogs and men come into close contact, is called hydatid disease, and the cysts are known as hydatid cysts. These cysts are formed principally in the liver, but may occur in any of the organs. They may attain a large size, and sometimes cause the death of the patient. The fluid of the cysts is clear and sterile, but it contains immature forms, which must not be allowed to escape during removal of the cysts. Intradermal injection of the fluid is said to give a specific skin reaction in cases of hydatid disease. Treatment is surgical removal of the hydatid cyst with appropriate precautions to prevent spillage of the infective agents. Hydrogen peroxide in dilute solution seems to be the agent of choice.

It seems that the history of echinococcal disease in the United States started early in this century. It was known in swineherds in the southeast, and by 1920 it had spread to the Mississippi Valley. Recently there have been serious outbreaks in western states, where the cycle involves sheep as intermediate hosts. Sheep-ranchers, Basque-Americans in California, Mormons in Utah, and the Navajo, Zuñi, and Santo Domingan Indians in Arizona and New Mexico are at risk wherever dogs are permitted to eat uncooked sheep offal.

Skin testing has shown a positive reaction in native populations of Alaska (22%), the Yukon (40%), and in Canadian Eskimos and Indians of British Columbia. To detect the presence of cysts, CT scans have become important and the Casoni test (intradermal injection of echinococcal antigen) is a useful diagnostic procedure.

TREMATODES OR FLUKES

These small, flat, leaf-shaped unsegmented worms include several varieties of flukes, infesting both animals and man in the Orient, of which the liver fluke in China and the lung fluke in China and Japan may be mentioned. The life cycle of trematodes cannot continue without an intermediate host, which is a water snail.

Schistosomiasis. This is the most common disease caused by flukes. Again, there are several varieties responsible. The only one we shall mention is *Schistosoma haematobium*, generally referred to as bilharzia. This fluke causes widespread disease in Egypt and in other parts of northern Africa. The flukes live in the veins of the pelvis and bladder, and the ova, which are armed with a sharp spine, are laid in the wall of the bladder where they produce an intense reaction with continual passage of blood in the urine and a marked predisposition to cancer of the bladder wall.

EXTERNAL PARASITES: ARTHROPODS

The parasitic arthropods, so called because they have joined legs, are numerous and cause many skin troubles, particularly in the tropics. Some are also carriers of disease. The commonest skin parasites are lice, fleas, and acarus, the "itch insect," which causes scabies. The bites of arthropods always itch to some degree, the itching being due to the development of hypersensitivity to the saliva deposited at the site of the bite. The hypersensitivity may be so extreme that the itching becomes almost intolerable.

Acarus scabiei. The itch insect, which is the cause of scabies, is shaped like a turtle, but is only 0.5 mm long. The impregnated female bores a tunnel into the skin between the fingers, at the wrists, or in the axillas, laying her eggs at the end of the tunnel where the young are hatched. These in turn bore new tunnels, so that the irritation and itching may be intense. The male remains quietly on the surface and causes no trouble. This parasite can be transmitted easily from person to person. The disease is common among school-age children, and, as with other diseases, it may find a comfortable reservoir among the adults at the home of the child. Because of its benign nature (recurrent itching and a mild rash), it is often undiagnosed and unsuspected.

Pediculi. Various pediculi or lice may infest the skin. The head louse (*Pediculus capitis*) lives on the scalp, and causes some irritation. The "nits" we observe are ova, minute bodies attached to the hairs. The body louse (*Pediculus corporis*) lives on the surface of the skin and breeds in clothing. Not only does the body louse produce much greater irritation than the head louse, but it is responsible for carrying the infection of typhus fever, relapsing fever, and trench fever. It does this by biting first a sick and then a healthy person.

Fleas. The common flea is of little significance in relation to disease. The rat flea, on the other hand, is of great importance, because it conveys plague not only from one rat to another, but also from rat to man.

Arthropods as Disease Carriers

In the course of our study of infection, whether of bacteria, rickettsiae, viruses, or protozoa, we have seen that an arthropod vector or conveyer, usually an insect, is necessary in many instances for the continuation of the infection. A vector may be mechanical or biologic. The mechanical vector merely picks up the infecting agent from the body or excreta and deposits it on exposed food (house flies in relation to typhoid, or to bacillary and amebic dysentery), or conveys infection through contamination of the biting organ (flies and mosquitoes in relation to anthrax). The biologic vector plays an essential part in the completion of the life cycle of the pathogen rather than merely offering it a free ride. In many instances it is only the female that transmits disease, an illustration of the old saying that the female of the species is more deadly than the male.

SYNOPSIS

Parasitism is an evolutionary process.
Alternate hosts are necessary for many parasites.
Control of vectors in the life cycle of many parasites is the means of disease control.
Protozoa and metazoa are 2 great classes of animal parasites.
Parasites are causative agents of classic disease processes such as anemia, cirrhosis, and cancer.

Terms

Definitive host	*Cestode*	*Schistosomiasis*
Intermediate host	*Trematode*	*Trichinosis*
Malarial parasite	*Arthropod*	*Scabies*
Nematode	*Hydatid cyst*	

FURTHER READING

Bourée, P., et al.: Outbreak of trichinosis near Paris. Br. Med. J., *1*:1047, 1979.

Bulla, L.A., Jr., and Cheng, T.C.: Pathobiology of invertebrate vectors of disease. Ann. N.Y. Acad. Sci., *266*:1975.

Cameron, T.W.M.: *Parasites and Parasitism.* London, Wiley, 1956.

Faust, E.C., Russell, P.F., and Jung, R.C.: *Clinical Parasitology*, 8th Ed. Philadelphia, Lea & Febiger, 1970.

Krick, J.A., and Remington, J.S.: Toxoplasmosis in the adult—an overview. N. Engl. J. Med., *298*:550, 1978.

Krogstad, D.J., Spencer, H.C., and Healy, G.R.: Amebiasis. N. Engl. J. Med., *298*:262, 1978.

Marcial-Rojas, R.A.: *Pathology of Protozoal Helminthic Diseases with Clinical Correlations.* Baltimore, Williams & Wilkins, 1971.

Marsden, P.D.: Leishmaniasis. N. Engl. J. Med., *300*:350, 1979.

Moser, R.H.: Trichinosis from Bismarck to polar bears. J.A.M.A., *228*:735, 1974.

Schantz, P.M.: Echinococcosis in American Indians living in Arizona and New Mexico. Am. J. Epidemiol., *106*:370, 1977.

Schantz, P.M., and Glickman, L.T.: Toxocaral visceral larva migrans. N. Engl. J. Med., *298*:436, 1978.

Teutsch, S.M., et al.: Epidemic toxoplasmosis associated with infected cats. N. Engl. J. Med., *300*:695, 1979.

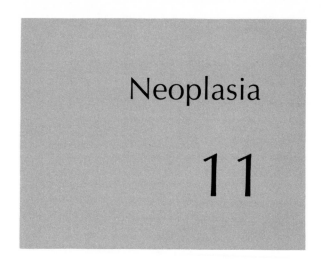

Neoplasia

11

It is death, not what comes after death, that men generally are afraid of.—SAMUEL BUTLER

Of all the disease processes we have to study in this book, none is more intriguing, more fascinating, and more perplexing than neoplasia. The term means new growth. There are, of course, various forms of new growth such as repair, the formation of granulation tissue, and compensatory hypertrophy of an organ. The term **neoplasm** is reserved for the formation of benign and, more particularly, malignant tumors or cancer. Tumor is a more general term signifying a swelling or lump, but there are many lumps that are not neoplasms, such as abscesses.

DISTURBANCES OF GROWTH

The normal organs and tissues of the body are made up of cells under the control of laws of growth. Unfortunately, these laws are not written down. An organ such as the liver or bone increases in size, usually, not by an increase in cell size (the cells of a whale are the same size as the cells of a mouse), but by an increase in the number of cells. In youth, this multiplication is rapid, partly because of the abundance of growth hormone, and partly because of the genetic programming of the tissue. However, in adult life, cell replication is sufficient only to replace what is lost by continual wear and tear. Occasionally, there is an increase in the number of cells in a tissue (**hyperplasia**) in the adult due to unknown or

nonspecific causes. This increase happens most often in tissues such as the endocrine glands, which respond particularly to growth-promoting hormones. In many instances the hyperplasia seems autonomous.

Another phenomenon of growth is the adaptive response to work demand (**hypertrophy**), which may be best demonstrated by physical training in skeletal muscle; this also occurs in cardiac muscle and other tissues. An increase in the size of an organ is usually due to an increase in the size of individual cells. With specific work training, muscle cells increase the number of cytoplasmic myofilaments and thereby enlarge. Today we can adapt the use of this term hypertrophy, which used to be applied only to tissues and organs, to the new world of the cell, and we can talk of hypertrophy of a mitochondrion. Equally, a cell, which by virtue of adaptation has increased its number of mitochondria, could be said to show hyperplasia of the mitochondria.

The converse of these adaptative responses is a loss of normal size or number of structural units, which results in **atrophy** of an organ or tissue. In muscle, this may be due to lack of use, to injury, to loss of innervation, or to interference with the normal blood supply, and in other tissues it may be due to a loss of endocrine stimulus, as in pituitary hypofunction. A decrease in size of the tissue or organ may, on the other hand, have a congenital

Table 11–1. Disturbances of Growth

Agenesis	Complete absence of growth of an organ or tissue.
Aplasia	Congenital disturbance in which there exist only primitive and usually small structures representative of an organ or tissue.
Hypoplasia	Congenital disturbance occurring during embryonal development of an organ or tissue, resulting in a smaller, and usually deformed, structure which may or may not function.
Atrophy	Decrease in size and/or number of cells of an organ or tissue after it has achieved normal size.
Hyperplasia	Increase in the number of cells.
Hypertrophy	Increase in the size of an organ. Cellular hypertrophy may occur.
Metaplasia	A change in type of adult tissue to a type which is not normal for that tissue.
Dysplasia	An abnormality in the maintenance or development of a tissue.

(From Perez-Tamayo, R.: *Mechanisms of Disease.* Philadelphia & London, W. B. Saunders, 1961.)

origin and may result from an abnormal blood supply or from a failure of development. The terms **agenesis, aplasia,** and **hypoplasia** have been applied to some of these conditions (Table 11–1).

A third general variation in the normal growth and structure of a tissue occurs frequently in response to different types of stimuli; some are irritative, some nutritional. These changes from normal are reflected in an unusual pattern of structure: the replacement of 1 type of epithelium by another, as occurs in the bronchi and trachea of long-term smokers. A change from ciliated columnar epithelium to squamous epithelium is called **metaplasia**, and is regarded with a high degree of suspicion as being potentially malignant. However, we know that some other substances (for example, vitamin A) help to maintain tissue integrity. Equally, in the tissue of the breast or cervix, there may be histologic and cytologic changes that warrant the use of the term **dysplasia**, and, as we shall discuss, this is interpreted as a warning sign that the normal controls over growth and development of the tissue may be lacking. These relationships are schematized in Fig. 11–1.

We know that if 1 kidney is removed, the other kidney will increase in size, and we talk of this as a compensatory mechanism. What is the stimulus to this response? Equally, if a portion of the liver is removed, the liver will regenerate. Unfortunately, few tissues in man can react in this way. The stimuli to new growth are poorly understood and the factors that signal the end of the new growth are even less clear. However, we know that cells in a tissue are in direct contact with each other.

When this contact is broken, as in a cut where cells are injured, the loss of contact may be the stimulus to new growth. When cells make contact with each other, there is cessation of movement. This process is called **contact inhibition.**

A neoplasm is a mass of new cells, which proliferate without control and serve no useful function. This lack of control is particularly marked in malignant tumors (cancer). Cancer cells are the anarchists of the body, for they know no law, pay no regard to the com-

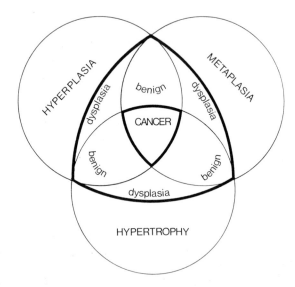

Fig. 11–1. This diagram shows the overlap of 3 different types of adaptive response, namely, hyperplasia, metaplasia, and hypertrophy. Cancer is represented at the intersection of these in the center, benign neoplasia at the periphery, and dysplasia at the tangential margins. This concept is not meant to be a literal representation of the events leading to cancer. It only suggests how these cellular responses may be interrelated.

monweal, serve no useful function, and cause disharmony and death in their surroundings. It used to be thought that cancer was a peculiarly human disease, but we now know that it occurs throughout the entire vertebrate animal kingdom. It seems to be a phenomenon of the extremes of age; most cancers seem to occur in the young and in the aged.

Cancer, including leukemia, is now a leading cause of nonaccidental death in children between the ages of 3 and 14 in the United States and Canada. These cancers differ from those in adults in clinical features, sites of origin, and types of tumor. Tumors of embryonic origin (embryonic tumors) are common in infants and young children, but correspondingly rare in adults. Four out of 5 of these tumors in children arise from the nervous system, the urinary system, or the lymphopoietic system, whereas in adults, 4 out of 5 cancers arise from the alimentary, respiratory, or genital systems.

Cancer has 2 characteristics that make it life-threatening, and put it in second place in the list of causes of death in North America. Cancer kills because of invasion of tissue, and by distant spread to vital organs, where it may compress, obstruct, or destroy vital functions by its metastases. In 1975 there were an estimated 380,000 deaths in the United States from cancer. The types of tumors that caused these deaths are shown in Table 11–2.

This pattern may change with earlier diagnosis and treatment, but it may also change with social and occupational exposures.

NATURE OF NEOPLASIA

There is much talk about the mystery of cancer, as if it were the only mysterious process in the entire realm of disease. But in-

Table 11–2. Sites of Cancer in Order of Frequency as Cause of Death

	FEMALE	MALE
1.	Breast	Lung
2.	Colon/Rectum	Colon/Rectum
3.	Uterus	Prostate
4.	Ovary	Stomach
5.	Lung	Pancreas

flammation is mysterious, and we have not solved the mystery by inventing such words as irritation and chemotaxis; diabetes is a mystery that has not been solved by the discovery of insulin; multiple sclerosis and schizophrenia remain mysteries without even the suggestion of a solution. A normal cell seems concerned more with function than with growth, but the cancer cell is concerned more with growth, in the sense of reproduction of itself, than with function. The capacity for growth seems to have supplanted that for function. The nerve cells of the human brain represent the highest in specialization of function, but they have lost the power of reproduction. Neoplasms of the brain consist not of nerve cells, but of neuroglia (supporting cells).

Cancer Cells

Cancer is a disorder of cell growth, and the cancer cell appears to be a modified cell. An electron micrograph of a cancer cell is shown in Fig. 11–2A and a drawing illustrating some of its features in Fig. 11–2B. Another scheme (Fig. 11–3) shows the many differences between cancer and normal cells that have been identified in recent years, but not all these differences occur in all tumors, nor are any of them necessarily diagnostic. Unfortunately, we do not know the mechanism of normal growth and its regulation, so it is small wonder that we do not understand cancer. The cancerous modification comprises loss of the more specialized functions in addition to the acquisition of increased growth function, an increase that results in invasion of the surrounding tissue and the formation of the secondary growths at a distance known as **metastases**. We have already seen that normal function is the result of chemical activity governed by enzymes situated for the most part in the mitochondria and endoplasmic reticulum in the cytoplasm, these enzymes in turn being under the control of the chromosomes in the nucleus with their associated genes. Since cellular growth is a chemical process, it would appear that the abnormal growth we call cancer must reflect some basic alteration in this chemical process. The question is: What is the basic alteration?

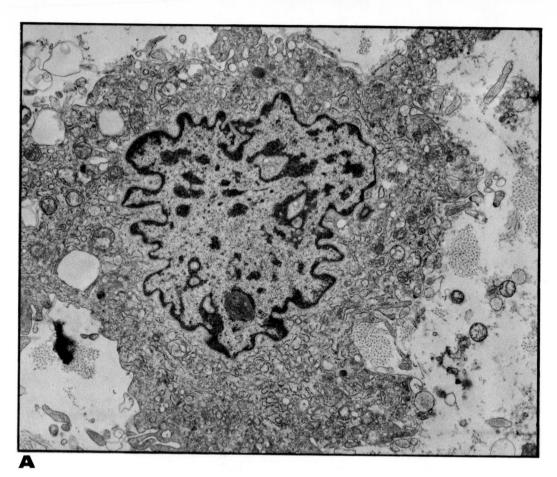

A

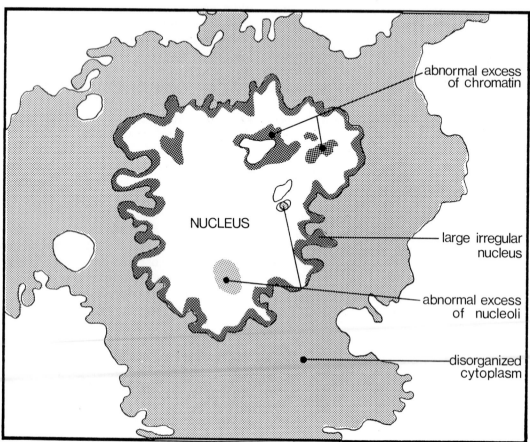

abnormal excess
of chromatin

NUCLEUS

large irregular
nucleus

abnormal excess
of nucleoli

disorganized
cytoplasm

B

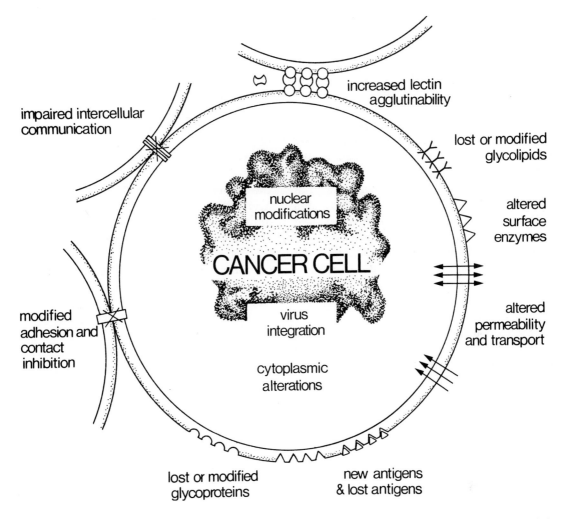

increased lectin
agglutinability

impaired intercellular
communication

lost or modified
glycolipids

altered
surface
enzymes

nuclear
modifications

CANCER CELL

altered
permeability
and transport

virus
integration

modified
adhesion and
contact
inhibition

cytoplasmic
alterations

lost or modified
glycoproteins

new antigens
& lost antigens

Fig. 11–3. This drawing shows peripheral and central abnormalities in the cancer cell, namely, impaired intercellular communications, increased cell surface substances, altered permeability and transport mechanisms, and modifications in the nucleus. (Adapted from Nicolson, G.L.: Transmembrane control of the receptors on normal and tumor cells. II. Surface changes associated with transformation and malignancy. Biochim. Biophys. Acta, *458*:1, 1976.)

←

Fig. 11–2. *A,* This electron microphotograph of a liposarcoma cell shows the irregular appearance of the cytoplasm and nucleus. The normal cell of this type is an adipose cell, which has a small and unremarkable nucleus, a large storage depot of triglyceride, and active but peripheral mitochondria. *B* specifically illustrates the abnormalities in the electron microphotograph.

Some 50 years ago, Warburg introduced a generalization concerning tumor growth. The carbohydrate metabolism of a normal cell consists of 2 processes, glycolysis (splitting of the sugar molecule) and respiration (use of oxygen for further breakdown of the carbohydrate into carbon dioxide and water). Warburg showed in the laboratory that the cancer cell derives its energy mainly from anaerobic glycolysis, whereas the metabolism of the normal cell depends mainly on oxidation. The normal cell breathes; cancer cells do not breathe, but ferment. It was suggested that a difference in chemical behavior might explain differences in morphology and function. Unfortunately Warburg's thesis, although true for some tumors, proved to be an overgeneralization, for anaerobic glycolysis is both absent in some tumors and present in many normal tissues.

Another concept is concerned with enzyme systems normally involved in regulating the synthesis of substances essential to cell division. Loss or disruption of such systems would make normal regulation of cell division impossible, with resulting unrestricted growth, that is to say, neoplasia. Carcinogens, or cancer-producing agents, whether chemicals or radiation, could be responsible for damage to enzyme systems. The result would be loss of function and an increased ability to multiply.

Early steps on the path to cancer probably occur all the time in our bodies, but the path is most often aborted. Cancers that do establish themselves are the "successful ones," those most effective in growth, invasiveness, and metastasis. There are a variety of strategies employed in these processes. Tumor cells may well produce **proteases** (enzymes that digest proteins) that facilitate the crossing of barriers into adjacent tissues. They also produce **angiogenesis** factors, which promote the growth of local circulatory vessels to feed the tumors. Finally, these cells alter metabolic and surface characteristics: some of these changes must surely be advantageous in tumor establishment.

A difference between the metabolism of cancer cells and that of normal cells may explain why a cancer, given sufficient time, kills its host unless treated promptly and effi-

ciently. Of course, it may do this by blocking a natural passage such as the esophagus, or by causing ulceration of a mucous membrane with fatal hemorrhage. But apart from these complications, cancer causes loss of weight, wasting, emaciation, and, finally, death. A large neoplasm acquires nitrogenous building blocks from the body stores to satisfy the continual demand for protein synthesis, but the supply of these blocks is not unlimited. Cancer cells appear to exercise priority over the demands of normal tissues for amino acids, thus constituting a nitrogen trap. If amino acids marked with radioactive isotopes are fed to animals with rapidly growing neoplasms, the nitrogen trap can be observed in operation. Small wonder that wasting and cachexia are a characteristic feature of the later stages of malignancy.

Much recent research has focused on the properties of cancer cells. There are experimental analogs of cancer cells, cultivated in tissue culture, known as **transformed** cells, which exhibit similar biochemical changes to cancer cells, and often cause tumors *in vivo*. Several conclusions can be drawn about the important changes in transformed cells. Cell shape and cytoskeletal architecture are affected; transformed cells are rounder than their normal counterparts, and the ordered array of actin/myosin filaments and microtubules is disrupted. Transformed cells are less fastidious in their nutritional requirements. "Normal cells" in tissue culture often grow attached to a support such as glass; their transformed counterparts will grow in suspension or in semisolid agar ("anchorage independence"). This property correlates strongly with their ability to cause tumors *in vivo*. Transformed cells also seem to have reduced nutritional requirements as compared with normal cells. When normal cells completely cover the culture dish surface and make contact with one another, they usually enter a resting phase ("contact inhibition" or "density-dependent control of growth"), whereas transformed cells overgrow these boundaries. Normal cells placed in culture usually grow for a short time and then die; transformed cells are immortalized and will grow indefinitely. Finally, normal cells form gap junctions at points of membrane contact, through which small molecules can pass as a means of cell-to-cell communication. Transformed cells do not display such junctions.

Cancer cells display a different set of metabolic and surface characteristics from their cells of origin, combining traits of diverse cell types in a novel arrangement. Reappearance of embryonic marker proteins has been observed in a variety of cancers. Rather than suggesting a source of origin for tumor cells, these shared traits of embryonic and cancer cells may be those most conducive to their similar "lifestyles." Although there are profound differences, the 2 populations share steady growth, migration to new body sites, and a relatively undifferentiated state.

It is worth remembering that cancer is probably not a single disease, with a predictable cause and a predictable program, but rather that it represents the visible manifestations of those errors in cell behavior that produce cells capable of division, invasiveness, and metastasis beyond the control of host regulation. The changes involved are stable and are passed on to the offspring of the formative tumor cells. One reasonable interpretation is that mutational changes in the DNA program are responsible for the inheritable alterations. An examination of differentiation suggests a model for the evolution of a cancer. It is known that all the cells in the body have virtually the same sequence of DNA. It is the control of this DNA that differs among tissues: only a small segment is selected for expression in each cell type. It may be the regulation of expression of DNA that is disarrayed in cancer. Perhaps genes can be altered to produce "cancer proteins"—modified proteins capable of inducing neoplastic transformation by altering the choice of active cell functions. Alternatively, the disturbance in gene expression could result from mutagenesis of regulatory DNA sequences with a resultant interference with their function. The observed significance of mutagens in experimental and natural carcinogenesis is discussed later in this chapter.

There is evidence from an experimental system for an "epigenetic" change in gene expression. Such a model proposes a change in the specificity, timing, or stimulus requirements of existing regulatory factors with no

irreversible change in the DNA. This is presumably the type of change that accompanies normal tissue differentiation. Cells from a murine teratocarcinoma have been mixed into an early mouse embryo, and the fetus matured in a foster mother. Normal offspring develop, having many of their somatic cells in many tissues derived from the teratocarcinoma cells. The conclusion is that in a normal environment, the tumor cells are induced to reverse their phenotype and to behave and differentiate as normal cells. One interpretation is that the teratocarcinoma DNA was unaffected in any irreversible fashion during transformation, but rather suffered an epigenetic alteration in its pattern of expression. The possibility of mutation is certainly not excluded, but these experiments suggest that a strictly epigenetic model of carcinogenesis may be relevant in some systems.

Cancer can be thought of as a change in cell metabolism. The regulator of cellular activity, the governor of the engine, is nucleic acid. The intricate mechanism of chromosomes and genes with their nucleic acid, which controls cellular reproduction as well as metabolism, can be upset in various ways. The interference may lead to permanent changes or "mutation" in the genes, and if the change is such as to permanently speed the rate of mitotic division, the result will be cancer. Just as the

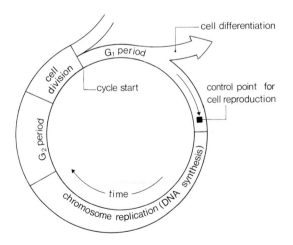

Fig. 11–4. This diagram of the cell cycle illustrates the point in the cycle at which alterations that may pervert the cell function are likely to take place. (From Thorn, G.W., et al. (Eds.): *Harrison's Principles of Internal Medicine*, 8th Ed. New York, McGraw-Hill, 1976.)

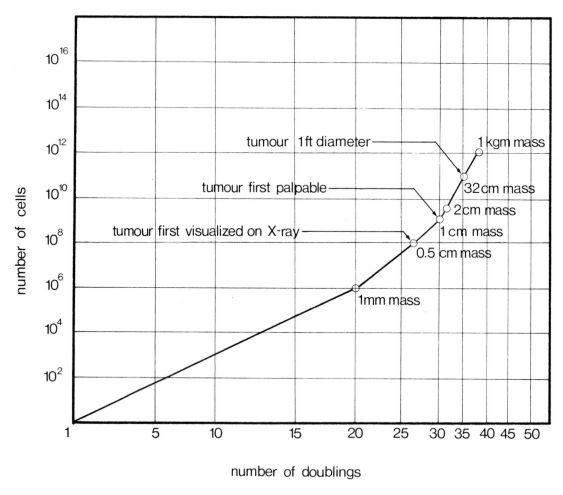

Fig. 11–5. This graph shows the number of cells, the number of doublings, and the size of the mass. It illustrates that a tumor may be first visible only after 25 or more doublings. The rapid growth from that point is indicated in the change in the slope of the curve. (From Thorn, G.W., et al. (Eds.): *Harrrison's Principles of Internal Medicine*, 8th Ed. New York, McGraw-Hill, 1976.)

regulator of a watch may be moved to fast or slow, so may the mitotic rate be permanently accelerated by carcinogens or retarded by radiation and colchicine. The time at which cells are most susceptible to alterations in their growth controls is in the G1 period, shown in Figure 11–4. As one cell will produce 60,000 daughter cells after 16 divisions, it is apparent that even a slight increase in the rate and rhythm of cell division will soon produce a tumor. The rate of growth of a tumor is dramatically demonstrated in Figure 11–5, in which the number of doublings and the number of cells are related to the size of the mass of tumor.

CAUSES OF CANCER

The exact cause of cancer is not known. It is doubtful, indeed, whether there is any single universal cause of all cancers, any more than we would expect to find any single universal cause of all inflammations. Both inflammation and cancer are processes, not diseases, whereas inflammation of the appendix and cancer of the stomach are diseases in the ordinary sense of the term. Again, just as it would be absurd to expect to discover a single method of treatment that would cure all infections, so it is probably useless to hope for a single cure of all cancers. The alliteration of "the cause of cancer" and "the cure of cancer" is unfortunate, because it has implanted deep in the mind of the public the fixed idea that there must be 1 cause and 1 cure, so that persons tend to reject the information that great advances have been made both in our knowledge of the causation and in the treatment of malignant disease. As a matter of fact, there are many chronic pathologic conditions, such as cirrhosis and emphysema, that are far less curable than cancer. Tumors form a group, just as do the infectious diseases, and each has to be considered by itself. We do know a good deal about certain factors that play a part in the production of cancer, just as we do know a good deal about treatment of the disease. Important factors in carcinogenesis are: (1) chemical carcinogens, (2) ionizing radiation, (3) viruses, (4) hormones, (5) heredity, (6) environment, and (7) chronic irritation. This does not mean that there may not be others, or that only 1 is responsible in a given case. It will be noticed that some of the factors may be termed external, others internal. Cancer, like inflammation, is a fire that burns continuously, and there are many methods of starting a fire, some physical and some chemical.

Chemical Carcinogens

The first observation on chemical carcinogenic agents was that of Sir Percival Pott in 1775, who made the association between the frequent appearance of cancer of the scrotum in chimney sweeps and the extraordinary amount of soot and coaltar in their clothing and on their bodies. This observation and recognition is widely quoted as the first instance of occupational cause of cancer.

In 1915, 140 years after Pott's paper, Yamagiwa in Japan put this idea to the test by painting tar on a rabbit's ear every day for 6 months, and succeeded in producing cancer of the skin. This was an epoch-making discovery, because for the first time it was possible to produce a malignant tumor in an experimental animal. It may be noted that if Yamagiwa had used a rat instead of a rabbit he would have failed, because, for unknown reasons, these species do not respond in the same way to the same stimulus. Eventually,

the mouse proved to be a much more suitable animal than the rabbit for this kind of promotion.

Tar is a complex substance that contains many chemical agents. Again, a number of years had to pass before the first carcinogen was isolated from the tar. This was the hydrocarbon benzpyrene. Soon it was discovered that a number of hydrocarbons synthesized in the laboratory were also powerfully carcinogenic, 1 of the most commonly used being 1:2:5:6 dibenzanthracene. These synthetic carcinogenic hydrocarbons all have a benzene six-membered ring structure. It is perhaps significant that a slight change in the chemical structure of a substance may convert it from a noncarcinogen into a carcinogen. Any of these carcinogens can produce carcinoma (epithelial cancer) or sarcoma (connective tissue cancer) at the site of application. Some can even convert a tissue culture of fibroblasts into a culture of cancer cells.

The application of a chemical carcinogen to a tissue is not followed by the presence of a tumor in a matter of days. The time between the exposure to a carcinogen and the appearance of a tumor is called the latent period, which is variable, but may be as long as years.

Berenblum and Shubik studied these phenomena and found that the development of such tumors could be enhanced by the application of a noncarcinogen, a mildly irritating substance such as croton oil. They described thus 2 stages in experimental tumor production: **initiation**, in which the conversion to neoplastic potential is effected by exposure to a carcinogen, and **promotion**, or chronic irritation, which may accelerate the rate at which the tissue has a chance to become malignant. This process is schematically illustrated in Figure 11–6.

Initiators are virtually always mutagens. Promoters are usually not, although they may establish some association with cellular DNA. First, promoters most often enhance cell division. A number of interpretations have been suggested: cell division provides chances for generating errors during DNA replication, either primary mutations or chromosomal rearrangements or missegregations. Alternatively, cycles of cell growth provide for changes in gene expression that may expose

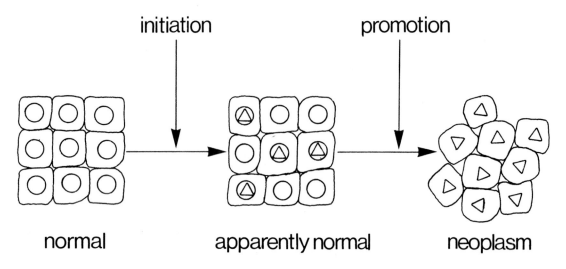

initiation   promotion

normal   apparently normal   neoplasm

Fig. 11–6. Normal cells are shown at the left. Following initiation, some of these cells may have changes in their nucleic acids, as indicated by the presence of triangles within the nucleus. Following repeated exposure to agents, which is promotion, a tumor may appear.

the regions of DNA previously affected by the initiator. Moreover, the stimulation of division causes a selection for cells more successful at multiplication, with a subsequent amplification of clones of cells with neoplastic tendencies. Second, the binding of promoters to DNA may itself trigger changes in gene expression; these epigenetic events may pair with the earlier somatic mutagenesis and may supply the necessary changes to produce a cell with neoplastic behavior. It should be emphasized that neoplastic transformation is not a switch to a preprogrammed, well-defined "other state." Tumors undoubtedly evolve continuously. At each stage (primary growth, invasion, metastasis), few cells survive, and the result is the natural selection of the most "successful" neoplastic behavior. The new environments encountered with tumor progression provide different stimuli and different selective pressure. Surrounding cells are pushed away, nutritional supplies may be different, new changes in gene expression may continue to be dictated by chromosomal rearrangements. The "spontaneous" metabolic and karyotypic (chromosome structure) alterations that are well adapted to tissue culture support this notion of change in response to a changed environment.

Many aromatic compounds have a resemblance to and/or an affinity for DNA and its building blocks. Increased accuracy and

feasibility in identifying and in characterizing carcinogenic compounds has resulted from the recently developed bacterial testing system (Ames test). Bacterial mutants, with a single error in their DNA that renders them unable to grow in a given medium, are plated in the presence of a test compound; any mutagenic compound causes some mutations at the site of the original error that render the compound wild-type and so allow growth of a bacterial colony. Thus different compounds can be evaluated for their mutagenic potency. Almost all known carcinogens have been so found to be potent mutagens, and some newly tested compounds found to be mutagenic have been then shown to be carcinogenic in animals. This is a powerful way of screening our environment for hazards and of testing new compounds before their use. It also has made clearer the relationship of mutation to carcinogenesis. Some compounds tested are found not to be mutagenic in their pure state; however, after incubation with an extract of liver containing a sampling of metabolic enzymes, they tested positive. Thus some compounds are metabolized to carcinogens by our bodies. In fact, there are now known to be detoxifying enzymes that are designed to reduce the toxicity of ingested organic compounds; some of the intermediates in these reactions are carcinogenic. The rapidity of the various steps in the cascade varies and determines the amount and duration of carcinogens in our system. These enzymes are inducible with a number of different types of compounds. Thus intake of a chemical or a drug may elevate the level of a person's detoxifying enzymes and so make that person more likely to accumulate carcinogens metabolized from the diet. It is possible as well that there are inherited variations in the level and rate of detoxification steps that yield hazardous intermediates.

Epidemiologic evidence has shown synergistic interactions between 2 environmental factors in cancer causation: for example, cigarette smoking and asbestos exposure in the etiology of lung cancer. The incidence of cancer after exposure to both smoking and asbestos is the sum of the incidence of the disease following exposure to either factor alone. Experimentally, 2 chemicals may not be carcinogenic when administered alone or in a given order, but with the correct protocol in the correct sequence are highly active. Chemical carcinogenesis is interpreted as requiring 2 types of events: initiation and promotion.

There is also evidence of **physical carcinogenesis**: the implantation of a plastic barrier, interrupting normal communication between cells, has been shown to cause tumors. The normally tight interrelatedness of cells selects for mutual dependency and coregulation. Changing that status quo will select for something different, which in some cases may be for cells that grow autonomously and outgrow the local signals, i.e., neoplasia. Further changes may have additional effects on tumor development; there is evidence in 1 neuroblastoma system that tumors can be induced to further differentiation along the normal pathway of their original cell type. Application of the appropriate hormone or inducer causes the cells to respond, to differentiate, and to lose their malignancy.

Ionizing Radiation

That ionizing radiations are important and powerful carcinogens became clear soon after Roentgen's discovery in 1895, when many early experimentalists received skin burns and developed tumors of the bones of their

Table 11–3. Neoplasms of Various Types and Sites in Irradiated Populations, Tentatively Quantified as in Excess or Not

NEOPLASM CATEGORY	ATOMIC BOMB SURVIVORS	OCCUPATIONALLY EXPOSED WORKERS	THERAPEUTICALLY IRRADIATED PATIENTS	
			ADULTS	CHILDREN
Bladder	−	−	+	−
Brain	−	−	−	+
Cervix uteri	+	−	+	−
Connective tissue	−	−	+	+
Cranial sinuses	−	+	+	−
Liver	−	−	+	−
Lymphoma	+	+	−	−
Multiple myeloma	+	+	−	−
Ovary	−	−	+	−
Pancreas	−	−	+	−
Pharynx	−	−	+	−
Rectum	−	−	+	−
Salivary glands	+	−	+	+
Skin	−	+	+	+
Vagina	−	−	+	−

Data from Albert and Omran (1968); Upton (1968); ICRP (1969); McIntyre and Pointon (1971); BEIR (1972); Pochin (1972); UN (1972); Nishiyama et al. (1973); Modan et al. (1974); Matanowski et al. (1975); Smith and Doll (1976).

(From Upton, A. C.: Radiation effects. In *Origins of Human Cancer, Book A.* Edited by H. H. Hiatt, et al. New York, Cold Spring Harbor Laboratory, 1977.)

hands. Even today, leukemia has a greater incidence than normal in radiologists (Table 11–3).

A single dose of 600 r is followed by benign and malignant tumors of the skin, connective tissue, and viscera in the experimental animal. The early workers with x rays developed cancer of the skin of the hand many years later, because they were unaware of the danger. This long latent period is of particular interest. The survivors of the first Hiroshima and Nagasaki atomic blasts show a tenfold increase in leukemia in the heavily exposed group. The miners in Schneeberg and Joachimsthal, Germany, for centuries have suffered from a high incidence of carcinoma of the lung; this is now known to be due to radioactive uranium. Ultraviolet light radiation is also carcinogenic, which explains the high incidence of cancer of the skin and lip among field workers in the white population of the tropics, Australia, and the southern United States. This form of cancer is rare in the Negro, who is protected by a high pigment content of the skin.

Hormones

Although hormones can also act as carcinogens, they differ from other carcinogens in 2 respects: (1) they induce tumors only in those organs on which the hormone has a physiologic effect, and (2) prolonged exposure of the susceptible tissue is required. Moreover, the cancer is at first hormone-dependent on the endocrine imbalance that initiated the process. Sex hormones provide the most striking example of a carcinogenic action. Indeed, the structural resemblances between the carcinogenic hydrocarbons and the female sex hormones might suggest similar physiologic activities. Estrogens frequently require the cooperation of 1 or more additional agencies, the most important of which is heredity. Thus removal of the ovaries at an early age in mice of a high cancer strain will prevent the occurrence of spontaneous mammary cancer, but hormonal administration will cause cancer to develop. In the prostate there seems to be little doubt that an endocrine dysfunction is an etiologic factor

in the production of cancer in man; the hormones may be gonadal or adrenal in origin.

The subject of hormone-dependent tumors has come to assume great clinical importance in relation to the treatment of cancer of the breast in women by removal of the ovaries, and of cancer of the prostate in men by the administration of estrogens, by adrenalectomy, or, as a last resort, by hypophysectomy, i.e., removal of the hypophysis or pituitary, which stimulates the adrenals to activity. The whole outlook in these cancers has been changed for the better to a remarkable degree by the adoption of 1 or more of these measures. Benefit from hormone therapy or removal of endocrine tissue can only be expected when the tumor is still hormone-dependent.

Viruses

One of the most exciting modern discoveries relating to carcinogenesis is that of the role of viruses. As far back as 1911, Rous showed that a cell-free filtrate of a sarcoma of fowl could produce a new tumor when injected into another fowl of the same breed. This experiment was the breakthrough, but it aroused no enthusiasm, for the only similar tumors were confined to birds. Then in 1932 a tumor due to a filter-passing viral agent was described in a wild rabbit by Richard Shope. A short time later, Bittner proved that cancer of the breast in mice can be transmitted to the newborn by an agent in the mother's milk. The agent was known as the Bittner milk factor. At present, the production of malignant tumors of a variety of types by cell-free filtrates in laboratory animals has become commonplace. It is even possible to induce cancer in cultures of human cells by the addition of the polyoma virus.

There is ample evidence for the induction of cancer by viruses in experimental animal systems. Among the DNA viruses, the polyoma, adenoviruses, and some herpesviruses are tumorigenic; among the RNA viruses, only the retroviruses induce cancer. It should be recalled that the latter form a DNA copy of their genome, which is then stably integrated into the host chromosome. It is probably this property of intimate and long-lasting association with host DNA that allows viruses to cause cancer. *In vivo*, in the wild, most DNA virus infections are lytic: infected cells are killed. This life cycle is incompatible with neoplastic transformation, and so most DNA viruses are not normally carcinogenic. Under other conditions, these viruses have been shown to be capable of stable, persistent infection. Only the herpesviruses have been seen to establish such a pattern of nonlytic growth with accompanying modification of cellular growth patterns in natural, *in vivo* infections.

A major advance in our thinking on the subject of the viral origin of cancer is represented by Gross's concept of vertical transmission. A laboratory animal suffering from a bacterial or viral disease will readily spread the infection to its neighbors of the same generation. This spread may be termed "horizontal transmission." However, the same is not true of a viral neoplasm, such as leukemia or mammary carcinoma in the mouse. Leukemia in mice is an example of a latent virus infection that produces a neoplastic disease that develops in an inbred strain when the mice reach early adult life. Gross has shown that the carcinogenic agent is transmitted vertically, that is to say, from 1 generation to another, through the germinal cells. In the case of mammary gland carcinoma in the mouse, the virus is transmitted through the mother's milk. The agent may remain latent throughout the life span of the host, which remains healthy, and yet carries and transmits the seeds of disease.

That the seeds are there can be shown by the inoculation of cell-free filtrates into newborn mice of a low-leukemic strain (which would not develop the disease spontaneously) with the subsequent production of leukemia when the animals reach adult life. The reason the newborn animal is used is that the fetus is unable to make antibodies against antigens to which it is exposed, an inability that persists for a few hours or days after birth. We have already examined this subject in connection with autoimmunity. When the virus of leukemia or the Bittner milk virus is inoculated later in life, it is destroyed by an-

tibodies, so that no neoplasm develops. This phenomenon suggests that a virus present in the body at birth may live in the cells for years until some external factor combines with it to turn it into a true carcinogen. If the reader wishes to become really confused, he may like to learn that some of the low-leukemic strain mice injected with cell-free extracts of leukemic tissue did develop not leukemia, but rather carcinoma of the parotid gland or fibrosarcoma of connective tissue. Still more startling was the discovery by Stewart that, when the same leukemic agent was grown in tissue culture, and when a cell-free extract was injected into newborn mice, the animals developed a broad spectrum of more than a dozen apparently unrelated tumors. The agent was named the polyoma (multiple tumor) virus.

It will be recalled from the virology chapter that EBV (Epstein-Barr virus), a herpesvirus, causes mononucleosis in man, and that the EBV genome is thought to persist in a small population of transformed lymphocytes in the host after the acute infection. EBV was also said to be closely associated with 2 human cancers, nasopharyngeal carcinoma and Burkitt's lymphoma. It is currently thought that these cancers are multicausal, with transformation by EBV as the first step. A number of additional events are implicated with Burkitt's lymphoma, including environmental factors such as holoendemic malaria, physiologic changes in the immune system, and molecular events, such as the characteristic chromosome rearrangement observed in the tissue of patients with Burkitt's lymphoma as well as in other lymphomas. In this case, then, EBV transformation is the initiator, and cancer follows after a long latency, if the appropriate promoters are supplied. Another herpesvirus, HSV-2 is implicated in the etiology of cervical cancer; the accompanying cofactors are not completely understood.

There is recent evidence implicating another DNA virus in human cancer: hepatitis B virus (HBV) and primary hepatocellular carcinoma. The distribution of hepatocellular carcinoma coincides with that of chronic HBV. HBV causes a chronic infection that often follows a typical course in an asymptomatic carrier—chronic hepatitis, cirrhosis, and finally, carcinoma. Neonatal or infantile infection with HBV is common in such persons. In patients with primary hepatocellular carcinoma, evidence of HBV infection and expression has been reported in 70 to 95% of cases examined, and integrated HBV DNA has been detected in the hepatoma cell chromosomes. The factors involved in activating the chronic HBV or in promoting the change from hepatitis or cirrhosis to a hepatoma are as yet unknown. However, this correlation is new, and trial vaccinations of pregnant women and of newborns are in progress. It is significant that there is another virus similar in genomic and protein components, the woodchuck hepatitis virus, which is also associated with chronic hepatitis and hepatoma in its natural host.

Finally, let us discuss the role of retroviruses and cancer. We owe a good deal of our understanding of the nature of neoplastic transformation in murine and avian systems to studies of leukemia-inducing and sarcoma-inducing retroviruses. Their relevance to carcinogenesis in the wild is less certain. Endogenous retroviruses are inherited as stable genes in most species of mammals. Sometimes these are expressed, sometimes not. Unexpressed viruses can sometimes be experimentally activated, and occasionally they are naturally activated at a certain stage of the animal's life. Highly tumorigenic endogenous viruses would certainly be deleted if they exerted their effect before or during the reproductive years.

The mechanism by which the leukemia viruses induce transformation of their target cells is unknown, but perturbations of the normal process of selection and amplification of cells within the immune system have been postulated. Viruses are specific to cell types (Table 11–4). It has become clear that viruses can evolve and display changed properties by recombination with cellular genes or with other endogenous viral genes. Many of the sarcoma viruses are defective and need a helper retrovirus for growth; they have replaced a crucial gene with a transforming function known as **src**. Viral studies show that the src protein is directly necessary for transformation; recent analysis indicates that it is an enzyme that phosphorylates proteins. The significance of this fact is as yet unknown, although it is a common cellular mode of regulating and modifying enzymatic activities. The src protein seems to be related to a cellular protein found in some normal tissues; the normal role of the protein, and why it becomes carcinogenic in the presence of the retrovirus, is unclear. However, carcinogenesis due to integration of the gene in another chromosomal site, or to the altered control of its expression in the new environment, is a model consistent with our earlier discussion of carcinogenesis. Selection of viruses from tumors will certainly yield those vectors that successfully trigger a neoplastic change, and may not represent an accurate picture of the average viral potential. The relative inactivity of most wild retroviruses as compared to the potency and breadth of host range of laboratory strains is a testament to virus-host plasticity and to the role of natural selection.

The mammary tumor virus of mice is another case. This virus is inherited as a single Mendelian gene, but, when expressed, is only active in mammary cells where it induces a carcinoma, usually

Table 11–4.   Neoplasms of Viral Etiology

TYPE OF NEOPLASM	ANIMAL SPECIES	REFERENCES
Chicken leukoses	Fowl	Ellerman and Bang (1908)
Chicken sarcomas	Fowl	Rous (1911)
Chicken sarcomas	Fowl	Fujinami and Inamoto (1914)
Mill-Hill endothelioma	Fowl	Foulds (1934)
Chicken fibrosarcomas	Fowl	Duran-Reynals (1946)
Mammary cancer (adenocarcinoma)	Mice	Bittner (1936)
Maxillary gland tumors	Mice	Gross (1953)
Leukemia	Mice	Gross (1952)
Papillomatosis	Rabbit, cattle, horse	Shope (1932), Olson (1941)
Adenocarcinoma of kidney	Leopard, frog	Lucke (1934, 1938)
Papilloma (warts)	Humans	Green, et al (1940)
		Strauss, et al (1950)

(From Perez-Tamayo, R.: *Mechanisms of Disease.* Philadelphia & London, W. B. Saunders, 1961.)

late in the mouse's life. Its activation has been shown to be sensitive to hormone stimulation. When activated, the virus can be transmitted through the milk to nursing offspring; most early mammary carcinomas in mice stem from this mode of exogenous infection.

Leukemia in the feline and bovine populations is known to be caused by retroviruses. In animals, it is thought that the horizontal transmission of retrovirus is significant in disease, and that the endogenous viruses are silent remnants of long-ago infection of cells. The role of horizontal spread of animal retroviruses to humans is unknown, although evidence of primate viruses has been detected in selected human tissues. Human retroviruses have never been found with absolute certainty. However, DNA or proteins similar to retroviruses of other species have been detected by many investigators in human cells. Whether these are involved in human malignancy is unknown. New breakthroughs in virology promise an understanding and control of cancers where viral infection is a causal agent.

Genetic Factors

In the experimental animal, of which pure strains can be bred with ease, the genetic constitution may be a factor of paramount importance. Thus we have high-cancer strains and low-cancer strains of mice for a particular tumor and organ. It is not possible to apply the results of breeding experiments in mice to men for obvious reasons, but a few human tumors show such a familial tendency that every member of the family may die of the disease if he lives long enough. Such tumors are neuroblastoma of the retina and malignant polyp of the large bowel. An historic example of a familial tendency is that of Napoleon, who died at St. Helena of cancer of the stomach. His father, his grandfather, his brother, and his 3 sisters all died of the same disease.

Several types of evidence make it clear that the genetic component of human cancer is relatively small. Studies on identical twins show that their experiences with cancer are no more similar than those of nonidentical twins. Most convincing are the studies on

migrating populations in the context of worldwide epidemiology. The relative incidence of specific cancers varies greatly from country to country; this finding is consistent with the significance of environmental factors: diet, soil, water, air, industrial by-products. Japan has high levels of stomach cancer, but relatively lower levels of breast, large intestine, and prostate cancer as compared with the United States. When Japanese immigrants migrate to California, their cancer profile looks similar to that of native Californians within 2 generations. As breeding within the group remains prevalent, the dominant force here is environmental. Since the shift is not immediate, the environmental factors probably include elements, such as diet, that change slowly with cultural assimilation rather than automatic stimuli, such as air quality. Studies of other migrant populations illustrate the same point. Epidemiologists have attempted to define the environmental factors that correlate with the relative international frequencies of given cancers. For example, it appears that the increased incidence of cancer of the large intestine correlates well with the high meat consumption in a society or, alternatively, with low cereal intake.

There are some situations, however, in which a genetic predisposition for a given cancer is apparently involved. Women whose sisters or mothers have suffered from breast cancer have a far greater likelihood of having breast cancer than do women in general. However, this is clearly not a simple, one-factor system. In all women, the incidence of breast cancer increases as the age at first pregnancy increases. Whether there is a change in breast tissue at pregnancy that deters cancer or whether there is a hormonal effect at work is unclear.

A hereditary disorder known as xeroderma pigmentosum illustrates the role of inherited and somatic (not in the germ-line, but rather occurring independently in body cells) mutation. Therefore, persons who inherit this mutation are more susceptible to DNA damage effected by environmental radiation, for example the ultraviolet irradiation of sunlight. Persons so affected have a significantly increased level of skin cancer, especially those living in tropical climates with plentiful sunshine. Ultraviolet-induced damage to DNA remains unrepaired in affected persons, and these accumulated mutations obviously exert a carcinogenic effect.

Environment

It is certainly the case that some forms of occupation bear a striking relation to cancer in particular sites. This is a subject of increasing importance in the industrial age in which we live, and in which workmen's compensation claims a corresponding degree of attention. Mere mention need be made of workers with coal tar and petroleum distillates, aniline dyes, x rays and radioactive material, and many other raw materials and products. The truth is that throughout life we seem to swim in a sea of carcinogens, and it is more by good fortune than by good management that some of us escape to die from causes other than cancer. Chronic irritation used to be a favorite scapegoat, but it is seldom heard of now, although a few examples come to mind. Cancer

of the gallbladder is usually associated with gallstones, cancer of the urinary bladder is common in persons infected with *Schistosoma* ova, and cancer may develop in the edge of a chronic ulcer in which prolonged destruction of tissue demands constant replacement of parts with disturbance of the normal growth mechanism.

Environmental exposure to industrial hazards or simply to contaminants of the household has gained increasing attention as a possible etiologic factor in the rising tide of our ills (Table 11–5). It is now clear that asbestos, an insulating and fireproofing material, offers real hazards to the industrial worker, whether a miner or a fitter engaged in using the material. It even appears the the worker's family is at increased risk, because when he returns home, his clothing may carry sufficient asbestos particles to expose those who wait daily for the worker's return. The role of asbestos in producing cancer of the pleural surfaces is clearly recognized, although the latent period may be long.

Other recent connections between occupa-

Table 11–5.   Occupational Cancers

AGENT	OCCUPATION	SITE OF CANCER
Ionizing radiations radon	certain underground miners (uranium, fluorspar, hematite)	bronchus
X rays, radium	radiologists, radiographers	skin
radium	luminous dial painters	bone
Ultraviolet light	farmers, sailors	skin
Polycyclic hydrocarbons in soot, tar, oil	chimney sweepers	scrotum
	manufacturers of coal gas	skin
	many other groups of exposed industrial workers	bronchus
2-Naphthylamine; 1-naphthylamine	chemical workers; rubber workers; manufacturers of coal gas	bladder
Asbestos	asbestos workers; shipyard and insulation workers	bronchus pleura and peritoneum
Arsenic	sheep dip manufacturers; gold miners; some vineyard workers and ore smelters	skin and bronchus
Benzene	workers with glues, varnishes, etc.	marrow (leukemia)
Mustard gas	poison gas makers	bronchus; larynx; nasal sinuses
Vinyl chloride	PVC manufacturers	liver (angiosarcoma)
(Chrome ores)	chromate manufacturers	bronchus
(Nickel ore)	nickel refiners	bronchus; nasal sinuses
(Isopropyl oil)	isopropylene manufacturers	nasal sinuses
*	hardwood furniture makers	nasal sinuses
*	leather workers	nasal sinuses

* Specific agent not identified.

(From Doll, R.: Introduction. In *Origins of Human Cancer, Book A.* Edited by H. H. Hiatt, et al. New York, Cold Spring Harbor Laboratory, 1977.)

tional exposure and cancer have been made. For example, in the plastics industry, exposure to vinyl chloride has been shown to produce a tumor of blood vessels in the liver. It has been known for decades that workers in the heavy metals industries (nickel, copper, cobalt) all may have significantly increased risks for different cancers, and it has even become clear that sawmill workers have an extraordinarily high risk of cancer of the sinuses.

The incidence of different forms of cancer certainly varies greatly in different parts of the world. Sometimes we know the reason for this, but in most instances we do not. Cancer of the bladder is common among Egyptian farm workers, and we have already seen that this is related to the high incidence of *Schistosoma haematobium* infection in Egypt, although how the presence of the ova of the parasite in the wall of the bladder causes cancer we do not know. We have already seen that cancer of the skin is common in white-skinned persons living in the tropics, because

of ultraviolet light radiation. Endless other examples could be given, usually with no explanation. Cancer in Africa provides one of the most exciting and challenging examples of the geographic pathology of the disease. The pattern of cancer in that continent differs profoundly from that in both Europe and North America. There must be good reasons for these differences, but, with a few exceptions, we are ignorant of them. Two of the most striking examples are cancer of the liver and tumors of the jaw. China also offers many examples of cancer which to most of us are bizarre.

Burkitt's lymphoma provides the newest and most dramatic feature of the exciting story of cancer in Africa. A young English observer, armed only with a pencil, a notebook, and the power to draw conclusions from what he saw, pointed out that great numbers of children in Africa on the line of the equatorial belt running from coast to coast suffered from a neoplasm of the lymphoid tissue, most frequently in the jaws, but also in

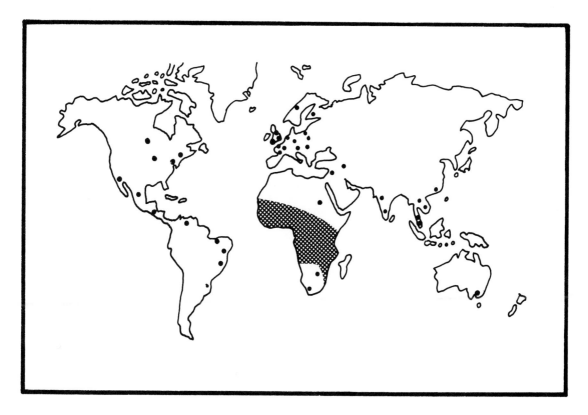

Fig. 11–7. This map shows the distribution of Burkitt's lymphoma (From Burkitt, D. In *Proceedings of the International Conference on Leukemia-Lymphoma.* Edited by C.J.C. Zarafonetis. Philadelphia, Lea & Febiger, 1968.)

many of the abdominal and thoracic organs. The most probable cause is a virus, which is also found in the mosquitoes that abound in this zone (see Chap. 8). Figure 11–7 shows a world map illustrating the distribution of this tumor. In many respects, the tumor resembles the multiple neoplasms produced by the polyoma virus when injected into newborn mice.

Occupational hazards, which affect a significant fraction of the population, and the fascinating observations on geographic pathology have less significance for the North American population than the increasing interest in environmental factors in general. Our air is heavily polluted, as are our water sources. The use of preservatives in foodstuffs, filters for preparing beverages, additives to make or to suppress foam in beer, hormones to increase growth rates in cattle, antibiotic additives in poultry feed, and organic pesticides on fruit all suggest that we are surviving in a sea of potential carcinogens. It is hard to know what to do as an individual and even more difficult to give ad-

vice when faced with such a confused and increasingly complex environment.

In summary, the cause of cancer is unknown. The range of variation in incidence is remarkable (Table 11–6). From the foregoing discussion, we can talk of different etiologies—radiation, viruses, chemical carcinogens—all of which have as their final common pathway the nucleic acid of the target cells. Alteration in the mechanism of normal replication has been demonstrated for most carcinogens. Lewis Thomas has suggested, "I think you'll find that cancer is the result of a single mechanism. Earlier diseases that troubled us, like syphilis, had the appearance of many separate diseases too. The skin, bones, and blood vessels were all involved. The brain and heart were disabled years after the initial infection. It looked like a multifactorial disease with environmental aspects—that is, a disease with many causes, the way cancer looks today. But syphilis turned out to be a host of reactions to a single mechanism, an organism known as a Spirochete. I think Nature is simple and dis-

Table 11–6. Range of Variation in the Incidence of Common Cancers

TYPE OF CANCER	HIGH-INCIDENCE AREA	CUMULATIVE RISK[a] (%)	RANGE OF VARIATION[b]	LOW-INCIDENCE AREA
Skin	Australia, Queensland	>20	>200	India, Bombay
Esophagus	Iran, N.E.	20	300	Nigeria
Bronchus	England	11	35	Nigeria
Stomach	Japan	11	25	Uganda
Cervix uteri	Colombia	10	15	Israel, Jewish
Liver	Mozambique	8	70	Norway
Prostate	USA, black	7	30	Japan
Breast (♀)	USA, Connecticut	7	5	Uganda
Colon	USA, Connecticut	3	10	Nigeria
Buccal cavity	India, part	>2	>25	Denmark
Rectum	Denmark	2	20	Nigeria
Bladder	USA, Connecticut	2	4	Japan
Ovary	Denmark	2	8	Japan
Corpus uteri	USA, Connecticut	2	10	Japan
Nasopharynx	Singapore, Chinese	2	40	England
Pancreas	New Zealand, Maori	2	5	Uganda
Penis	Uganda, part	1	300	Israel, Jewish

[a] By 75 years of age in absence of other causes of death.
[b] At ages 35–64 years.

(From Doll, R.: Introduction. In *Origins of Human Cancer, Book A.* Edited by H. H. Hiatt, et al. New York, Cold Spring Harbor Laboratory, 1977.)

eases which look so mysterious today will turn out to have a single core. I don't think nature is that tricky as to use a hundred different mechanisms to produce a single disease." (*New York Times Magazine*, July 4, 1976.)

CHARACTERISTICS OF TUMORS

An operational and reasonable definition for all tumors is that of Willis: "A tumor is an abnormal mass of tissue, the growth of which exceeds and is uncoordinated with that of normal tissues, and persists in the same excessive manner after the cessation of the stimuli which evoked the change."

Tumors can be divided into 2 general classes: the one innocent or benign, the other malignant. Sometimes a benign tumor may develop into a malignant one. A malignant tumor differs from a benign one in the following particulars.

1. A malignant tumor, if untreated, will kill the patient wherever it occurs, even in the hand or foot. A benign tumor may only cause death if it happens to grow in a vital organ such as the brain.

2. A malignant tumor infiltrates the surrounding tissue. It sends claws into it like a crab. The word cancer means a crab. A benign tumor grows by expansion, as a toy balloon does when blown up, and is usually separated from the surrounding tissue by a capsule so that it can be shelled out, or at least readily removed.

3. When a malignant tumor is excised, it may recur. This is because some of the outlying parts have not been completely removed; they are so minute that they cannot be seen by the surgeon, but they may soon grow to the size of the original tumor. When a benign tumor is removed, it usually does not recur.

4. Generally, a malignant tumor grows more rapidly than a benign one, although some cancers are remarkably slow in growth, especially in old people. The rapid growth is because tumor cells divide rapidly. The presence of numerous mitotic figures, particularly abnormal mitotic figures, indicates to the pathologist that the tumor is almost certainly malignant.

5. A malignant tumor sets up secondary growths (metastases) in lymph nodes and in distant organs. This is because the cancer has invaded the lymph or blood vessels, and the tumor cells are carried to other parts of the body, where they settle down and form new tumors. This is the single most obvious criterion of malignancy: the presence of **metastases**.

There are microscopic differences of great importance to the pathologist in the task of determining whether the tumor removed by the surgeon is or is not cancer, but they need not be detailed here. Suffice it to say that a benign tumor tends to reproduce the structure of the organ from which it grows, whereas a malignant tumor fails to do so. This is a histologic distinction, a failure in arrangement. In addition, the individual cells of the malignant tumor may show a lack of normal differentiation, a reversion to a more primitive and undifferentiated type, which is known as **anaplasia**. Both the histologic and cytologic changes may be so great that the pathologist can diagnose the case as one of cancer the moment he looks down the microscope. In other cases, a decision may be difficult, and different pathologists may disagree in their interpretations of the microscopic picture.

Carcinoma-in-situ. An important step in the fight against cancer is the recognition by the pathologist of the earliest beginnings of the malignant process. When metastases have occurred, it is too late. When invasion of the deeper tissues can be recognized, it may be too late. However, when the malignant change is still cytologic rather than histologic, the disease is curable. This state of affairs is known as *carcinoma-in-situ* or preinvasive carcinoma. The cells appear restless, as if looking for a way to get out. The condition may be reversible, but in many cases, the *in-situ* state develops into an invasive one. It is in carcinoma of the cervix uteri that recognition of preinvasive carcinoma is of the greatest practical importance and has already saved the lives of countless women (see Fig. 11–8). A drawing to illustrate this concept is shown in Figure 11–8, in which *A* represents normal cells in a tissue, and *D* represents

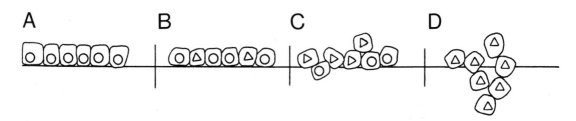

Fig. 11–8. *A* illustrates normal cells, *B* shows cells with some atypia that could be considered dysplastic. *C*, Carcinoma-in-situ is represented by the change of the basement membrane, and *D*, frank invasion, or carcinoma, is shown. The triangles for nuclei rather than circles symbolize an altered genome, whatever the cause.

Table 11–7. Characteristics of Benign and Malignant Tumors

CHARACTERISTICS	BENIGN	MALIGNANT
1. Growth	Slow, expansive, often encapsulated	Rapid, invasive, nonencapsulated
2. Metastases	Absent	Frequent
3. Recurrence after removal	Absent	Frequent
4. Histology	Relatively normal	Abnormal to a varying degree
5. Cytology	Normal	Varying degrees of anaplasia
6. Mitoses	Absent	Often numerous and abnormal
7. Constitutional effects	Rare, apart from endocrine adenomas	The rule

malignant cells invading the surrounding tissue.

Some of the principal distinguishing features between benign and malignant tumors are given in Table 11–7. It must be understood that these are generalizations to which there are frequent exceptions.

Spread of Tumors

This subject has already been referred to. An innocent tumor increases in size but can hardly be said to spread. A malignant tumor, on the other hand, spreads locally and to distant parts. The local spread is due to the invasive character of the growth, the cancer cells worming their way into the surrounding tissues and growing along the lymphatics. This permeation of the lymphatics is particularly well seen in cancer of the breast (Fig. 11–9).

The other method of spread is by **tumor embolism**, the cancer cells forming emboli and being carried by the blood stream to distant parts in the same way as thrombi may become detached and converted into emboli. If the lymphatic vessels are invaded, the tumor cells are carried to the nearest (regional)

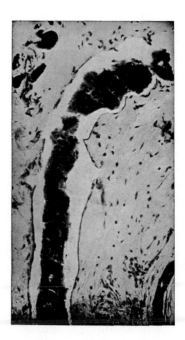

Fig. 11–9. Lymphatic permeation by carcinoma. × 125. (Boyd, W.: *Textbook of Pathology.* Philadelphia, Lea & Febiger.)

lymph nodes, where they are arrested and form new tumors similar to the primary one. In the surgical treatment of cancer of the breast, the lymph nodes in the axilla, which receive the lymph from the breast, are removed together with the breast. This is done even though they are not enlarged, for they may contain cancer cells that have not yet had time to form a visible tumor.

In embolism by the blood stream, the tumor cells are carried to some other organ, where they are arrested in the capillaries and start secondary growths or metastases. In abdominal organs such as the stomach, the secondary growths are usually in the liver, because the blood from the digestive tract is carried first to the liver. In the case of other organs, the metastases commonly occur in the lungs, but any organ in the body may be involved.

Having reviewed some of the general aspects of tumor pathology, we may now briefly consider a few of the more important varieties of tumors. Many of these are described in more detail in connection with the organs in which they occur. It is difficult to give an interesting or even intelligible account of tumors without reference to the microscopic structure and the use of a large number of technical terms, but this is avoided as far as possible, for microscopic descriptions are nothing but a mass of words unless one has the opportunity to study the microscopic sections themselves.

Benign Tumors

The general characteristics of a benign tumor have already been outlined so they need not be repeated here. In describing benign tumors, and the same is true of malignant tumors, we name them after the tissue from which they arise, adding the suffix -oma, which indicates tumors, just as -itis indicates inflammation. Some of the principal tissues are as follows: (1) **epithelium**, which makes up the skin, the mucous membranes that line the mouth, stomach, intestine, and uterus, and the glandular organs, such as the breast, liver, and uterus; (2) **fibrous** or **connective tissue,** which forms a general framework of the body and therefore occurs in all organs; (3) **fat**; (4) **bone** and cartilage; (5)

muscle; (6) **blood vessels**; (7) **nervous tissue**; (8) **lymph nodes**.

Epithelioma. This benign epithelial tumor grows as a projecting mass from an epithelial surface. Its common site is the skin, but it also occurs in the mouth, large intestine, and bladder. Sometimes a papilloma, especially when irritated, may become malignant. A wart is an epithelioma caused by a virus.

Adenoma. This benign epithelial tumor is glandular in structure, that is to say, the cells are arranged around secretory spaces. It occurs most commonly in organs that are themselves glandular, such as the breast and thyroid gland.

Fibroma. This is a tumor of fibrous tissue, and therefore dense and hard. As fibrous tissue is universally present, a fibroma may occur in practically every part of the body, and yet strangely enough fibromas are distinctly uncommon tumors. Perhaps the most common site is under the skin.

Lipoma. A soft fatty tumor growing from fat (adipose tissue), lipoma may occur wherever fat is present, but is most common in the neck, shoulders, back, and buttocks, and other places where fat is abundant.

Osteoma and Chondroma. An osteoma arises from osseous tissue or bone, and consists of bone; a chondroma arises from cartilage and consists of that tissue. In the embryo, the bones consist of cartilage that is gradually converted into bone. As long as bone is growing in length, some cartilage remains at each end. It is natural, therefore, that both osteomas and chondromas should grow from the ends of bones.

Myoma. This tumor is composed of muscle, of which there are 2 kinds: (1) voluntary or striated muscles, which are under the control of the will and form the ordinary muscles of the limbs and trunks; (2) involuntary or unstriated (plain) muscles, which are not under the control of the will and are found in the walls of the stomach and intestine, the blood vessels, and the uterus. Curiously enough, myomas are a rarity in voluntary muscles, but they are common in the uterus, where they are frequently called fibroids, because of the large amount of fibrous tissue that is mingled with the muscle. The correct name for such smooth muscle tumors is **leiomyoma**.

Angioma. This tumor is composed of vessels, usually blood vessels, but sometimes lymph vessels. It is therefore generally of a bright or dark red color, although a lymph angioma is colorless. Its common site is the skin, especially of the face or neck, where it forms a red patch known as a port-wine stain or birthmark. The latter term is used because the tumor is usually present at birth. An angioma may form an unsightly swelling of the lip in children.

Nevus. A tumor of the skin, a nevus is composed of epidermal cells filled with melanin pigment, being usually dark in color and sometimes jet black. It is therefore a melanoma. There are 2 varieties of melanoma, benign and malignant. The nevus is a **benign melanoma**, its common name being a mole, which simply means a mass. Moles are so common that nearly everyone has at least a tiny one, and many people have a large number. A nevus is a congenital condition, but it may not be apparent at birth. The common sites are the face, neck, and back. They are probably under hormonal influence, for they tend to increase in size at puberty. They may grow slowly for a time, remain quiescent for a long period, and then gradually atrophy. The beginning of a malignant change in later life is indicated by an increase in size and pigmentation, the presence of a pink halo due to congestion, and itching. The tumor has now become a **malignant melonoma**. It is customary to refer to the benign form as a nevus. The designation of the cancerous tumor is malignant melanoma. The dangerous sites are the palm, the sole of the foot, the fingers and toes, the genitals, and places exposed to continued trauma. The transformation is often slow and insidious, for melanoma enters by stealth like a thief in the night, but any sudden increase in the rate of growth should arouse a suspicion of malignancy, and the tumor should be removed at once. A mole that shows no change need not be touched except for cosmetic reasons, but chronic irritation and trauma must be avoided at all costs.

Malignant Tumors

For every tissue of the body that can give rise to a benign tumor, a malignant tumor also may arise. In practice, however, nearly all malignant tumors can be divided into 2 great groups, **carcinoma** and **sarcoma**, both of which are included under the common term cancer. This simplification of nomenclature is possible because the epithelial tumors are called carcinoma, whereas the name sarcoma is applied not only to connective tissue tumors but also to tumors of bone, cartilage, fat, and muscle, which are derived from or closely related to connective tissue. The carcinomas form a more uniform group, the sarcomas a more diverse one.

Carcinoma. The commonest of malignant tumors spreads principally by the lymphatics, so that secondary involvement of the regional lymph nodes is common and has to be considered by the surgeon in every case. Spread by the blood stream is also common, and it sometimes happens that the first indication of cancer in an organ such as the lung is the development of a secondary tumor in the brain, the secondary tumor naturally being mistaken for the primary one until the original is discovered. It is evident that when tumors are present in 2 organs, it may be difficult to say which is primary and which secondary.

Carcinoma may arise either from the skin or from glandular organs (breast, thyroid), including the secreting glands in the mucous membranes of the stomach, intestine, and uterus. The microscopic structure differs in the 2 cases. In skin cancer, there is some attempt at reproducing the normal arrangement of the epithelial cells in layers, so that this tumor is known as **epidermoid carcinoma** (resembling the skin or epidermis). In glandular cancers, there is an attempt at arrangement of the cells around gland spaces, so that the tumor is known as **adenocarcinoma** (Greek *aden*, gland). In both forms of the disease, masses of tumor cells invade the deeper structures.

The degree to which carcinoma can resemble the normal skin or glandular structure varies greatly. There may be absolutely no approximation to the normal arrangement of cells; such a tumor is said to be **undifferentiated** or **anaplastic**. These anaplastic tumors are usually highly malignant, and as they are rapidly growing they may be sensitive to radiation. Conversely, the tumor may reproduce the normal structure with a fair degree of success, and is then said to be **differentiated**. It is evident from what has been said previously that, if a tumor is highly differentiated, the pathologist may have difficulty in distinguishing it from a benign epithelial tumor (adenoma, papilloma). The degree of differentiation is expressed in 4 grades, grade 1 being the most differentiated, grade 4 the most anaplastic.

The common sites of carcinoma are the skin, mouth, lung, stomach, breast, and uterus. Skin cancers as a rule are not highly malignant, and early removal is followed by a high percentage of cures. A special type of skin cancer used to be called rodent ulcer (Fig. 11–10); this is confined almost entirely to the face, is of slow growth, long duration, and low malignancy, and is therefore very amenable to treatment. The microscopic picture is called **basal cell carcinoma**, because the tumor is composed of cells resembling the basal cell layer of the epidermis and differing from epidermoid carcinoma, in which the cells tend to become cornified or keratinized as are those of the superficial layers of the normal skin. Mouth cancer occurs chiefly on the lower lip and tongue, usually on the basis of some previous site of irritation. Cancer of the lip is usually of low-grade malignancy and has a good prognosis, whereas cancer of the tongue tends to be of a higher grade, with a

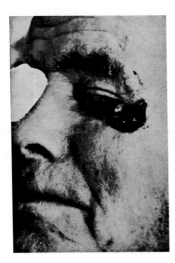

Fig. 11–10. Rodent ulcer; at the outer angle of the eye.

correspondingly bad prognosis. Cancer of the other organs is described when the diseases of those organs are considered.

Sarcoma. This is a malignant tumor of connective (fibrous) tissue and of those structures such as bone and cartilage that are derived from connective tissue. Although we say that a sarcoma is a tumor of connective tissue, we must keep in mind that it is a tumor of connective tissue cells, not of connective tissue fibers. The term is sometimes applied loosely and incorrectly to certain other malignant tumors. Sarcomas may occur in any part of the body, as connective tissue is present everywhere, but the principal sites are bone, subcutaneous tissue, and muscle. These tumors are uncommon as compared with carcinoma. A sarcoma infiltrates the surrounding tissue, just as does a carcinoma, but it seldom spreads by the lymphatics to the local lymph nodes. Distant spread is by the blood stream, and metastases are usually in the lungs.

Lymphosarcoma. This is a malignant tumor of the lymph nodes. Its chief characteristics are its wide distribution and its sensitivity to radiation. The response to radiation is remarkable, large masses of tumor melting away in a few days or weeks as snow before the sun. Some cases can be cured and many held in check for a long time by means of radiation.

Malignant Melanoma. We have already encountered this neoplasm as a malignant development of a nevus. The change from nevus to melanoma seldom takes place before puberty, suggesting that hormonal stimulation plays an important part in the development of the malignancy. As the name implies, the tumor cells are usually loaded with black melanin pigment. The great danger of malignant melanoma is not local destruction, as is seen in carcinoma and sarcoma, but early invasion of the lymphatics and blood vessels, causing widespread dissemination and the formation of metastases throughout the body. Perhaps the most dangerous site of origin is the foot. A pigmented lesion is less likely to attract attention there than on the hand or face. The melanoma, unfortunately, is resistant to treatment with radiation, but early surgery and new chemotherapeutic and immunologic approaches offer the patient some hope. Occasionally, the tumor arises from the pigment cells not of the skin, but of the eye.

Glioma. This is a malignant tumor of the glia or neuroglia of the brain that separates the nerve cells from one another and acts as a kind of connective tissue. Brain tumors are common, but such tumors practically never arise from nerve cells, always from neuroglia. The gliomas vary much in malignancy, but even the least malignant ones show no attempt at encapsulation and merge with the surrounding brain tissue. This makes the task of the brain surgeon peculiarly difficult, because even when the tumor has been exposed, it is difficult to know how much of the surrounding brain to remove. Oddly, brain tumors do not metastasize outside the skull.

DIAGNOSIS OF CANCER

The final diagnosis of cancer, that is to say, whether a lump is a neoplasm, and whether that neoplasm is innocent or malignant, must be made in the laboratory. The clinician can be suspicious, but not certain. The laboratory, or rather the person who works in the laboratory, can employ a number of techniques.

Biopsy. When a tumor is removed by a surgeon in the operating room it is sent to the pathology laboratory where it is fixed, sectioned, and stained. It is on the microscopic examination of these sections that the final diagnosis is made by the pathologist as to whether or not the lesion is malignant. Under some circumstances, particularly in the case of lumps of the breast, it may be desirable for the surgeon to have a report on the nature of the lesion during the course of the operation, so that he may determine the extent of the subsequent procedure. For this purpose, the frozen section on unfixed tissue stained with polychrome methylene blue enables a "rush diagnosis" to be made on a "rapid section" in the course of a few minutes. The responsibility on the pathologist is heavy. If he says that the lesion is benign, nothing more need be done. If he says that it is malignant, the entire breast and regional lymph nodes may be removed. If the lesion is in a limb, the

pathologist's opinion may decide whether or not the patient will lose an arm or a leg.

Exfoliative Cytology. Cancer cells tend to lose the adhesiveness characteristic of normal cells, so that they may be cast off or exfoliated from a surface early in the disease, even in the preinvasive stage. These cells are found in exudates, secretions, washings, and scrapings. This diagnostic method, often referred to loosely and inaccurately as cytology, has opened up new vistas in the early diagnosis of cancer. Its greatest value at present is in cancer of the cervix and bronchus, where it is easy to obtain fresh cells that have not yet autolyzed. By this means it is possible to detect early cancers. Curiously enough, in advanced cancer the test may be negative, because the cells have become necrotic and therefore unrecognizable. The test is associated with the name of Papanicolaou, although he first introduced his smear method for the study of cells in animal vaginal secretions, and not for cancer.

In the laborious task of "screening" large numbers of presumably normal persons for carcinoma, more particularly for cancer of the cervix uteri, fluorescence microscopy has proved a time-saving measure. This procedure has an additional advantage in that it can be done by physicians or technicians without special training in exfoliative cytology. The method employs cytochemistry, with special relation to the cytoplasm, whereas the conventional method depends on cytomorphology, with particular attention to the nucleus. When the fluorescence dye acridine orange is used, the deoxyribonucleic acid (DNA) of the nucleus appears green under the fluorescence microscope, whereas the ribonucleic acid (RNA) of the cytoplasm appears brown, orange, or flaming red. Malignant cells usually contain large amounts of cytoplasmic RNA, associated with active protein synthesis, so that they display brilliant orange or red cytoplasmic fluorescence, and are readily distinguished from the normal cells, which display green or brown fluorescence. Study of the cells by the standard method is essential in the cases showing a suggestive fluorescence reaction.

Chemical Tests. Enormous amounts of time

and money have been spent on the search for a chemical test of the blood or of the secretions that would indicate that neoplasia was in progress. We need a method such as the Wassermann test for syphilis or the test for hyperglycemia (high blood sugar level) in diabetes. The results have been generally disappointing. It is true that in individual instances, some tests may be of clinical value, as in carcinoma of the prostate, in which increased acid phosphatase levels may suggest that diagnosis. Recently, with newer knowledge of the biologic behavior of different tumors and with the elegant methods of immunology that permit the detection of molecular amounts of material, some hope for cancer detection has come forward. The liver synthesizes many things, but it has been discovered that, early in its development, it synthesizes a protein that later is no longer made. Tumors partake of many characteristics of embryonic tissue. It is now clear that tumors may synthesize substances that are not the product of normal cells. One such product, alpha-fetoprotein, normally made by the fetal liver, is also produced by some liver tumors, so patients suspected of liver cancer can be tested for alpha-fetoprotein.

Another example of this is the recognition of an antigen produced in embryonic bowel. Some patients with cancer of the large bowel have carcinoembryonic antigen (CEA) in their serum, which usually arises from cancer of the bowel.

An exciting, recent development of the CEA marker (which turns out not to be entirely specific for either bowel or cancer) is that the presence of CEA can be identified in the living patient by means of radioactively labeled antibody to CEA with nuclear scanning techniques. This means that areas of tumor that secrete CEA can be identified in the living patient, and promises to guide the surgeon, radiotherapist, or chemotherapist to a better attack on the cancer. If the preliminary studies with the method are confirmed, it gives hope that other tumor-specific antigens may be identified and will also permit *in vivo* localization, and even the likelihood that tissue-specific chemotherapy or radiotherapy will follow soon. These prospects are hopeful,

and if they are only limited to the present data on tissues positive for CEA, they still provide knowledge that has not been available before.

For the few tumors known to secrete hormones (parathyroid, adrenal), it is possible to determine the site of the excess production by cannulating the venous drainage to establish the location on the right or the left, so to guide the surgeon in exploration.

Staging of Tumors

The treatment and prognosis of cancer has been modified by new insights into the variability of different types of cancer and by their response to different protocols or types of therapy. One important factor in treating cancer has been to determine its extent in a given patient before beginning treatment. This is called staging of cancer. By staging we mean defining the extent of the cancer in a patient, that is, whether the tumor involves only a small part of an organ or whether it is widespread and involves regional lymph nodes and other organs at anatomically remote sites. The implications of this widespread distribution are that the tumor not only is great in total mass, and therefore both burdens the body metabolically and is likely to involve critical sites, but that it is likely as well to continue to metastasize because of multiple foci that have become sites for tumor growth. The staging procedure has allowed comparisons to be made among groups of patients treated at widely different centers and groups of patients treated by radically different methods for the same cancer (chemotherapy versus surgery, or surgery versus radiotherapy). The system for staging has been called the TNM system, after the abbreviations for *t*umor, lymph *n*odes, and *m*etastases. The tumor is considered in terms of its size and extent at the primary site, it is appraised in terms of the presence and extent of lymph nodes involved, and it is judged by the presence of metastases.

The classification is based on involvement of different anatomic sites and is shown in the accompanying Table 11–8. The oldest staging procedure is Duke's classification of cancer of the bowel shown in Table 11–9.

Table 11–8. The TNM System

T:	PRIMARY TUMOR
N:	REGIONAL LYMPH NODES
M:	DISTANT METASTASES

TUMOR

T_0	No evidence of primary tumor
T_{IS}	*Carcinoma-in-situ*
T_1, T_2, T_3, T_4	Ascending degrees of increase in tumor size and involvement

NODES

N_0	Regional nodes not demonstrable
N_{1a}, N_{2a}	Demonstrable regional lymph nodes; metastases not suspected
N_{1b}, N_{2b}, N_3	Demonstrable regional lymph nodes; metastases suspected
N_x	Regional lymph nodes cannot be assessed clinically

METASTASES

M_0	No evidence of distant metastases
M_1, M_2, M_3	Ascending degrees of metastatic involvement of the host including distant nodes

(From Thorn, G. W., et al. (Eds.): *Harrison's Principles of Internal Medicine,* 8th Ed. New York, McGraw-Hill, 1977.)

Table 11–9. Duke's Classification of Colorectal Cancer

Type A.	Growth confined to the rectum. No extrarectal spread, no lymphatic metastases.
Type B.	Spread by direct extension into extrarectal tissues; no lymphatic metastases.
Type C.	Lymphatic metastases present.

A second and important aspect in understanding the biologic behavior of cancer, both treated and untreated, is called grading. This can be done approximately by the gross appearance, or more frequently by the histologic appearance, of a tumor. Tumors are graded according to the degree of anaplasia or undifferentiation, which has come to imply the rate of growth. Tumors are usually graded 1 to 4, with the lower numbers implying a lesser degree of malignancy. Unfortunately, one tumor may differ histologically in different parts of the body, so such attempts to predict the biologic behavior of a given cancer have not always been valuable.

Symptoms of Cancer

The most important single fact about the clinical picture of cancer is that, in the early stages, the disease is often painless. If it were as painful as toothache, far fewer people would die from the disease. The symptoms vary with the location of the tumor, but in most cases there are likely to be such general constitutional symptoms as weakness, loss of weight, anemia, and pain later in the disease. In a superficial part, such as the lip or breast, a lump may be felt. When the affected organ communicates with the surface, there may be a discharge or bleeding, as in cancer of the uterus. In cancer of the stomach the first evidence may be loss of appetite; in the case of the kidney, there may be blood in the urine. There may be no symptoms of any kind for a considerable period, as is shown by the fact that a malignant tumor of some size may be discovered incidentally at autopsy, although the patient presented no evidence suggestive of any malignant disease.

Finally, it must be remembered that the symptoms may not be due to the primary tumor, which may remain latent, but to metastases. One of the best examples of this confusing occurrence is that of a silent carcinoma of the lung that metastasizes to the brain, so that the patient comes to the doctor with symptoms of a brain tumor, but no cough, shortness of breath, pain in the chest, or spitting of blood.

So far we have spoken of the clinical effects of cancer as those due to the local lesion and to metastases. But the most puzzling, indeed mysterious, effects are those known as systemic manifestations. These effects are too multiform to be enumerated, but they may be dermatologic, including various inflammations of the skin; vascular, more particularly thrombophlebitis migrans; hormonal disturbances involving many hormones; and neuromuscular symptoms suggesting lesions of the nerves and muscles. For some of these, the term **paraneoplastic syndrome** has been coined. It has become clear that some tumors secrete peptides and other substances that may act like hormones.

There is, for example, a syndrome, albeit

rare, in which patients complain of marked weakness and fatigue of large muscle groups, particularly those of the thighs, arms, and girdle, and may have, as well, difficulty swallowing, slurred speech, and blurred vision. All these findings suggest a disorder of the neuromuscular junction, and a disease called myasthenia, or weakness of muscle. Whereas examination of the tissue by microscopy does not show any specific abnormalities to date, electrical stimulation of muscle (electromyography) shows a distinctive change that allows the diagnosis to be made. This syndrome, named after the 2 men who first described it (Eaton-Lambert), is most frequently seen in persons with small cell carcinoma of the bronchus.

TUMOR IMMUNITY

Recently there has been a growing awareness of the defenses that the body often mobilizes against cancer cells. For many years it has been recognized that some malignant tumors are surrounded by lymphocytes and evoke a substantial inflammatory response. Now we know that patients with defective immune mechanisms often are visited by cancer. The commonest example of this phenomenon today is the person who has received steroids and radiation or drugs to depress the immune response after receiving a kidney transplant, for instance. In fact, a few patients have received both a transplant, such as a kidney, as well as a tumor that was inapparent in the donor. Other patients taking immunosuppressive drugs have an unusually high rate of new cancers. In addition, it is currently held that tumor cells often become viable when a person's normal defense mechanisms have been impaired. We now believe that the lymphocytes around the new tumor represent T cells attacking the immunologically recognizable nonhost cancer. This has been called **immune surveillance.**

These observations have led to therapeutic attempts to stimulate the host defenses by using such nonspecific stimulants as attenuated tubercle bacilli (BCG). It may be that our older notions of therapy, using cytocidal drugs and radiation, impair the defenses even more than they destroy the tumor cells.

Before the discovery of the chemical carcinogens, all the experimental work consisted of transplanting malignant tumors that occurred spontaneously in animals into other animals. The second animal had to be another member of the same species (homotransplantation). The tumor would not grow in an animal of another species (heterotransplantation), because the tumor tissue acted as a foreign antigen, which stimulated the formation of specific antibodies that destroyed the antigenic tumor tissue. For this reason it was impossible to transplant successfully human cancer to laboratory animals. Resistance of heterotransplantation has now been overcome in 2 ways: (1) preliminary radiation of the animal, and (2) administration of cortisone. Both methods appear to depress antibody production to heterologous antigens in the transplanted tumor, probably owing to a great reduction in the number of lymphocytes known to produce antibodies. The result of these procedures has been exciting, for it is now possible to transplant human cancer to such animals as the rat, guinea pig, and rabbit, and to maintain the disease over successive generations.

Spontaneous Regression. Of all the words with ugly connotations, none is more repellant than cancer. When we think of cancer in general terms, we are apt to conjure up a process characterized by a steady, remorseless, and inexorable progress in which the disease is all-conquering, and which none of the immunologic and defensive forces that help us to survive the onslaught of bacterial and viral infections can serve to arrest the faltering footsteps to the grave. The idea that antibodies may be produced against neoplastic tissue has aroused fresh interest in the subject of the spontaneous regression of cancer. We are apt to think of a cancer as growing continuously and at a uniform rate. This is true of a tissue culture of cancer cells, but it is not true of neoplasia either in the experimental animal or in man. A cancer often grows by fits and starts, and it may apparently stop growing for a period. The arrest is almost certainly due to something in the environment rather than to a change in the cancer cells. We have already seen the control that hormones exert on neoplasia. The accelerated growth of breast cancer during pregnancy has long been recognized. Cancer in man may be made to regress either by the administration of hormones or by removal of endocrine glands. In rare instances this regression may be spontaneous, the tumor not only ceasing to grow, but actually disappearing. I (William Boyd) have collected and reported a series of such cases, in all of which the diagnosis of cancer had been confirmed previously by microscopic examination. In many of them there has been a history of partial surgical removal, palliative radiation therapy, or the occurrence of some acute bacterial infection. In all of these instances there seems to have been some change in the immunologic relationship between the tumor and the host, which may be regarded as the converse of the depression of immunologic resistance induced by the use of cortisone.

The object of this brief discussion of tumor immunity is to suggest that the cancer problem is not so hopeless as it is customary to believe, and that the body can develop some degree of resistance, either local or general, to the neoplasia that threatens its life. If I (William Boyd) may be excused for quoting my own case, I may say that I have the great good fortune to have a partial resistance to cancer, enough to keep it in check for 31 years. Early in 1948, when I was 63 years old, I noticed a small lump on the left side of my face. It was removed some time later and proved, to my surprise, to be an adenocarcinoma of the parotid gland. Surgical excision was followed by radiation therapy. The same tumor spread to my neck in 1967 and was removed in December of that year; again in July, 1970, and once more in April, 1976. In September, 1969, a small basal-cell carcinoma (rodent ulcer) was removed from my right cheek. Thus I have had cancer for 30 years or more, but during that time it has never caused me pain or other symptoms. I mention this to encourage other patients with cancer and to emphasize the need for probing the cause of such resistance.

CANCER THERAPY

At the present time, cancer can be treated effectively by surgical removal, by radiotherapy, and by hormonal therapy or chemotherapy. Unfortunately, it is impossible to avoid the destruction of normal tissue both by the surgeon's knife and by the even

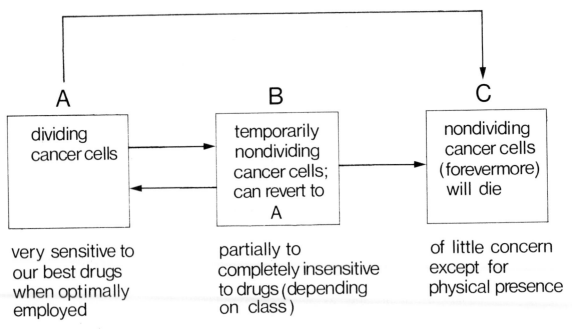

Fig. 11–11. This drawing shows when cells may be susceptible to chemotherapy. (From Thorn, G.W., et al. (Eds.): *Harrison's Principles of Internal Medicine*, 8th Ed. New York, McGraw-Hill, 1976.)

more lethal agent of radiation. The ideal therapeutic agent would be one with a selective action on malignant cells that leaves normal cells untouched, just as antibiotics lead to the destruction of bacteria, but do not interfere significantly with the metabolism of normal tissues (Fig. 11–11).

Innocent tumors are treated with complete success by local removal, that is to say, only the tumor itself needs to be removed and none of the surrounding tissue. With malignant tumors, the reverse is the case. Not only the tumor, but as much of the surrounding tissue as is feasible, must be excised, for it may harbor cancer cells that cannot be detected by the eye or hand, but only by the microscope. A cancer of the breast may be no larger than a pea in size, yet the whole breast may be removed. Depending on the part of the body affected, the regional lymph nodes also may have to be removed, but cancer of each organ must be considered as a separate entity, and what is true of one is not necessarily true of another. Thus the regional lymph nodes, although apparently normal, are always removed in cancer of the breast, but not necessarily in cancer of the lip. The presence of distant metastases implies that surgical treatment offers small hope of cure.

It should be emphasized that we believe every cancer is curable in the early stage before it has begun to spread. This is particularly true of cancer of the skin, lip, and other places where it can be readily seen. Other tumors may eventually recur after, say, 5 years, but to give a man or woman of 60 years another 5 years of life is surely something worthwhile.

The concept we put forward is that cancer has a single focus in which the neoplastic cells originate, and that if that focus is removed soon enough, the cancer will not disseminate. However, there is abundant evidence that some tumors (skin cancer in those exposed to sunlight for many years, carcinoma of the bowel in families with polyposis, alveolar cell carcinoma of the lung, to name a few) occur in multiple foci and are called multicentric in origin. Thus the paradigm of a single site of origin may be a fiction of our way of looking at most cancers. In fact, we have been impressed recently with the concurrence of 2 or more cancers in a single patient; that is, 2 histologically different cancers such as carcinoma of the breast and of the bowel, arising in the same patient, each with or without distant metastases. A review of the literature suggests that this concurrence of multiple carcinomas occurs in about 3% of the autopsy population.

Radiation is a well-tried and valuable method of treating certain forms of cancer. This treatment is made possible because radiations have a greater destructive action on rapidly growing cells than on normal cells. They therefore have a selective action on cancer cells compared with that on the surrounding tissue. It is possible, however, to kill all the tissue by radiation, and this danger has constantly to be borne in mind by the radiotherapist. His aim is to use the maximum amount of radiation on the cancer, but to stop just short of damaging the normal tissue. This requires as much skill and special training as it does to cut the tumor out with a knife.

Radium gives off radiations (gamma rays) that are similar in nature to x rays and that have a similar action on tumor tissue. Both may be used for attacking some tumors, but, in most cases, one or the other is preferable. X rays may be of low voltage (50,000 to 100,000 volts) or of high voltage (usually around 220,000 volts, although from some machines much higher). The low-voltage rays are known as soft; they have only slight penetrating power and are therefore suitable only for surface tumors. High-voltage rays are known as hard; they have great penetrating power, which makes them ideal for treating deep-seated tumors. However, even with 200,000 volt radiation, there were often superficial radiation burns, so even more powerful, high-energy generators have been developed (2×10^6 volts to 25×10^6 volts). These generators avoid the radiation burns of skin and deliver tumoricidal doses deep to tissues such as lymph nodes around the aorta. It may be necessary to press the treatment until a marked and sometimes painful inflammatory reaction is produced.

Tumors vary tremendously in their response to radiation (Table 11–10). Some, such as the malignant growth of lymph nodes

Table 11–10.   Radiosensitivity of Human Tumors

GROUP I	GROUP II	GROUP III
(Sensitive tumors: disappearance of tumors with doses less than 2500 r; normal tissues unaffected)	(Intermediate tumors: regression with doses of 2500 to 5000 r)	(Resistant tumors: more than 5000 r with irreversible changes in normal tissues)
Lymphosarcoma	Basal cell carcinoma	Carcinoma of the breast
Lymphoepithelioma	Some epidermoid	Carcinoma of the stomach
Ewing's sarcoma	carcinomas of the skin	Osteogenic sarcoma
Chronic leukemia	and uterine cervix	Chondrosarcoma
Some parotid tumors	Carcinoma of the thyroid	Malignant melanoma

(From Perez-Tamayo, R.: *Mechanisms of Disease.* Philadelphia & London, W. B. Saunders, 1961.)

known as lymphosarcoma, are highly radiosensitive; others, such as malignant melanoma, are as highly radioresistant. An intimate knowledge of tumor pathology is therefore necessary before treatment of cancer by radiation can be attempted. The tumors most sensitive to radiation are those in which the cells are dividing most rapidly, which are furthest removed from normal structure, and which are therefore the most malignant. The rays have no discriminating action on innocent tumors, as these resemble normal tissues in structure. Speaking generally, roentgen rays are used for the treatment of widely diffused tumors such as lymphosarcoma, as well as for deep-seated tumors such as cancer of the lung. Radium, on the other hand, is planted directly into the tumor and kills all the cancer cells within reach. Cancer of the cervix

of the uterus, one of the most common and most dreaded forms of cancer in women, has proved particularly susceptible to treatment by radium. Frequently, the various forms of treatment are combined, e.g., surgery and radiation (Table 11–11).

Some tumors may be treated successfully by various types of radiation. The source of the radiation may be an x-ray tube, a naturally occurring isotope such as radium, or a man-made isotope such as cobalt-60. There is no difference between the gamma rays that come from a radioactive source and the x rays that come from an x-ray machine.

With the development of nuclear reactors, a host of new radioactive isotopes has been produced. Some of these, such as cobalt-60 and cesium-137, can replace the x-ray tube as the source of gamma rays, and isotope units

Table 11–11.   Choice of Treatment in Localized and Regional Tumors and Hematologic Malignancies

DIAGNOSIS	SURGERY	TREATMENT RADIOTHERAPY	CHEMOTHERAPY
Carcinomas			
Breast	P	Alt/adj	T
Uterine cervix	P	P	T
Choriocarcinoma	Alt	—	P
Lung	P	Alt	T
Stomach	P	—	T
Pancreas	P	—	T
Leukemias and Lymphomas			
Leukemia			
Acute myeloblastic	—	—	P
Hodgkin's disease	Alt	P	T

P   —Primary method of treatment
Alt —Alternative method of treatment, or one useful in special situations
Adj—Used as adjunctive therapy
T   —Currently under clinical investigation as adjunctive treatment
—   —No data available on this form of treatment

(From Thorn, G. W., et al. (Eds.): *Harrison's Principles of Internal Medicine,* 8th Ed. New York, McGraw-Hill, 1977.)

may be used in place of an x-ray machine. For example, the rays from a cobalt-60 unit treating at a distance of 80 cm are equivalent to the rays from a 3,000,000-volt x-ray machine. Most deep-seated tumors today are treated with some type of cobalt-60 unit. For an interesting account of radiotherapy, one might read the novel *Cancer Ward* by A. I. Solzhenitsyn.

A word about so-called cancer cures and quack remedies. Most of these remedies are in the form of cancer pastes that are applied to external growths. They contain powerful irritants such as arsenic, which may kill the superficial part of the cancer and irritate the deeper part to increased activity, so that by the time the surgeon is consulted, the case has become hopeless. Sometimes one hears of cancers that have been cured by such remedies. In every case it will be found that no microscopic examination of the tumor has been made. Unless a biopsy is done, and a microscopic examination of the piece removed is made, it is impossible to be certain whether the supposed cancer is really a tumor or is merely an inflammatory mass.

Our awe of cancer as a mortal problem dims our expectations of ready solutions, but the trend to earlier cures of several specific malignant processes raises our hopes that persistence will be rewarded.

SYNOPSIS

Cancer is a process in which multiple factors play a role.

Chemical carcinogenesis has been interpreted in terms of initiation, promotion, and a variable latent period.

Viral carcinogenesis has been identified and vertical transmission of latent virus explains some animal cancers.

Hormonal dependence of some tumors has been shown and is used therapeutically in some human cancer.

Hereditary factors are poorly understood in all but a few human tumors.

Environmental carcinogens may be difficult to incriminate because of a long latent period (decades).

The distinctions between benign and malignant tumors are clear on theoretic, histologic, and cytologic grounds in most cases.

The recognition that immune mechanisms play a role in resistance to tumors offers new modes of therapy.

Spontaneous regression of histologically proven cancer has been shown in a few instances.

Serologic tests for cancer may become valuable, but cytologic and biopsy methods form the backbone of diagnosis.

We teach that cancer arises in 1 focus, but there are abundant examples of multicentric origin for cancers, and multiple cancers in a single human being are becoming more apparent.

Cancer may produce a syndrome of fever, weight loss, and nonspecific signs. Some cancers secrete hormones that mimic other diseases.

Terms

Neoplasia	*Anaplasia*	*Carcinoma*
Contact inhibition	*Dysplasia*	*Sarcoma*
Metastases	*Carcinoma-in-situ*	*Exfoliative cytology*
Cachexia	*Immune surveillance*	*Biopsy*
Carcinogen	*Epithelioma*	*Carcinoembryonic antigen*
Polyoma virus	*Adenoma*	*Paraneoplastic syndrome*
Bittner factor	*Nevus*	
Burkitt's lymphoma	*Melanoma*	

FURTHER READING

Editorial: Is cancer irreversible? Br. Med. J., *1*:585, 1978.

Berenblum, I.: The co-carcinogenic action of croton resin. Cancer Res., *1*:44, 1941.

Bittner, J.J.: Milk factor in mammary mouse cancer. Science, *84*:162, 1936.

Bodel, P.: Tumors and fever. Ann. N.Y. Acad. Sci., *230*:6, 1974.

Burkitt, D., and Hutt, M.S.R.: Geographic pathology in developing countries. Int. Pathol., *7*:1, 1966.

Burton, A.C.: Why do human cancer death rates increase with age? A new method of analysis of the biology of cancer. Perspect. Biol. Med., *20*:327, 1977.

DeVita, V.T., Jr.: The evolution of therapeutic research in cancer. N. Engl. J. Med., *298*:907, 1978.

Effron, M., et al.: Nature and rate of neoplasia found in captive wild mammals, birds and reptiles at necropsy. J. Natl. Cancer Inst., *59*:185, 1977.

Eilber, F.R., et al.: Adjuvant immunotherapy with BCG in treatment of regional lymph node metastases from malignant melanoma. N. Engl. J. Med., *294*:237, 1976.

Everson, T.C., and Cole, W.H.: *Spontaneous Regression of Cancer.* Philadelphia, W. B. Saunders, 1966.

Friedman, H., and Southam, C.: International conference on immunobiology of cancer. Ann. N.Y. Acad. Sci., *276*, 1976.

Gold, P., and Freedman, S.O.: Demonstration of tumor-specific antigens in human colonic carcinomata by immunological tolerance and absorption techniques. J. Exp. Med., *121*:439, 1965.

Gusberg, S.B.: The changing nature of endometrial cancer. N. Engl. J. Med., *302*:729, 1980.

Henderson, B.E.: Observations on cancer etiology in China. Natl. Cancer Inst. Monogr., *53*:59, 1978.

Henle, W., Henle, G., and Lennette, E.T.: The Epstein-Barr virus. Sci. Am., *241*:48, 1979.

Linos, A., et al.: Low dose radiation and leukemia. N. Engl. J. Med., *302*:1101, 1980.

Markert, C.L.: Cancer: the survival of the fittest. In *Cell Differentiation and Neoplasia.* Edited by G. F. Saunders. New York, Raven Press, 1978.

Maugh, T.H., II: Biochemical markers: early warning signs of cancer. Science, *197*:543, 1977.

Miller, R.W.: Cancer epidemics in the People's Republic of China. J. Natl. Cancer Inst., *60*:1195, 1978.

Morrison, A.S., and Buring, J.E.: Artificial sweeteners and cancer of the lower urinary tract. N. Engl. J. Med., *302*:537, 1980.

Pitot, H.C.: *Fundamentals of Oncology.* Basel, Marcel Dekker, 1978.

Roizman, B.: The structure and isomerization of herpes simplex virus genomes. Cell, *16*:481, 1979.

Rous, P.: Transmission of a malignant new growth by means of a cell-free filtrate. J.A.M.A., *56*:198, 1911.

Shope, R.E.: A filterable virus causing a tumor-like condition in rabbits and its relationship to virus myxomatosum. J. Exp. Med., *56*:803, 1932.

Solzhenitsyn, A.I.: *Cancer Ward.* New York, Dial Press, 1968.

Stewart, S.E., et al.: Viral production of cancer. Virology, *3*:380, 1957.

Strong, L.C.: Genetic etiology of cancer. Cancer, *40*:438, 1977.

Wagoner, J.K.: Occupational carcinogenesis: the two hundred years since Percival Pott. Ann. N.Y. Acad. Sci., *271*:1, 1976.

Warren, S.: Radiation carcinogenesis. Ann. N.Y. Acad. Sci., *46*:133, 1970.

Inherited Disease

12

Heredity is nothing but stored environment. —BURBANK

Although it has been suspected for hundreds of years that some diseases are transmitted from parent to child, knowledge of the patterns of inheritance has become defined only recently. Archibald Garrod is generally acknowledged as the man who proposed that errors of metabolism may be inherited. He identified not only the mode of inheritance for some disorders (he worked at a time when Mendel's observations were rediscovered), but also the biochemical abnormalities responsible for several hereditary disorders (alkaptonuria, albinism, cystinuria, and pentosuria) in his Croonian lecture of 1908. Garrod notices that some diseases occur in clusters of a single family, and whereas the parents did not show any stigma of the disorder, they were discovered to be cousins or closely related. This consanguinity, of course, facilitates the expression of a recessive gene. Garrod's insights are a good example of the value of cross fertilization in science; without his chemical background and the opportunity to discuss genetic matters with Bateson, a geneticist, the explanation of a recessive transmittance of a biochemical disorder might not have been made for many years.

A brief overview of some elements of modern genetics will set the stage for an outline of

hereditary diseases. The reader is referred to such contemporary texts as Goodenough and Levine, *Genetics,* for a more complete review of genetics in general, and such matters as organization of DNA, coding, recombination, linkage, transcription, translation, point mutations, and the elegant subjects of genetic mapping. For detailed information on inborn errors of metabolism, see *The Metabolic Basis of Inherited Disease,* by Stanbury, Wyngaarden, and Fredrickson.

All hereditary information is contained in nucleic acid, DNA (deoxyribonucleic acid), which resides entirely within the nucleus of every cell (except for less than 1%, which is in the mitochondria) in a disperse and "invisible" material while cells are resting (interphase). As a cell undergoes preparation for division (mitosis), the DNA and a lot of other material (histones) become assembled in the long, thin structures called chromosomes, which can be visualized with the light microscope and recently have been studied with new dyes to bring out their many bands (Fig. 12–1). Each plant and animal cell has a species-specific number of chromosomes: man has 46 (23 pairs), of which 2 are the sex chromosomes responsible for our gender. A person's chromosomes can be visualized

271

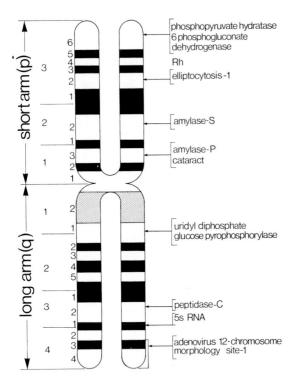

phosphopyruvate hydratase
6 phosphogluconate
dehydrogenase

Rh

elliptocytosis -1

amylase-S

amylase-P
cataract

uridyl diphosphate
glucose pyrophosphorylase

peptidase-C

5s RNA

adenovirus 12-chromosome
morphology site-1

Fig. 12–1. This drawing of a chromosome shows the banding that is now visible with modern staining techniques. The drawing shows the loci for the determination of a variety of enzymes on a human chromosome. (From Thorn, G. W., et al. (Eds.): *Harrison's Principles of Internal Medicine,* 8th Ed. New York, McGraw-Hill, 1976.)

(karyotype) from photographs of dividing cells from our body. A drawing of such a preparation is called an idiogram (Fig. 12–2).

The gene, not the chromosome, is the unit of heredity, however, and a structural gene is now defined operationally as a functional unit of inheritance, situated on a chromosome and

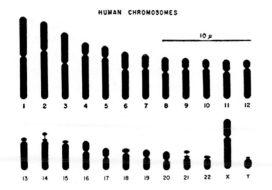

HUMAN CHROMOSOMES

10 µ

Fig. 12–2. Idiogram of human chromosomes. (D. Yi-Yung Hsea: N. Engl. J. Med.)

responsible for the synthesis of a specific polypeptide. This synthesis results most commonly in the production of proteins of 2 general classes, namely, those concerned with the framework of cells (structure proteins) and those concerned with intermediary metabolism, or the rate of protein synthesis (regulatory proteins). Genes therefore have been considered in the same way, i.e., those that control the amino acid structure of proteins, and those that govern their regulatory functions. Genes could, in the concept of Monod and Jacob, be either active or inactive, that is, derepressed or repressed.

This general concept was enunciated more than 40 years ago in the dictum "1 gene—1 enzyme," which was subsequently amplified to "DNA makes RNA which makes protein." These ideas can be better understood in the following propositions: (1) All biochemical processes in all living organisms are under the control of genes. (2) Each biochemical reaction can be resolved into different steps, governed by the availability of substrate and enzyme. (3) Each step of any reaction is under the control of a different gene. (4) Mutations of single genes affect single steps of a reaction. (5) Mutations may affect either the structure of the product of a reaction or the amount of the product of the reaction.

Mutations may have several effects on this set of pathways. In general, it seems that a mutation leads to decreased protein synthesis. The mutation may affect either the regulatory genes or the structural genes, and the effect is most often lethal. In unicellular organisms, the effect is commonly on regulator genes, but the existence of regulatory mutations in man is not well documented. Mutations of structural genes may also affect the rate of synthesis of abnormal proteins. One well-known example in which a mutation leads to a different conclusion is the biosynthesis of a structurally abnormal molecule, such as sickle cell hemoglobin, discussed in Chapter 1.

Endless attempts have been made to relate the bands of chromosomes to different genes, and now new methods to uncover the coding mechanisms of DNA in relation to specific genic functions in man are directed at the same goal. It seems clear, at least for bacteria, that the genetic material behaves as a single group for each gene, and it is possible to isolate the macromolecule of DNA as a continuous loop from bacteria. The mapping of the function of bacterial genes is much simpler than writing a geography of man's genetic apparatus, but only 20 years ago a voyage to the moon seemed a remote prospect.

For man, the effect of genes is probably greater than simple control over structure and biochemical function. There is evidence to support the idea that our very behavior may be genetically preordained. Wilson comments in *On Human Nature:*

In 1977 the geneticists Victor McKusick and Francis Ruddle reported in *Science* that twelve hundred genes had been distinguished; of these, the position of 210 had been pinpointed to a particular chromosome, and at least one gene had been located on each of the twenty-three pairs of chromosomes. Most of the genes ultimately affect anatomical and biochemical traits having minimal influence on behavior. Yet some do affect behavior in important ways, and a few of the behavioral mutations have been closely linked to known biochemical changes. Also, subtle behavioral controls are known that incorporate alterations in levels of hormones and transmitter substances acting directly on nerve cells. The recently discovered enkephalins and endorphins are protein-like substances of relatively simple structure that can profoundly affect mood and temperament. A single mutation altering the chemical nature of one or more of them might change the personality of the person bearing it, or at least the predisposition of the person to develop one personality as opposed to another in a given cultural surrounding.

Comprehension of the chain of events starting with the mechanisms of heredity and ending in an abnormal protein led to the enunciation by Pauling of the idea of molecular disease.

Recently, attention has been focused on practical details of how lesions may occur in the genetic mechanism. There have been strenuous objections to experimentation with hybridization of different cells, and to attempts with synthetic nucleic acids to develop models that will reveal the nature of genetic controls, because of fears that man is tampering with the essence of creation. However, we have gained much useful knowledge about how agents that are causally related to cancer affect the genetic apparatus. For example, we

know that x rays damage DNA indirectly by producing free radicals in the vicinity of DNA, perhaps by creating peroxides, such as H_2O_2 from H_2O. Ultraviolet light, the most common cause of skin cancer, acts directly on DNA by causing breaks in chain continuity due to alteration in the base pairing. Some chemicals, such as acridine orange or proflavine, cause errors in replication by producing distortions in regularity of base pairing, because the dye molecules become wedged in the spaces of the nucleic acid and change the angle of pitch of the helix. Other agents that cause mutations may do so because their size and shape are similar to those of the natural base, but they are analogs and are not able to function in exactly the same way. They function similarly to the way in which the body accepts strontium or lead instead of calcium, and deposits them in bone as if they were calcium. These molecular mechanisms of mutation become increasingly important as we recognize the extent to which we can accept or adapt to such exposure.

The majority of new mutations are harmful or even lethal, because in a delicately balanced system such as the gene complex, as in the engine of a motorcar or circuitry of a television set, almost any change is likely to be for the worse.

Wilson points out again,

One analysis of American and French populations produced the estimate that each person carries an average of four lethal gene equivalents: either four genes that cause death outright when in the homozygous state, eight genes that cause death in fifty percent of homozygotes, or other, arithmetically equivalent combinations of lethal and debilitating effects. These high numbers, which are typical of animal species, mean that inbreeding carries a deadly risk. Among 161 children born to Czechoslovakian women who had sexual relations with their fathers, brothers, or sons, fifteen were stillborn or died within the first year of life, and more than forty percent suffered from various physical and mental defects, including severe mental retardation, dwarfism, heart and brain deformities, deaf-mutism, enlargement of the colon, and urinary-tract abnormalities. In contrast, a group of ninety-five children born to the same women through nonincestuous relations were on the average as normal as the population at large. Five died during the first year of life, none had serious mental deficiencies, and only five others had apparent physical abnormalities.

The manifestations of inbreeding pathology constitute natural selection in an intense and unambiguous form. The elementary theory of population genetics predicts that any behavioral tendency to avoid incest, however slight or devious, would long ago have spread through human populations. So powerful is the advantage of outbreeding that it can be expected to have carried cultural evolution along with it.

On the other hand, mutation can be regarded as the masterword in evolution, for helpful mutants are inherited just as are normal genes, and without them life would never have advanced. Animals with protective coloration owe their protection to a helpful mutation, although the black sheep of a white flock may blame its color on mutation, and the same might be said of the black sheep of a human family. In addition to the spontaneous variety, mutation may be induced by external influences, of which the best example is radiation.

Table 12–1 lists some relatively common hereditary disorders of man. Table 12–2 lists the frequency of some chromosomal aberrations.

MODES OF INHERITANCE

Dominant inheritance is naturally the easiest type to recognize, for each affected person has an affected parent and grandpar-

Table 12–1.   Some Relatively Common Mendelian Disorders

AUTOSOMAL DOMINANT	AUTOSOMAL RECESSIVE	X-LINKED
Familial monogenic hypercholesterolemia	Cystic fibrosis	Hemophilia A
Marfan's syndrome	Deaf mutism	Classic agammaglobulinemia (Bruton)
Adult polycystic disease	Phenylketonuria and other hereditary aminoacidurias	Pseudohypertrophic muscular dystrophy
Huntington's chorea	Wilson's disease	Testicular feminization
Neurofibromatosis	Homocystinuria	Vitamin D-resistant rickets
Osteogenesis imperfecta	Albinism	
von Willebrand's disease	Emphysema (due to alpha-1 antitrypsin deficiency)	
Achondroplastic dwarfism	Friedreich's ataxia	

(From Bearn, A. G.: Pedigree analysis in inherited disease. In *Cecil Textbook of Medicine*, 15th Ed. Edited by P. B. Beeson, W. McDermott, and J. B. Wyngaarden. Philadelphia, W. B. Saunders, 1979.)

Table 12–2.   Frequency of Selected Chromosomal Aberrations

	A SPONTANEOUS ABORTIONS	B LIVE-BORN
Sex chromosome abnormalities:		
Turner's syndrome (all types)	1/18	1/3,500 "females"
Klinefelter's syndrome (all types)	Probably same as in live-born	1/500 "males"
Extra X chromosomes (females mainly XXX)	Probably same as in live-born	1/1,360 "females"
Autosomal abnormalities:		
Trisomy G	1/40	1/600
Trisomy 18	1/200	1/4,500
Trisomy D	1/33	1/14,500
Trisomy 16	1/33	Almost 0
Triploidy	1/22	Almost 0

(From Wintrobe, M., et al. (Eds.): *Harrison's Principles of Internal Medicine*, 7th Ed. New York, McGraw-Hill, 1974.)

ent. The character can be transmitted by a parent of either sex to a child of either sex. If 1 parent has the dominant gene, 2 out of 4 children will inherit this gene, and, although the condition is heterozygous, they will show the trait (Fig. 12–3). The other 2 children will not receive the dominant gene and are homozygous for the recessive gene, so that they will appear normal. Examples are brachydactyly (short fingers and toes), which has been traced through many generations; polydactyly, in which there are too many digits on the hands and feet; multiple polyps of the colon; sickle cell anemia; diabetes insipidus; and countless other conditions.

Recessive inheritance is much more difficult to recognize. The defect is only obvious in a homozygous person, in whom a double dose of corresponding genes determines the same defect (Fig. 12–4). It must therefore have been inherited from heterozygous parents, neither of whom exhibited the defects, but who merely acted as carriers. A lethal recessive gene may be paired with a normal dominant gene, but its possessor goes through life happily unaware that genetically he carries a program for information that may be devastating for his offspring. The condi-

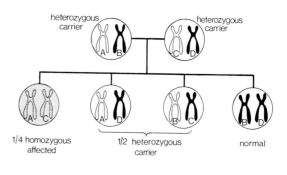

1/4 homozygous affected   1/2 heterozygous carrier   normal

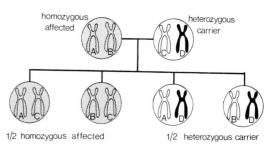

1/2 homozygous affected   1/2 heterozygous carrier

Fig. 12–4. This diagram shows the proportions of affected persons and of carriers in recessive inheritance.

tion may thus remain unsuspected for many generations, until a homozygous mating brings 2 recessive genes together. This is most likely to happen with a marriage of first cousins. If 2 people, each carrying the same abnormal recessive gene, happen to marry, the offspring have 1 chance in 4 to be abnormal, 1 to be normal but to carry the trait. The most striking example of recessive inheritance is the disease with the tragically descriptive name, amaurotic (blind) family idiocy. A moving account of this condition will be found in H. G. Wells' short story, "The Valley of the Blind," written many years ago. The parents are always normal, although both must carry the recessive gene. No affected person ever grows up to be a parent, as the disease is fatal in early life (lethal). Another example of recessive inheritance is albinism, a startling defect in pigmentation that leaves the skin, eyes, and hair a varying degree of white. An albino will usually marry someone who does not carry that particular and unusual gene; all the children will be heterozygous carriers. If an albino marries someone who is a heterozygote, half the children will be albinos and half unaffected heterozygotes.

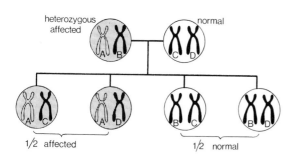

1/2 affected   1/2 normal

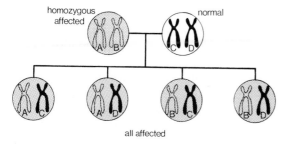

all affected

Fig. 12–3. This diagram shows the proportions of affected children in dominant inheritance.

If 2 albinos marry, all the children will be albinos.

The 5 possible results of mating dominant with recessive autosomal genes are shown as follows (D represents a dominant gene and r a recessive one):

1. DD × DD = DD
2. rr × rr = rr
3. DD × rr = Dr
4. DD × Dr = ½DD + ½Dr
5. Dr × Dr = ¼DD + ½Dr + ¼rr

Sex-linked inheritance is much less frequent than other mutations. Both autosomes and sex chromosomes are arranged in pairs, 1 member of each pair being maternal and the other paternal in origin. Each of the 44 chromosomes (autosomes) contributed by a male gamete is homologous with a corresponding chromosome contributed by a female gamete. In addition, there are 2 chromosomes that determine the sex of the individual; these are known as the X and Y sex chromosomes. In the female somatic cells there are 2 homologous X chromosomes, whereas in the male the arrangement is heterologous, with 1 X and 1 Y chromosome. With a stretch of the imagination, it might be said that the essential difference between Romeo and Juliet was that Romeo has a Y chromosome in place of a double X. The Y chromosome is as small as the smallest of the autosomes and carries few genes. The distinction between the 2 is easy to recognize in the giant chromosomes of the salivary gland of the fruit fly.

In the reduction division (meiosis), which precedes the formation of a gamete, there are naturally 2 kinds of spermatozoa, a set with 1 X chromosome, which on fertilization will result in a female offspring, the other with 1 Y chromosome, which will result in a male. The father passes on the Y chromosomes received from his father to all his sons, and the X chromosomes received from his mother to all his daughters. In the unusual circumstance in which a family has 6 daughters in a row, it may be that the father is chromosomally abnormal and unable to create a male child. Both sex chromosomes carry additional nonsexual genes known as sex-linked genes. As the female has 2 X chromosomes, she will be heterozygous and therefore a carrier for a mutant gene in a single X chromosome, whereas the male with a single X chromosome will be homozygous for the mutant gene, so that the trait will become apparent. The gene in question may be passed from father to daughter and from mother to son, but if it is recessive it is only in the male, in which it is unmasked, that it will become apparent (Fig. 12–5). The abnormality is thus confined to the male, but is transmitted by the female. In the female, the recessive abnormal gene (X) will be masked by the dominant normal gene on the other X chromosome. This explains what is at first sight the peculiar sex distribution of hemophilia, "the bleeding disease," which is the most famous example of a sex-linked inherited dis-

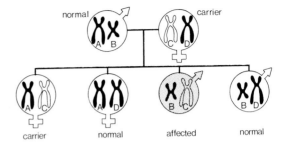

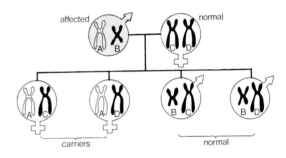

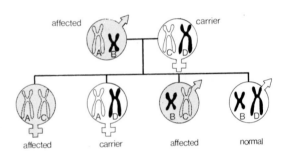

Fig. 12–5. This figure shows the effect of sex-linked inheritance on the numbers and carriers of the offspring.

ease. Only the male is affected and only the female transmits the disease, another illustration of the old saying that the female of the species is more deadly than the male.

The matter of sex chromatin has already been discussed. This simple method of determining the true sex by the examination of cells is of particular value in doubtful cases of intersex, and also in the determination of the chances of fertility.

Sex anomalies due to errors of development are uncommon, fortunately, although of great importance to the person involved. Even in the most normal person, neither sex represents a state of absolute unisexuality. Usually 1 sex predominates to such an extent that no doubt exists. Again, from Wilson, there is increasing evidence that chromosomal constitution also affects behavior. This is particularly true of the difference in genders.

One of the most controversial but informative examples is the XYY male. The X and Y chromosomes determine sex in human beings; the XX combination produces a female, XY a male. Approximately 0.1 percent of the population accidentally acquires an extra Y chromosome at the moment of conception, and these XYY individuals are all males. The XYY males grow up to be tall men, the great majority over six feet. They also end up more frequently in prisons and hospitals for the criminally insane. At first it was thought that the extra chromosome induced more aggressive behavior, creating what is in effect a class of genetic criminals. However, a statistical study, by Princeton psychologist Herman A. Witkin and his associates, of vast amounts of data from Denmark has led to a more benign interpretation. XYY men were found neither to be more aggressive than normal nor to display any particular behavior pattern distinguishing them from the remainder of the Danish population. The only deviation detected was a lower average intelligence. The most parsimonious explanation is the XYY men are incarcerated at a higher rate because they are simply less adroit at escaping detection.

Although the genitalia are an important criterion of sex, they are often unreliable indicators of chromosomal sex. True hermaphroditism (Hermes, messenger of the gods, and Aphrodite, goddess of love), in which testes and ovaries are both present, is rare. In pseudohermaphroditism, only testes or ovaries are present, but there is intersexual anatomy of the rest of the reproductive system. Two examples are described later in this chapter in connection with chromosomal abnormalities.

In discussing hereditary disease, we should define some terms that are often used congruently and casually. Congenital disease refers to those that are recognized as a result of occurrences during development and are present at birth, but do not have a hereditary (genetic) cause, i.e., there is no chromosomal or genetic origin for the disease. The best examples of congenital disease are the deafness and the cardiovascular lesions that are formed in the infant born to a mother who was infected with rubella virus during her first trimester of pregnancy. Recently, it is estimated that more than two-thirds of mothers so exposed to rubella have children

with severe defects. This information has made strong arguments for abortion in the first trimester.

It is nonetheless necessary to recognize that it is not always possible to be certain about the origin of a given defect that is apparent at birth. Since some abnormalities are associated with genetic factors, it is appropriate to discuss briefly some frequent and important structural defects that appear at birth and are generally called congenital malformations. They are listed in Table 12–3 with their approximate frequency and sex ratio.

It has been stated that congenital malformations account for 25% of total infant mortality, and for more than 10% of all deaths up to age 15. One fact that sheds some doubt on the importance of environmental factors as a causative agent in congenital disease is an increased risk of congenital malformations in subsequent pregnancies. The recurrence rate is only 4% in subsequent children for anencephaly, spina bifida, and hydrocephalus, but it is much higher after 2 malformations, implying a genetic cause in these instances. For such disorders, a polygenic mode of inheritance seems the most likely explanation. At this time, it is difficult to distinguish between congenital and genetically determined disease, and it is probably wise to use the purest definition: **congenital disease is considered to be one in which there is no recognized genetic determinant.**

We can classify hereditary diseases in a number of ways. One way of looking at hered-

Table 12–3. Approximate Frequency and Sex Ratio of Common Congenital Malformations

MALFORMATION	FREQUENCY/1000 BIRTHS	M:F
Congenital heart disease	2.5	1:1
Talipes equinovarus (club foot)	2.0	2:1
Myelomeningocele	1.5 (0.5–4.4)	1:1
Anencephaly	2.0	1:2
Down's syndrome (mongolism)	1.6	1:1
Cleft lip ± cleft palate	1.0	2:1
Klinefelter's syndrome	1.0	1:0

(From Bearn, A. G.: Congenital malformations. In *Cecil Textbook of Medicine*, 15th Ed. Edited by P. B. Beeson, W. McDermott, and J. B. Wyngaarden. Philadelphia, W. B. Saunders, 1979.)

itary diseases is to consider them in terms of their seriousness. We can talk about asymptomatic or trivial disorders that may be of interest to the geneticist but that may not cause discomfort to the patient. Pentosuria and inherited disorders of tasting or color blindness may fall into this group. A second group of genetic disorders, such as glucose 6-phosphate deficiency, porphyria, and even the disorders of clotting mechanisms (hemophilia) may only be significant or even detectable if there is an accident that evokes the bleeding or exposure to an unusual chemical that initiates the hemolysis. Then there are those genetic disorders, such as the lipid storage or glycogen storage diseases, that are associated with irreversible and often lethal consequences in the central nervous or cardiovascular system. However, this type of classification is not useful, because we now recognize that the same genetic disease may be more serious in different persons (case-to-case variability in the expression of the disease depending on the rest of the patient's genome), an idea that has been particularly emphasized by McKusick, a pioneer in contemporary human genetics.

Finally, we could classify human genetic disorders on an anatomic basis, according to which system (cardiovascular, renal, or respiratory) is involved, or on a biochemical basis, according to which pathways are modified. You may expect to find genetic disorders for every system, and may anticipate lesions in every biochemical pathway. In fact, once we thought hemophilia was a single entity; now we have discovered 2 or more types of X-linked hemophilia whose genes are far apart on the X chromosome. For the purposes of this chapter, the concepts and general types of lesions are more important than a catalog of genetic disorders.

Perhaps the conventional and most satisfactory approach to a classification of genetic disorders is to group hereditary diseases into 3 subsets:

1. Those that have been shown to be due to abnormalities in the number of chromosomes, or to abnormalities in their arrangements. These diseases are therefore designated **chromosomal disorders.** They may be due to changes in chromosomal number or to changes in chromosomal structure, such as deletions or translocations.

2. Those disorders in which there is clear-cut genetic evidence of a disorder, but no chromosomal abnormality; therefore, they are **disorders that result from mutations.** The lesion resides in the gene and cannot be seen with the conventional methods of study, and is usually determined retrospectively or by pedigree analysis only.

3. Those disorders in which all evidence supports a genetic etiology, but the data are not explicable on the basis of a defect in a single gene. These disorders, such as some forms of gout and diabetes mellitus, are called **polygenic,** requiring the interaction of several genes to make their effect known.

DISORDERS OF CHROMOSOMAL ABERRATIONS

Chromosome anomalies fall into 2 general categories: changes in the number of chromosomes, and changes in the structure of individual chromosomes. The incidence of chromosome anomalies in live births is generally estimated at about 6.5 per 1,000 live births.

The Klinefelter syndrome is the most common of the sex anomalies (Fig. 12–6). The basic feature is the addition of a sex chromosome, so that the sex chromosome complex is XXY. The testes are small, with resulting infertility, the breasts may be enlarged, there are eunuchoid features, and the presence of sex chromatin (female) in smears of the buccal mucosa serves to clinch the diagnosis. The gonads of the early embryo have developed into testes rather than into ovaries, as they would normally. Mental deficiency is a common feature of the Klinefelter syndrome, as it is in other sex reversals.

In Turner's syndrome (Fig. 12–7), fortunately a rare condition, there is a single X chromosome, often written as XO. It forms an interesting contrast to the sex anomaly just described, for just as Klinefelter's syndrome may be regarded as feminization of the male, so Turner's syndrome is a masculinization of the female. The nuclei therefore lack sex chromatin. The nuclear sexing test shows that the majority of these "girls" are really males

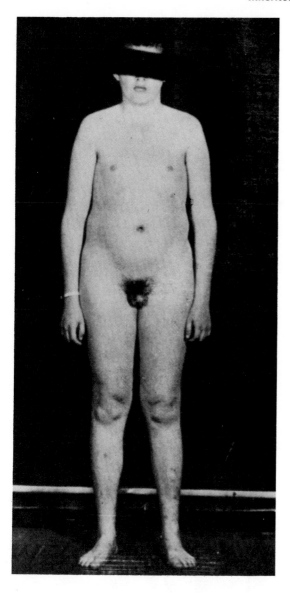

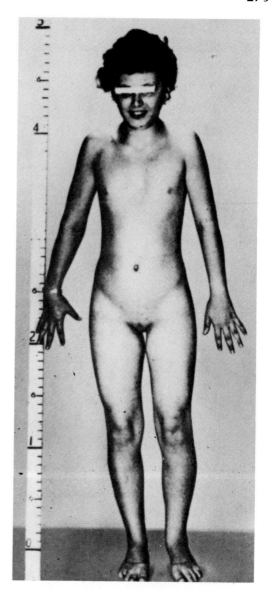

Fig. 12–6. This photograph shows the phenotypic appearance of a Klinefelter patient. Note the long extremities, narrow shoulders, and relatively wide hips. (By permission of the Upjohn Company, Kalamazoo, Michigan, monograph on cytology.)

Fig. 12–7. This photograph shows the phenotypic appearance of Turner's syndrome. The chest is relatively wide and the neck is short. (By permission of the Upjohn Company, Kalamazoo, Michigan, monograph on cytology.)

with absence of testicular tissue, so that secondary sex characters fail to develop at puberty, as does menstruation.

Loss of an entire chromosome, known as monosomy because only 1 of a pair remains, is nearly always fatal. One exception is sex chromosome monosomy, discussed in the foregoing paragraph, in which there is a single X or, as it is expressed, XO. Trisomy, the presence of 3 chromosomes of a kind in-

stead of the normal pair, is also damaging, but is not nearly as bad. Again, nearly all the cases with more than 1 extra chromosome have involved the sex chromosomes. There are 4 well-established and fairly common syndromes, 3 involving sex chromosomes, and 1 an autosome, 3 being trisomies with 47 chromosomes, 1 a monosomy with 45. Table 12–4 shows the correlation of phenotype sex chromatin and sex chromosomes.

Table 12–4.   Correlations of Phenotype, Sex Chromatin, and Sex Chromosomes

	SEX PHENOTYPE	BARR BODIES (MAXIMUM NUMBER PER CELL)	SEX-CHROMOSOME CONSTITUTION
Normal male	Male		XY
Testicular feminization syndrome	Female (with testes)		XY
Double Y (or XYY) male	Male		XYY
Turner's syndrome	Female		XO
Normal female	Female		XX
Klinefelter's syndrome	Male		XXY
Klinefelter's syndrome	Male		XXYY
Triple X syndrome	Female		XXX
Triple X-Y syndrome	Male		XXXY
Tetra X syndrome	Female		XXXX
Tetra X-Y syndrome	Male		XXXXY
Penta X syndrome	Female		XXXXX

(From Wintrobe, M., et al. (Eds.): *Harrison's Principles of Internal Medicine.* New York, McGraw-Hill, 1974.)

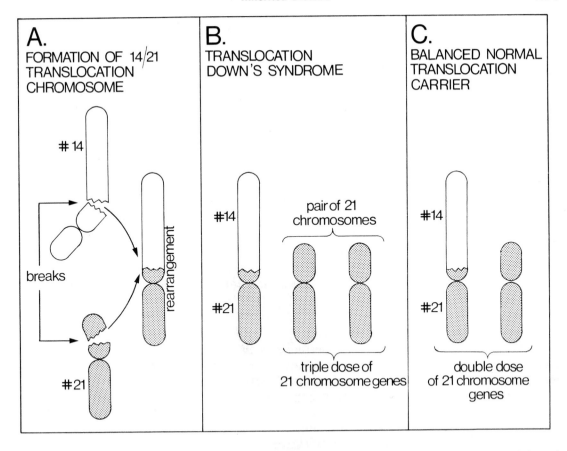

A.
FORMATION OF 14/21
TRANSLOCATION
CHROMOSOME

14

breaks

#21

rearrangement

B.
TRANSLOCATION
DOWN'S SYNDROME

#14

#21

pair of 21
chromosomes

triple dose of
21 chromosome genes

C.
BALANCED NORMAL
TRANSLOCATION
CARRIER

#14

#21

double dose
of 21 chromosome
genes

Fig. 12–8. These drawings show the mechanism of translocation (A) resulting in Down's syndrome at B, and in a balanced, normal translocation at C. (From Thorn, G. W., et al. (Eds.): *Harrison's Principles of Internal Medicine,* 8th Ed. New York, McGraw-Hill, 1976.)

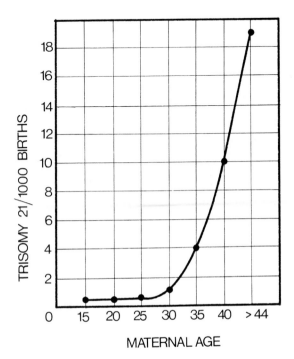

Fig. 12–9. This graph shows the relative frequency of Down's syndrome with increasing maternal age. (Adapted from Thorn, G. W., et al. (Eds.): *Harrison's Principles of Internal Medicine,* 8th Ed. New York, McGraw-Hill, 1976.)

TRISOMY 21/1000 BIRTHS

MATERNAL AGE

Table 12–5. Chromosomal Changes in Leukemias and Lymphomas

	NORMAL KARYOTYPES	CHROMOSOMAL CHANGES
Acute leukemia	40%	7,8,9 and 21
Chronic lymphocytic leukemia	75%	trisomy 9,17,21
Plasma cell leukemia	25%(?)	14q⁺
Polycythemia vera	80%	20q⁻; trisomy 8,9,21
Myeloproliferative disorder	10%	7,8,9
Burkitt's lymphoma	15%	t(8; 14)
Malignant lymphoma	?	isochromosome 17; 14q⁺; trisomy 7

Trisomy-21 is that condition in which autosome No. 21 is in triplicate, and the newborn child has mongoloid (slanted) eyes, hyperextensibility of the finger joints, imbecilic facies, and, as becomes apparent only too soon, an imbecilic mind, Down's syndrome. The trisomy is believed to be due to the failure of a pair of homologous chromosomes to segregate or to undergo disjunction at a meiotic division during the formation of gametes, a condition known as nondisjunction (Fig. 12–8). Other examples of trisomic syndrome are coming to light, some of them incompatible with life. They often occur with increasing maternal or paternal age (Fig. 12–9).

Recently there has been increasing interest in the relationship of chromosomal disorders to cancer. The best-known relationship has been the chromosomal changes in acute leukemias (Chromosome 21). More recently, other leukemias and lymphomas have also been shown to have chromosomal changes (Table 12–5). Accumulating evidence shows that other human neoplasms are associated with additional chromosomal disorders, and Table 12–6 illustrates those associations uncovered to date.

DISEASES DUE TO MUTATIONS

The gene acts as a biochemical carrier of biologic information from 1 generation to the next. As in the case of the chromosomes, the genes are in pairs known as allelomorphs or alleles (Greek *allelon,* one another), 1 member of the pair being maternal, the other paternal in origin. Allelic genes from father and mother are situated at the same spot or locus on the 2 members of the same pair of homologous chromosomes.

Both genes or a pair producing a similar trait and occupying the same locus on the homologous chromosomes may be dominant or both may be recessive, a homozygous condition, or one may be dominant and the other recessive, the resultant being heterozygous. If the gene is **dominant,** the individual will show the corresponding characteristic, whether the arrangement is homozygous or heterozygous, because the strong gene does not need to be reinforced. When the gene is **recessive** and single, the corresponding character is not evident, and the individual plays the part of a passive carrier. The single recessive gene holds its place on the chromosome, biding its time in obscurity. It may have to wait for many generations (a short time in the case of the fruit fly, but in the case of human beings, hundreds of years) before it gets its chance by being freed of suppression by a dominant gene. It is small wonder that some hereditary diseases of man are not recognized as such.

Dominance may not be as pure as suggested by what has just been said. It is not necessarily a matter of all or nothing. The degree of dominance, the grade of potency, is expressed by the term **penetrance.** When a dominant gene fails to manifest itself in the individual carrying the gene, there is said to be partial penetrance. A dominant gene with 80% penetrance will express itself in only 80% of cases; the remaining 20% carrying it will skip a generation.

The number of disorders that have been traced to mutant genes, dominant or recessive, is increasing daily as our studies are more refined by biochemical knowledge of errors in product quality and amount, and as our interest in human pedigrees increases. Such disorders as the hemoglobinopathies (disorders in the biosynthesis of the protein chains of hemoglobin), disorders of connective tissue (osteogenesis imperfecta, Marfan's disease), and tumors that occur in families

Table 12–6. Chromosome Changes Most Common in Human Neoplasms

1	2	3	4	5	6	7	8	9	10	11	12	13	14	15	16	17	18	19	20	21	22	XY
						AL	AL	AL				R	BL			CLL			PV	AL	CML	
						BL	BL	CLL					CP			CML				CLL	M	
						MD	CML	CML					ML			ML						
						ML	CP	MD					PL									
							M	PV														
							MD															
							PV															

| | | | | | | SV40 | | | | | | | | | | AdV12 | | Polio | | | | |

(Adapted from Mitelman, F., and Levan, G.: Clustering of aberrations to specific chromosomes in human neoplasms. II. A survey of 287 neoplasms. Hereditas, 82:167, 1976.)

(familial polyposis, multiple neurofibromas) are all autosomal dominant disorders. In several instances, it is apparent that these mutations vary widely in their gene product. For example, up to 1975 at least 30 different abnormal hemoglobins have been identified in man that carry varying risks for morbidity.

Autosomal **recessive** mutants, more difficult to identify, represent the largest number of hereditary diseases, and they normally occur in unsuspecting, unaffected parents. Such diseases as Gaucher's, a disorder of storage of lipid (lipoidoses), in which the absence of essential enzymes has been identified; the glycogenoses, disorders of enzymes responsible for structuring the glycogen molecule, and Wilson's disease, in which a copper-carrying protein (ceruloplasmin) is absent, are all recessive traits. This list can be lengthened considerably to include such diseases as cystic fibrosis and sickle cell anemia, which are discussed elsewhere.

Sex-linked mutants are best exemplified by the hemophilias, which have been so notorious in the royal families of Europe. A striking account of the effect of hemophilia on the patient and his family can be read in the account of the Czar of Russia and his family in *Nicholas and Alexandra,* by Robert Massie.

DISEASES WITH POLYGENIC INHERITANCE

Defined as those traits for which many genes contribute a minor effect, polygenic inheritance is best understood in those traits that show a continuous variation, such as the distribution of height in man. This type of inheritance is illustrated in Figure 12–10. The term multifactorial disease has occasionally been used in the same context, but this usage seems inappropriate, since it implies that factors other than heredity also play a role in bringing out the abnormal pattern or disease. In fact, **multifactorial disease,** as a term, should be defined as **those conditions that are brought out by the interaction between hereditary and environmental factors,** such as the anemias that occur when certain people eat fava beans, or the diarrhea that happens when lactase-deficient persons are placed on a milk regimen. We prefer to use the term polygenic for certain conditions and to define

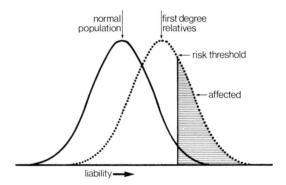

Fig. 12–10. This graph shows the effect on the appearance of disease of multiple factors. The normal population is shown in the curve at the left. Persons with a hereditary risk, which depends on several genes being present and working together to make a particular disease evident, move the curve to the right. Not all persons with a particular complement of genes will necessarily show the disease, as the manifestation of disease may depend in addition on some environmental factors. Thus those who show the disease are represented on the right-hand part of the right curve. (From Bearn, A. G.: Polygenic and multifactorial inheritance. In *Cecil Textbook of Medicine,* 15th Ed. Edited by P. B. Beeson, W. McDermott, and J. B. Wyngaarden. Philadelphia, W. B. Saunders, 1979.)

them as the collaboration of many genes at different loci as distinct from traits that are determined by a single gene. This is different from disease with a multifactorial etiology.

Polygenic disease should be considered when the illness in question is known to exist in several generations.

Finally, there are diseases, such as diabetes mellitus, hypertension, rheumatoid arthritis, and gout, that are best explained not in terms of a single-gene effect (and no chromosomal abnormality has been identified), but on the basis of multiple-gene dosage. In fact, the whole concept of health and disease should be reviewed with this background of multiple genic factors in mind to help to explain why some family groups seem singularly successful, live to ripe old age, and are relatively free of mortal disorders, whereas other families seem fated to a short and ailing life. Rene Dubos, in *The Mirage of Health,* has interesting and important things to say in this respect.

Although the reader can review the diseases hypertension and diabetes mellitus in the chapter on disturbances of blood flow, and the pancreas, respectively, this is as good a place to discuss gout as the chapter on the musculoskeletal system.

Gout is produced by an elevated serum uric acid level, which in turn may develop in a variety of different ways. Chronic gout is a good example of multifactorial disease.

Gout is an example of a **multifactorial** disease, because there are many ways to develop an elevated serum uric acid level (hyperuricemia). Gout may appear in persons who have acute leukemia, for example, since there is an increased production of uric acid due to rapid death of the leukemic cells. In theory, an elevated serum uric acid level can be produced in 1 of at least 3 ways: (1) by an increased production of uric acid, (2) by an increased absorption of precursors, (3) by a decreased excretion or decreased breakdown of uric acid. Recent evidence points to increased uric acid production and reduced excretion by the kidneys as the principal causes of elevated serum levels.

What is gout and what does this serum uric acid level have to do with the exquisitely painful big toe, or other joint?

Gout is a most intriguing disease that may involve any joint and many other areas of connective tissue. Its prevalence varies widely and is said to occur in 9% of men and in 1% of women, usually in the fourth or fifth decade (Fig. 12–11). An attack of acute gouty arthritis is usually unheralded, and the patient is often awakened in the middle of the night by a severe pain, often in the great toe. The slightest disturbance of the bed or the bed clothes may cause intense pain. The pain is attributed to the presence of crystals of sodium urate in the tissue of this afflicted part. One proposed mechanism of onset of this disease is a cycle of crystallization of urate from supersaturated body fluids that evoke an inflammatory response (Fig. 12–12). The white blood cells (leukocytes) that are called in consume oxygen, produce lactate, and produce a lower pH; more urate is then crystallized, causing more inflammation.

Gout has been known since the earliest times under the name podagra (Greek *pous*, foot, and *agra,* attack). Colchicine, the autumn crocus, was used 1,500 years ago as a specific drug and is still used. We now think its effectiveness is due to its ability to prevent mobilization of white blood cells into the area of precipitation, because colchicine interferes with the mobility of the white blood cells by disrupting microtubules. More modern therapy is directed toward increasing the uri-

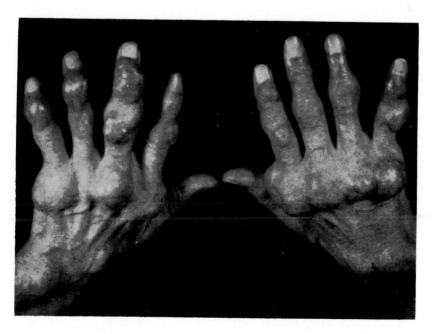

Fig. 12–11. Marked formation of gouty tophi in the hands of a man who was supposed for years to have rheumatoid arthritis, and was treated as such. (Boyd, W.: *Pathology for the Physician*).

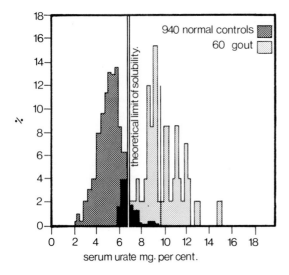

Fig. 12–12. This graph illustrates the range of serum urate levels in 940 normal persons and in 60 persons with gout. The limit of solubility of uric acid ranges around 6.5 mg%. Thus those who have higher levels of uric acid precipitate crystals. (From Seegmiller, J. E.: Diseases of purine and pyrimidine metabolism. In *Duncan's Diseases of Metabolism,* 7th Ed. Edited by P. K. Bondy, and L. E. Rosenberg. Philadelphia, W. B. Saunders, 1974.)

nary excretion of uric acid. Strict dieting with sanctions against all meats and good things have proved unnecessary. There is also a better understanding of the age-old belief that alcohol is an important predisposing factor in the production of gout. With considerable consumption, there is an excess of lactate produced that may suppress the renal excretion of uric acid, thereby elevating the serum level and contributing to the production of urate crystals.

Chronic gout is due to the formation of masses of crystals in connective tissues of the joint and other sites, where they appear as chalky white deposits, rather like drops of paint, an appearance from which the name gout is derived (Latin, *gutta*, a drop). These crystal deposits may have a destructive effect on the cartilage of the joint and cause an arthritis similar to osteoarthritis. Tophi are masses of crystals that accumulate in the soft tissues and joints and that may cause marked deformities. These accumulations may also appear in the ear. The kidneys may accumulate deposits in the collecting system, and urate crystals here may lead to serious and

chronic renal dysfunction. It is of interest that deposits of uric acid in tissues are soluble in the conventional fixatives and storage solutions, so that if you wish to demonstrate the urates, the tissue should be preserved in alcohol. The occurrence of kidney stones should always suggest gout as a possible cause in men over 40 years of age. Renal failure is a serious and sometimes fatal complication of gout.

As implied by placing a consideration of gout in this chapter, and as stated in the first sentence of this section, gout is a disorder of metabolism, associated with a high serum uric acid, in which the error may be either hereditary or acquired. We may speak of primary gout, those cases in which there is no predisposing cause other than an inborn error of metabolism, and secondary gout, in which we can relate the disease to some other cause of hyperuricemia.

The familial and hereditary nature of gout has been known since earliest times, and many pedigrees have been analyzed to determine the mode of inheritance. The disease is also of interest because of the extraordinary number of outstanding intellectuals who have been afflicted with it, such as Martin Luther, the Pitts of Great Britain, Isaac Newton, Benjamin Franklin, and Samuel Johnson, to name a few. Although it has been suggested that gout was an autosomal dominant trait, it is reasonable on the basis of all the current data to suggest that the serum uric acid level is controlled by multiple genes, any one of which may appear dominant in any selected population. This theory implies that whereas multiple metabolic defects may be responsible for hyperuricemia, a single defect may be characteristic of a particular family. This important concept is relevant to other diseases that can be considered multifactorial and/or polygenic.

Gout is of additional interest because of the association of hyperuricemia with academic achievement in males. Several studies have shown that mean levels of uric acid are higher in supervisors than in laborers, in medical students than in high school students, and there is a significant positive correlation between the serum uric acid level and aptitude or intelligence tests in a large series of army inductees. One suggestion is that, during the course of evolution, serum uric acid has had a beneficial effect as a cerebral stimulant!

Regardless of the relevance of these findings, it is generally conceded that the defect in primary (hereditary) gout is due to both overproduction and underexcretion of uric acid, and both processes are present in differing degrees in gouty patients. One might note that, just to confuse the matter further, there are a few cases in which a sex-linked inheritance has been established; a rare disorder of overproduction of uric acid is associated with cerebral palsy, mental deficiency, and self-mutilation (Lesch-Nyhan syndrome).

As alluded to earlier, in some disorders of the hematopoietic system, there may be an accelerated turnover of nucleic acid, which may lead to overproduction of uric acid, which in turn may become chemically apparent with urate deposits. Most other instances of secondary gout are traced to decreased excretion of uric acid, as in chronic renal diseases (polycystic kidney, chronic glomerulonephritis, and pyelonephritis). There are also specific interferences with renal tubular function, which may result in uric acid accumulation (e.g., lead poisoning, use of therapeutic drugs, e.g., chlorothiazide). However, the important thing to recognize is that, although the expression of the disorders may be the same (arthritis, tophi), these vastly differing causes can be elucidated and the patient successfully treated by the use of drugs to aid in the excretion of the uric acid and depression of its symptoms.

We might mention here a new area of study, a territory that is relatively unexplored but that has already yielded rewards for the careful worker, i.e., the field of **behavioral genetics,** in which early results indicate that the dualism of environment and heredity is just as important as in the more obvious areas of nutrition and infectious disease. Gene effects for aggressive behavior, maze-learning, susceptibility to seizures, and avoidance learning performances, have all been described. For example, studies on mice show that dominant males emit more than 70% more 70 kHz ultrasounds in response to females than do subordinates. Such inhibition of behavior by social subordination early in the mating sequence could be a major factor that contributes to Darwinian fitness of such dominant males. This area will certainly receive more attention in the years to come.

TREATMENT OF GENETIC DISORDERS

In order to be effective, the treatment of genetic disorders requires a clear knowledge of the nature of the defect. Despite rapid

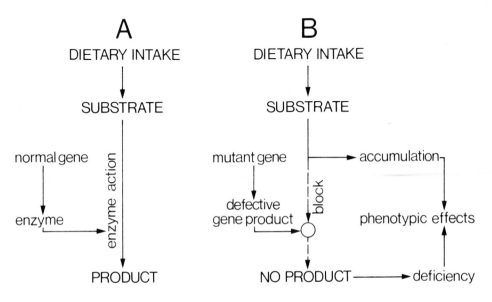

Fig. 12–13. This figure shows the effect on the accumulation of substrate in a person with a mutant gene, which results in the defective gene product. The treatment of this problem is to remove the accumulation of material, or to substitute a normal gene for a defective one. (From Whaley, L. F.: *Understanding Inherited Disorders.* St. Louis, C. V. Mosby Co., 1974.)

growth in our knowledge of many disorders, we are not yet able to modify many inborn errors of metabolism although for a few (phenylketonuria, cystinuria) there are impressive statistics to show a change in prognosis. Reverting for a moment to conceptual expression, we may list several approaches to

metabolic diseases, provided we have relevant biochemical data. We may: (1) supply the missing product or metabolite (as with insulin for the diabetic); (2) limit the precursor of the abnormal material (which, in the case of such a disease as phenylketonuria, has a cumulative toxic effect) (Fig. 12–13); (3) ad-

Table 12–7.   Risks for Rare Mendelian Disorders in Families

MODE OF INHERITANCE	FIRST DEGREE RELATIVES AT RISK	RISK	OTHER RELATIVES AT RISK	RISK
Autosomal dominant	Sibs, parents, children (both sexes)	50%	Uncles, aunts, nephews, nieces	25%
			First cousins	12.5%
Autosomal recessive	Sibs (both sexes)	25%	Uncles, aunts, nephews,	
	Children	Negligible*	nieces, cousins	Negligible
X-linked recessive	Brothers	50%**	Maternal uncle	50%**
	Sisters (carriers)	25%**	Maternal aunt (carrier)	50%**
			Maternal male cousin	25%**
			Maternal female cousin (carrier)	25%**

*Risks for children of patients affected with common autosomal recessive diseases depend on gene frequency (highest risk [2%] for sickle cell anemia [0.08 × 0.25]).

** Risks are negligible when the disease in an affected patient is caused by a new mutation. Recent work suggests that the proportion of new mutations may be much less than the expected 33% in X-linked lethal diseases.

(From Motulsky, A. G.: Genetic counseling. In *Cecil Textbook of Medicine,* 15th Ed. Edited by P. B. Beeson, W. McDermott, and J. B. Wyngaarden. Philadelphia, W. B. Saunders, 1979.)

Table 12–8.   Genetic Diseases-Carrier Detection* Advisable for Reproductive Decisions

DISORDER	MODE OF INHERITANCE	METHOD OF CARRIER DIAGNOSIS	PREVENTIVE MEASURES IN CARRIERS	POPULATION AFFECTED
Duchenne muscular dystrophy	X-linked	CPK level	Amniocentesis for male sex	All
Hemophilia	X-linked	AHG level and AHG cross-reactive material	Amniocentesis for male sex	All
Lesch-Nyhan syndrome	X-linked	HGPRT assay	Amniocentesis— HGPRT assay	All
Translocation Down's syndrome	Empirical recurrence risks apply	Chromosomal tests for balanced carrier	Amniocentesis— chromosomal study	All
Sickle cell anemia	Autosomal recessive	Hemoglobin electro-phoresis	Genetic counseling	Blacks
β-Thalassemia major	Autosomal recessive	Red cell abnormalities Hb A_2 increased	Genetic counseling	Mediterranean and tropical population
Tay-Sachs disease	Autosomal recessive	Hexosaminidase A assay	Amniocentesis— hexosaminidase assay	Ashkenazic Jews

* Limited to translocation Down's syndrome, X-linked, and *frequent* autosomal recessive diseases. Detection of carriers for many rare inborn errors associated with enzyme deficiency is possible, but the risk for normal sibs of affected patients to have affected offspring is small, because the frequency of the carrier state for such inborn errors is low in the population.

(From Motulsky, A. G.: Genetic counseling. In *Cecil Textbook of Medicine,* 15th Ed. Edited by P. B. Beeson, W. McDermott, and J. B. Wyngaarden. Philadelphia, W. B. Saunders, 1979.)

minister a metabolic inhibitor (using allopurinol, which regulates uric acid metabolism in patients with gout and prevents stone or tophus formation); (4) deplete the body of the inappropriately stored material (such as using phlebotomy in iron storage disorders); (5) use genetic counseling (Tables 12–7 and 12–8). Unfortunately, there are not many situations to date in which clear evidence of the carrier state is available from chromosome maps or biochemical data (such as an elevated creatine phosphokinase in a family known to have the trait for muscular dystrophy).

Outside of these theoretical and specific considerations, supportive therapy and treatment of the complications of the disorder are the same as for all human disease.

SYNOPSIS

Genetic controls of subcellular, cellular, tissue, organ, and integrated mechansims may often be abnormal. Mutations may affect either the structure or the amount of a cellular product.

Genetic diseases may be inherited as dominant, recessive, or with differing degrees of penetrance. They may be classified anatomically, in relation to their importance, or as diseases of chromosomal aberration, due to mutations, or of polygenic etiology.

Klinefelter's, Turner's, and Down's syndrome are examples of chromosomal disorders. Hemoglobinopathies and familial polyposis are examples of mutation. Gout is an example of a disease process of both multifactorial and polygenic etiology.

Genetic disorders can be treated by supplying the missing product, by limiting the abnormal precursor, by administering an inhibitor, by depleting the body of the abnormal stores, and by using family counselling.

Terms

Gene	*Turner's syndrome*	*Trisomy*
Chromosome	*Recessive*	*Down's syndrome*
Mutation	*Dominant*	*Gout*
Klinefelter's syndrome	*Sex-linked*	

FURTHER READING

Ash, P., Vennart, J., and Carter, C. O.: The incidence of hereditary disease in man. J. Med. Genet., *14*:305, 1977.

Caspersson, T., et al.: Identification of human chromosomes by DNA-binding fluorescent agents. Chromosoma, *30*:215, 1970.

Defries, J.C., and Plomin, R.: Behavioral genetics. Annu. Rev. Psychol., *29*:473, 1978.

Dubos, R.: *Mirage of Health: Utopias, Progress, and Biological Change*. New York, Harper and Row, 1979.

Fraser, F. C., and Nora, J. J.: *Genetics of Man*. Philadelphia, Lea & Febiger, 1975.

Goodenough, U., and Levine, R. P.: *Genetics*. New York, Holt Rinehart & Winston, 1979.

Holmes, L. B.: Congenital malformations. N. Engl. J. Med., *295*:204, 1970.

McKusick, V. A., and Ruddle, F. H.: The status of the gene map of the human chromosomes. Science, *196*:390, 1977.

Mitelman, F., and Levan, G.: Clustering of aberrations to specific chromosomes in human neoplasm. II. A survey of 287 neoplasms. Hereditas, *82*:167, 1976.

Motulsky, A. G.: The genetic hyperlipidemias. N. Engl. J. Med., *294*:823, 1976.

Rakic, M. T., et al.: Observations on the natural history of hyperuricemia and gout. Am. J. Med., *37*:862, 1964.

Rimoin, D., and Shimke, R. N.: *Genetic Disorders of the Endocrine Glands*. St. Louis, C. V. Mosby, 1971.

Spaeth, G. L., and Barber, G. W.: Homocystinuria and the passing of the one gene—one enzyme concept of disease. J. Med. Philos., *5*:8, 1980.

Stanbury, J. B., Wyngaarden, J. B., and Fredrickson, D. S.: *The Metabolic Basis of Inherited Disease*, 3rd Ed. New York, McGraw-Hill, 1972.

Wilson, E. O.: *On Human Nature*. Cambridge, Harvard University Press, 1978.

The Organs and their Diseases

2

The Heart

13

The physics of a man's circulation are the physics of the waterworks of the town in which he lives, but once out of gear you cannot apply the same rules for the repair of one as of the other.—W. OSLER

From the earliest of times, our ancestors have realized the importance of the heart to life itself. Our language testifies to this, particularly in the language of the poets. We say that a man is brokenhearted, or wounded to the heart, or that he wears his heart on his sleeve, or that it is in his throat, or in his boots. Our knowledge of the anatomy and physiology of the heart has advanced incredibly in recent years. We pass catheters into its cavities, measure the electrical changes in its muscle, record pressures and gradients, estimate the degree of injury by enzyme assays, and probe it by sound waves (echocardiography) and by computer-assisted radiology. We also cool it for operations and shock it to make it beat again. We still do not understand how it is that one person may have extensive myocardial scarring without suffering unduly, whereas another dies of sudden heart failure without adequate explanation.

Structure. The average weight of the human heart is 300 grams in the male, 250 grams in the female, about the size of a person's fist, but the heart is considerably larger in a big, muscular laborer, or smaller in a tiny, fragile woman. It is composed of muscle and valves (Fig. 13–1). Viewed with routine roentgenograms, the important structures of the cardiovascular system are shown in posterior/anterior and lateral views in Figure 13–2. The valves consist of thin and delicate membrane, the endocardium, which also lines the

cavity. Although so thin as to be translucent, the valves prevent a single drop of blood from leaking through when closed. On the right side of the heart, the tricuspid valve divides the chamber into

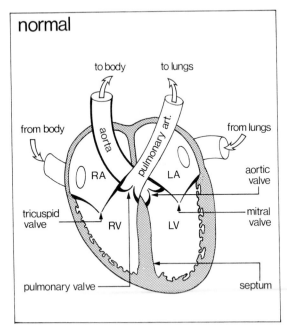

Fig. 13–1. This diagram of the normal heart shows the relative proportions of the sizes of the ventricles and the atria, RV, LV, RA, LA, that is, right and left ventricles and right and left atria. It also illustrates the relative wall thicknesses of the aorta and pulmonary artery, and the placement of the respective atrial ventricular valves, the tricuspid on the right and the mitral on the left, the pulmonic valve, and the aortic valve. IVC is the inferior vena cava.

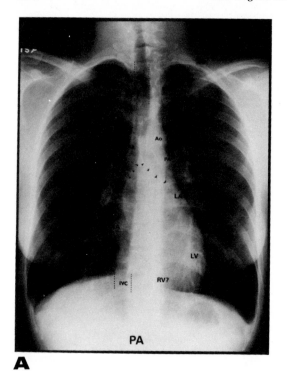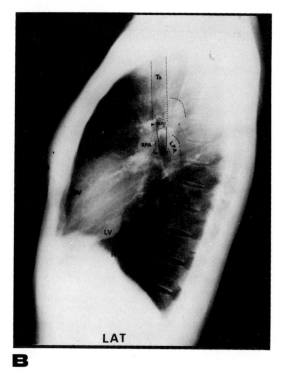

Fig. 13–2. *A,* This figure shows a normal chest roentgenogram in PA (posteroanterior, or back to front) projection. The cardiac silhouette is seen in the center of the chest, with left ventricle (LV), right ventricle (RV), left atrium (LA), right atrium (RA), aortic knob (AO), left and right pulmonary artery (LPA and RPA), azygous vein (AZ). The trachea is shown at T, and the remainder of the chest film is unremarkable. IVC is inferior vena cava and the arrows outline the mainstem bronchi which contain air. *B,* In the lateral projection, the left pulmonary artery is seen at LPA, the right pulmonary artery at RPA, and the main stem bronchus to the right upper lobe at RUL.

an atrium or auricle, which receives the venous blood from the body, and a ventricle, which sends blood to the lungs by the pulmonary artery, whose mouth is guarded by the pulmonary valve. The left side of the heart is divided by the mitral valve into an atrium, which receives blood from the lungs, and a ventricle, which sends this blood out into the great artery, the aorta, whose opening is controlled by the aortic valve. The function of the valves is to prevent backflow of blood between the beats.

Just as the interior of the heart is lined by the endocardium, so its outer surface is covered by another delicate membrane, the epicardium. The part of the chest in which the heart is situated is lined by a second layer of pericardium, so that between the 2 layers there exists a space, the pericardial cavity, in which the heart can contract and expand. This cavity normally contains a small amount of serous fluid (20 ml), which lubricates the sliding surfaces. After injury or infection in the pericardium, fibrin can accumulate and can roughen these pericardial surfaces, even causing a noise similar to that of sandpapering (friction rub).

The heart muscle or myocardium has an abundant blood supply. It is much more important than in the case of other muscles, because, unlike them,

the heart does not rest for long. This blood supply is provided by 2 arteries, the right and left coronary arteries, which arise from the aorta immediately above the aortic valve and carry blood to every part of the heart muscle; the maximum flow is during the filling phase or diastole.

These arteries are different from others of the same size in the body, having an extra layer of longitudinal smooth muscle, perhaps because they are subject to the intermittent stretching that takes place with each contraction of the heart.

Coronary sinus catheterization now enables us to look into the physiology of the myocardium and cardiac metabolism in a way never before possible. Physiologists have begun to explore the electric activity of single heart muscle cells by inserting a microelectrode into the interior of a cell, and to map the function of heart muscle during open heart surgery.

Function. The heart is a hollow muscular pump whose function is to circulate the blood through the body. It is a common misconception to think that the heart is the master of the body; the reverse is more reasonable—that the heart is the servant of the body and is subject to many forces, as shown in Figure 13–3. It sends venous blood to the lungs,

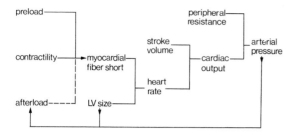

Fig. 13–3. This diagram illustrates interactions between components that regulate cardiac activity. (From Braunwald, E.: Regulation of the circulation. N. Engl. J. Med., *290*:1124, 1974.)

where oxygen is taken up and carbon dioxide given off, and then pumps oxygenated blood to the tissues, where the oxygen is used.

The heart can be trained or will adapt to training. With regular exercise, the amount of blood that is expelled with each contraction can be increased, and the rate of the heart will be lowered. An Olympic athlete may have a heart rate as low as 40 beats per minute, half the resting rate of a sedentary office worker.

We do not know actually what makes the heart beat, although we know a lot about what regulates its rate. What we call the beat is a contraction, similar to that of other muscles, but, unlike other muscles, the beat can go on after the nerves that

supply the heart are cut, and even after the animal (or person) is dead. I (Huntington Sheldon) was once much startled to feel the heart begin to beat in my hand on the autopsy table, the patient having been dead a number of hours. The contraction of the myocardium, which drives the blood out of the ventricles into the arteries, is known as systole. The succeeding relaxation during which the cavities become refilled with blood from the veins is called diastole (Fig. 13–4). In health, valves prevent a backflow of blood from the arteries into the right and left ventricles, and from the ventricles into the atria. The sinoatrial (auricular) node, a small area of specialized tissue in the upper part of the right atrium close to the entry of the superior vena cava, is called the pacemaker. A current of electricity passes through the myocardium from the sinoatrial node each time the heart beats. Impulses pass out in all directions, reaching the ventricle, where they are carried by a specialized branch of muscular and nervous tissue called the atrioventricular bundle of His. If this bundle is interfered with by disease, the result is known as heart block, which is characterized by a much slower rate of contraction, because the impulses are generated separately in atria and ventricles.

There are many ways in which medical treatment can influence the pacemaker, some old, such as digitalis, originally an infusion or brew made from the leaves of the purple foxglove, *Digitalis purpurea* or ladies' fingers, and some new, such as the electric pacemaker. When the heart is diseased,

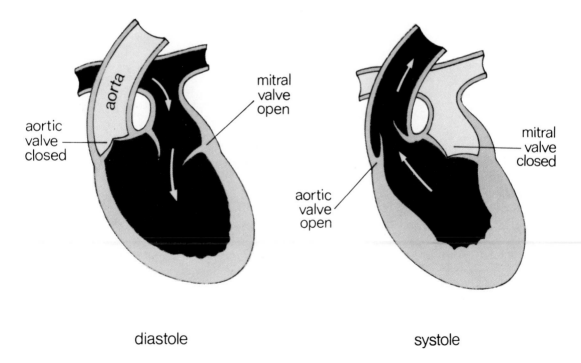

diastole   systole

Fig. 13–4. This drawing shows the relative sizes and positions of the mitral valve, left ventricle, aortic valve, and aorta in diastole and systole, illustrating that the pump depends not only on contractions but the integrity of the valves.

a quivering of the atria in place of a regular beat often sets in, known as atrial or auricular fibrillation. Impulses now pass into the bundle of His so rapidly that the ventricles respond irregularly and ineffectively.

The electric pacemaker has been used in those serious cases of heart block known as Adams-Stokes disease (also called Stokes-Adams disease) with a slow pulse rate, which may be associated with severe congestive heart failure. The condition may be a later aftereffect of myocardial infarction involving the bundle of His. A tiny transistorized pacemaker driven by a long-life battery is placed under the skin of the abdominal wall and is con-

nected to electrodes implanted in the heart muscle. The heart block is now overcome and a new rate is established. The cardiac output may be best at induced rates different from that of the natural sinoatrial pacemaker.

An electric current is normally generated in the contracting myocardium, and this is recorded on the electrocardiogram. This device shows a series of waves, known by the letters Q, R, and S, by contraction of the ventricles (Fig. 13–5). The accompanying diagram relates the electrical activity to the pressures in the aorta and to the venous system as well (Fig. 13–6). In heart disease, the waves may show a change in shape and position,

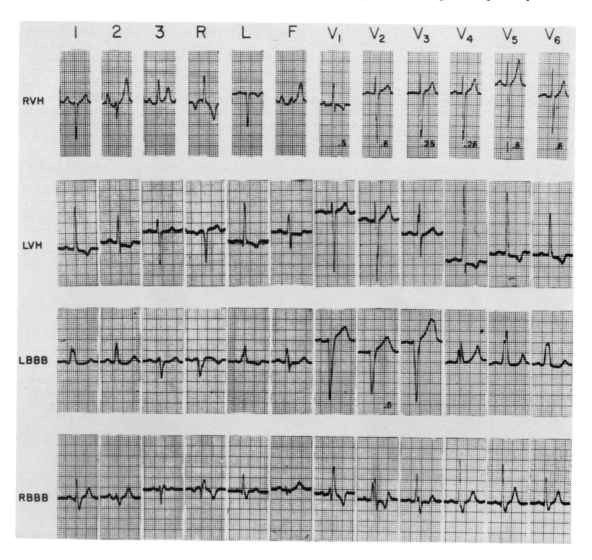

Fig. 13–5. Shown here is the typical appearance of electrocardiograms in a variety of abnormal conditions, namely, right ventricular hypertrophy (RVH), left ventricular hypertrophy (LVH), left bundle branch block (LBBB), and right bundle branch block (RBBB). The numbers at the top of the illustration are the numbers of the electrocardiographic leads. Compare the direction and amplitude of the QRS complex in lead 1 in RVH and LVH. Their opposite direction results from the different ventricular mass; hypertrophy of the right ventricle in one instance, the left in the other. (From Wintrobe, M., et al. (Eds.): *Harrison's Principles of Internal Medicine*, 7th Ed. New York, McGraw-Hill, 1974.)

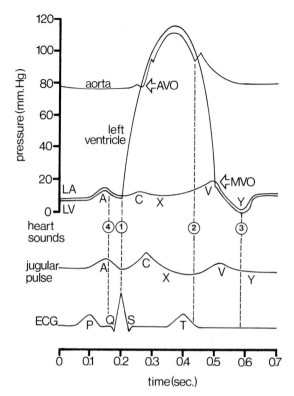

Fig. 13–6. Simultaneous ECG, pressures obtained from the left atrium, left ventricle, and aorta, and the jugular pulse during one cardiac cycle. For simplification, right heart pressures have been omitted. Normal right atrial pressure closely parallels that of the left atrium, and right ventricular and pulmonary artery pressures correspond closely to their left heart counterparts, except that the former are reduced in magnitude. The normal mitral and aortic valve closures precede tricuspid and pulmonic closures, respectively, whereas valve opening reverses this order. The jugular venous pulse lags behind the right atrial pressure.

During the course of one cardiac cycle, the electrical events (ECG) initiate and therefore precede the mechanical (pressure) events, and the latter precede the auscultatory events (heart sounds) that the mechanical events themselves produce. Shortly after the P wave, the atria contract to produce the A wave; a fourth heart sound may succeed the latter. The QRS complex initiates ventricular systole, followed shortly by left ventricular contraction and by the rapid build-up of left ventricular (LV) pressure. Almost immediately, LV pressure exceeds left atrial (LA) pressure. This imbalance closes the mitral valve and produces the first heart sound. When LV pressure exceeds aortic pressure, the aortic valve opens (AVO), and when aortic pressure is once again greater than LV pressure, the aortic valve closes, which produces the second heart sound and terminates ventricular ejection. The decreasing LV pressure drops below LA pressure to open the mitral valve (MVO), and a period of rapid ventricular filling commences. During this time, a third heart sound may be heard. (From Andreoli, K. G., et al.: *Comprehensive Cardiac Care*, 4th Ed. St. Louis, C. V. Mosby Co., 1979; modified with permission from Hurst, J. W., et al.: *The Heart, Arteries, and Veins*, 3rd Ed. New York, McGraw-Hill, 1974.)

which may help the physician to arrive at a correct diagnosis (Table 13–1).

When the normal heart is listened to with the assistance of a stethoscope applied to the chest wall, 2 hearts sounds are heard. The first sound is longer, softer, and of deeper pitch than the second sound. The first sound, which is caused partly by contraction of the heart muscle and partly by closure of the valves (mitral and tricuspid) between the atria and ventricles, is likened to "lubb;" the second sound, short, hard, and of a higher pitch, is represented by "dup." A change in the quality of these sounds is an indication of disease of the valves.

The rate of the heartbeat, i.e., the pulse, varies. The normal rhythm of the heart depends on the balance of 2 sets of nervous impulses, 1 tending to slow, the other to accelerate the heart's action. Both nerves belong to the involuntary or autonomic nervous system. The vagus nerve is responsible for the retarding impulses; acetylcholine is liberated at the nerve endings of the vagus and acts on the heart muscle. The accelerating impulses pass along the sympathetic nerve fibers, and another substance is liberated at their nerve endings. The quickening of the heartbeat that results from emotion, the feeling that your heart is in your mouth or in your boots, is due to an upset of the exquisite balance that normally exists between these 2 sets of influences.

The rate of the heart also depends on the demand of the tissues for oxygen. The runner's heart beats faster and he breathes more quickly in response to an increase in this demand. Muscular work is an expenditure of energy, and energy is obtained from the burning of food. As food cannot be normally burned without oxygen, the heartbeat is quickened and breathing becomes deeper and faster to supply this need.

The condition of the blood vessels must also be taken into account in any consideration of the heart's action. When the heart pumps blood into the arteries, it does so against a certain amount of resistance (peripheral resistance). This resistance may become too high or too low in pathologic conditions; in hypertension, narrowing of the arterioles increases the peripheral resistance, whereas in shock, there is little or no peripheral resistance. No organ works continually at its maximum capacity; the heart has a large amount of reserve force in order to cope with emergencies. When hypertension develops, the heart adapts to the increased work load by hypertrophy or increase in the muscle mass. We call this compensation. In the course of time or because of disease of the heart muscle, this power may fail and decompensation sets in.

The amount of blood that the heart puts out is determined by several factors (Fig. 13–7). We can organize them under 4 headings. Many years ago, the English physiologist Starling observed that the heart responded as any other muscle to stretch. He stated that the strength of contraction was propor-

Table 13–1.   Elements of Electrocardiography

	PATHOLOGY/ABNORMALITIES
P Wave Represents spread of electrical impulse from atria (activation or depolarization of atria)	Increase in amplitude usually indicates atrial hypertrophy in atrioventricular valve disease, hypertension, cor pulmonale, congenital heart disease
P–R Interval Measures time taken by impulse to travel all the way from SA node to ventricular muscle fibers	PR interval may be increased in congenital disease, rheumatic heart disease or from drugs (digitalis) as well as in heart block (ischemic)
QRS Complex Represents spread of impulse from ventricular muscle (activation or depolarization of ventricles)	(1) an increase in duration indicates abnormal intraventric conduction, usually meaning block of 1 of the bundle branches (2) if the amplitude is too low, it may indicate cardiac failure, widespread myocardial damage
T Wave Represents recovery period of ventricles when they recruit their spent electrical forces (repolarization)	Unusually tall T waves suggest myocardial infarct or K^+ intoxication, or myocardial ischemia without infarction. Low T wave indicates low K^+
Q–T Duration From beginning of QRS to end of T represents total duration of ventricular systole	(1) Prolonged Q–T occurs in congestive heart failure, myocardial infarction, hypocalcemia (2) Q–T can be shortened by digitalis, Ca excess, K^+ intoxication.

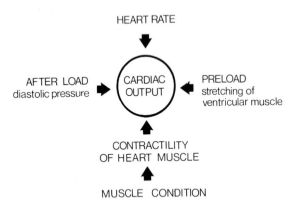

Fig. 13–7.   This diagram illustrates the relationship between cardiac output and several different factors. Cardiac output depends on the interrelationship of all the factors shown. If the heart rate falls below 40/min or exceeds 180/min, the cardiac output cannot support normal metabolic requirements. If the ventricular muscle is not slightly stretched, the ventricle will not contract with sufficient force to provide an adequate systolic pressure to maintain the circulation. If the myocardial muscle is deprived of oxygen or if it is subject to either an excess or a deficiency of potassium, the muscle will not be able to contract, regardless of the rate per minute or of the stretch of the muscle. Thus all the factors shown are important in the maintenance of cardiac output.

tional to the filling of the heart. This concept, that stretching the ventricular musculature results in increased cardiac output, is referred to as **preload.**

Clearly, the effectiveness of each contraction of heart muscle depends on the state of health of the muscle, which in turn depends on its nutritional supply, e.g., the correct amount of intracellular potassium and calcium. The well-being of cardiac muscle governs the strength of contraction and is a determinant of cardiac output. This state is called the **contractility** of heart muscle.

Within the hydraulics of the vascular system, the pressure for continuous perfusion of the capillaries (diastolic pressure) and the size of the left ventricle, which dictates the pressure that is developed by the muscle fibers (wall tension), are factors that govern how much blood can be delivered with each systole into the aorta. This notion is expressed as **afterload** in contemporary nomenclature.

Finally, the rate at which the heart beats naturally affects the circulatory efficiency, so that heart **rate** is important in a consideration of the mechanics of the circulation.

Clinical symptoms of heart disease may be caused by lesions in any of the anatomic subdivisions of the heart. We have **endocardial** diseases (which include valvular diseases), **myocardial** diseases, and **pericardial** diseases. The patient's medical history and the physical examination should give much insight into the possible reasons for a particular patient's heart failure.

LABORATORY INVESTIGATIONS. The myocardium is rich in enzymes, the most important of which, from the clinical standpoint, is an enzyme specific for muscle, creatine phosphokinase (CPK). Another enzyme found in heart muscle is glutamic oxaloacetic transaminase, called GOT or SGOT (S for "serum") for convenience. The normal serum level is low, from 4 to 40 units, but in myocardial infarction a large amount is released into the blood, so that the serum level is a sensitive and valuable index of recent necrosis of the myocardium (Fig. 13–8).

Chest roentgenograms and specific techniques for outlining the chambers of the heart, as with the use of barium in the esophagus, may demonstrate right ventricular enlargement. Angiography (contrast

media injected into veins or arteries) and cardiac catheterization are special techniques done in diagnostic centers. Modern use of isotopes allows us to visualize areas of heart muscle that do not function (Fig. 13–9). At least 2 different techniques are used for imaging of infarcts with modern methods. Some isotopes are taken up by the normal myocardium, so that an infarct of any age or an area of hypoperfusion is shown as an area of absent or reduced activity (cold spot). Other isotopes are taken up by the damaged tissue, so that an acute infarct is shown as a positive image (hot spot). The mechanisms by which isotopes are taken up are debated but it may be related to the deposition of calcium in or near mitochondria of damaged cells. The optimal time for these scans is between 24 and 48 hours after the beginning of the infarct, scanning 1 to 2 hours after injection of the isotope, and viewing in 3 projections. A positive result with a technetium scan, for example, may be obtained up to 6 days after the infarct. The use of such scans is being developed day by day, and as we learn more about the value of such methods, they may be put to greater use. At the present time, most scans are not reliable for assessing the size of an infarct, because the uptake of radioactivity depends greatly on the blood flow and may not be proportional to the volume of the infarct itself. These methods are currently used to confirm the presence of infarcts rather than to make the original diagnosis. Routine electrocardiography is helpful, particularly when tracings can be compared with earlier records. Precordial leads detect the sequential passage of electrical impulses and help to show which parts of the ventricular muscle are not functioning (Fig. 13–10A,B). Echocardiography allows direct estimate of ventricular wall thickness and competence of valves (Figs. 13–11 and 13–12).

Heart disease heads the causes of death. Its mortality is twice that of cancer, its nearest rival. The statistics of the Metropolitan Life Insurance Company show that 700,000 people die of heart disease in the United States every year. The incidence has been steadily rising over the last hundred years until very recently, partly, at least, because of the increased number of older people. Arbitrary classifications of subsets of heart disease show some

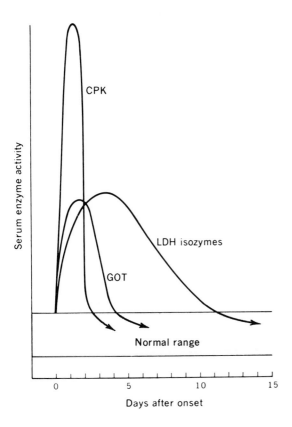

Fig. 13–8. This graph shows the time relationships between the CPK, LDH (lactic dehydrogenase) and GOT enzymes following myocardial infarction. (From Wintrobe, M., et al. (Eds.): *Harrison's Principles of Internal Medicine*, 7th Ed. New York, McGraw-Hill, 1974.)

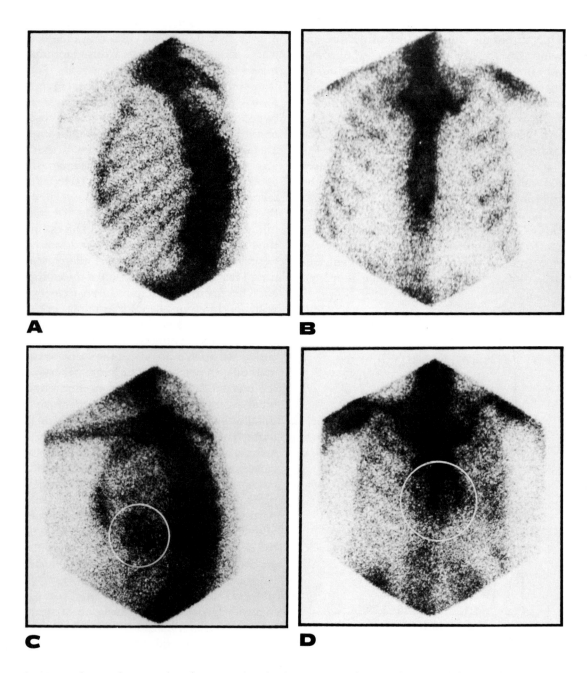

Fig. 13–9. These nuclear scans show the pattern of uptake of TC99mPP, a calcium-seeking agent in the normal person *(A & B)* and in a patient with a myocardial infarct *(C & D)*. *A*, lateral view of the heart and chest, *B*, frontal view of the heart and chest. *C* and *D* show an area of increased uptake in the area of the infarction, which is shown within the circle. The resolving power of this new method allows one to see areas that are comparatively large; a very small lesion (1 centimeter square) will not be visible. However, one can identify the presence of the isotopes which are concentrated in the necrotic area

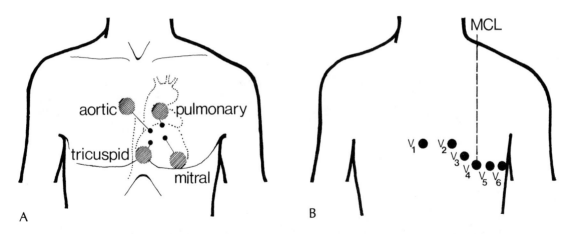

Fig. 13–10. *A* shows the location of the heart sounds. The small black dots in the center are the anatomic location of the heart valves; the larger shaded areas are the points to which the valve sounds are usually referred. *B* illustrates the electrode positions of the precordial leads for an electrocardiogram: V_1 and V_2 are placed at the fourth intercostal space on either side of the sternum; V_3 halfway between V_2 and V_4; V_4 at the midclavicular line (MCL) and fifth intercostal space; V_5 and V_6 directly lateral to V_4. (Adapted from Andreoli, K. G., et al.: *Comprehensive Cardiac Care,* 4th Ed. St. Louis, C. V. Mosby Co., 1979.)

changes with time of the incidence of different diseases. These changes can be credited both to changes in life-styles (different eating and exercise habits) and to changes in medical treatment (open heart surgery), as well as to artificial differences because of new diagnostic methods and different diagnostic classifications.

The principal categories of heart disease that we consider in this chapter are: (1) coronary artery disease, (2) hypertensive heart disease, (3) congenital heart disease, (4) valvular heart disease, (5) infectious heart disease (endocarditis), and (6) rheumatic heart disease. Of these, by far the most common are hypertensive heart disease and coronary artery disease, then rheumatic heart disease; much less common are bacterial endocarditis and congenital heart disease. Table 13–2 shows the relative frequency of different types of heart disease in the population, but it is important to remember that regardless of the overall rarity or abundance of any particular disease, to the person afflicted there is no more important type of disease than the one from which he suffers.

CORONARY ARTERY DISEASE

In a previous chapter, we studied the effect of cutting off the arterial blood supply to an organ not provided with good collateral circulation, and we found that the effect usually depended on whether the closure of the artery was slow or sudden. Gradual closure due to narrowing of the lumen of the artery by atherosclerosis led to atrophy and death of the specialized cells of the part (e.g., heart muscle) and their replacement by scar tissue. Sudden closure by embolism or by thrombosis caused the formation of an infarct, an area in which all the tissue was killed by the sudden ischemia.

Unfortunately, the coronary arteries are frequently affected by atherosclerosis. This process narrows the lumen of the vessels and predisposes a person to thrombosis and occlusion. Coronary artery narrowing seems to accompany old age, but it is more severe in men than in women at earlier ages. Many factors predispose a person to atherosclerosis in general, and we think of coronary artery disease as having multifactorial etiology. Heredity, obesity, metabolic disease such as diabetes mellitus, hypertension, abnormalities of lipid metabolism, and personal and social factors such as smoking and stress all play a role.

Traditionally, whenever there is pain in the chest, we jump to the conclusion that there is an impending "heart attack." Ischemia (lack of oxygen) of the myocardium is heralded by

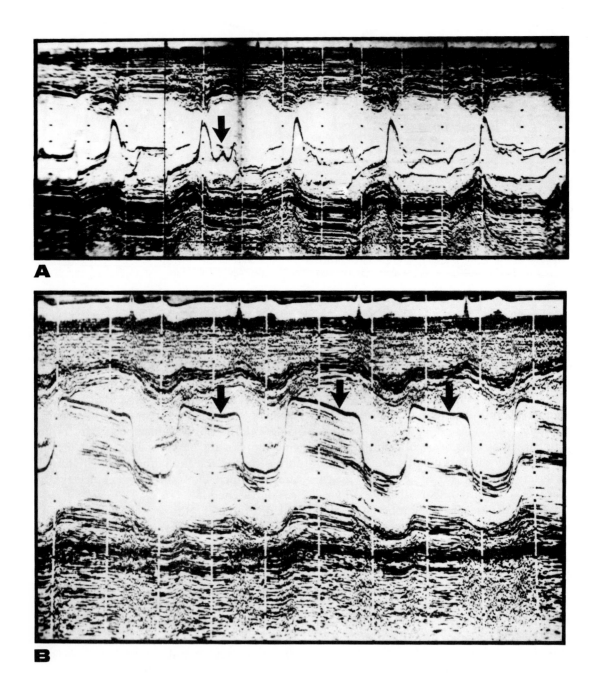

Fig. 13–11. These are M-mode echocardiograms showing *A,* the normal M-shaped motion of the mitral valve, reflecting the opening and closing of a normal valve during diastole and atrial systole. The valve motion is seen at the arrow. *B,* A similar echocardiogram showing the restricted motion of a stiffened stenotic valve at the arrows.

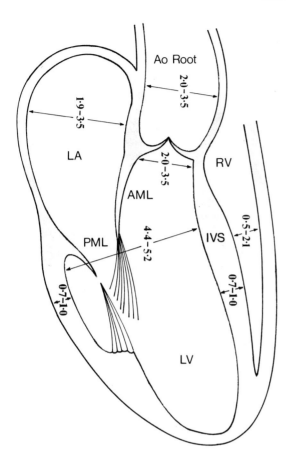

such pain; the most common cause of ischemia is arterial narrowing or occlusion. Narrowing of the coronary vessels by atheromatous plaques (which may be only segmental) and the occurrence of thrombi with or without plaques are the most common findings at autopsy in cases of acute myocardial infarction. We know that thrombi are constantly forming and being broken down by fibrinolysins; an additional etiologic factor, then, may be changes in our fibrinolytic mechanisms. In some instances, no anatomic lesion of the coronary artery can be found, but the monitor in the intensive care unit clearly records acute ischemia. In such cases we speak of "spasms" of the vessels, but are no better able to explain their etiology than in those rare cases of "sympathetic" death, when sudden death occurs on hearing bad news or following bereavement.

To recapitulate, although the public speaks of a "coronary" (at best an inaccurate and slangy term), from the standpoint of the patient the essential feature is the presence or absence of a myocardial infarct. An infarct may occur without thrombosis, the lumen of the coronary artery being greatly narrowed by atherosclerotic thickening of the inner coat (intima), and the final obstruction produced occasionally by rupture of the soft atheromatous material into the lumen. Or thrombosis may occur without the production of an infarct, because the area of cardiac muscle is supplied with blood from one of the other coronary arteries (collateral circulation). It is

Fig. 13–12. This scheme illustrates the appearance of the chambers and wall thicknesses of a heart as determined by **echocardiography.** This should be compared with Figure 13–1 to show the dimensions of the chambers and their walls. The **echocardiogram** is used as a direct measurement of wall thickness and chamber size. LA is left atrium, LV left ventricle, PML posterior mitral leaflet, AML anterior mitral leaflet and IVS interventricular septum.

Table 13–2. Age-Adjusted Death Rates by Cause in the United States, 1968 and 1973

| | RATES PER 100,000 POPULATION | | |
CAUSE OF DEATH	1968	1973	PERCENTAGE OF CHANGE
All deaths	743.8	692.9	− 6.8
All cardiovascular diseases	372.1	336.6	− 9.5
Ischemic heart disease	241.6	218.9	− 9.4
Cerebrovascular disease	71.3	63.7	−10.7
Hypertensive disease	9.5	6.3	−33.7
Rheumatic heart disease	7.2	5.4	−25.0
Congenital heart disease	3.7	3.4	− 8.1
Other cardiovascular disease	38.9	38.9	0.0
All other diseases	371.7	356.3	− 4.1

(Source: The National Heart and Lung Institute, Bethesda, Md., from unpublished data from the National Center for Health Science.)

the infarct of the heart muscle, not the thrombosis of the coronary artery, that produces the symptoms and distress from which the patient suffers. The infarct is a soft, yellow area of dead muscle in the wall of the left ventricle, varying greatly in size (Fig. 13–13). The softness of the dead tissue makes it a weak spot in the wall of the ventricle which may rupture during the first week.

In myocardial infarction, enzymes are liberated from the dying cells and pass into the blood. Both the CPK and SGOT levels may rise from 2 to 20 times the normal within 24 hours of an infarction, not returning to normal for 3 to 6 days. The level of CPK is more specific for muscle damage—there are specific muscle isozymes that can be tested for—and rises more rapidly than transaminase; CPK levels also fall more quickly. In response to necrosis, the white blood cell count will rise (leukocytosis) as will the body temperature (fever), and we may be able to detect changes in the cellular function of the muscle by changes in the wave of repolarization (EKG). Today, radioisotope scans may be used to

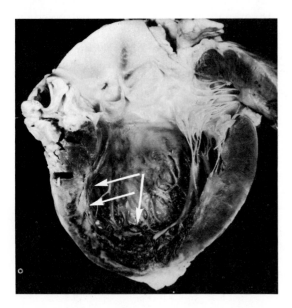

Fig. 13–13. This photograph of the inside of a left ventricle of a recently infarcted heart shows a dilated chamber with a massive infarction. The variegated appearance of the ventricular myocardium at the arrows on the left shows the hemorrhage and necrosis. The arrow at the right shows mural thrombus material. (McGill University, Department of Pathology Museum.)

show the infarct in a questionable case. Ancillary methods to support the diagnosis are determinations of the central venous pressure and the pulmonary wedge pressure by catheters that demonstrate the loss of functional capability of the ventricular muscle.

The prognosis in coronary artery occlusion varies greatly, depending on the functional importance of the artery that is blocked, the extent of the damage to the heart muscle, and the question of collateral circulation. The annual mortality rate of patients with disease of 1 coronary artery is 2.2%; with two-vessel disease it is 6.8%; and with three-vessel disease it is 11.4% per year. Patients with left main artery disease have the same life expectancy as those with three-vessel disease. The patient may die instantaneously; this, indeed, is the most classical cause of sudden death. However, if the heart survives the shock, as is frequently the case, a collateral circulation is in time established. When this occurs, the patient may make a reasonably satisfactory recovery. The recent development of cardiopulmonary resuscitation methodology, which is being taught at every level, and the availability of emergency mobile resuscitation equipment, all leading to intensive care units, is changing the pattern of survival from acute infarctions (Fig. 13–14). The immediate mortality of coronary artery thrombosis is believed to be around 10%.

Considerable emphasis today is placed on early support and treatment of the patient with acute myocardial infarction. If he can be brought to an intensive care unit alive within the first hour, his chances of survival are greatly improved over 5 years ago, because of modern pharmacotherapy with drugs such as propranolol and lidocaine. If the patient survives the attack, the infarcted area needs at least 6 weeks to become strengthened by scar tissue. The patient should therefore be kept at rest for this period. Once the infarct has healed, the patient may live for 15 to 20 years in good health.

Recently, it has become possible to identify as the principal cause of death 2 major, different types of pathophysiology. Ventricular fibrillation is the first and most common. This process has been managed increasingly suc-

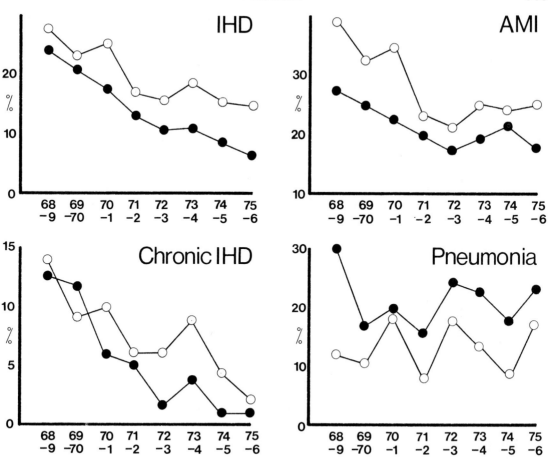

Fig. 13–14. These graphs show the decreasing mortality from ischemic heart disease (IHD), acute myocardial infarction (AMI), and chronic ischemic heart disease, as compared with pneumonia. Clearly, there has been a remarkable decline in mortality from ischemic heart disease and from chronic ischemic heart disease. The dark dots represent the female population and the light circles, the male. (From Craig, I. H., et al.: Changing mortality from ischemic heart disease and acute myocardial infarction. Med. J. Aust., 2:463, 1978.)

Fig. 13–15. This scheme illustrates the outcome at the present time, following a myocardial infarct. The rate of recovery of 85% of afflicted persons as a result of early and effective treatment, which is based largely on the widespread use of cardiopulmonary resuscitation and on rapid hospital support, represents a radical change from 10 years ago, when as many as 60% of the patients with an infarct died before reaching a hospital. (From Robbins, S., and Angell, M.: *Basic Pathology.* Philadelphia, W. B. Saunders, 1976.)

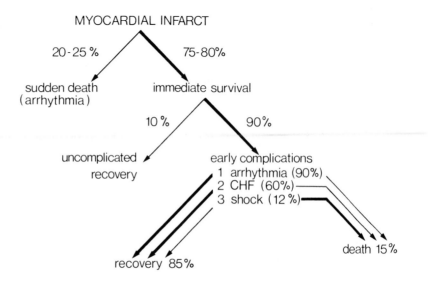

cessfully with electrical shock and drugs such as lidocaine, which decreases the irritability of the ischemic muscle. In-hospital deaths from acute fibrillation used to account for 30% of cardiovascular deaths; this figure has been halved by recognizing that arrhythmias occur most commonly soon after symptoms are present. The greatest success in managing heart disease is the salvage of 65% of male patients who used to die within the first hour of symptoms. Today, up to 85% of first-attack patients seen within the first 30 minutes leave the hospital alive (Fig. 13–15). The second type of pathophysiology is represented by patients with significant pump failure. These persons are managed better now with diuretics, vasodilator agents, inotropic drugs, and pacemakers.

Attempts have been made to categorize and to classify heart failure in order to assess the effectiveness of different management protocols, as shown in Table 13–3.

In angina pectoris, which refers to pain in the chest due to relative ischemia, the patient should be advised to live within his exercise tolerance, i.e., he should do no more activity than can be performed without production of anginal pain. The use of nitroglycerin may give relief to the anginal pain at the time of its occurrence.

More attention should be paid to decreasing the risk factors in coronary artery disease. In addition, diabetes mellitus, overweight, smoking, a sedentary life, high serum lipids, and hypertension all materially increase a person's predisposition to coronary artery thrombosis.

Table 13–3.   Classes of Heart Failure

		HOSPITAL MORTALITY
Class I.	No pulmonary edema	0.5%
Class II.	Moderate failure: rales, S3 gallop, tachypnea, right heart failure, jugular venous distension	10 to 20%
Class III.	Severe pulmonary edema	35 to 45%
Class IV.	Shock with systolic pressure less than 90 mm, peripheral constriction, cyanosis, mental confusion, decreased urine output	85 to 95%

Table 13–4.   Classic Complications of Myocardial Infarct

Arrhythmias
Rupture
Mural thrombus
Embolism
Aneurysm
Intractable failure

Apart from "sudden death," the complications of an infarct include chronic heart failure, about which more will be said later. During the time when the necrotic muscle is weakest, a rupture may occur. Frequently, this is accompanied by hemorrhage into the pericardial space (tamponade), which interferes with cardiac filling and causes death. Sometimes the necrotic area is replaced by scar that does not contract, and a bulge or aneurysm of the ventricle is formed. In this area, or in any area where the endocardium has been injured, thrombus material may accumulate. This thrombus on the wall of a ventricle (mural thrombus) may then break off and embolize to remote organs such as brain, kidney, or extremities, resulting in loss of function. But the most common complication of these is heart failure, which has been increasingly well managed with new drugs. Finally, of course, 1 infarction may be followed by another, the risk of which is always enhanced in someone who has experienced a first infarction. Table 13–4 shows the classic complications of infarction, and Table 13–5 lists the classic anatomic and histologic changes found at intervals after the acute event has taken place. These patterns seem to be changing today as newer ways of managing infarcts are used (vasodilators, *beta* blocking drugs, and pacemakers).

To summarize, the **complications of an infarct include arrhythmia, shock, rupture, tamponade, aneurysm, thrombus, embolism, and chronic heart failure.**

HYPERTENSIVE HEART DISEASE

If the heart has to work for years against a greatly increased resistance in the form of high blood pressure, it will gradually become exhausted and fail. The strain falls

Table 13–5. Sequence of Changes in Myocardial Infarction

TIME	GROSS CHANGES	LIGHT MICROSCOPE	HISTOCHEMISTRY	ELECTRON MICROSCOPE
0 to 2 hours	None	?Waviness of fibers at border. Contraction bands and wavy lines	↓ Glutaminase I and β-hydroxybutyrate dehydrogenase; ↓ K and ↑ Na⁺ and Ca⁺⁺	Mitochondrial swelling and granules; distortion of cristae
4 to 12 hours	Swollen area	Beginning coagulation; edema; hemorrhage; marginal neutrophils	Succinic dehydrogenase negative	Relaxation of myofibrils (prominent I-bands); aggregation and margination of nuclear chromatin
18 to 24 hours	Pallor	Continuing coagulation (pyknosis of nuclei; shrunken eosinophilic cytoplasm)	Succinic dehydrogenase negative	
24 to 48 hours	Pallor, sometimes hyperemia	Total coagulative necrosis with loss of nuclei and striations; heavy interstitial infiltrate of neutrophils and mononuclear leukocytes	Succinic dehydrogenase negative	
2 to 4 days	Hyperemic border; central yellow-brown softening; pericarditis (11%)	Beginning fatty change		
10 days	Maximally yellow and soft; beginning scarring at margins	Beginning fibrosis		
Seventh week	Scarring complete	Collagenization		

(From Robbins, S. L., and Angell, M.: *Basic Pathology*, 2nd Ed. Philadelphia, W. B. Saunders, 1976.)

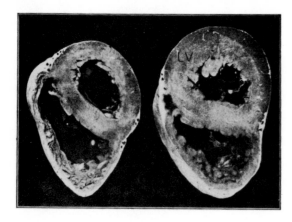

Fig. 13–16. This photograph shows, on the right, marked concentric left ventricular hypertrophy compared with a normal left ventricle on the left. (McGill University, Department of Pathology Museum.)

principally on the left ventricle, and in a while, the wall of this ventricle becomes thicker, or hypertrophied (Fig. 13–16), so as to be able to overcome the increased resistance. When the heart is grasped at post mortem examination, it feels like a closed fist. Finally, however, its power is lost, the heart fails, the ventricle becomes dilated, and the end picture is much like that of other forms of heart failure. This condition is known as hypertensive heart disease. The symptoms are similar to those of heart failure from other causes, such as valvular disease and coronary artery disease. It must be pointed out, however, that many persons with hypertension live vigorous lives for decades without developing signs of heart failure. Such persons would be happier if they were ignorant of their high blood pressure. There is some evidence, however, that the treatment of hypertension is changing the pattern of this disease, but the evidence is not overwhelming.

It should be stated here that there is an important difference between hypertension with a slightly elevated systolic pressure and a diastolic of 95 mm Hg and a diastolic pressure of over 120 mm Hg which represents a medical emergency. All hypertension is not the same.

The principal causes and varieties of hypertension are discussed in the next chapter. In the most common form, known as essential hypertension, the small arteries throughout the body are contracted with narrowing of their lumen, and this leads to increased peripheral resistance to the blood flow, so that the diastolic pressure of the blood in the large arteries rises. The patient with hypertension may not die of heart failure, but rather as the result of the rupture of a blood vessel in the brain (cerebral hemorrhage). The narrowing of the small arteries to the kidneys may lead to dysfunction of these organs, and the patient may die of renal failure. Death in hypertension may therefore be due to disease of the heart, the brain, or the kidneys.

CONGENITAL HEART DISEASE

Heart disease may be congenital rather than acquired. A child is born with cardiac defects due to failure in the process of development. One important predisposing cause is German measles in the mother during the first 3 months of pregnancy. This condition has assumed practical importance, because surgical operations are available for the treatment of several of these defects. Many congenital abnormalities of the heart may occur, some rare, others incompatible with life. Table 13–6 shows the relative frequency of each of the more important congenital anomalies. Those amenable to current surgical treatment will be described.

The key to most of the defects lies in variations in the formation of the septum, which divides the heart into a right and a left side. The most important feature of congenital heart disease is the possibility of a mixing of the blood in the systemic and pulmonary circulations as the result of a shunt. Three common causes of shunts are (1) atrial septal defect (Fig. 13–17), (2) ventricular septal defect (Fig. 13–18A,B), and (3) patent ductus arteriosus (Fig. 13–19). In all of these defects, the lungs become overloaded with blood. Another distinction may be made between cases with cyanosis and those without cyanosis. Cyanosis (a bluish color due to inadequate oxygen saturation of the arterial blood) is caused by a right-to-left venous-arterial shunt, because poorly oxygenated venous blood then enters the systemic circulation.

Congenital defects also commonly predis-

Table 13–6.   Common Congenital Heart Diseases

ANOMALY	MALE TO FEMALE RATIO	DEFINITION	% OF INCIDENCE OF CHD IN INFANTS	DISORDERS ASSOCIATED WITH INCREASED INCIDENCE
Ventricular septal defect	1:1	Abnormal opening between the ventricles	28.3	Down's syndrome
Patent ductus arteriosus	1:3	Persistence of the fetal connection between the aorta and pulmonary artery	12.5	Rubella syndrome
Atrial septal defect	1:3	Abnormal opening between the atria	9.7	Down's syndrome
Coarctation of the aorta	4:1	Stricture in the thoracic aorta	8.8	Turner's syndrome
Tetralogy of Fallot	1:1	Ventricular septal defect, pulmonic stenosis with right ventricular hypertrophy and aorta overriding the ventricular septum	7.0	Thalidomide ingestion

(Adapted from Whaley, L. F.: *Understanding Inherited Disorders*. St. Louis, C. V. Mosby, 1974.)

pose a patient to endocardial infections with bacteria for reasons that remain obscure. Sometimes the patient with congenital heart disease dies of bacterial endocarditis.

At least 90% of the patients with congenital disease of the heart and great vessels fall into 1 of 4 groups. These are, in their order of frequency, although not in their order of discussion: (1) septal defects, (2) coarctation of the aorta, (3) patent ductus arteriosus, and (4) the tetralogy of Fallot. All of these are treatable by surgery.

Septal Defects. Atrial septal defects may be trivial or serious. Patency of the foramen ovale, the opening in the septum between the 2 atria that is normally present at birth, is the most common and the least important of congenital cardiac anomalies. As the opening is small and oblique, little blood usually passes from 1 side to the other. A true septal defect due to failure of development is another matter. The opening may be large, and blood passes readily from the left to the right side where the pressure is lower, so that both the right atrium and the right ventricle become greatly dilated and hypertrophied. There is no cyanosis until cardiac failure sets in; the patient may live from 30 to 50 years.

Ventricular septal defects may be uncomplicated by other cardiac anomalies. The opening is usually small, situated in the membranous part of the septum, and causes little disturbance. Here again cyanosis will be absent except as a terminal phenomenon. Bacterial endocarditis, however, occurs at the margin of the opening in many cases, so that surgical closure of the defect is appropriate. When the defect is small, the characteristic physical sign is a loud systolic murmur. Defects smaller than 5 mm are of little physiologic significance.

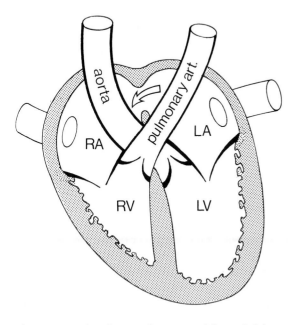

Fig. 13–17. This diagram shows an atrial septal defect. Since pressure in the left atrium is higher than in the right, blood is shunted into the right atrium. This creates extra work for the right side of the heart, resulting in right atrial and ventricular hypertrophy.

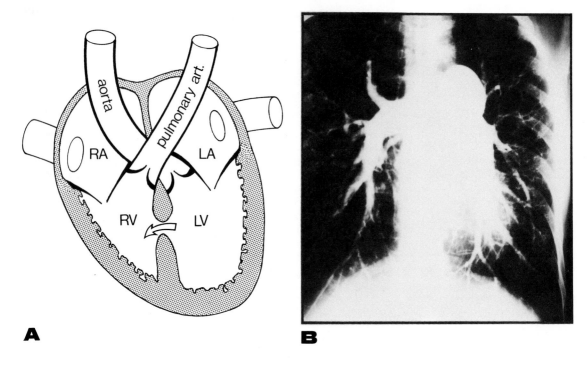

A   **B**

Fig. 13–18. *A,* This figure shows a defect in the ventricular septum. Blood is shunted into the right ventricle, which results in right ventricular hypertrophy and in increased pulmonary blood flow. Life expectancy depends on the size of the defect. *B,* This arteriogram shows a remarkably enlarged pulmonary artery with all of its branches dilated.

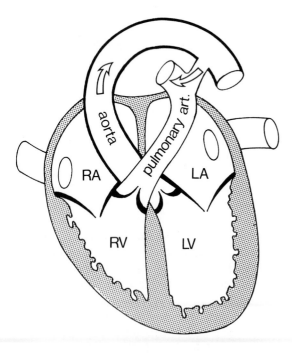

Fig. 13–19. Patent ductus arteriosus. Shunting of blood from the aorta into the pulmonary artery results in right ventricular hypertrophy and in increased blood flow and pressure in the pulmonary arterial system.

Tetralogy of Fallot. This is a most important congenital lesion of the heart, and the most common of the lesions causing cyanosis, for reasons that will soon become obvious. The most significant physiologic part of this condition is pulmonary valve stenosis. The pulmonary valve is narrowed, so that the blood is unable to pass in sufficient quantity from the right ventricle to the lungs. Fallot described 3 other changes in addition to the pulmonary stenosis. (1) The aorta, which normally receives blood only from the left ventricle, overrides the right ventricle. (2) There is incomplete closure of the interventricular septum (a high septal defect exists). (3) As a result of the increased resistance to outflow, the right ventricle becomes hypertrophied. So the 4 defects that constitute the tetralogy are: pulmonic stenosis, ventricular septal defect, overriding aorta, and right ventricular hypertrophy (Fig. 13–20). The tetralogy of Fallot is the most common cause of the condition known as the "blue baby," a name given because of the extreme degree of cyanosis, the blue color

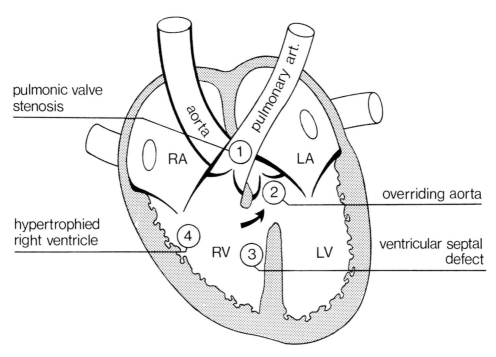

Fig. 13–20. This drawing shows the anatomical anomalies of the Tetralogy of Fallot. They are pulmonary valvular stenosis, which leads to right ventricular hypertrophy, a ventricular septal defect, and an overriding aorta. The principal physiologic problem is the failure of blood to flow through the lungs for oxygenation, which leads to the classic "blue baby."

being most marked on the lips, ears, cheeks, and hands. The principle of the operation is to bypass the obstruction at the opening of the pulmonary artery. This is done by anastomosing (connecting) the left subclavian artery, a branch of the aorta, to the pulmonary artery beyond the obstruction, so that the blood now reaches the lungs, although from the left ventricle instead of from the right. Reference to Figure 13–20 may make the matter clearer, although the branches of the aorta are not shown in the diagram. The improvement in the child's condition is immediate and dramatic, the cyanosis and shortness of breath often being improved by the time the patient is returned to bed from the operating room.

Patent Ductus Arteriosus. The ductus arteriosus is a short vessel that passes from the pulmonary artery to the aorta. During intrauterine life, the blood from the right side of the heart passes along this channel into the aorta without passing through the lungs, as these organs are not used for respiration while the child is still *in utero*. The ductus should become closed a few weeks after birth. It may, however, remain open or patent. Thus

the blood continues to flow from the aorta into the pulmonary artery because the pressure is higher in the former than in the latter. Blood therefore receives sufficient oxygen from the lungs, and there is no cyanosis except in cases complicated by other congenital defects. Although the condition is compatible with a long and active life, in most cases life expectancy is considerably shortened. This is because the increased flow and increased pressure in the pulmonary arterial system eventually causes a thickening of the walls of the pulmonary arterioles and raises the pulmonary arterial pressure. In turn, the right ventricle must do more work, and, as the resistance increases, the right ventricle may fail. Another danger is the development of bacterial endocarditis at either end of the ductus. The treatment is surgical division of the ductus, a relatively simple operation.

Coarctation of the Aorta. This condition is a narrowing of the aorta (Latin *coarctare*, to press together) in the region where it is joined by the ductus. It is usually beyond the origin of the large arteries to the head and arms, so that there is an abundant flow of blood to

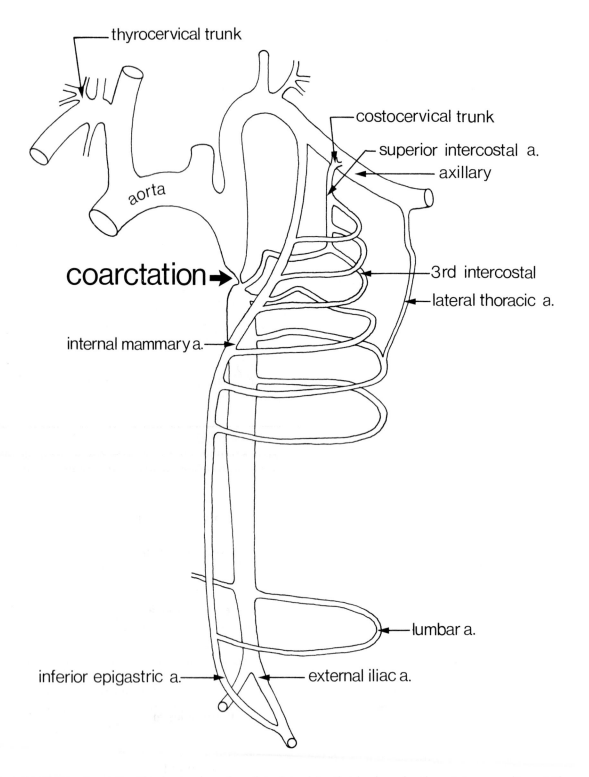

thyrocervical trunk

costocervical trunk

superior intercostal a.

axillary

aorta

coarctation→

3rd intercostal

lateral thoracic a.

internal mammary a.

lumbar a.

inferior epigastric a.

external iliac a.

Fig. 13–21. Coarctation. This drawing shows the collateral circulation that develops when the aorta is narrowed (arrow). The collateral circulation causes the intercostal arteries to become enlarged. They in turn enlarge the inferior surface of the ribs, which can be visualized on routine chest films. Coarctation is characterized by hypertension proximal to the narrowing and hypotension (absent pedal pulses) distal to the narrowed segment.

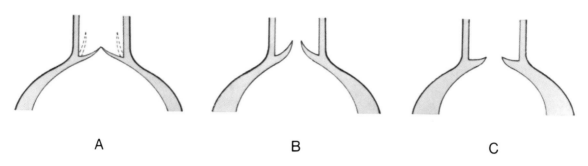

A   B   C

Fig. 13–22. *A,* This drawing shows the appearance of a normal valve, which may open widely or close completely. *B,* This valve is unable to open completely, and is considered stenotic. *C,* This valve is unable to close and is considered insufficient.

these parts and the blood pressure in the arm is high. Little blood passes through the narrowed aorta to the abdomen and legs, where the blood pressure is low, and the pulse can hardly be felt. Usually enough blood manages to bypass the obstruction through abundant collateral vessels that open up (Fig. 13–21). Recognition of this collateral circulation by means of radiography greatly assists the physician in making a correct diagnosis. The surgical treatment consists of clamping the aorta above and below the obstruction, excising the narrowed segment, and sewing the divided ends of the aorta together. This dramatic operation is usually attended with complete success.

VALVULAR DISEASE

Although this form of heart disease used to be a sentence of limited life, since the early 1950's, with the development of intrathoracic surgery and techniques for intracardiac operative procedures, the valvular heart diseases have been operated on with increasing success. Nowhere is the illustration clearer that progress in medicine depends on technical developments as much as on the particular skill of a single physician. Extracorporeal circulation machines, cardioplegic drugs, which bring the heart to a standstill, and the evolution of new valvular prostheses have effected a revolution in the management of these disorders. We have already seen that there are 4 valves in the heart, 2 on the left side and 2 on the right. We shall confine our attention to the valves on the left side, namely the mitral and

the aortic. Either of these may be too narrow (stenosed) or too wide (insufficient or incompetent) (Fig. 13–22). There are thus 4 possibilities.

Mitral Stenosis. Most, if not all, cases of mitral stenosis are rheumatic in origin. The condition is much more common in women than in men. The valve opening may be a mere buttonhole, which will hardly admit the tip of the little finger (Fig. 13–23), whereas the normal opening should admit 2 fingers with ease. The valve looks like a deep funnel, the walls of which are formed by the fused cusps. The blood rushing through this rigid funnel on its way from the left atrium to the ventricle causes a vibration of its walls, which is responsible for the characteristic diastolic murmur heard and the thrill felt. If the reader

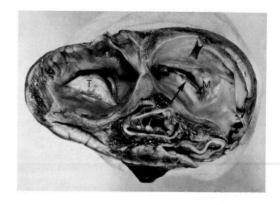

Fig. 13–23. This photograph shows the mitral valve as seen from above the tricuspid valve at T, the aortic valve at A, and the mitral valve at M. The arrow shows the free margin of this fish-mouth stenotic valve, which is unable to open adequately. (McGill University, Department of Pathology Museum.)

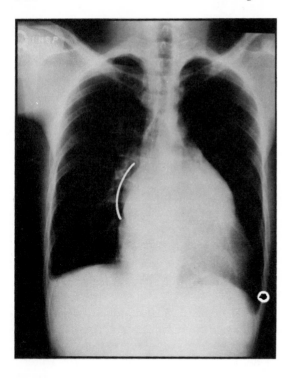

Fig. 13–24. This posteroanterior film of the chest shows the typical configuration of the heart in mitral valvular disease, in which there is both stenosis and insufficiency of the mitral valve. The prominent finding at the white line is the presence of an enlarged left atrium. The cardiac silhouette is of a globular shape, reflecting the hypertrophy of the right heart which may have a ventricular wall as thick as the normal left ventricle.

will pause to think of the anatomy of the heart and of the direction of the blood flow, he will not need to be told that, owing to the obstruction, the left atrium and eventually, the right side of the heart become greatly dilated (Fig. 13–24). A thrombus may form in the dilated left atrium, and this may become detached and give rise to cerebral embolism. The general effects of mitral stenosis are those of chronic venous congestion.

The stenosis can now be treated surgically by valvotomy and reconstruction of the valve or by replacement with an artificial valve. Figure 13–25 shows two x-ray studies of the chest of a patient whose diseased mitral valve has been replaced by a Starr-Edwards ball-in-cage prosthesis. The ball is a Silastic, long-lasting structure kept in an open or shut position by 3 metal struts, as shown in the accompanying photograph. The two x-ray studies

show the ball's position in systole and diastole. In assessing the value or desirability of the operation, it must be remembered that the condition is not necessarily progressive, and that well over 50% of the patients survive without operation for 20 years or more, many showing little change in their clinical condition.

Mitral Insufficiency. This is the least well defined of the 4 principal valvular lesions. Incompetence is caused by sclerosis and contraction of the cusps or by dilatation of the valve ring. One common cause is rheumatic endocarditis, but bacterial endocarditis may also cause incompetence. Although it is convenient and appropriate to speak of stenosis or incompetence as if they were discrete and specific entities, and whereas it is important to learn the signs and symptoms of these particular forms of valvular disease, it is also true that even if the physiologic lesion is predominantly stenotic, there is usually a measure of incompetence, and if the physiologic abnormality is predominantly insufficiency, there is some measure of stenosis.

Aortic Stenosis. Pure aortic stenosis usually occurs in men over 50 years of age, whereas mitral valve stenosis is commoner in women at an earlier age. The stenosis is of the calcified nodular type, best called calcific aortic stenosis. The cusps adhere together to form a kind of diaphragm as in mitral stenosis, but the most striking feature is the presence of warty calcified masses, which may cover the cusps (Fig. 13–26). The entire valve is incredibly hard and rigid. This stenosis has 3 accepted causes: it may be rheumatic in origin, it may occur on congenital bicuspid valves, or it may be an expression of atherosclerosis without known contributing factors. Calcific aortic stenosis is certainly being encountered more frequently than formerly. The heart shows a perfect example of pure or concentric hypertrophy of the left ventricle (Fig. 13–27A,B). The most characteristic physical sign is a rough rasping systolic murmur and thrill at the aortic area. Cardiac surgery offers relief with a reasonable degree of safety. The radiologic demonstration of calcification in the area of the aortic valve may serve to confirm the diagnosis. It must be noted that calcific aortic stenosis is often well tolerated

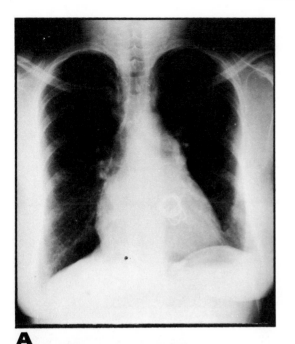

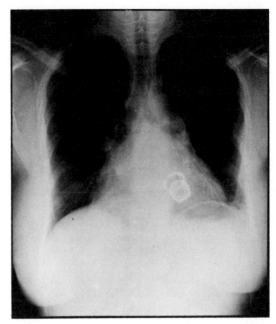

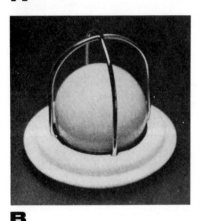

Fig. 13–25. *A,* These two chest roentgenograms show an artificial (Starr-Edwards) ball-in-cage mitral valve. The roentgenogram on the left shows the ball of the valve closing the orifice in left ventricular systole. On the right, the ball or poppet is in the cage and the left ventricle is filling. *B,* A Starr-Edwards prosthetic mitral valve.

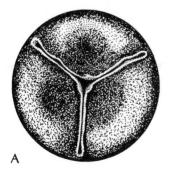

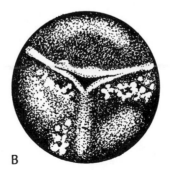

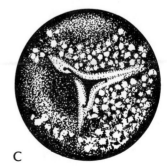

Fig. 13–26. These drawings show the appearance of the aortic valve, normal in the left area, a severly stenotic valve with only two cusps on the middle, and an even more severely stenotic atherosclerotic valve in the right view.

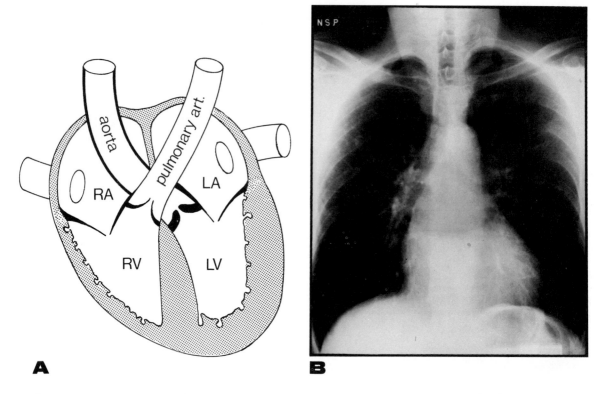

Fig. 13–27.   *A,* Aortic stenosis and resulting left ventricular hypertrophy. *B,* This posteroanterior chest film shows a prominent, straight left cardiac silhouette, which is usually seen in left ventricular hypertrophy.

into old age, even after evidence of severe obstruction to the aortic outflow has been noted, but once heart failure occurs, the prognosis is poor.

Aortic Insufficiency. Insufficiency or incompetence of the aortic valve may be due to endocarditis of the valve cusps or to dilatation of the aorta and the aortic ring. The former may be caused by rheumatic endocarditis or by bacterial endocarditis. The latter used to be a common result of syphilitic aortitis before the days of modern treatment of syphilis. It was the syphilitic form that used to give the classic picture of the disease, which was well known to French poets, but this is now becoming rare.

In this condition, the heart is all left ventricle, which is greatly hypertrophied as well as dilated, on account of the regurgitant flow of blood from the aorta into the ventricle through the incompetent valve during systole (from the dilated ventricle), and of too little blood during diastole (owing to the backward

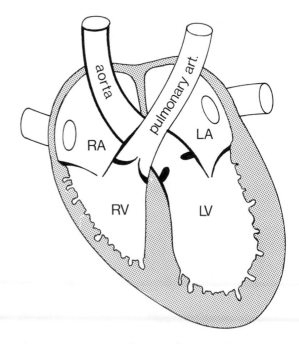

Fig. 13–28.   Aortic insufficiency. The aortic valve is incompetent. Blood flows back into the left ventricle in time and causes it to dilate and to become hypertrophied.

flow) (Fig. 13–28). This process accounts for the "water-hammer pulse" of leaping character felt at the wrist. The loud diastolic murmur, which is the most characteristic physical sign, is due to the rush of blood back into the ventricle during diastole.

RHEUMATIC HEART DISEASE

This disease is not nearly so common today as it used to be. The simple reason may be that its origin as a reaction to the antigens of a streptococcal sore throat has been modified by the frequent and extraordinary use of antibiotics. Rheumatic heart disease is attributed to an inflammatory process with an immunologic etiology, as demonstrated by the rise in titer of antistreptolysin antibodies (antibodies to group A hemolytic streptococci) that occurs about 3 weeks after a streptococcal sore throat. At this time, all parts of the heart may be inflamed in a pancarditis.

As a result, the valves (commonly the mitral) become inflamed, and from the blood flowing over them, blood platelets and fibrin are deposited on them. These deposits form little nodules called vegetations, each about the size of a pin's head, which form a row along the margin of the cusps. The inflamed cusps, normally almost as thin as gossamer, become markedly thickened, and tend to adhere to one another, just as do inflamed loops of bowel when brought in contact. As the inflammation subsides, fibrous tissue takes the place of the inflammatory exudate, and this slowly contracts, causing retraction of the cusps. This process takes months or years.

The effect of all this on the function and use of the valve may be 1 of 2 kinds, although often both result. Owing to the adhesions between the thickened cusps, they are unable to open properly when the blood flows through the valvular opening, so that this opening becomes permanently narrowed (stenosis). This narrowing may become so extreme that finally the opening is no larger than a buttonhole, whereas normally it should admit 2 fingers. The mitral valve is the common site of rheumatic endocarditis, and mitral stenosis is one of the most serious forms of heart disease, for not enough blood can flow from the left atrium into the left ventricle, and so is dammed back first in the lungs, then in the right side of the heart, and finally in the veins of the body (Fig. 13–29A,B). The left atrium may become greatly dilated behind the obstruction (Fig. 13–30). Mitral stenosis is 3 times more common than all other rheumatic heart lesions. The second result is incompetence of the valve. Here the retraction of the cusps is much more marked than their self-adhesion. The result is that the cusps are unable to meet when the valve tries to close, and the blood escapes back from the ventricle into the atrium in the case of the mitral valve, and from the aorta into the ventricle in the case of the aortic valve.

It is important to realize that a person with chronic valvular disease of the heart is not necessarily an invalid, nor should such a person be encouraged to consider himself to be as one. The evidence of a valvular lesion is a murmur heard by the stethoscope over the heart, but a person with a cardiac murmur may lead a full and vigorous life. If the heart muscle is healthy, it is able to compensate for the valvular lesion, unless the latter is marked and progressive. Today, thoracic surgery offers valve replacements with ingenious plastic and metal devices that function as well as normal valves, and hundreds of patients have their symptoms relieved by surgical intervention.

In addition to causing inflammation of the valves, rheumatic fever also damages the heart muscle and pericardium. Small areas of inflammation and destruction, known as Aschoff bodies or nodules, are scattered through the muscle, and later these become converted into scar tissue. Such a scarred myocardium cannot fail to be weakened. On account of the damage to the wall of the atrium, the peculiar condition known as atrial fibrillation is apt to develop, especially in mitral stenosis. Normally the atria beat at the same rate as the ventricles; this is natural, because normally the wave of muscular contraction starts in the atria and passes on to the ventricles; it is the beat of the ventricles that produces the pulse. In atrial fibrillation, the atria no longer contract in a regular manner; they seem to be trembling instead of contracting. The result is that the ventricles contract in a rapid and ir-

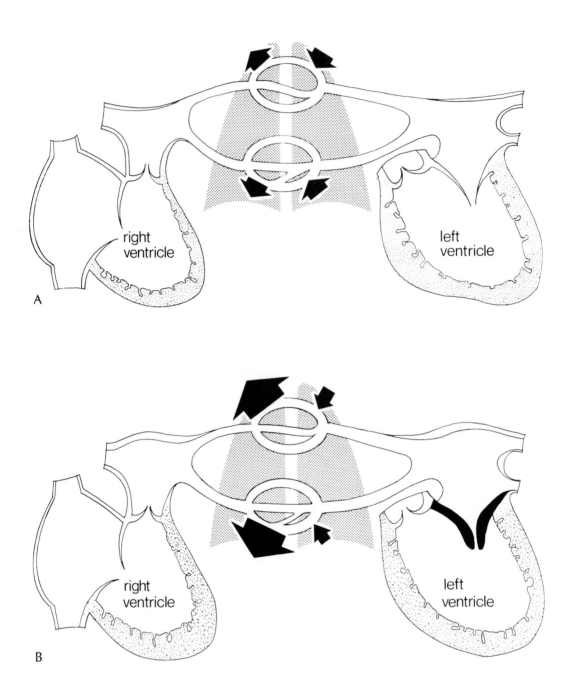

Fig. 13–29. A illustrates schematically the appearance of a normal right ventricle, pulmonary vascular bed, left ventricle, and mitral valve. The arrows indicate the traditional balance in the Starling hypothesis. B shows the effect of mitral valve stenosis on the pulmonary vascular bed; the large black arrows represent the extravasation of fluid into the interstitial space, which is greater because of the increased hydrostatic pressure due to the failure to empty the left atrium. This pulmonary edema then causes the patient to feel short of breath. The right ventricle is shown as hypertrophied in this drawing; it is a compensatory hypertrophy. (From Edwards, J.: Pathology of chronic pulmonary hypertension. Pathol. Annu., 9:1, 1974.)

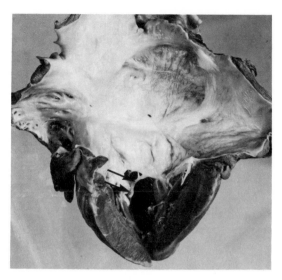

Fig. 13–30. This photograph of the left atrium, mitral valve, and left ventricle shows the remarkable dilatation and hypertrophy of the left atrium in a representative case of prolonged mitral stenosis. The thickened, shortened, chordae tendinae so typical of rheumatic heart disease are shown at the arrow. (McGill University, Department of Pathology Museum.)

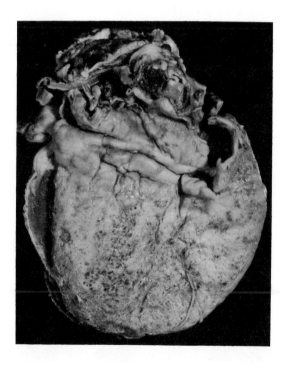

Fig. 13–31. This photograph of the epicardial surface of the heart shows the ragged fibrinous adhesions which have been described as bread and butter, that may be seen in chronic uremic disease, in persistent rheumatic injury, or even in a purulent pericarditis. (McGill University, Department of Pathology Museum.)

regular manner, this irregularity being reflected in marked irregularity of the pulse. The ventricles tend to become exhausted, with resulting heart failure, the symptoms of which are palpitation and dyspnea. The administration of drugs prevents the irregular impulses from the atria from reaching the ventricles, which then commence to beat in a much slower and more regular manner, with immediate relief to the patient.

The pericardium also becomes inflamed, a condition known as pericarditis (Fig. 13–31), and the 2 inflamed layers of pericardium may stick together and form adhesions that may seriously hinder the heart's action. The truth of the remark made in the general discussion of rheumatic fever will now be evident, that it is a disease that licks the joints but bites the heart, for the patient is left with permanent lesions that may cripple his heart to the day of his death, although the day may be far removed. "The moving finger writes, and having writ moves on."

INFECTIOUS ENDOCARDITIS

In the continually changing picture of disease, it would be difficult to name a condition that has altered its appearance more completely in recent years than infectious endocarditis. It used to be a malady in which the heart beat a muffled march to the grave, in quick time in the acute form, with a slower but just as deadly rhythm in the subacute variety. Now, thanks to antibiotics, it has become a curable disease when treated early. This, indeed, is one of the great triumphs of antibiotic chemotherapy and cardiovascular surgery. A sharp distinction has been drawn in the past between the acute and subacute forms of infectious endocarditis. The importance of this distinction has faded, and more emphasis is laid on the infecting agent and on whether the patient can have the infected valve replaced by a prosthesis. It is, however, still convenient to speak of acute and subacute varieties.

Subacute Bacterial Endocarditis. This form of endocarditis is much less common than the rheumatic form, but it used to be much more fatal. Until the introduction of antibiotic therapy, the mortality was practically 100%.

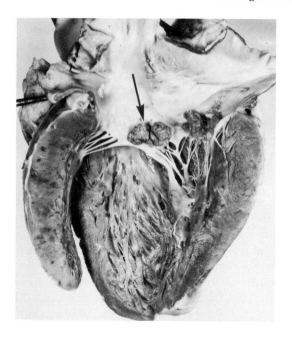

Fig. 13-32. This photograph shows large vegetations attached to the mitral valve at the arrow. These are present in endocarditis. (McGill University, Department of Pathology Museum.)

The disease used to run its course in a number of months, sometimes a year. It is commonly caused by a variety of nonhemolytic streptococcus *(Streptococcus viridans).* One peculiarity is that the disease is usually superimposed on an old rheumatic endocarditis, healthy valves being seldom affected. The bacterial colonies are called vegetations and are large and extremely friable (Fig. 13–32). The cusps of the valve are sometimes destroyed. The vegetations are teeming with streptococci, and these are discharged into the blood stream where they can be detected by blood culture. This procedure is of great value in the diagnosis of difficult or suspected cases.

The most striking feature of the disease is the formation of large numbers of emboli due to the breaking off of fragments of the friable vegetations. These sail off into the blood stream and come to rest in various organs, where the emboli give rise to characteristic symptoms of the disease. Some of the emboli are large, and if these lodge in the brain, they may cause paralysis or abscesses, whereas in the kidney they may cause blood to appear in

the urine. Sometimes they are minute, but if these tiny emboli should lodge in the smallest vessels of the skin, they will cause these vessels to rupture, with the formation of multiple pinpoint hemorrhages known as petechiae. Petechiae in the skin, blood in the urine, and streptococci in the blood culture, together with enlargement of the spleen and long-continued fever, are principal clinical features that point to the correct diagnosis. The low-grade fever combined with any known valvular heart lesion or heart murmurs should clinch the diagnosis.

Acute Infectious Endocarditis. This is a much rarer form of endocarditis caused by enormous numbers of pyogenic bacteria such as *Staphylococcus aureus* and *Streptococcus hemolyticus.* The cusps of the valves are rapidly destroyed (hence the term acute) (Fig. 13–33), and the patient used to die in less than 6 weeks without antibiotic therapy. Today, early surgical removal of the infected valve, together with antibiotic therapy, has improved the life expectancy of such patients.

Five types of disease of the heart have been outlined, together with the 4 principal valvular lesions. Practically nothing has been said about diseases of the myocardium, apart from the effect of coronary artery occlusion, nor about the pericardium, which may be involved in various forms of inflammation in addition to rheumatic pericarditis. Such discussions would be out of place in this *Intro-*

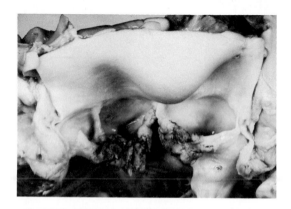

Fig. 13-33. This is a photograph of destructive bacterial endocarditis, destroying the noncoronary cusp of the aortic valve. This leads to aortic valve insufficiency and left ventricular failure. (McGill University, Department of Pathology Museum.)

duction. It may be mentioned, in addition, that tumors of the heart, both benign and malignant, do occur, but fortunately are rare.

CLINICAL PATTERNS OF HEART DISEASE

The chief symptoms of heart disease are pain, palpitation, and dyspnea or shortness of breath. Pain has already been discussed in connection with coronary artery occlusion. Palpitation, a condition in which the patient becomes aware of the forcible beating of the heart, may be a symptom either of valvular or myocardial disease. Frequently, however, it does not indicate any organic heart disease, but rather is caused by anxiety, too much stress (often associated with too much tea or coffee), or perhaps by such a disorder as hyperthyroidism. Disorders of rhythm may take the form of increased rate (tachycardia) or irregularity of rhythm, occasional beats being missed. Murmurs, which may be heard with the stethoscope, are caused by the blood leaking back through an incompetent valve or forcing its way through a stenosed one. Heart block is a condition in which the pulse rate drops to about one-half the normal, and is caused by scars due to coronary artery disease

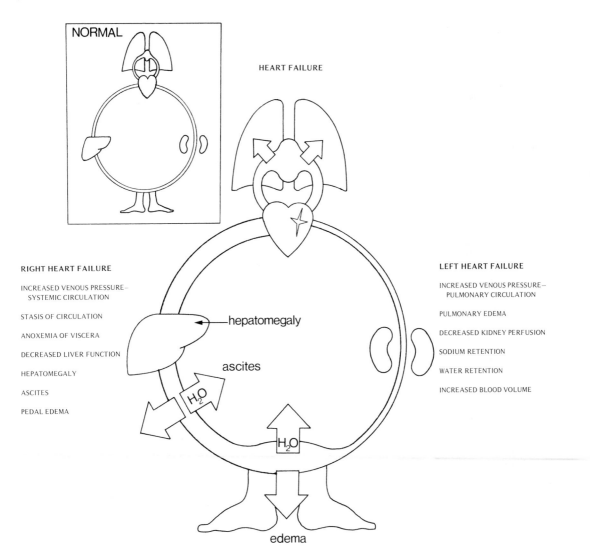

Fig. 13–34. This diagram illustrates end-stage congestive heart failure and many of its complications. The primary lesion is in the heart, whose ability to pump blood forward becomes severely compromised. This leads to venous congestion and to reduced arterial blood flow. The inset shows the *normal balanced circulation.*

interfering with the "conduction bundle," which carries the electric impulse necessary for muscular contraction from 1 part of the heart to the other.

Dyspnea is the most common symptom of heart failure. The shortness of breath is caused by the inability of the failing heart to move blood through the lungs. Fainting attacks (syncope) may occur in aortic valvular incompetence because part of the blood, instead of going to the brain, escapes back into the left ventricle. This causes cerebral ischemia, which is the essential cause of all fainting attacks. Congestive heart failure is a picture presented by patients, the right side of whose heart is becoming exhausted, and is particularly well seen in mitral stenosis. There is damming back of the blood in the veins that empty into the right atrium, so that the veins in the neck stand out prominently; the liver is enlarged and tender because the blood accumulates in its substance (Fig. 13–34). The lips, ears, and fingers are cyanosed or blue because of insufficient oxygenation of the blood flowing through them, for it is the presence of oxygen that imparts to the blood in the arteries its bright red color.

Edema is generally evidence of congestive heart failure, although it may also be caused by other conditions, such as kidney disease. In heart disease, it occurs because the hydrostatic pressure of the venous end of the capillary circulation is raised, and the interstitial fluid gradually increases in volume and collects in the tissues; it is most marked in the feet and legs, where it causes a swelling in which a depression can be made by steady pressure of the finger (pitting on pressure). The reason for this transudation of fluid from the blood vessels is partly the increased pressure in the microcirculation caused by the back pressure from the heart, and partly damage to the vessel walls with an increase of their permeability owing to an insufficient supply of the oxygen that is necessary for their own health.

Congenital heart disease has its own special symptoms. Cyanosis is the most characteristic of these symptoms, sometimes being present from the moment the blue baby makes its appearance in the world, but usually developing later. Dyspnea on exertion is equally common, but may range from the slightest to the most severe. Polycythemia (increased number of red blood cells), which is compensatory in nature, serves for a time to offset the deficiency in oxygen. Clubbing of the fingers, one of the most striking of the physical signs, is due to a disturbance of nutrition of the tissues that affects both the terminal phalanges and the nails, the latter being thickened and curved. Cerebral symptoms such as faintness, dizziness, and even syncope are frequent owing to the anoxia.

Perhaps the most important fact to remember is that the majority of people with structural heart disease are able to lead useful lives. The discovery that a cardiac murmur is present does not mean that the patient's whole mode of life has to be changed. Someone with valvular disease of the heart may live comfortably for many years due to the compensatory ability of the heart muscle.

Sometimes one can do little about the underlying heart disease, but the occurrence of the edema can be treated in most cases. The most important part of the treatment is the use of a diet that is low in salt. In heart failure, salt tends to accumulate in the body fluids. This concentration results in the retention of water and edema in various regions. Salt and water can also be eliminated from the body by the use of diuretics. After an episode of heart failure, the patient may again be able to resume activity, but may be instructed to limit exertion until he has acquired a tolerance for physical activity. This may be done with a supervised rehabilitation program. Education of the patient with heart disease as to the mode of life best suited to him is a most important item in the treatment. Too great solicitude can be as unfortunate as too great recklessness.

Finally, it must be remembered that no organ is influenced to so marked a degree by nervous stimuli and the emotions. The simple everyday words of our language testify to the truth of this statement. We say that the person is heavyhearted, hardhearted, heartless, good-hearted, that his heart aches with loneliness, flutters with alarm, or stops with fear. It is evident that many cardiac symptoms may have an emotional rather than an organic basis, and to confuse one with the other is a

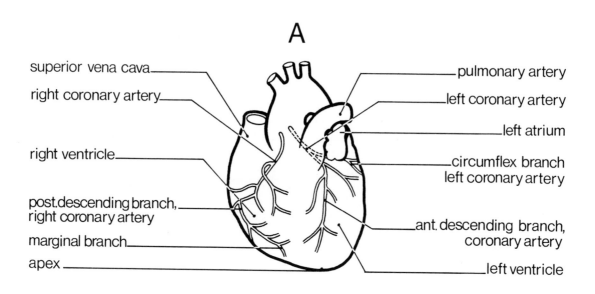

A

superior vena cava ——
right coronary artery ——

right ventricle ——

post. descending branch, ——
right coronary artery

marginal branch ——
apex ——

pulmonary artery
left coronary artery
left atrium
circumflex branch
left coronary artery

ant. descending branch,
coronary artery
left ventricle

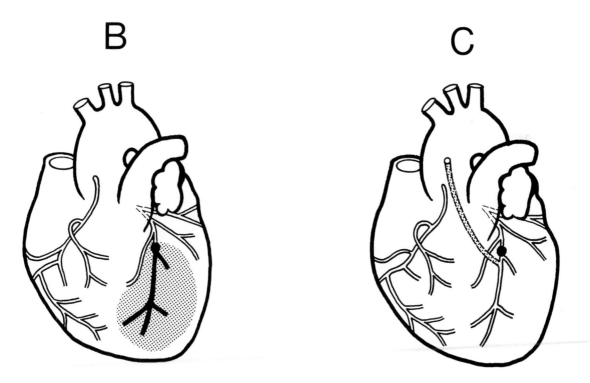

B

C

Fig. 13–35. *A* shows the normal coronary circulation, which supplies blood to the heart. (Reprinted with permission of the American Heart Association.) In *B*, an infarct has occluded the anterior descending branch of the left coronary artery. This has cut off the blood supply to that portion of the left ventricle that is supplied by this vessel. The infarct results in tissue damage or death. *C* illustrates an aortocoronary bypass. A vein graft (usually from the patient's leg), is attached to the aorta at one end and to the coronary artery at the other, beyond the occlusion.

serious matter for both the physician and the patient.

a last resort, if you will, rather than a panacea for most pains in the chest.

HEART TRANSPLANTATION

The general subject of tissue transplantation has already been discussed. Transplantation of the heart has naturally aroused keener interest and greater excitement than in the case of any other organ. The principal problem is rejection of the transplanted heart, a problem that has not yet been solved, in spite of the use of many immunosuppressive drugs. Indeed the heart seems more vulnerable to rejection than the kidney. The rejection may be early, in 1 to 4 weeks, or late, in weeks or months, with occlusion of the coronary arteries. It is evident that immunosuppressive therapy must become more efficient without destroying the patient's resistance to infections if the future is to be as bright as we hope. By 1979, 2 patients have survived 9 years with heart transplants.

Over 400 transplants will have been carried out in the 12 years since the first. The cost effectiveness of this procedure will always be debated; it is currently 3 times as expensive as routine valve replacement or as aortocoronary bypass procedures. Lack of suitable donors remains a major obstacle; one-third of patients accepted into a program die before a donor heart becomes available. In the best hands, however, there is nearly a 70% one-year survival rate, and nearly a 60% five-year survival rate (Shumway). The considered opinion today, however, is that heart transplantation offers therapy for only a few carefully selected patients with end-stage heart disease who would surely die without it. It is

AORTOCORONARY BYPASS SURGERY

The surgical approach to the treatment of vascular disease of the coronary arteries has now developed to the point where it is being demanded by almost every anxious man over 40 with pain in the chest. The existence of the technical feasibility does not obscure our ignorance of its real value in prolonging life. As this is written, it is not clear that this expensive procedure ($15,000), which now has an acceptable operative mortality (0.5 to 3%) does improve prognosis. It does seem to alleviate the disabling angina in most cases (80%), and exercise testing shows that more than half the patients who have the procedure gain benefit. In this domain, however, psychogenic factors have been recognized as playing a major role for at least 3 decades. A comparative study of the effects of medical versus surgical management of coronary artery disease has demonstrated though, for one class of patient, the A–C bypass (Fig. 13–35A,B,C) offers better results than more conservative medical treatment. The present indications for surgery are stable angina pectoris, which is disabling, unstable angina which is medically uncontrolled, or symptomatic patients with angiographic evidence of left main coronary artery stenosis. It is felt by most conservative and thoughtful physicians that each case must be decided on its own merits, and the decision for operation should be made on factors other than prolongation of life.

SYNOPSIS

Heart muscle supplies blood for 2 circulations: the systemic and pulmonary.

Preload, afterload, contractility, and heart rate are the principal determinants of cardiac output.

Heart function can be assessed by measuring pressure, flow, size, sounds, electrical activity, and the presence of muscle enzymes in the serum.

The heart has a limited adaptability to work, but its effectiveness can be improved by training.

Heart diseases may be classified by several different methods, e.g., endocardial, myocardial, pericardial or congenital, vascular, metabolic, infectious, inflammatory, iatrogenic, idiopathic, or on some other taxonomic basis.

Complications of ischemic heart disease are: failure, arrhythmias, rupture, thrombus, embolism, and aneurysm.

Complications of congenital heart disease include: failure, shunts, compensatory hypertrophy, pulmonary hypertension, polycythemia, and endocarditis.

Complications of valvular heart disease depend on the valve or combinations of valves involved and include: failure, arrhythmias, dilatation, hypertrophy, sudden death, thrombosis, embolism, and endocarditis.

Terms

Myocardium	*Essential hypertension*	*Pancarditis*
Endocardium	*Septal defect*	*Endocarditis*
Pericardium	*Coarctation*	*Syncope*
Systole	*Valvular stenosis*	*Angina pectoris*
Diastole	*Valvular insufficiency*	*Aortocoronary bypass*
Tamponade		

FURTHER READING

Editorial: Myocardial imaging. Br. Med. J., 2:717, 1978.

Adolph, E. F.: The heart's pacemaker. Sci. Am., 216:32, 1967.

Anturane Reinfarction Trial Research Group: Sulfinpyrazone in the prevention of cardiac death after myocardial infarction. N. Engl. J. Med., 298:289, 1978.

Braunwald, E.: Regulation of the circulation. N. Engl. J. Med., 290:1124, 1974.

Braunwald, E., Ross, J., Jr., and Sonnenblick, E. H.: Mechanisms of Contraction of the Normal and Failing Heart. Boston, Little, Brown, 1968.

Connolly, J. E.: The history of coronary artery surgery. J. Thorac. Cardiovasc. Surg., 76:733, 1978.

Darsee, J. R., Heymsfield, S. B., and Nutter, D. O.: Hypertrophic cardiomyopathy and human leukocyte antigen linkage. N. Engl. J. Med., 300:877, 1979.

Frick, M. H.: Coronary bypass surgery. An overview. Ann. Clin. Res., 10:235, 1978.

Gould, S.E.: Pathology of the Heart, 3rd Ed. Springfield, Ill., Charles C Thomas, 1968.

Hartung, G. H., et al.: Relation of diet to high-density lipoprotein cholesterol in middle-aged marathon runners, joggers, and inactive men. N. Engl. J. Med., 302:357, 1980.

Hillis, L. D., and Braunwald, E.: Coronary-artery spasm. N. Engl. J. Med., 299:695, 1978.

Hillis, L. D., and Braunwald, E.: Myocardial ischemia. N. Engl. J. Med., 296:971, 1977.

Isom, O. W., et al.: Does coronary bypass increase longevity? J. Thorac. Cardiovasc. Surg., 75:28, 1978.

Jude, J. R., Kouwenhoven, W. B., and Knickerbocker, G. G.: Cardiac arrest: report of application of external cardiac massage of 118 patients. J.A.M.A., 178:1063, 1961.

Kannel, W. M.: Coffee, cocktails and coronary candidates. N. Engl. J. Med., 297:443, 1977.

Kaye, D.: Changes in the spectrum, diagnosis and management of bacterial and fungal endocarditis. Med. Clin. North Am., 57:941, 1973.

Kuller, L., Cooper, M., and Perper, J.: Epidemiology of sudden death. Arch. Intern. Med., 129:714, 1972.

Lemire, J. G., and Johnson, A. L.: Is cardiac resuscitation worthwhile? A decade of experience. N. Engl. J. Med., 286:970, 1972.

Marx, J. L.: Sudden death: strategies for prevention. Science, 195:39, 1977.

Michaelson, S. P., et al.: Recurrent myocardial infarction with normal coronary arteriography. N. Engl. J. Med., 297:916, 1977.

Paffenbarger, R. S., Jr., and Hale, W. E.: Work activity and coronary heart mortality. N. Engl. J. Med., 292:545, 1975.

Shumway, N. E., and Stinson, E. B.: Two decades of experimental and clinical orthotopic homotransplantation of the heart. Perspect. Biol. Med., 22:S81, 1979.

Silver, M. D.: Late complications of prosthetic heart valves. Arch. Pathol. Lab. Med., 102:281, 1978.

Stary, H. C.: Regression of atherosclerosis in primates. Virchows Arch. [Path. Anat.], 383:117, 1979.

Taussig, H. B.: Congenital Malformations of the Heart, 2nd Ed. Cambridge, New York Commonwealth Fund, 1960.

Weinblatt, E., et al.: Relation of education to sudden death after myocardial infarction. N. Engl. J. Med., 299:60, 1978.

Yano, K., Rhoads, G. G., and Kagan, A.: Coffee, alcohol and risk of coronary heart disease in Japanese-Americans. N. Engl. J. Med., 297:405, 1977.

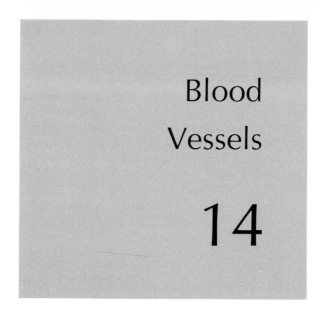

Blood Vessels

14

A man is as old as his arteries.—SYDENHAM

This chapter should be regarded as a direct extension of the preceding, just as the arterial tree and vascular system are in continuity with the heart, and cannot be separated from it, speaking from a functional point of view. In this section we discuss the arterial tree (Figs. 14–1 and 14–2) and its diseases, review the relationship of atherosclerosis to hypertension, and then go on to discuss disorders of the venous circulation. In earlier chapters, we considered such disorders of the circulation as thrombosis, embolism, edema, and shock; there is no need to include them here.

ARTERIES

A sound heart is greatly to be desired, since it has to pump from 9 to 10 tons of blood every day, but if it must do so into a diseased arterial tree, it will have its work greatly increased. The aorta acts not just as a tube, such as a garden hose or a piece of plumbing, but as an elastic reservoir, which receives each cupful of blood from each heartbeat by distending in an elastic way so as to cushion the body from this jolting shock. The effect of each heartbeat can be visualized by crossing 1 leg over the other knee and watching the movement made with each heartbeat by the foot

that hangs as a pendulum. As the arteries lose their elasticity with age or disease, or if the aortic valve loses it competence, the shock of each heartbeat becomes more abrupt, until the whole head will shake with the force of each beat. The value of the elastic recoil of the aorta is to provide a reservoir of energy that permits continuous flow through the capillary bed during the intervals between each beat, much as one builds up pressure in a better-grade garden sprayer, which permits the vapor to continue to cover foliage between pumping actions. To achieve this important facility of continuous perfusion, we have evolved blood vessels that consist of 3 layers, an inner coat (intima), which includes the nonwettable lining cells, the endothelium; a middle coat composed mainly of muscle (media), which includes elastic tissue in the arteries and arterioles; and an outer coat of connective tissue, the adventitia (Figs. 14–3 and 14–4).

We must not forget, however, that the 100,000-km network of the blood vessels of the body is composed largely of capillaries (Figs. 14–5 and 14–6), which form connecting links between the arteries and veins and which allow all the exchange to take place within a tissue. These links are about 10

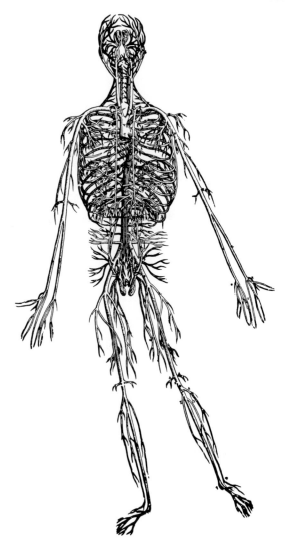

Fig. 14–1. This drawing from Vesalius shows the distribution of the arterial tree of the whole human body. Wood engraving from Andreas Vesalius, *De Humani Corporis Fabrica.*

people of middle age and later life. These diseases belong to 2 groups: those that are sometimes called degenerative and are represented principally by arteriosclerosis, and those that are inflammatory and are often grouped under the heading of arteritis. Numerically, instances of arteritis are uncommon, whereas arteriosclerosis is so universal in the western world that we usually consider it to be a concomitant of aging. In fact, we exclaim when an elderly person is found to exhibit little arteriosclerosis at autopsy.

Arteriosclerosis

Before describing arteriosclerosis (Fig. 14–8), it may be well to mention that the arteries can be divided into 3 main groups: (1) the large or elastic arteries, such as the aorta and its main branches; (2) the medium-sized distributing or muscular arteries, which carry the blood from the main trunks to the various organs and tissues; (3) the small arteries and arterioles, which extend from the ends of the distributing arteries to the capillary beds. Arteriosclerosis is a general term that really signifies hardening of the arteries; arterio**lo**sclerosis is a medial and intimal hyperplasia of arterioles.

Atherosclerosis is a term best reserved for the local lesion in the wall of the artery. It is a focal process—composed of fat-laden cells, smooth muscle cells, collagen, and fibrin and platelets—that affects principally the large arteries, especially the aorta and its main branches, but also the small arteries, particularly the coronary and cerebral arteries. This is the form of arteriosclerosis that commonly predisposes a person to thrombosis, which lends to atherosclerosis a sinister significance.

This patchy or nodular thickening of the intima of the artery, with accumulations of lipid, often results in narrowing of the lumen (Fig. 14–9). The blood supply may be cut down to the danger point, and a thrombus is apt to form on the diseased wall and to obstruct the narrowed lumen. It is worth recognizing, however, that an artery may be lined with atheromas or plaques and still be functional. The normal perfusion does not fall off until more than two-thirds of the diameter

microns in diameter, and their walls are only 1 micron thick, an ideal structure for the passage of substrates and oxygen between the circulating blood and the tissues.

The principal site of resistance or cause of work for the heart is the arteriolar bed, the small precapillary muscular arterioles, which respond to pressor agents, such as angiotensin, and to the increase of salt and water that occurs in heart and kidney failure (Fig. 14–7).

Diseases of the arteries are among the most common causes of morbidity and mortality in

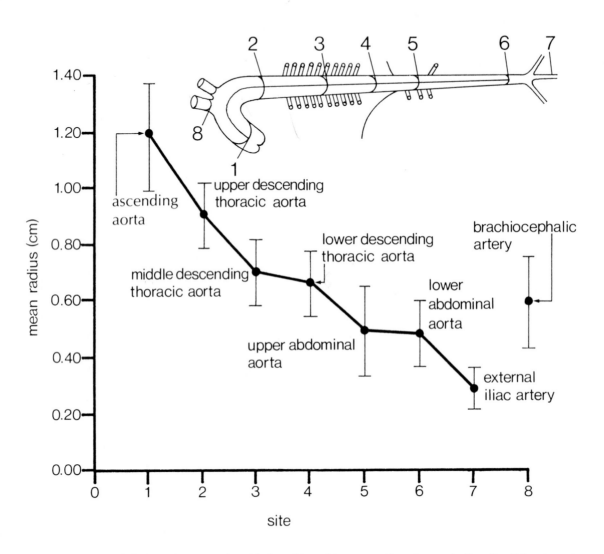

Fig. 14–2. This graph illustrates the mean radius of the branchings of the aorta and its major vessels. (From Fry, Griggs, Jr., and Greenfield, Jr.: In vivo studies of pulsatile blood flow. In *Pulsatile Blood Flow*. Edited by Attinger. New York, McGraw-Hill, 1963.)

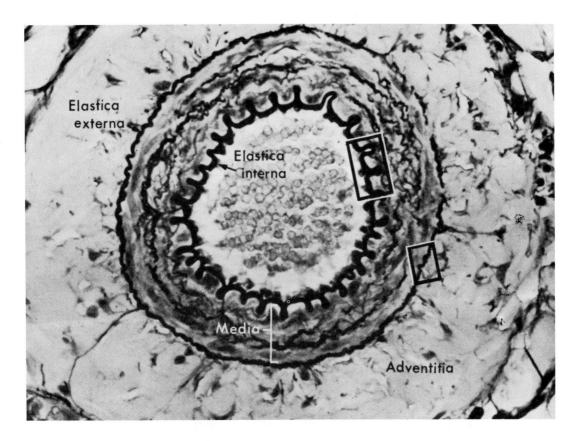

Fig. 14–3. A cross section of a small muscular artery showing the internal and external elastic lamellae, and the relative thickness of the wall. (From Bloom, W., and Fawcett, D. W.: *A Textbook of Histology,* 9th Ed. Philadelphia, W. B. Saunders, 1968.)

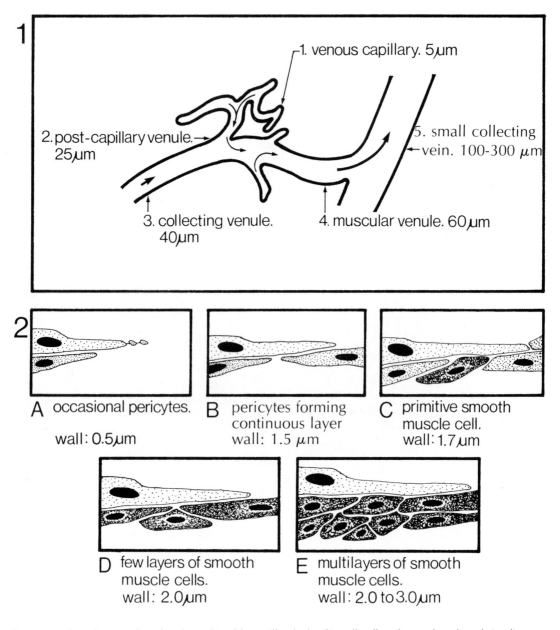

1

1. venous capillary. 5μm

2. post-capillary venule. 25μm

5. small collecting vein. 100-300 μm

3. collecting venule. 40μm

4. muscular venule. 60μm

2

A occasional pericytes.

wall: 0.5μm

B pericytes forming continuous layer

wall: 1.5 μm

C primitive smooth muscle cell.

wall: 1.7μm

D few layers of smooth muscle cells.

wall: 2.0μm

E multilayers of smooth muscle cells.

wall: 2.0 to 3.0μm

Fig. 14–4. These drawings show the relationship of the capillary bed and its cell walls to the venule and its relative diameters. (From Rhodin, J. A. G.: Ultrastructure of mammalian venous capillaries, venules and small collecting veins. J. Ultrastruct. Res., 25:452, 1968.)

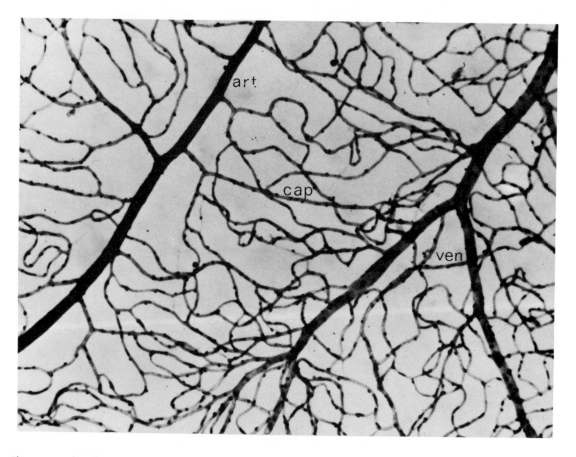

Fig. 14–5. This whole mount preparation of the retinal vessels shows an artery (art), the adjoining capillary bed (cap), and a venule (ven), to illustrate the relative proportions of the microcirculation. (Courtesy of T. Kuwabara.)

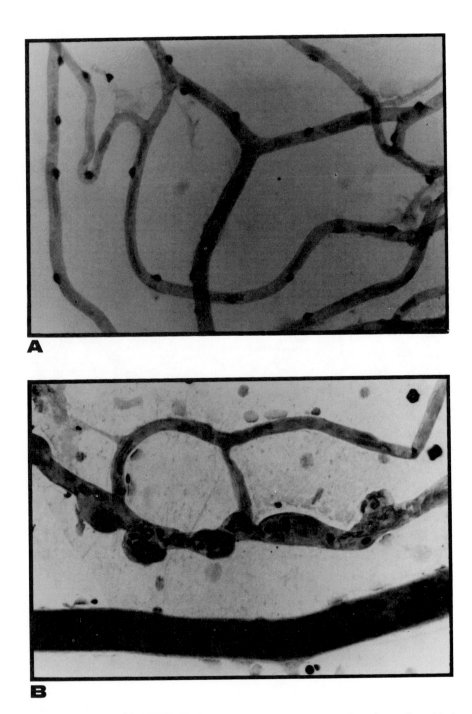

Fig. 14–6. These photographs of the microcirculation of the retina show *A*, the normal capillary cells and *B*, the presence of microaneurysms in a diabetic patient. (Courtesy of Dr. S. Brownstein.)

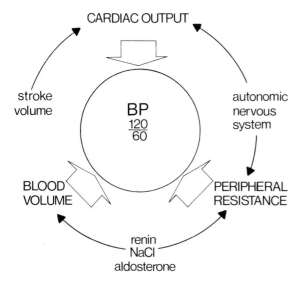

CARDIAC OUTPUT

stroke
volume

BP
120
60

autonomic
nervous
system

BLOOD
VOLUME

PERIPHERAL
RESISTANCE

renin
NaCl
aldosterone

Fig. 14–7. This figure shows the major factors that affect the blood pressure.

of any vessel lumen is occluded. If obstruction has been gradual, as sometimes occurs in the femoral artery, even complete occlusion may not cause symptoms, because a collateral circulation has had time to develop. This presupposes that the demand for arterial oxygen remains relatively constant and that a collateral circulation is available to compensate for the obstruction. Unfortunately, in some situations (some hearts) collateral circulation is not available, and sometimes the demands are unusual and excessive (as in snow shoveling), and the narrowing due to atheromatous plaques is sufficient to result in serious or fatal ischemia. This is the mechanism of production of coronary thrombosis, cerebral thrombosis, and thrombosis in the arteries of the leg. Atherosclerosis is an extremely common condition and is the chief cause of ischemia of the heart muscle, the brain, and the extremities.

At different times, emphasis has been placed on different aspects of the anatomic lesions: on the abundance of lipid, on the presence of fibrous tissue, on the smooth muscle hyperplasia, on the intimal injury, and on the deposition of platelets and thrombus material. The significance of atherosclerosis lies in its potential to (1) obstruct, (2) weaken the wall of the vessel, and (3) predis-

pose a person to thrombus formation and all its complications.

Etiology. It is remarkable that, in spite of the frequency of atherosclerosis and the enormous amount of time and money expended in its investigation, we know as little about its cause as about the cause of cancer. That is to say, we know a great deal, but the pieces of the puzzle are not yet in place to reveal the pattern. This lack of comprehension has proved to be an obstacle to devising some method of preventing this crippling and often fatal condition, which is the curse of the declining years of life. It is perhaps better to speak of the pathogenesis of atherosclerosis, rather than of its etiology, which implies a causal agent. The large amount of experimental work has brought forth several lines of thought, but unfortunately the natural condition is almost exclusively a human disease, and does not occur spontaneously in the laboratory animal.

There have been many attempts to create a unifying hypothesis to explain all the observations, but before we enter the realm of hypotheses, it is better to record some of the observations themselves.

First, atherosclerosis increases with age. It is significantly more noticeable in those who live to 60, but there are exceptions and some octogenarians die with arteries a 30-year-old would be proud of.

Second, it apparently progresses more rapidly in women after the menopause and seems to be more severe in men than in women under the age of 40.

Third, there are worldwide differences in the severity of atherosclerosis, and many studies testify to the changing prevalence of the disease in homogeneous genetic pools as people move, for example, from Japan to Hawaii, or from Asia to North America. The disease has been characterized as being of affluent societies.

Fourth, the disease is more severe in those with hypertension. Other risk factors of significance are obesity, cigarette smoking, high fat intake, an intense "achiever" personality, and coincidental disease such as diabetes mellitus.

In 1974, for the first time in 2 decades, the United States statistics showed a decline in

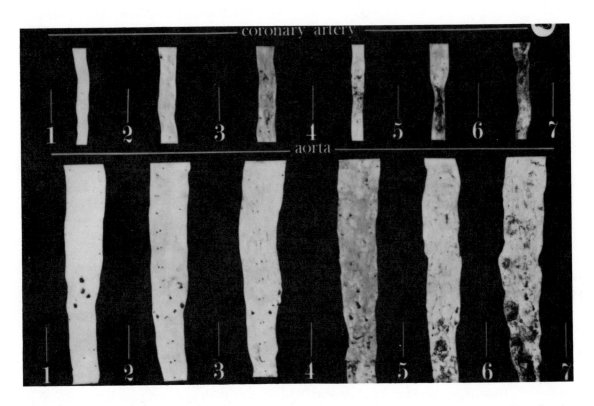

Fig. 14–8. These whole preparations of the coronary arteries and aorta illustrate the relative amounts of atherosclerosis, ranging from 1 to 7. Seven is severe and involves thrombosis and ulceration.

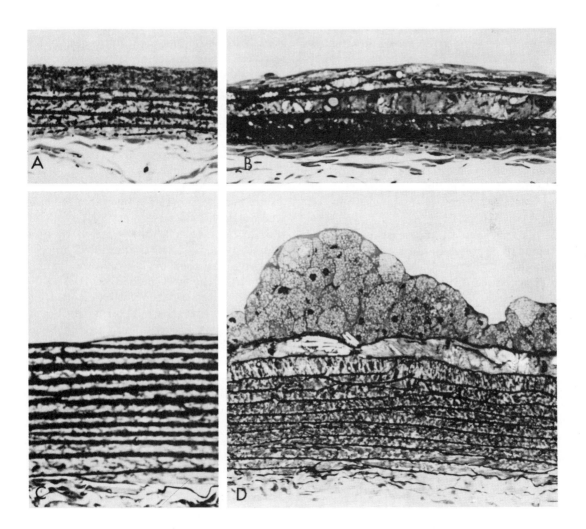

Fig. 14–9. This set of photographs from experimentally induced atheromas of the carotid arteries and aortas of rats shows: *A*, some thickening in a carotid artery that has been injured; *B*, a more marked degree of atheroma in a cholesterol-fed animal; *C*, the thoracic aorta of the control animal; and *D*, the foam cells from the addition of cholesterol to the diet of a rat. (From Clowes, A. W., et al.: Regression of myointimal thickening following carotid endothelial injury and development of aortic foam cell lesions in long term hypercholesterolemic rats. Lab. Invest., *36*:73, 1977. Copyright 1977 by the U.S./Cdn. Div. of the International Academy of Pathology.)

the deaths attributed to coronary artery disease, atherosclerosis, and its complications.

A factor, the significance of which is undetermined, but that may be extremely relevant to our understanding of atherosclerosis is exercise. A sedentary occupation is clearly a risk factor, and the rise in participation in physical work/exercise may be partly responsible for the leveling off in premature deaths attributable to atherosclerosis.

There is also the observation that populations that reside in areas where the water is "soft" have a higher incidence of ischemic heart disease attributable to coronary artery atherosclerosis than populations that drink "hard" water. An imbalance with respect to zinc and copper in the diet has been shown to play a role in the experimental production of atherosclerosis. Table 14–1 shows some of these relationships.

Perhaps ischemic heart disease might even be regarded as a disorder of zinc and copper metabolism.

A final comment is to note that atheromas are reversible. Baboons shown to have atherosclerosis from an atherogenic diet lose their plaques when placed back on a normal diet. This holds out hope for the millions of people who may regard atherosclerosis as a necessary consequence of living beyond their 20's.

Thus, the list of factors that have been identified as contributing to premature atherosclerosis is long, and their interrelationships are difficult to disentangle.

These, then, are the principal observations: epidemiologic, clinical, and experimental.

How do they relate to the diseased blood vessel?

The classic theories have been (1) the lipid theory, (2) the encrustation theory, and (3) the insudation theory.

The lipid theory, based principally on the presence of lipid in the wall of the aorta, and on the identification of the similarity of such lipids with those that occur in the serum, has received wide attention. It has been suggested that these lipids, which are stored or possibly synthesized by cells in the aorta, interfere partly through sheer bulk and partly because of the inflammation that they may elicit with the normal elastic nature of the aorta. The inflammatory cells secrete enzymes that destroy the elastica; the lipid merely makes it inelastic.

Other suggestions have been that the lipid accumulates (a) because of a caloric overload, and (b) because cells in the vessel wall are injured by some other unidentified process, implying that atheroma is a symptom but not the agent of the arterial change.

The second classic theory is based on (a) the observations that atheroma forms most commonly at sites of turbulence in the blood stream, where arteries divide, or at parts where smaller subdivisions arise, (b) the fact that the intima is the target for much of the injury, and (c) the similarities between the organization of a thrombus and atheromatous plaques, a fact that proposes that arteriosclerosis is the result of surface injury in which platelets and fibrin are laid down. It supposes that the lipids are the result of degradation processes that digest and deposit the

Table 14–1. Epidemiology of Ischemic Heart Disease (IHD)

ENVIRONMENTAL CHARACTERISTICS	IHD RISK*	POSSIBLE EXPLANATION
Diets low in fat & sucrose & high in vegetable fiber	<	Have low Zn/Cu; or contain phytate, a protective chelate
Nursing of infants	<	Human milk has low Zn/Cu
Cirrhosis of the liver	<	Increased loss of Zn
Exercise	<	Zn/Cu of sweat = 16; or synthesis of muscle & bone traps Zn
Chronic kidney disease	>	Bone loss releases Zn; or Zn infused during treatment
Availability of hard water	<	Decreased absorption of Zn

* < decreased; > increased

(From Klevay, L. M.: Elements of Ischemic Heart Disease. Perspect. Bio. Med., 20:186, 1977.)

materials in macrophages or in pools of cholesterol crystals.

The third popular hypothesis has a little of both of the other 2 theses and states that the materials of the bloodstream enter the wall of the aorta by insudation, and that they enter the wall more rapidly under increased pressure (hypertension). The serum proteins and lipids are sequestered there, if they cannot be metabolized by the resident cells, and thereby lead to the fibrin or lipid-containing plaques that we recognize.

A fourth theory, currently popularized by Benditt, suggests that atherosclerosis really is the product of a clone of new smooth muscle cells, akin to a tumor. The new smooth muscle cells proliferate and have an abnormal metabolism, which preferably synthesizes lipids or secretes fibrin.

All these theories have 1 thing in common: none explains all of the observations, and each is partly valid.

To summarize, we must acknowledge that we do not have any single explanation for this widespread disorder of blood vessels. The recognition that many factors may contribute

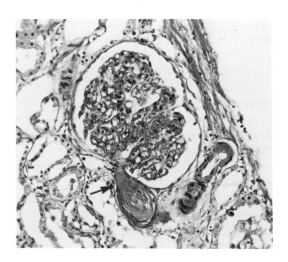

Fig. 14–11. This photomicrograph shows the arterioles entering a glomerulus that had been subject to hypertension for many years. The lumen of the arteriole is narrowed and the wall is hyalinized. This is **arteriolosclerosis.** (McGill University, Department of Pathology Museum.)

to its development has been the greatest contribution of the last 2 decades (Fig. 14–10).

Arteriolosclerosis. The smaller arteries of the visceral organs such as the kidney have been designated the "intimate vasculature," or, more recently, the microcirculation. These vessels may participate in changes similar to the changes of the aorta, with thickening of the wall and narrowing of the lumen. However, lipid deposits are seldom seen and the changes are not so dramatic. Intimal hyperplasia and medial hypertrophy, even with accumulations of fibrin, are common reactions to hypertension and are designated as arteriolosclerosis (Fig. 14–11). In cases of accelerated hypertension, there may be necrosis of these arteries, and the entity then goes by the name of arteriolonecrosis.

Vascular Disease and Hypertension

We might review hypertension and underscore its relationship to vascular disease at this point. Earlier, we defined hypertension as having 2 components, systolic (elevations over 150 mmg Hg), and diastolic (elevations over 90 mm Hg), and recognized that blood pressure readings are variable in the same person, depending on such different factors as the patient's anxiety, whether the patient is

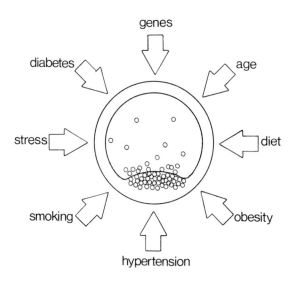

Fig. 14–10. There are no clear-cut "causes" of arteriosclerosis, but several factors are known to increase the risk of this disease. Those shown here increase the concentration of lipid in the blood as well as in the artery wall. Many of these factors are interrelated; for example, high-fat diets lead to obesity, obesity and smoking raise blood pressure. The coexistence of more than one factor increases a person's risk of arteriosclerosis and of myocardial infarction.

supine or standing, or whether the blood pressure cuff is appropriate to the task. For practical purposes, because the diagnosis of "hypertension" carries with it such a dread connotation, it is wise to determine the blood pressure on 3 separate occasions (days) and to check the results both sitting and lying, because the anxiety of the visit to the doctor's office alone may cause a falsely high reading. After all, what one is trying to determine is the measurable level of work that the heart is called on to do during the daily life of the individual patient in question. It is important to recognize that a constant pathologic elevation of the blood pressure carries with it a considerable risk for stroke, accelerated atherosclerosis, and heart failure (Fig. 14–12).

The diagnosis of essential hypertension, as we have stated earlier, is a diagnosis of exclusion. Of all causes of hypertension, only about 6% are surgically curable (4% being due to renovascular disease, 1% to coarctation of the aorta, 1.5% to aldosterone-secreting tumors, 0.2% to Cushing's syndrome, and 0.2% to pheochromocytoma). The remainder are considered "essential."

Hypertension, however, must be put in a perspective of general occurrence. It is important to recognize that the incidence of hypertension increases with age, is higher in relatives of people with hypertension, is lower in people with active jobs (as opposed to sedentary), and is higher in people who are obese or have severe atherosclerosis.

In primitive societies, for instance, in the Solomon Islands, there are 2 populations; 1 cooks its vegetable diet in sea water, the other lives nearby, a few kilometers from the sea, and uses stream water for cooking. Those with the diet enriched with salt have significantly higher blood pressures. Similarly, a group of Kenyans with low blood pressure left their farms and entered the army, where they ate a diet containing as much as 18 gm of salt per day. They all developed hypertension; this took about a year to occur. This effect of salt on blood pressure is probably one of the most important environmental factors in producing hypertension, and our diets are routinely rich in salt. It seems clear from studies on rats that not all individuals in any population are susceptible to such a factor as increased salt in the diet.

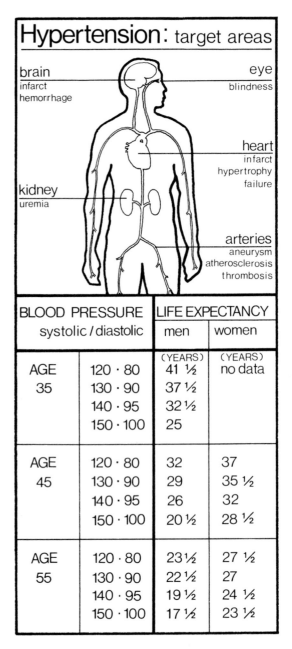

BLOOD PRESSURE		LIFE EXPECTANCY	
systolic / diastolic		men	women
AGE 35	120 · 80	(YEARS) 41 ½	(YEARS) no data
	130 · 90	37 ½	
	140 · 95	32 ½	
	150 · 100	25	
AGE 45	120 · 80	32	37
	130 · 90	29	35 ½
	140 · 95	26	32
	150 · 100	20 ½	28 ½
AGE 55	120 · 80	23 ½	27 ½
	130 · 90	22 ½	27
	140 · 95	19 ½	24 ½
	150 · 100	17 ½	23 ½

Fig. 14–12. This diagram illustrates the changes in life expectancy with elevations in blood pressure and shows the sites of complications of hypertension. (From Metropolitan Life Insurance Co.)

Hypertension is clearly known to accelerate the process of arteriosclerosis in the aorta and the arteries. How it does so, whether by enhancing the permeability of the cells of the wall, by loosening junctions, by the effect of direct pressure (pressure necrosis), which may lead to cell death in the intima or media, or by increasing the likelihood of thrombus formation by increasing the mechanical interaction between platelets and endothelium, is not known. However, a rapid rise in blood pressure alone may cause injury to the arterioles and create a sequence of lesions in these vessels that is called **malignant hypertension.** This disease of unknown etiology is best remembered because of the clinical pattern. Usually a person so afflicted may complain of headaches and visual difficulties. Examination shows that, in addition to the elevated systolic and diastolic pressures (200/140), there is an abnormal protrusion of the optic nerve (papilledema), and microscopic hemorrhages and exudation can be seen in the retina with the ophthalmoscope. These same changes are probably occurring in the microvascular bed throughout the body. They have particularly damaging effects in the kidney (leading to renal failure) and brain (giving intracerebral hemorrhages and coma, eventually).

Perhaps nowhere is the relationship of arteriosclerosis and hypertension better illustrated than in the blood vessels of the pulmonary circulation. Usually this system, a low-pressure (20/10 mm Hg), low-resistance circulation, shows no atheromas even in persons who have high serum lipids and who develop severe atherosclerosis in their aorta and systemic vessels. Even in obese, sedentary smokers (provided they have not developed severe lung disease), atheromas of the pulmonary circulation are rare. When, however, owing to a shunt or some other cause, pulmonary hypertension occurs, then one can expect to see and usually finds atheromas and arteriosclerosis in the pulmonary arteries, just as they appear in the systemic circulation.

Although multiple factors that contribute to atherosclerosis have been enumerated, it is not clear yet how each of them is related to the etiology of this ubiquitous disorder. However, the role of hypertension in promoting atherosclerosis cannot be doubted.

Arteritis

So far we have been considering the conditions to which the arteries and arterioles are liable. We may now turn to the much less common inflammatory lesions. A number of these appear to be manifestations of allergy or of hypersensitivity, although little or nothing is known about the substances to which the person is allergic.

Polyarteritis Nodosa. This is one of the diffuse collagen diseases (the collective phrase collagen diseases or collagen vascular diseases represents an attempt to group diseases of unknown etiology that manifest morphologic changes in the histologic appearance of connective tissue), and is also known as periarteritis nodosa, by reason of the periarterial inflammatory exudate that is often a prominent microscopic feature. It is an acute inflammation that involves the small arteries of the viscera. The cause is unknown, but strong evidence suggests that this disease represents a type of hypersensitivity. The disease often runs an acute course with fever, ending fatally in a few weeks or months. Symptoms vary widely, depending on which arteries are involved. The principal vessels affected are those of the gastrointestinal tract, the kidney, and the heart. There may be acute abdominal symptoms due to involvement of the mesenteric arteries, acute cardiac symptoms from coronary artery involvement, or neuritic pains due to lesions of the arteries supplying the peripheral nerves.

Disseminated Lupus Erythematosus. In this confusing name, the word "lupus" originally signified wolf, but is now taken to denote the distribution of the facial rash mentioned below. This is another of the collagen diseases, similar in many ways to polyarteritis nodosa, for it involves the small vessels of the viscera. The heart, kidneys, skin, and serous membranes are also involved. A butterfly-like red rash over the bridge of the nose and both cheeks is a common and striking feature. A peculiar occurrence is the finding of what are known as LE (lupus erythematosus) cells. These are polymorphonuclear leukocytes containing a large homogeneous inclusion mass. The inclusion has been shown to be altered DNA and the presumed antigen is believed to be the patient's own DNA. The LE cells were first found in the bone marrow of patients suffering from the disease, but it is now known that the phenomenon depends on the presence of some factor in the patient's blood serum that acts on the cells. When a test is made for the LE phenomenon, the patient's blood serum is mixed with his white blood cells, and a smear is made and searched for the development of LE cells. It must be realized that the test is *in vitro,* not *in vivo.* Today, the outlook for patients with SLE (systemic lupus erythematosus) is greatly improved because of new ways of using immunosuppressive and anti-inflammatory drugs.

Thromboangiitis Obliterans. A thrombotic occlusion (obliteration) of the vessels of the legs in relatively young men, this disease results in gangrene of the toes and then the feet. Buerger, in 1908, brought this condition to the attention of the medical profession, so that it is commonly referred to as Buerger's disease. The sex incidence is striking, for the disease is practically confined to men. The cause is unknown, but it is believed that there is a condition of allergic hypersensitivity in the arterial wall, as a result of which an acute inflammatory reaction develops. Patients seem to be specially hypersensitive to tobacco, and the sufferer is often found to be a heavy cigarette smoker. In the treatment of the disease, one of the most important points is to give up tobacco. Buerger called the lesion angiitis, meaning an inflammation of vessels, both arteries and veins, but at the present time thrombosis is coming to be regarded as the dominant feature of the disease.

Syphilis. This disease attacks 2 important sets of vessels: (1) the thoracic aorta, including the coronary artery ostia, more especially the ascending portion, and (2) the cerebral arteries.

Syphilitic Aortitis. Formerly one of the most common and most important of the lesions of syphilis, modern antibiotic therapy has made this condition a rarity. The destruction caused by the *Treponema pallidum* in the wall of the aorta may produce aortic valvular insufficiency or aneurysm. Aortic insufficiency or incompetence is caused by destruction of the aortic ring to which the cusps of the aortic valve are attached. This destruction occurs by ischemic injury to the elastic tissue that forms a chief constituent of the wall, so that gradual stretching and dilatation occur and the valve becomes incompetent. The 3 cusps of the valve are shrunken and show a characteristic cord-like thickening, becoming separated from one another, and thus further adding to the incompetence. The smooth intimal surface of the aorta becomes pitted, scarred, and wrinkled like the bark of a tree. An aneurysm is a localized or diffuse dilatation of the wall of the thoracic aorta caused by damage to the elastic tissue of the wall. Syphilitic aneurysm is considered in the next section, together with other varieties of aneurysm. The common mechanism of injury was said to be occlusion of the vasa vasorum or the small vessels that supply the aortic wall itself. However, the spirochete itself may have initiated some of the injury. It is important to recognize that only one-third of all people with primary syphilis ever suffered this type of cardiovascular syphilis (see Chap. 7).

Aneurysms

This localized dilatation of an artery may be saccular, an outpouching of the vessel at a single point (Fig. 14–13), or fusiform, a uniform dilatation of an entire segment of the artery. Every aneurysm is due to weakening of the arterial wall. As a rule, it is the media that is damaged. Syphilis used to be the most important cause of aneurysm of the aorta and its main branches. With the modern control of

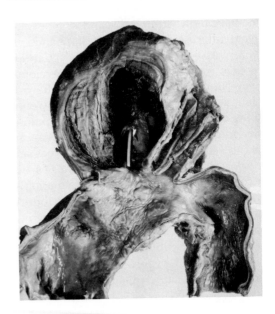

Fig. 14–13. This photograph shows the arch of the aorta in a patient who had syphilis several decades ago. The bulging protruding mass at the top of the picture is an **aneurysm** that is lined with thrombus material. This aneurysm has ruptured, causing the death of the patient. (McGill University, Department of Pathology Museum.)

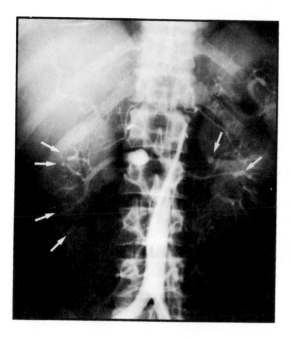

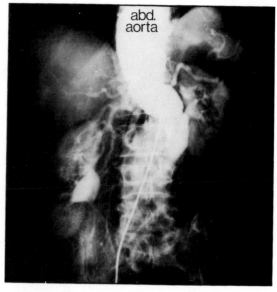

Fig. 14–14. This aortogram shows multiple small aneurysms, seen at the arrows, in a case of periarteritis nodosa, a rare disease of arteries.

Fig. 14–15. This arteriogram shows a markedly dilated atherosclerotic aorta, in which the dilatation extends from the diaphragm to the level of the internal iliac arteries.

syphilis and with the increasing age of the population, atherosclerosis has come to replace it. Polyarteritis nodosa may weaken the artery and lead to the formation of multiple small aneurysms (Fig. 14–14). Finally, congenital weakness of the media in the arteries at the base of the brain has been suggested as a cause of so-called congenital aneurysms in this region. We shall confine our attention here to aneurysms of the aorta.

Aortic Aneurysm. Aneurysm due to atherosclerosis occurs at a later age than the syphilitic form; it generally affects the abdominal aorta, and it usually causes diffuse dilatation of the vessel (Fig. 14–15). The site of the involvement is the lower part of the aorta below the origin of the renal arteries. This is singularly fortunate, because it makes possible the replacement of the aneurysm by an aortic homograft or a plastic tube that may be a lifesaving procedure. Unfortunately, the aneurysm may press on the lower dorsal and lumbar vertebrae, with disastrous results. A syphilitic aneurysm usually involves the ascending aorta or the arch, is usually saccular, and presses on the surrounding structures, causing pain in the back, dyspnea, and

difficulty in swallowing. It may rupture on the surface or internally, killing the patient at once.

Dissecting aneurysm is not a true aneurysm, as the vessel is not dilated. A hemorrhage occurs in the media of the aorta at a point of weakness, and spreads along the vessel dissecting the media into 2 layers (Fig. 14–16). The usual pattern may be: a sudden sharp or excruciating pain in the chest or the abdomen, accompanied by prostration. The patient often experiences what he describes as a tearing sensation. The pain passes, but in a typical case death occurs some days later from the rupture of the aneurysm into the chest or the abdominal cavity. This clinical pattern is not the only one, since the dissection may take a number of routes. It may separate the walls of the aorta and narrow the renal arteries; it may close off the mesenteric supply to the bowel; or it may dissect retrograde to narrow the coronary arteries. The aneurysm may also rupture into the pericardium, thereby preventing normal ventricular filling and killing the patient because of the effect of what is called tamponade. Studies of collected cases show that 3% of patients with a dissecting aneurysm die immediately; 20% die

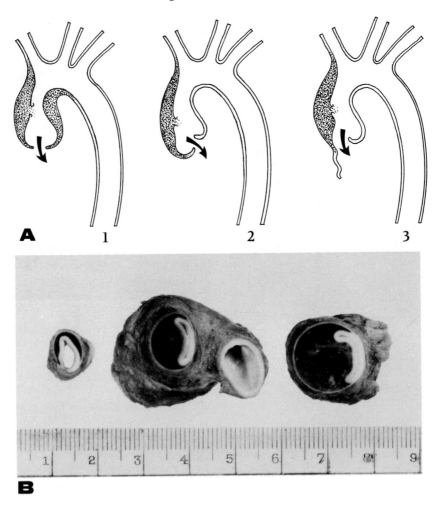

Fig. 14–16. *A,1,2,3,* The drawings show different routes for the accumulation of blood within the wall of the aorta in different types of dissecting aneurysms. (From Slater, E. E., and DeSanctis, R. W.: Dissection of the aorta. Med. Clin. North Am., 63:146, 1979.) *B,* This cross section of a carotid artery shows the effect of hemorrhage in the wall of the aorta. It narrows the lumen and thus obstructs blood flow. (McGill University, Department of Pathology Museum.)

within a day; 60% die within 2 weeks; and 90% die within 3 months. In a few lucky cases, the person may survive many years. It is important to make the diagnosis as distinct from a myocardial infarction with which it is usually confused, because there is some hope from an early surgical approach to the aneurysm. Hypotensive agents certainly seem to have increased the short-term outlook for patients with dissecting aneurysms.

VEINS

The pathology of the veins is entirely different from that of the arteries. Veins differ from arteries in 2 respects, both of which have a bearing on the development of disease. (1) They have valves (Fig. 14–17). Failure of the valves is one of the important features of varicose veins. (2) They have lymphatics, which explains why malignant growths invade veins with the greatest ease, but seldom invade the walls of arteries, which are lacking in lymphatics. Bacteria from without can also readily penetrate the vein wall by way of the lymphatics.

Phlebitis or inflammation of the veins used to be of great importance, but antisepsis and chemotherapy have changed the picture completely. The danger of phlebitis used to be

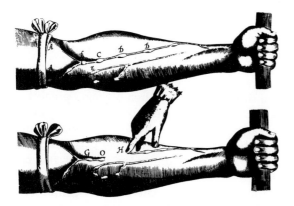

Fig. 14–17. This illustration from William Harvey's *De motu cordis* (1628) shows how Harvey demonstrated valves in the venous system and the direction of the blood flow in veins by applying pressure from below.

an associated thrombosis, often septic in character. This has disappeared, but venous thrombosis unassociated with phlebitis still remains a threat and an unsolved problem. Two conditions that affect veins in which thrombosis is common and sometimes serious, namely varicose veins and hemorrhoids, will be considered here. The 2 really belong to the same group, for hemorrhoids are merely varicose veins at the lower end of the intestinal canal.

Varicose Veins. These are veins that are dilated and tortuous (Fig. 14–18). The dilatation may be extreme, so that the valves that normally guard veins and prevent a backflow because of gravity become incompetent and cease to function. As a result of this failure, the stagnation and accumulation of blood in the vein greatly increase. The common site of varicose veins is in the superficial veins of the leg, just under the skin. Bluish knuckles of veins can be seen pushing the skin in front of them. These nodules are liable to injury, with resulting hemorrhage into the surrounding tissue. Thrombosis may occur due partly to the slow blood flow in the dilated vessels, partly to the frequency of injury to the vessel wall. The circulation in varicose veins is interfered with, the legs become swollen, and varicose ulcers are formed in the lower part of the leg. These ulcers used to be chronic and difficult to treat, but the outlook has been changed by modern methods of treating the varicose veins by surgical removal.

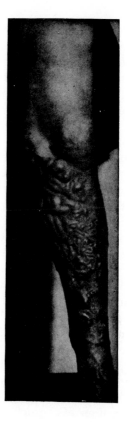

Fig. 14–18. Varicose veins. (Boyd, W.: *Pathology for the Surgeon.* Philadelphia, W. B. Saunders Co.)

The causes of varicose veins are obscure. Heredity undoubtedly plays a part, and the condition may run in a family. The active factor is increase of pressure in the vein. This may be due to prolonged standing, intermittent, increased venous pressure (in the case of hemorrhoids), or the pressure of a tumor in the pelvis, a pregnant uterus, or even a continually loaded rectum.

The treatment of varicose veins is directed to the relief of the congestion, the accumulation of stagnant blood, in the dilated vessels. This may be accomplished by the application of a uniform support to the leg in the form of an elastic bandage or stocking which should extend to the groin rather than to the knee, as is more often the case. If this method fails to relieve the condition, the veins may be removed. The varicosity only affects the superficial veins, and as these communicate with the deep veins of the leg by small collateral channels, the circulation is reestablished through the leg veins. For the same reason, there is no danger of emboli passing from the superficial veins into the general circulation.

Hemorrhoids. The condition in which the veins at the lower end of the rectum become varicose and enlarged is known as hemorrhoids. Internal hemorrhoids are those covered by the mucous membrane of the lower end of the rectum; they may "come down" through the anal opening and appear on the surface, although they can be replaced by pressure. External hemorrhoids are covered by the skin in the neighborhood of the anus.

The causes are those of varicose veins, i.e., heredity and increased pressure in the venous system. The most common cause of increased pressure is chronic constipation accompanied by undue muscular straining while the bowel is being emptied. A condition that must always be borne in mind, especially in a man past middle age, is cancer of the rectum, which may produce hemorrhoids by causing pressure on the veins coming from the lower end of the bowel. In this case hemorrhoids are merely a symptom of a much more serious condition. This is also true of the presence of hemorrhoids in patients with cirrhosis of the liver, in which the rise in portal pressure makes the collateral circulation of the esophagus and rectum anatomically important but susceptible to rupture.

The possible effects that may render the condition serious are hemorrhage, phlebitis, and thrombosis. Hemorrhage when the bowels are moved is usually small in amount, but may be continued over a long period, so that anemia may be produced without the patient's suspecting its cause. Phlebitis or inflammation of the dilated veins together with inflammation of the surrounding tissue is commonly referred to as an "attack of the piles." Its danger is that it may lead to the formation of an infected thrombus, which readily becomes converted into an embolus.

The treatment of hemorrhoids is partly indirect, partly direct. By indirect treatment we mean keeping the bowels loose by means of bland laxatives and suitable food. Direct treatment is aimed at the dilated veins. These veins may be closed by the injection of sclerosing solutions, and no more may need to be done. In more severe cases, operative removal of the hemorrhoids may be necessary.

SYNOPSIS

Arteriosclerosis is common in persons over 50 years of age.

Arteriosclerosis is likely of multifactorial etiology.

Arteriosclerosis is reversible.

The pathogenesis of arteriosclerosis is debated, but hypertension, platelet aggregation, turbulent flow, intimal injury, hyperlipidemia, and damage to smooth muscle cells have all been implicated.

Arteriolosclerosis may both result from and contribute to hypertension.

The presence of arteriosclerosis contributes to systolic hypertension, arteriolosclerosis to diastolic hypertension.

Collagen vascular diseases are a group of diseases that share clinical features of fever, connective tissue and serosal involvement, pathologic features of uncertain etiology, and aspects of hypersensitivity reaction.

Terms

Arteriosclerosis	*Atherosclerosis*	*Aortitis*
Arteriolosclerosis	*Arteritis*	*Aneurysm*
Arteriolonecrosis	*Collagen vascular disease*	*Phlebitis*

FURTHER READING

Editorial: Regression of atheroma. Br. Med. J., *2*:1, 1977.

Benditt, E. P.: The origin of atherosclerosis. Sci. Am., *236*:74, 1977.

Clowes, A. W., Breslow, J. L., and Karnovsky, M. J.: Regression of myointimal thickening following carotid endothelial injury and development of aortic foam cell lesions in long-term hypercholesterolemic rats. Lab. Invest., *36*:73, 1977.

Dobrin, P. B.: Mechanical properties of arteries. Physiol. Rev., *58*:397, 1978.

Heptinstall, R. H.: Malignant hypertension: a study of fifty-one cases. J. Pathol. Bacteriol., *65*:423, 1953.

Hirst, A. E., Jr., Johns, V. J., and Kime, S. W.: Dissecting aneurysms of the aorta: a review of 505 cases. Medicine, *37*:217, 1958.

Keith, N. M., Wagener, H. P., and Kernohan, J. W.: The syndrome of malignant hypertension. Arch. Intern. Med., *41*:141, 1928.

LeQuesne, L. P.: Relationship between deep vein thrombus and pulmonary embolism in surgical patients. N. Engl. J. Med., *291*:1292, 1974.

Mann, G. V.: Diet-heart: End of an era. N. Engl. J. Med., *297*:644, 1977.

Marx, J. L.: Hypertension: a complex disease with complex causes. Science, *194*:821, 1977.

Murdoch, J. C., et al.: Down's syndrome: an atheroma-free model? Br. Med. J., *2*:226, 1977.

Stamler, J.: Dietary and serum lipids in the multifactorial etiology of atherosclerosis. Arch Surg., *113*:21, 1978.

Walker, W. J.: Diet-heart era: Premature obituary. N. Engl. J. Med., *298*:106, 1978.

The Respiratory Tract

15

One enlarges science in two ways; by adding new facts and by simplifying what already exists.
—C. BERNARD

STRUCTURE AND FUNCTION

The principal function of the lungs is oxygenation of the blood, a business in which the heart and lungs are partners. Blood laden with the waste products of the body in the form of carbon dioxide is brought to the lungs, where carbon dioxide is given off and fresh oxygen is taken up. Respiration is essential to life; when it ceases, so does life. Deoxygenated blood returns directly to the heart and is then sent through the arteries to supply the needs of the body. The lungs constitute the great mixing place of air and blood. Each lung is a honeycomb, with air in place of honey in the cells of the comb, and an infinite number of capillaries in their walls. These walls are virtually only 2 plasma membranes; gases (carbon dioxide and oxygen) readily pass through in either direction (Fig. 15–1). During inspiration, air is carried to the alveoli by the bronchi and their terminations, the bronchioles, which subdivide and ramify throughout the entire lung. The partial pressures of oxygen in the different compartments dictate the availability of this essential fuel. Under conditions of respiration at sea level (standard temperature and pressure) in a normal lung, hemoglobin will approach max-imal saturation. With decreased ventilation, or at high altitudes, or with disease in the lung, there will be a departure from normal values as shown in Figure 15–2.

The lung differs from most other organs in that it is supplied by 2 circulations: the pulmonary, a low-pressure, low-resistance system that perfuses the lung for purposes of oxygenation and excretion; and the bronchial circulation, which is a part of the high-pressure systemic circulation, mainly directed to keeping the branches of the bronchi alive. The differing pressures in the 2 circulations, the systemic and pulmonary, are shown in Figure 15–3. Before birth and before the lungs expand, the 2 circulations are joined by the ductus arteriosum, which normally closes within a few hours or days of birth. Should it remain open permanently, there will be a shunt of blood and pressure into the pulmonary circulation that eventually results in injury to the pulmonary arteriolar bed and causes a rise in pulmonary arterial pressures or **pulmonary hypertension.** Other shunts between the circulations may do the same, depending on the size and duration of the shunt (ventricular septal defect, atrial septal defect).

The quantity of oxygen that could be carried in the fluid part of the blood, the plasma, would not maintain life for a second. Red blood cells (25,000,000,000,000 in the blood of a man of average size) carry the oxygen because of the binding capabilities of hemoglobin. Carbon dioxide (CO_2), on the other hand, is carried mainly in the plasma combined with sodium as sodium bicarbonate

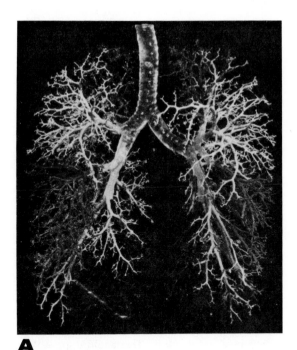

A

Fig. 15–1. *A,* This cast of the lung shows the extensive branching of the airways that starts at the junction of the left and right main stem bronchus and continues for as many as fourteen divisions before the alveoli are reached. (From West, J. B.: *Respiratory Physiology.* Baltimore, Williams & Wilkins, 1974.) *B,* This drawing of the microscopic appearance of the lung shows the terminations of the respiratory bronchioles in the alveolar ducts and spaces. Note the communication (pore) between alveoli. Both air and inflammation can use these portals for transalveolar spread. (From Sorokin, S.: In *Histology,* 2nd Ed. Edited by R. O. Greep. New York, McGraw-Hill, 1966.)

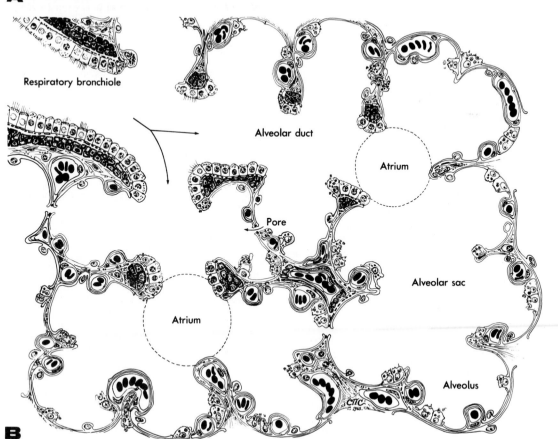

Respiratory bronchiole

Alveolar duct

Atrium

Pore

Atrium

Alveolar sac

Alveolus

B

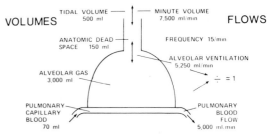

Fig. 15-4. This diagram illustrates the relationship between air exchange and blood flow in the lung. It shows the volumes and flows on which we depend for normal respiratory exchange of oxygen and CO_2. (From West, J. B.: *Respiratory Physiology*. Baltimore, Williams & Wilkins, 1974.)

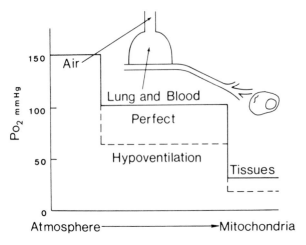

Fig. 15-2. This scheme illustrates the function of the lung by showing the gradient of oxygen from the atmosphere to the intracellular sink (mitochondria) where oxygen is used. (From West, J. B.: *Respiratory Physiology*. Baltimore, Williams & Wilkins, 1974.)

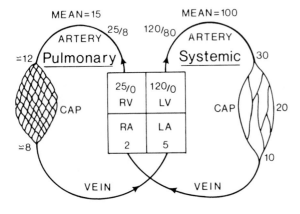

Fig. 15-3. This scheme illustrates the relationship of the systemic and pulmonary circulations and shows the difference in pressures in the two. (From West, J. B.: *Respiratory Physiology*. Baltimore, Williams & Wilkins, 1974.)

($NaHCO_3$). CO_2 is dissolved and combined with water to form carbonic acid (H_2CO_3). This process is greatly speeded by an enzyme in red blood cells known as carbonic anhydrase. The same enzyme also acts when the blood reaches the pulmonary capillaries, to break down H_2CO_3 into CO_2 and H_2O, the gas being eliminated in the expired air. The most remarkable feature of this beautiful mechanism is that it is the CO_2 in the blood flowing through the respiratory center in the medulla at the base of the brain that provides the stimulus for the

muscles of respiration. Even a slight increase in the amount of CO_2 in the blood will increase the rate and depth of breathing, as becomes evident whenever you exercise. Thus a waste gas that must be removed from the body stimulates the mechanism required for its removal, surely a *tour de force* of precise automation. The amount of air exchanged and expired to blood is shown in Figure 15-4.

Each of the alveoli is lined by a film of lipoprotein called **surfactant,** so named because it lowers the surface tension and thus prevents collapse of the alveoli. The ability of the lungs to retain air depends on the special properties of this film. In the absence of surfactant, the lungs readily collapse (atelectasis) and become unable to act as a surface for exchange.

It must not be supposed that respiration is the only function of the lungs, any more than excretion is the only function of the kidneys. Both are concerned also with maintenance of the acid-base balance. When that balance is temporarily upset, it can be restored to normal much more quickly by blowing off CO_2 than by the excretion of acid by the kidneys.

Owing to the rhythmic movements of the chest during respiration, air is being continually sucked into and expelled from the lungs. One great disadvantage of this arrangement is that the interior of the lungs is in communication with the outside air, so that infectious agents are liable to enter and to cause inflammation, although most of them are held back in the nose and throat. This is not the case with any of the other organs of the body, and, for this reason, bacterial infections are far more common in the lungs than in the heart or brain.

The barriers to infection in the respiratory tract are: (1) the presence of protective enzymes in the upper respiratory tract (lysozyme); (2) the integrity of the respiratory epithelium that lines the trachea, bronchi, and bronchioles; (3) the mucous blanket that covers this epithelium; and (4) the action of cilia, which constantly move this blanket toward the oral cavity, where the trapped particles and mucous are shed into the gut. At the level of the alveolus (should a bacterium get that far) there is another protector, (5) the alveolar macrophage, which acts as a kind of Cerberus to tax any pneumococcus that wishes to gain access to the interstitial or vascular sanctum. Commonly, small particles and bacteria are phagocytosed and carried to regional lymph nodes if they reach the alveolar space. At the junction between the terminal respiratory epithelium and the alveolar sac is a no-man's-land, in which the protective forces seem unable to cope with the stress of pollution. This zone is where diseases of pollution often strike and cause their destruction of lung tissue, resulting in emphysema. Another reason for this localization may be that the junction of the bronchiole and alveolus is poorly supplied by clearance mechanisms (lymphatics), so that pollutants accumulate here. Alcohol and smoking have been shown to inhibit macrophages and ciliary motility, respectively, thereby allowing bacterial invaders to gain a foothold.

The lung, like the heart, is also covered by a thin membrane, the **pleura,** and a similar membrane lines the chest wall. Although a potential space, the pleural cavity, exists between the layers, in health these layers are in contact with each other. It is evident that inflammation of the lung may easily extend to the pleura and set up inflammation in that space.

TECHNIQUES FOR STUDYING LUNG DISEASE

In medicine, the examination of the chest is one of the most challenging clinical adventures. By viewing the respiratory excursions, the use of accessory muscles, the rate and rhythm of breathing, much can be adduced about the effectiveness of the physiology of ventilation. Indirect examination of the anatomy of the lungs is now a changing art, as percussion and auscultation of the chest give way to newer radiographic methods (scans) (Fig. 15–5A,B) and to the measurement of blood gases. It used to be that the diagnosis of pneumonia or abscess was made by hearing dullness to percussion or tubular breath sounds, or by hearing a pressure splash or egophony. This clinical observation was confirmed by the chest roentgenogram and culture.

Today, we depend on tomograms, technetium scans, and serial studies to make the

diagnosis as well as transtracheal biopsies for culture, fiberoptic scopes for intrabronchial biopsy, and vast experience in 2 decades of exfoliative cytology. The first diagnosis has always been anatomic, and in this chapter we attempt to show both the radiographic and morbid anatomic representations of most of the lesions we discuss.

INFECTIOUS DISEASES

The limits of this book make it impossible to consider all diseases of the nose, throat, larynx, and trachea, which form the upper part of the respiratory tract, but brief mention must be made of the universal ailment, the common cold.

Although this is the most common of all infectious diseases, it is only during the last few years that we have become certain of its cause. The causal agent is a **filterable virus,** which can be grown in tissue of human and monkey embryo kidney, in which it produces recognizable degenerative changes. The virus is spread with extreme readiness from 1 person to another, so that epidemics of colds are frequent. Unlike most other filterable viruses, it fails to confer any immunity on the infected person, so that he may suffer from several attacks in the course of a winter. Several groups of viruses may be involved in different epidemics. It is little wonder, then, that a first attack does not immunize a person against a second. Predisposing or contributing factors probably play an important part, such as the chilling of the body as a result of sitting in a draft, wet feet, and the like.

This viral infection is acute, and, like other acute infections, it may clear up in the course of a few days. Too often, however, secondary invaders follow the primary infection and convert the acute into a chronic disease, which may drag on for many weary weeks. The most common of the secondary bacterial invaders are pneumococci, staphylococci, and streptococci.

The virus of the common cold and the secondary invaders attack first the nose and throat. Later they may spread down to the larynx, trachea, and bronchi, and up into the sinuses that open into the nose. For the first

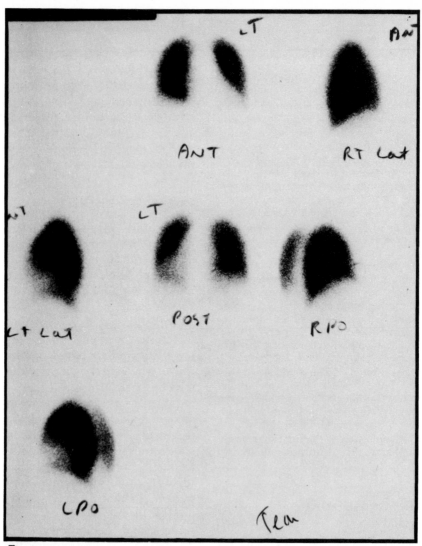

A

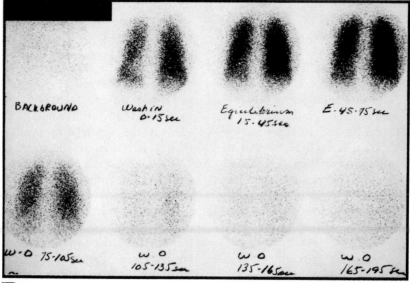

B

day or so, the mucous membrane lining the nose and throat is swollen, red, and dry, giving the well-known "stuffed-up" feeling, but soon a watery fluid is poured out that runs from the nose continually. If the secondary invaders gain a hold, the inflammation becomes suppurative in type, and the watery secretion is replaced by a purulent one, which may continue to be discharged for many weeks.

Bacterial Pneumonias

Pneumonia denotes an inflammatory condition of the lung caused by infection; a better name, therefore, would be pneumonitis. However, the term "pneumonia" is hallowed by tradition and will continue to be used and continue to have to be explained. Since the lung is an organ in the body that is in direct contact with the outside air, it is natural that bacterial infection is frequent. The most important causes of acute bacterial pneumonias are *Diplococcus pneumoniae, Streptococcus hemolyticus, Staphylococcus aureus,* and *Friedländer's bacillus.* The diffuse or lobar form of pneumonia is nearly always caused by the pneumococcus, whereas the patchy or bronchopneumonic form is likely to be due to 1 of the other organisms just enumerated.

Pneumococcal Pneumonia (Lobar). The normal habitat of the pneumococcus is the mucous membrane of the upper respiratory tract (nose and throat), from which it may pass down into the lungs. About 40% of healthy people carry pneumococci in their throat and nose. Infection is acquired from another person, usually someone who harbors pathogenic pneumococci in the throat (a carrier) rather than someone suffering from the acute disease. As in the case of other infections, predisposing causes are of great impor-

tance. Anything that lowers the resistance may act as a predisposing cause, but some of the most important are alcohol, malnutrition, congestive heart failure, and exposure or fatigue.

When a person with pathogenic pneumococci in the throat is exposed to a predisposing cause, the pneumococci pass down the trachea and bronchi and gain access to the alveoli, where they cause acute inflammation. As the thin-walled blood vessels in the walls of the lung are in such intimate relation with the alveoli, an abundant acute inflammatory exudate pours from the vessels into the air spaces. This exudate consists of the various elements that have already been described in the chapter on **inflammation,** but the predominating elements are polymorphonuclear leukocytes and serum, with formation of abundant fibrin from the latter. It is in essence a **fibrinopurulent exudate.** Many of the capillaries open up, so that red blood corpuscles are added to the exudate. The result of all this is replacement of the air in the alveoli by the exudate, so that the affected part of the lung is no longer air-containing, but is solid. This part of the lung is now said to be **consolidated.** The inflammation spreads throughout a lobe, and may involve the entire lung. Often, however, the consolidation is confined to 1 or 2 lobes, hence the term lobar pneumonia (Fig. 15–6). Such a consolidated lung is about as different from the normal spongy structure as it is possible to imagine and can be seen on chest film (Fig. 15–7). The infection reaches the pleura, and the beautifully smooth surface is now covered with a shaggy, fibrinous or fibrinopurulent exudate. This exudate may be detected because the 2 surfaces are now roughened as sandpaper and a noise similar to the rubbing together of the palms of your hand is audible with each breath. This is

Fig. 15–5. *A,* Normal lung **perfusion scan** using technetium 99m macroaggregates of albumin, which demonstrates areas of vascular perfusion. All areas that are dense are receiving blood. *B,* Normal lung **ventilation scan** using xenon 133, a radioactive gas, which fills all ventilated air spaces. Poor ventilation may be due to air space disease, chronic obstructive pulmonary disease, or obstructing lesions. Compare with the previous figure; if the airways are blocked, there will be no dark areas with xenon; if the blood vessels are blocked, there will be no dark areas from technetium.

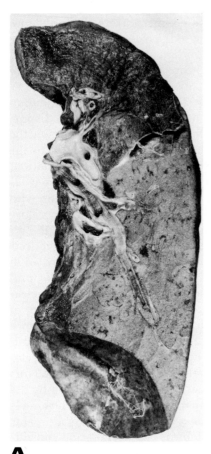

A

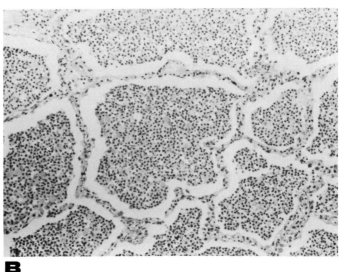

B

Fig. 15–6. *A,* Gross specimen of a lung shows the difference in color and consistency between the upper and lower lobe. The lower lobe contains no air due to replacement of the air space by pus. We call this pneumonia and refer to it as **lobar pneumonia,** when a whole lobe is involved. (McGill University, Department of Pathology Museum.) *B,* Microscopically the alveoli are filled with white blood cells.

called a **pleural friction rub** and is a sign of fibrinous pleurisy indicating underlying inflammation in the lung.

Lobar pneumonia usually runs its course in about a week. By the end of that time, provided the patient survives (which he usually does), the pneumococci are dead; the exudate dissolves and is finally removed by being coughed up in the sputum. The removal, which is called **resolution,** is extraordinarily complete, and in a few weeks, the lung is restored to its normal spongy condition, the alveoli being filled with air instead of with pus.

The foregoing description applies to the classic case of lobar pneumonia before the days of antibiotics. Naturally, if the infection is nipped in the bud by the administration of antibiotics, the lesions will not have time to develop, nor will the case come to autopsy.

Bronchopneumonia. This disease is usually caused by staphylococci, streptococci, or pneumococci. It is primarily a bronchitis, an inflammation of the bronchi, and is widespread throughout 1 or both lungs. Here and there the infection penetrates into the alveoli and produces a small patch of inflammatory consolidation. These patches may be seen throughout the lung, but they are separated by an abundance of air-containing lung tissue. Such a lung is not usually consolidated.

Bronchopneumonia is much more common than lobar pneumonia. It occurs at the extremes of age, being most frequent in young children and in the aged. It often accompanies the infectious fevers of childhood, and is so commonly found at postmortem examination as a terminal condition that it hardly attracts the attention of the pathologist unless it is unusually marked. Nevertheless, the disease must often serve as some ministering angel to snuff out the flickering flame when life is ebbing away.

In these days of prevalent staphylococcal

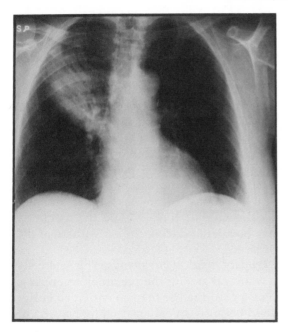

Fig. 15–7. This roentgenogram shows air space consolidation in the right upper lobe, consistent with lobar pneumonia. The dense material (inflammatory exudate) absorbs radiation, whereas normal alveoli do not.

hospital infections, bronchopneumonia has assumed a new twofold significance. (1) When admitted to hospital, persons suffering from some preexisting lung disease readily become infected with the antibiotic-resistant staphylococci residing in the hospital, and the resulting bronchopneumonia may prove fatal. (2) Such staphylococcal lesions, especially if they develop into lung abscesses (Fig. 15–8), may act as an important reservoir and source of infection, which can be widely disseminated by the coughing of the patient.

Viral Pneumonias

It is now recognized that viral pneumonias outnumber all other pneumonias, especially during epidemics. In addition to the pneumonitis complicating such viral infections as influenza and measles, there are many cases of primary lung infection caused by a variety of different viruses.

Influenzal Pneumonia. Influenza is an acute inflammatory disease of the upper respiratory tract (throat, trachea, and bronchi), associated with marked general debility. The special peculiarity of influenza is that usually it is the

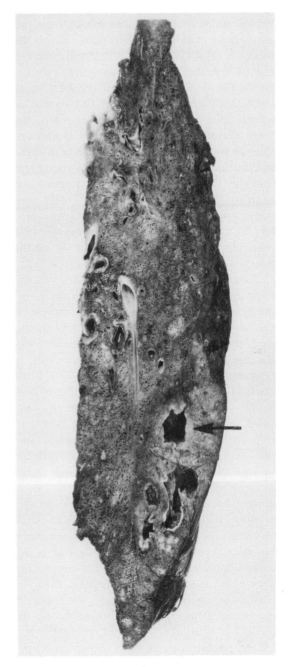

Fig. 15–8. This photograph of a lung shows (at arrow) abscess cavities with a thin wall. Frequently, such an abscess is the result of aspiration. (McGill University, Department of Pathology Museum.)

mildest of infections, lightly referred to as "a touch of the flu." At long intervals, it assumes a virulent form, and like "a blast from the stars," as an old writer said, great epidemics sweep across the world and kill millions of people. At such times, as in the pandemic of

1918 and 1919, it seems, as John Bright re-marked in another connection, that "the Angel of Death is abroad in the land; you can almost hear the beating of his wings." In the pandemic of 1918 and 1919, there were some 500,000,000 cases throughout the world, of whom 15,000,000 died. By comparison, the more recent (1957) pandemic of Asian influenza was comparatively mild. It is in these virulent outbreaks that pulmonary complications in the form of influenzal pneumonia acquire a fearful significance. These epidemics may spread with extraordinary rapidity. In a United States Army camp in 1918 there were 3 cases on one day and 3,000 on the next!

The cause of influenza is a filterable virus of various strains or groups. This virus is inhaled and sets up an acute inflammation in the nose and throat that may spread upward into the sinuses and downward into the trachea and bronchi, causing the feeling of rawness so familiar to everyone. The virus causes not only a characteristic feeling of profound weakness and lassitude, but in some cases lowers the resistance of the lungs, so that other bacteria, secondary invaders, like the 7 devils of Holy Writ, pass down into the lungs and produce pneumonia. This is much more likely to happen during the great epidemics, thus explaining the high mortality on these occasions. Influenzal pneumonia differs from the lobar variety in that both lungs are always involved, and, in place of being consolidated and dry as a result of containing a more or less coagulated exudate, they are wet and waterlogged. When the lung is examined at autopsy, it is found to be intensely congested with blood, so that it is a bluish-purple color. Under the microscope, the appearance of viral pneumonia differs from that of bacterial lobar pneumonia in that the interstitium is the principal site of inflammation, not the alveoli. The septums of the alveoli are thickened by the congestion and inflammation which increase the diffusing distance and may cause respiratory embarrassment.

Among the symptoms the dry, hacking **cough,** which is so common, is caused by acute irritation of the trachea and large bronchi. The profound **prostration** is due to a general toxemia. In influenzal pneumonia there may be marked **cyanosis** (blueness of lips and face) and **dyspnea. Fever** is present as in all acute infections. The most important complication of viral pneumonia is the frequent superinfection by bacteria. Viral infections typically cause cell death, and when the living cells of the bronchi are killed, the primary defense barrier to bacterial infection is broken, predisposing the patient to bacterial pneumonias. It is important to recognize that viral infections do not respond to conventional antibiotic therapy, and the diagnosis may be missed during the early phase of the disease.

Primary Atypical Pneumonia. This relatively new arrival among the pneumonias appears to be a group rather than an entity, so designated because it is not caused by bacteria or fungi. The disease may appear in small epidemics, usually in schools and army camps where young people are congregated. One of the most common causes of this disease is an organism called *Mycoplasma pneumoniae* (sometimes referred to as PPLO—pleuropneumonia-like organisms, or the Eaton agent). These organisms are smaller than bacteria and larger than viruses. There is an acute inflammation of the upper respiratory tract, only involving the lungs to a minor degree, so that, although the morbidity is high, the mortality is low. Even when pneumonia does develop, the physical signs are largely absent, a characteristic feature, but there is roentgenographic evidence of a patchy, ill-defined consolidation seldom involving more than a part of a lobe. The course is usually mild, with recovery occurring in 2 or 3 weeks.

Clinical Pattern. Lobar pneumonia will be taken as an example. Most of the symptoms can be explained by the pathologic lesions. The face is flushed, the breathing rapid, shallow, and painful; there is cough with blood-streaked sputum; fever and leukocytosis are present; and examination of the chest reveals changes in the lung. The dyspnea and rapid breathing are caused by interference with the free interchange of gases between the blood and air, owing to the exudate in the alveoli. The cough is due to irritation of the bronchi. The sputum is sticky, so that it can be pulled out in strings and is characteristically red or rust-colored. The stickiness is caused by the fibrin and mucus and the color by the red blood corpuscles in the exudate. The sputum consists largely of polymorphonuclear leukocytes (pus cells) and contains large numbers of pneumococci. The pain on breathing is an indication of pleurisy, the rough and inflamed surfaces of the pleura being rubbed together each time the patient takes a breath. Fever is caused by the toxins produced by the pneumococci. Leukocytosis is the natural result of the demand for enormous numbers of leukocytes to be poured into the alveoli of the lung. When the healthy chest is percussed, a resonant, drumlike note is heard, but when the lung is consolidated, there is dullness on percussion, owing to replacement of the air by exudate.

Abscess

In lobar pneumonia there is no true destruction; the walls of the alveoli are not destroyed. This phenomenon makes the complete structural recovery of the lung possible. Sometimes, however, especially when accessory factors are present that weaken resistance, the lung tissue is destroyed, and abscesses are formed. This complication is more likely to happen in bronchopneumonia, and, as we have already seen, staphylococcal infection is often responsible.

Abscess of the lung can be divided into 3 groups, depending on the method of causation. These are the aspiration, the embolic, and the pneumonic groups.

The aspiration group is the largest and most important. Lung abscess is a constant threat in operations on the mouth, nose, and throat, especially tonsillectomy and extraction of teeth. Infected material passes down the trachea and bronchi. Abscess is more frequent in the right lung, which has a more vertical bronchus, and in the lower lobe. Stomach contents may be vomited during general anesthesia and inhaled into the lungs. Foreign bodies, especially peanuts and coins, may pass from the mouths of children down the trachea and cause lung abscess.

The embolic group is due to a septic thrombus's being carried by the venous blood to the right side of the heart, and then through the pulmonary artery to the lung. Two sources of an infected blood clot that may be mentioned are the veins of the female pelvis and the lateral venous sinus of the skull, which becomes infected in inflammation of the middle ear and mastoid.

The pneumonic group represents a complication of pneumonia, usually streptococcal or influenzal in type; abscess formation is rare in lobar pneumonia.

The clinical pattern is fever, cough, copious expectoration of pus, foul breath, and foul sputum. An important complication of lung abscess is the development of an abscess of the brain, owing to infected material's being carried by the blood from the lung to the left side of the heart and thence to the brain. This process may also occur in bronchiectasis.

Pulmonary Tuberculosis

The general pattern of tuberculous infection has already been discussed, together with the observation of the decrease in the incidence of the disease from 700 deaths per 100,000 population in 1910 to 5 deaths per 100,000 today. As the infection is acquired in most cases by inhalation, it is natural that the lung should be by far the most common site of the disease. We have seen that tuberculosis is a struggle between attack and defense, usually on fairly even terms, but with the odds considerably in favor of the defense. When infection is established there are 3 possible courses: (1) **healing with scarring;** (2) **fibrocaseous tuberculosis;** (3) **acute tuberculous pneumonia.** The result depends on the size and frequency of the dose of tubercle bacilli on the 1 hand and on the natural powers of defense on the other. It is important to distinguish between primary infection and reinfection, often called secondary infection.

Primary Infection. The first infection usually occurs in childhood, but now, as the result of public health measures, it may be delayed until adult life. The primary lesion is a small caseous focus, seldom more than 1 cm in diameter, usually situated at the periphery of the lung. A consequence of this infection is the drainage of macrophages that contain the tubercle bacillus to a centrally located lymph

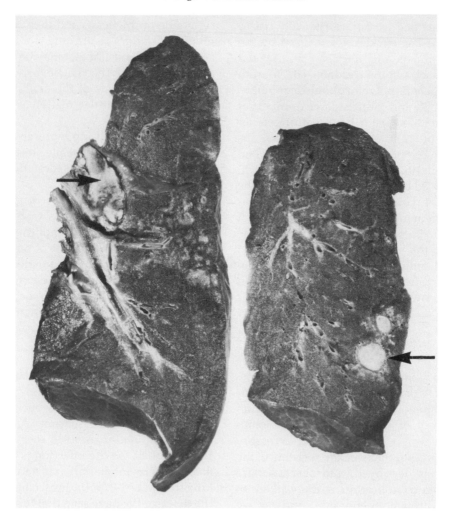

Fig. 15–9.   This photograph shows the peripheral lesion (round white mass) and the central lymph node with caseous necrosis (arrow) of the **Ghon complex,** the primary response to tuberculosis. (McGill University, Department of Pathology Museum.)

node. In the lymph node, further reaction takes place and leads to cellular hypersensitivity, but often the lymph node also shows a caseous lesion. This combination of the peripheral lesion (where the tubercle bacteria first gain their foothold) and the central lymph node lesion is called the **Ghon complex,** after its discoverer (Fig. 15–9).

In the Ghon complex, the primary infection contrasts sharply with the secondary lesion, which nearly always makes its first appearance at the apex of the lung. Infection spreads by the lymphatics, so that the regional lymph nodes become enlarged and caseous, again in contrast to what is found in secondary infection. The patient with primary infection

either recovers or dies; the disease does not become chronic, nor is there any cavity formation. Recovery is marked by disappearance of the pulmonary and lymph node lesions, or by their conversion into fibrous tissue with calcification. However, the patient is rendered hypersensitive or allergic to a subsequent infection, as shown by the tuberculin test. If healing fails to occur, there may be generalized septicemia with rapidly fatal bronchopneumonia.

Reinfection. The reaction of the now-allergic tissues to reinfection is different from that of the primary infection. The right lung is attacked much more often than the left, and the lesion is usually just below the apex. There are now 4 possibilities: (1) healing with fibrosis, (2) chronic fibrocaseous tuberculosis, (3) acute tuberculous caseous pneumonia, and (4) acute miliary tuberculosis. The result will depend both on the size and frequency of the dose of tubercle bacilli and on the patient's own resistance to disease. This may be expressed by the formula $D \propto \dfrac{V \times N \times H}{R^{n+a}}$, in which D is expression of the disease, V is virulence of organism, N is number of organisms, H is hypersensitivity of host, and R is resistance, both native (n) and acquired (a).

Healing with Scarring. This course, fortunately, is by far the most common for the infection to run, as shown by the frequent presence of old tuberculous scars at the apex of 1 or both lungs in persons who come to autopsy. The reason that tuberculosis localizes at the apex of the lungs is unknown. Two physiologic factors may play a role. First, the concentration of oxygen per unit volume of tissue at the apex is greater than elsewhere in the lung, and second, the venous and lymphatic pressures are less. Perhaps the tubercle bacillus thrives there because of the better environment and the potential difficulties of mobilizing adequate defenses. There is a limited amount of destruction of tissue, but if the bacterial dose is not large and if the person is in good health, the healing process asserts itself, the bacilli are overcome, fibrous tissue surrounds and invades the area, and finally only a scar is left, in which calcium salts are often deposited. Even during the active stage, the patient shows no symptoms, and is unaware that he has acquired tuberculosis, but the positive tuberculin test of the skin will show that this is the case.

Fibrocaseous Tuberculosis. This is the usual form in the person who shows active signs of tuberculosis. The name indicates that both main processes of the disease are at work. There is fibrosis, indicating healing, and caseation, indicating destruction. The basic lesion, as usual, is the tubercle. The tubercles coalesce to form caseous or cheese-like masses. The caseous material becomes softened, liquefied, discharged into a bronchus, and finally expectorated as tuberculous sputum filled with tubercle bacilli. A **cavity** is formed in the place formerly occupied by the

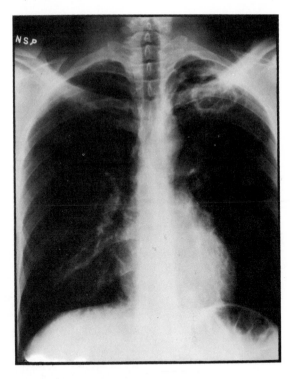

Fig. 15–10. This roentgenogram demonstrates a cavitary lesion in the left upper lobe, in this case due to a cavitated tuberculous abscess.

caseous material (Fig. 15–10). This cavity may be small, or it may be so large as to involve the greater part of a lobe. Sometimes an artery is left traversing a cavity. Should this vessel finally rupture, profuse hemorrhage may occur. In time, numerous cavities are formed. The intervening parts of the lung show tuberculous consolidation, the alveoli being filled with inflammatory cells and caseous material. If the progress of the disease is slow, fibrosis may be marked, especially around the cavities, but true healing does not occur. The disease spreads from the apex downward, so that the oldest and most advanced lesions are at the top. In a case with extensive lesions, there may be cavities in the upper part of the lung, consolidation in the middle, and separate tubercles at the base. Pleurisy is always present, and adhesions are formed between the 2 layers of the pleura.

Acute Tuberculous Pneumonia. Here the infection overwhelms the resistance, and runs through the lung like a forest fire, giving rise to the clinical picture of galloping consumption. There are no discrete tubercles, but in their place a diffuse pneumonic process. There is no fibrosis, no attempt at limitation of the infection. The disease may prove fatal in a few months or even weeks without therapy.

Acute Miliary Tuberculosis. This is a fourth possibility, which may be regarded as a com-

plication of any of the previous 3. The tuberculous process may penetrate the wall of a blood vessel or a lymphatic, which may effectively do the same thing—discharge large numbers of bacilli into the blood stream. These bacilli are carried throughout the body, where they cause an infinite number of miliary tubercles in all the organs. The lungs

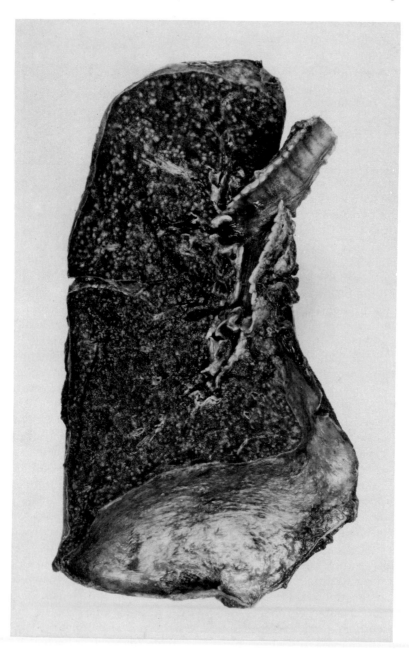

Fig. 15–11. This photograph shows lesions with the appearance of small white millet seeds scattered throughout the lung typical of **miliary tuberculosis.** Similar lesions can appear in the kidney, spleen, liver, and other organs. (McGill University, Department of Pathology Museum.)

are no exception, so that, in addition to a small lesion at the apex of 1 lung, both lungs may be peppered with fine tubercles. The term miliary is derived from the similarity of the tubercles seen with the unaided eye to millet seeds, small white grains. Miliary tuberculosis can be present in any or all organs, such as the liver, spleen, and kidney (Fig. 15–11).

Clinical Pattern. The cause of general symptoms, such as fever, loss of weight, and weakness, is uncertain. They become more marked when secondary infection with pyogenic bacteria is added to the pure tuberculous infection. **Cough** is due to irritation of the larger bronchi. **Pain in the side** is due to tuberculous pleurisy. The character of the **sputum** depends on the nature of the lesions. In acute miliary tuberculosis, there may be no sputum. Until cavities have formed, it is scanty and may contain no bacilli. After cavity formation, it is copious and purulent, often owing to secondary infection, and contains large numbers of bacilli. The more rapid the disease, the more bacilli will there be; the more stationary the disease, the fewer are their numbers.

Hemoptysis, the coughing up of blood, is due to erosion of a blood vessel. It has been said that hemoptysis marks the end of the beginning or the beginning of the end of the disease. At first, there may be erosion of a small vessel in the early process of softening, and the sputum becomes blood-streaked. In the advanced stage, a large artery or vein crossing a chronic cavity may give way and cause a severe and possibly fatal hemorrhage, as with the tragic heroine of Dumas, Camille *(La belle dame aux camélias).*

It must not be forgotten that the patient with pulmonary tuberculosis is a potential source of danger to those with whom he comes in contact. This danger may remain potential and not become actual if he is educated in the principles of hygiene. The 2 sources of danger are sputum and droplet contagion from coughing at close quarters. If sputum is safely disposed of and the danger of coughing infected droplets in the direction of another person recognized, the tuberculous patient need not be a source of infection to those with whom he lives. But the danger is always present, and precautions must not for a moment be relaxed. This is the reason that tuberculosis is so common in crowded living conditions of poor neighborhoods.

Bronchitis

Bronchitis may be acute or chronic. The acute form usually involves the trachea as well as the larger bronchi.

Acute Tracheobronchitis. The irritant responsible for the acute inflammation may be bacterial, mechanical (various dusts), or toxic (poisonous gases). The mucous membrane is red and swollen, and the lumen is filled with pus. When the irritant is removed, the inflammation is likely to subside.

Chronic Bronchitis. The definition of chronic bronchitis is "the presence of a productive cough for at least 3 months of the year over at least 2 consecutive years without other cause."

This inflammatory disease of the lung, characterized by cough and increased sputum production, is a common and serious disease in the middle-aged and older person. The disease occurs particularly in industrial areas and in heavy cigarette smokers. It has been identified in Great Britain as the most common chronic respiratory ailment, exceeded only by the common cold. The prevalence and seriousness of the disease was an incentive to clean up the endemic air pollution in the late 1960's in London. Although attempts to culture organisms have been made frequently, it is now accepted that environmental pollution, whether from the waste of factories or from the carbon and tars of smoke (household or tobacco), is the principal etiologic agent that leads to the hyperplasia of the mucous glands, the hypertrophy of the smooth muscle, and the increased thickening of the bronchial wall. The excess secretion of mucus as a response to irritants leads to plugging of the small airways (Fig. 15–12) and a loss of local ventilation. The residual lung volume becomes increased, the vital capacity reduced, and the patient complains of wheezing and shortness of breath (Fig. 15–13). Because some areas of the lung are well ventilated and perfused, the level of arterial oxygen may remain within normal limits for many

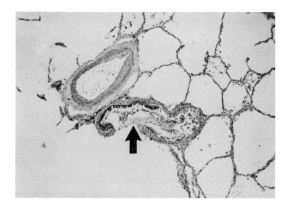

Fig. 15–12. This photomicrograph shows an area of lung in which a mucous plug obstructs a bronchiole *(arrow)*.

they may have bronchopneumonia, which is naturally much more serious than in a person with normal lungs. The outstanding feature of this disease is the obstructive element that leads to the general designation of **chronic obstructive pulmonary disease** for chronic bronchitis.

EMPHYSEMA

This extraordinarily common disease of the lung is also classified under the umbrella of chronic obstructive pulmonary disease (COPD), but is anatomically different from chronic bronchitis, although both processes often, or usually, exist in a patient at the same time. There is much discussion as to the possible relationships between them. Emphysema is characterized by an increase in the volume of the lung (Figs. 15–14 and 15–15), which is attributed to the overdistension and destructive changes that can be seen distal to the terminal respiratory bronchioles. In Figure 15–16A,B, the normal bronchial tree is contrasted with the dilated bronchial tree, and a dilatation, like a rotten apple on the branch of a tree, is seen at high magnification in Figure 15–16C. The alveolar spaces that are

years. When the obstruction becomes more widespread, CO_2 is retained, arterial hypoxemia results, and, because of reflex vasoconstriction in the arteriolar bed of the lung, the resistance of this circulation is increased. This change then leads to increased demands on the right heart and eventually to hypertrophy and failure (cor pulmonale).

In patients with chronic bronchitis, the plugging of bronchioles sets the scene for bacterial infections, and frequently in winter

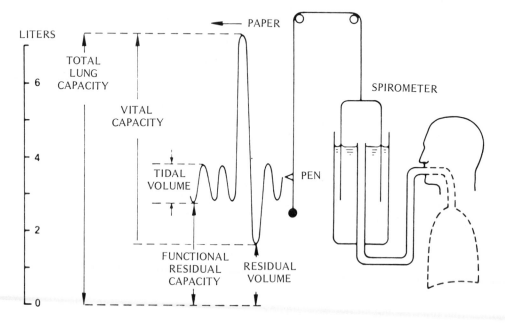

Fig. 15–13. This diagram illustrates the respective elements of ventilation which may be measured in normal and diseased states. Different lung diseases may affect different components of ventilatory function, as mentioned in the text. (From West, J. B.: *Respiratory Physiology*. Baltimore, Williams & Wilkins, 1974.)

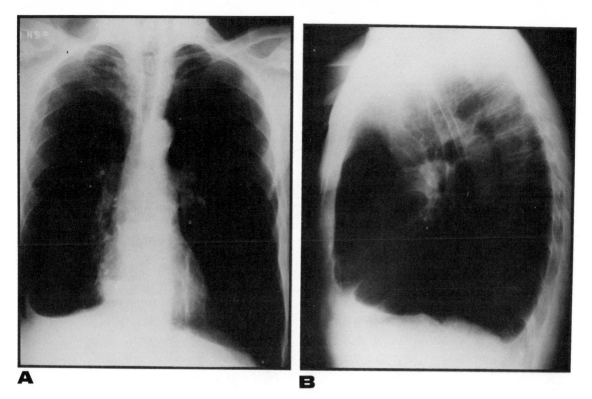

Fig. 15–14. *A* and *B,* These roentgenograms show the changes of chronic obstructive pulmonary disease. The lungs are overinflated, larger, and appear much less dense than normal because there is more empty space and less tissue. Note the increased diameter of the chest and the flattened diaphragm.

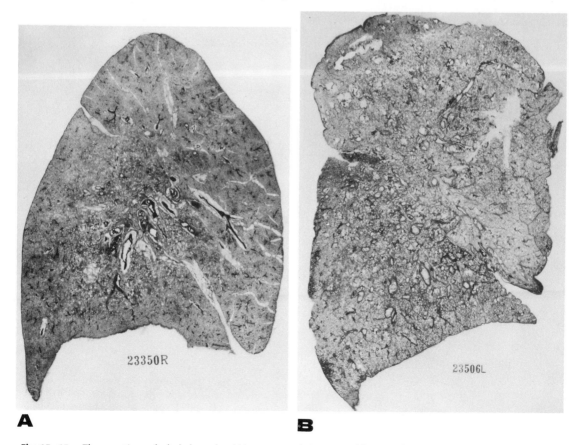

Fig. 15–15. These sections of whole lung should be compared: *A,* a normal lung, and *B,* a lung with extensive **emphysema.** Note the coarser texture of *B,* which is the result of destruction of the small airways and coalescence into large empty pockets. (Courtesy of Dr. J. Hogg, Department of Pathology, McGill University.)

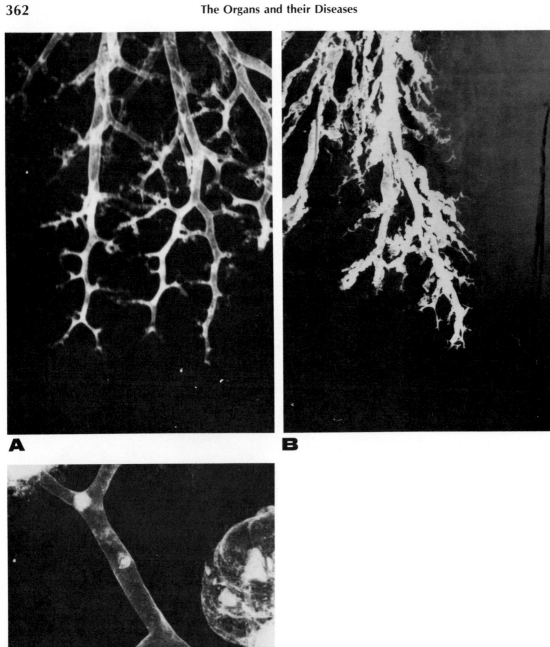

Fig. 15–16. These preparations demonstrate a normal bronchial tree, *A*, and a bronchial tree that is dilated saccular and distinctly pathologic, *B*. A higher magnification of an area of emphysema is shown in C. (Courtesy of Dr. J. Hogg, Department of Pathology, McGill University.)

normally delicate and uniform have been destroyed, and they coalesce in emphysema to create a large saccule. Typically, the injury may be limited to the center of a secondary lung lobule. The destruction frequently occurs together with chronic bronchitis. This type of emphysema is referred to as **central lobular.** Large balloons of lung may occur less commonly, and these are called **bullae.** Another type of change has been recognized, in which the injury involves more than just the central portion of the lung lobule, and this is referred to as **panacinar** emphysema. Typically, as may be seen in Figure 15–15, emphysema is more extreme in the upper lobes of the lung and in the apical segment of the lower lobe.

It should be remembered that, although the disease is primarily of the small airways and is associated with injury (pollution) and inflammation (bronchitis), and its association with injury and inflammation is well accepted, recently another association to explain the disease process has been made.

There is a rare hereditary form of emphysema in which a deficiency in a serum enzyme inhibitor (alpha-antitrypsin) has been found in members of a family who develop emphysema and chronic obstructive lung disease. It is suggested that the integrity of the lung depends on the presence of such an enzyme inhibitor. The lung destruction is explained in part by enzymatic damage to lung tissue. It has been suggested that the lack of antitrypsin may allow the trypsin, believed to come from bacteria and inflammatory cells, to digest the lung parenchyma and to cause the enlarged air spaces.

Emphysema is a crippling disease, feared because the patient does not die quickly, but drags out a miserable existence for many years, a trial and tribulation to himself, his family, and his physician. He has difficulty with every breath taken and breathes some 20,000 times every 24 hours. It has been said that perhaps the most compelling of human appetites is the need for air, and probably no distress is so agonizing as that which results from the inability to breathe adequately.

The effects of emphysema may be serious and far-reaching. The chest becomes barrel-shaped (Fig. 15–14), respiratory movements are diminished, and expiration is difficult and prolonged. Owing to the widespread atrophy and destruction of the alveolar walls, the small blood vessels that run in them are obliterated, with resulting obstruction to the pulmonary circulation.

CARCINOMA OF THE LUNG

At the present time, cancer of the lung is perhaps the most interesting and challenging of all malignant tumors. It is interesting because of the problems it presents with respect to: (1) **increased incidence,** (2) **possible relation to external carcinogens.** It is challenging because, of all the malignant tumors of internal organs, it is often readily seen by means of the bronchoscope, and yet the prognosis is among the worst.

When I (William Boyd) was a student in Edinburgh, the tumor used to be regarded as a rarity. In fact, I do not remember seeing a case either in the ward or in the autopsy room, but I do remember seeing many cases that were called "mediastinal lymphosarcoma" invading the lung. During the past 70 years, bronchogenic carcinoma has become the commonest of the killing cancers, especially in the male. One in 3 men with cancer has carcinoma of the lung. There can be little doubt that there has been a real increase (Fig. 15–17), but it is equally true that what we know we see. It was not until the beginning of the present century that coronary thrombosis and myocardial infarction were recognized. No one suggests that the disease started then, yet the lesions, which any medical student can now tell at a glance, were not appreciated by such masters as Virchow and Rokitansky, who may have given them different names.

If there were differences of opinion as to the question of an increased incidence of cancer of the lung, these differences are multiplied many times when we come to the matter of **causation.** The trouble is that there are so many possible carcinogens. The exhaust gases and soot from automobiles, especially when idling at stop lights in the city, are rich in carcinogenic agents. The same is true of radiation fallout, although that modern hazard can hardly be blamed for the development of cancer 40 or more years ago.

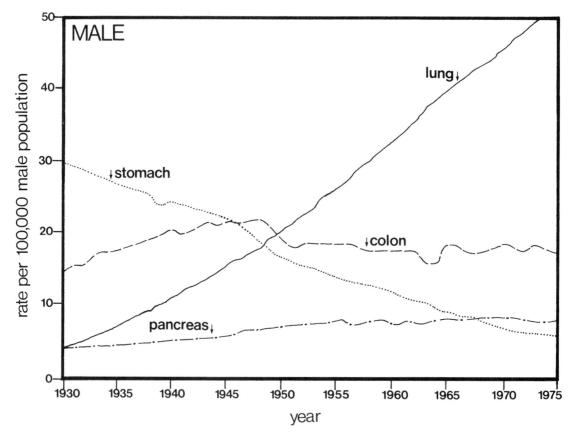

Fig. 15–17.   This graph shows the remarkable increase in the rate of lung cancer during the years 1930 to 1975. Compare with the rate for stomach (falling), and colon (relatively constant). (From Gilbert, E. F., and Huntington, R. W.: *An Introduction to Pathology.* New York, Oxford University Press, 1978.)

Cigarette smoking is the etiologic agent that has aroused the greatest interest and the most heated debates. Statistical evidence certainly supports the idea that excessive smoking is a factor of importance. If you do not smoke, the incidence of carcinoma of the lung is 3.4 per 100,000 population; if you smoke less than 1 pack per day, it is 59 per 100,000, and if you smoke more than 1 pack per day, it is 217 per 100,000. Statistics show that cigarette smokers have a greater risk of dying of lung cancer than have nonsmokers, and that the risk increases with the number of cigarettes smoked.

It is important to recognize that there are several distinct tumors of the lung that can collectively be called carcinoma, but at least 3 different subsets are distinguished by microscopic examination, by their behavior, and by their prognosis and response to

therapy. They probably are also different in that their cause may differ. Thus, we recognize 1 group of lung carcinoma as having a small cell pattern, arising in or around central bronchi and metastasizing early in the typical 50-year-old male patient. This type is called an "oat cell carcinoma" by popular designation, or, more correctly, **small cell carcinoma.** These cells have been shown to arise from cells other than those normally lining the respiratory tract. Instead, they are interstitial cells that stain with silver stains and contain secretory granules. These tumors sometimes are associated with syndromes of excess ACTH (adrenocorticotropic hormone) or ADH (antidiuretic hormone) production, and are responsible for the paraneoplastic syndrome, because of the ectopic hormones that these cells can secrete. It is important to recognize that this type of tumor (oat cell) ac-

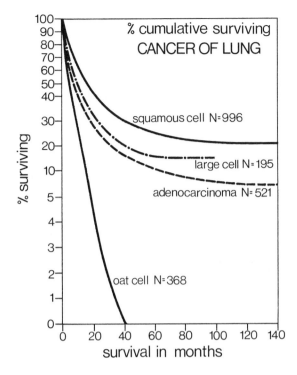

Fig. 15-18. This graph illustrates the survival rates for different histologic types of cancer of the lung. (From Mountain, C. F., et al.: A system for the clinical staging of lung cancer. Am. J. Roentgenol., *120*:130, 1974.)

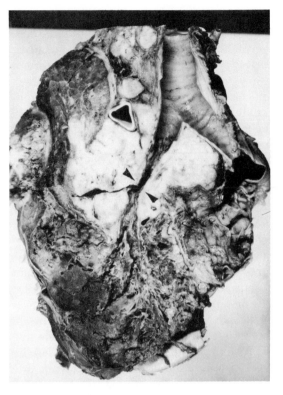

Fig. 15-19. The right lung is shown with a large area of **bronchogenic carcinoma** rising in the bronchus, which is narrowed (arrows). (McGill University, Department of Pathology Museum.)

counts for only about 15% of all lung cancers (Fig. 15-18).

The most common type is **squamous carcinoma** (40%), which arises in the metaplastic epithelium of the major bronchi. The tumor grows into and surrounds 1 of the major bronchi, gradually narrowing the lumen until it becomes partially blocked (Fig. 15-19). Two results follow from this blockage. (1) In the first place, the part of the lung supplied by the bronchus is cut off from a fresh supply of air, the air in this part of the lung is gradually absorbed into the blood, and finally the affected area of the lung undergoes collapse (atelectasis). This collapse can readily be recognized in the roentgenogram even though the tumor itself may be invisible, and by this means the correct diagnosis can be inferred. (2) The second possible outcome is recurrent infection beyond the obstruction, that is, an abscess, and pneumonia that does not resolve. This is because the secretions in the blocked part of the bronchus cannot escape and therefore stagnate and contribute a suita-

ble medium for infection. Cancer cells from the surface of the tumor that projects into the lumen of the bronchus are shed off and coughed up in the sputum. Examination of the sputum for these cells, either by making smears or by coagulating the sputum into a block of tissue and cutting microscopic sections, is an extremely valuable means of making an early diagnosis, especially in cases in which the tumor cannot be seen by the bronchoscope.

Other types of lung carcinomas are often thought of as subsets of this "bronchogenic" carcinoma. They may appear as large anaplastic cells (30%) or more poorly differentiated carcinomas. Another group that seems different comprises those carcinomas that show a glandular pattern (adenocarcinoma) (10%) and that arise in the periphery of the lung rather than in the larger central bronchi. Finally, there is another rare type (alveolar cell) (3%), which appears in many sites at once and resembles a disease in sheep attributed to a virus infection. Despite these morphologic differences, most lung cancers appear in persons who can give a history of heavy smoking for many decades; yet there are smokers who do not develop cancer, too!

One of the chief features of all carcinomas of the lung is the formation of metastases. Most frequently, carcinoma of the lung metastasizes to regional lymph nodes (80% at the hilum of the lung); then it is seen in the liver (40%), brain (15%), bone marrow (15%), and adrenal (15%). Even when the tumor in the bronchus is comparatively small, the cancer cells may spread by lymphatics to the lymph nodes in the chest, where they form a large tumor mass, or by the blood stream to distant organs such as the liver, brain, and bones. The first indication that the patient has cancer of the lung may be increase in girth due to metastases in the liver, severe headache due to a brain tumor, or a fracture caused by weakening of a bone from the presence of a secondary tumor. The adrenal and kidney are often involved. In addition to distant metastases, the tumor may spread widely throughout the lung and involve the pleura.

Clinical Pattern. The symptoms are due to metastases and obstruction. The **persistent cough** is due to irritation of the bronchus by a growth. When a patient in the cancer-prone age, particularly a man, has suffered from a cough and expectoration without obvious cause for more than a few weeks, it is always wise to suspect carcinoma and to examine the sputum for cancer cells or to pass a bronchoscope and inspect the lining of the bronchi. *Bloody sputum* is caused by the opening of a tumor in the bronchus into a blood vessel. **Dyspnea** may be due to the cutting off of air from the lung, to pressure by the enlarged glands, or to interference with the heart's action. **Pain** in the chest and back is caused by pressure on the nerves. Pleural effusion is common, and is due to irritation of the pleura by spread of the tumor. Other symptoms may be due to metastases in the brain and elsewhere.

Certain round, circumscribed benign tumors cannot be distinguished radiologically from inflammatory lesions (Fig. 15–20). These tumors are called **hamartomas** because

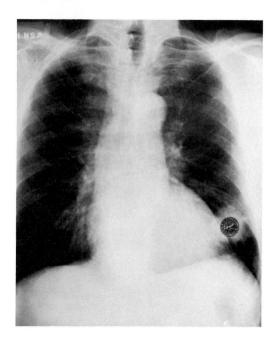

Fig. 15–20. This roentgenogram demonstrates a calcified "coin lesion" in the right upper lung, so-called because of its size and shape. The cause in this case was histoplasmosis.

they are attributed to developmental defect, and the problem of the cause of this **"coin lesion"** is best solved by surgical removal and histologic examination.

It is important, however, to realize that not all tumors that can be identified in the lung have arisen there. The lung is a favorite site for metastasis of tumor from other organs, particularly tumors of the breast, kidney, or colon. Often these tumors appear as solitary lesions, but sometimes they are multiple, as shown in Figure 15–21*A,B*. By the time such tumors are identified in the lung, it is usually too late to do much about them.

PNEUMOCONIOSIS

The long-continued irritation of certain substances may cause a chronic interstitial inflammation known as pneumoconiosis (Greek *konis*, dust). These dusts are encountered as the result of certain industrial processes. The most common dangerous element in the dust is silica.

Silicosis is the most widespread, the most serious, and the oldest of all occupational dis-

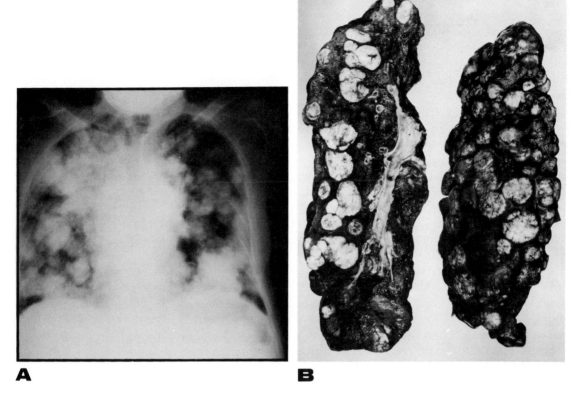

Fig. 15–21. *A,* The cloudy patches on this chest film are called "cannonball" lesions, and are consistent with multiple metastases to the lungs. *B,* The gross appearance of similar lesions throughout both lung fields, typical of metastatic tumor to the lungs from the kidney or bowel. (McGill University, Department of Pathology Museum.)

eases. It provides a serious hazard in the gold-mining industry in certain districts such as the South African Rand and northern Ontario. If, in coal mining, hard rock has to be drilled through, coal miners may also suffer. Other occupations in which there is danger are tin mining, stoneworking, metal grinding, and sandblasting. In all these cases, dust containing fine particles of silica may be inhaled over long periods of time.

The silica dust is carried by phagocytes from the bronchioles into the septums of the alveoli. There the dust acts as a stimulant to the formation of large amounts of connective tissue. This fibrosis goes hand in hand with destruction of the lung structure. At first there are discrete nodules of fibrous tissue, but in time these coalesce to form large fibrous areas, which are useless from the point of view of respiratory function. These fibrous areas give a characteristic roentgenographic picture, by

means of which an accurate diagnosis can be made.

We have spoken as if the silica particles explained everything. Another concept, the antigen theory, has come into fashion. Silica, instead of having a simple toxic effect on the tissue, is now believed to combine with body protein to form an antigen, so that there may be some element of an antigen-antibody reaction in the production of fibrosis.

The condition is progressive, and the patient continues to worsen even after he or she has been removed from the source of dust for a number of years. Many silicotics die of tuberculosis, because the presence of silica in the tissues favors the growth of tubercle bacilli to an astonishing degree. There is gradually increasing shortness of breath, with developing heart failure owing to the difficulty of the right ventricle in pumping blood through the densely fibrosed lungs.

This is one of the few conditions for which there is no treatment, and it is evident that in this case prevention is all-important. This can be done by adequately ventilating factories and by providing miners with masks that filter out the dust. Silicosis remains a great occupational hazard.

Anthracosis, sometimes called "black lung," is the name given to the lung filled with coal dust. All city dwellers have a degree of anthracosis, as they inhale heavily soot-laden air and filter out the soot that stains their tissues. If the coal is hard coal, damage will result, because the rock from which the coal was mined contains a certain amount of silica. **Asbestosis** is an important disease caused by the inhalation of asbestos dust. The disease may be acquired either during the crushing of asbestos rock, in the process of the manufacture of asbestos, or from handling building materials or insulation that is composed of asbestos. The simple act of sawing asbestos insulating board creates a fine dust that, when inhaled, can cause chronic injury to the lung. As the great bulk of asbestos comes from the province of Quebec, it is natural that many cases should be found in that locality. The lung shows the same airless and fibrous condition that is so characteristic of silicosis. Both in asbestosis and in silicosis there is a marked tendency to the development of pulmonary tuberculosis.

The most important aspect of asbestosis is not fibrosis, but rather the relation this material has to cancer of the lung and its covering, the pleura. We now recognize that the relatively rare tumor of the pleura, mesothelioma, is unequivocably associated with asbestosis. It now seems clear that occupational exposure to asbestos carries a risk for gastrointestinal cancers as well.

VASCULAR DISEASES OF THE LUNG

The most common pathologic state of the respiratory tract that causes serious symptoms, apart from the common cold, is **pulmonary edema.** This state arises when there is heart failure or, less commonly, when some other cause such as high altitude upsets the equilibrium in the capillary bed of the lung. By far the most common cause of pul-

monary edema, which causes marked **dyspnea,** is heart failure from any cause. The mechanism by which the edema occurs is simply an elevation in the pressure at the venous end of the capillary bed. Other mechanisms, such as valvular heart disease (aortic stenosis, mitral stenosis), which raise the left atrial pressure, result in pulmonary edema that can be recognized in the patient by the moist, bubbling sounds heard through a stethoscope. These sounds are called rales. The same rules, in general, govern the occurrence of pulmonary edema as dictate the presence of edema in other places in the body.

Emboli to the lung from leg veins or from areas of thrombophlebitis, or even from the right heart, are frequently life-threatening, if not fatal. The occurrence of pulmonary emboli is often overlooked clinically, particularly if they are small. One of the classic presentations is the occurrence of a sudden pain in the chest accompanied by blood-tinged sputum. This presentation is relatively easy to recognize, but in many instances there may be no hemoptysis, and the embolus may elicit no inflammatory reaction (Fig. 15–22 A,B). Therefore the patient may be unaware that it has occurred. Because the lung has a dual blood supply (bronchial vessels arising from the aorta and pulmonary vessels from the right heart), unlike other organs such as the kidney that have an endarterial supply, **infarction** does not inevitably accompany every embolus. It is only when the systemic circulation (bronchial arteries) is compromised and sluggish, as in cases of chronic heart failure, that occlusion of a branch of the pulmonary artery causes an infarct. These infarcts classically are wedge-shaped, reflecting the distribution of the smaller vessels, and reach to the pleural space. A fresh infarct in the lung is often visible radiologically, and, if you should examine it grossly, it will appear hemorrhagic.

Large pulmonary emboli often arrest at the bifurcation of the pulmonary arteries and are a cause of sudden death, presumably on a reflex basis. The most common predisposing cause to pulmonary emboli, big or small, are areas of thrombosis in the deep veins of the leg or pelvis. Prolonged bed rest, surgical operations, and immobilization following or-

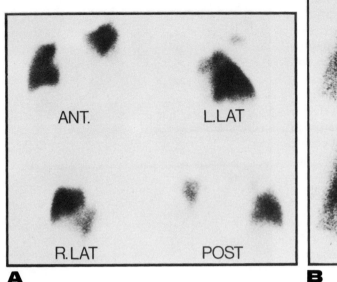

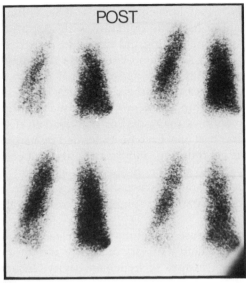

Fig. 15–22. These figures are lung scans. *A* shows multiple defects of perfusion due to pulmonary thromboembolism. Normal perfusion can be seen in *B*.

thopedic procedures are all significant predisposing causes to this serious vascular catastrophe.

A third but relatively rare disease of the pulmonary vasculature is prolonged and persistent hypertension. The pulmonary, as contrasted with the systemic, circulation is a low-pressure system in which the right ventricular pressure and main pulmonary artery pressure seldom exceed 30 mm Hg, about a quarter of the systolic pressure in the systemic circulation (120 mm Hg). It is a low-resistance, distensible system that receives the same volume of blood as the aorta, and even with exercise or after pneumonectomy there is only a slight increase in pressure. However, when there is narrowing of the pulmonary arteries due to chronic lung disease, or recurrent pulmonary emboli, or a reflex (vasomotor) constriction due to anorexia or acidosis, then the pulmonary artery pressure will rise and approach systemic values.

Increased resistance may be caused by increased flow, whatever the cause (congenital defects of the heart or great vessels), by increased pressure in the left atrium (mitral stenosis, left heart failure), or by reflex vasoconstriction (chronic lung disease). Many conditions may lead to a rise in pulmonary arterial pressure and may eventually result in right heart failure **(cor pulmonale),** but they are beyond the scope of this chapter.

An even rarer disease is **primary pulmonary hypertension,** which is also referred to as idiopathic. This simply means that all the recognized causes of pulmonary hypertension, such as recurrent pulmonary emboli, have been excluded as contributing to the disease, and this particular case has no known explanation for the hypertension and failure.

ASTHMA

This difficult and distressing disease is well named, for it is derived from the Greek word for panting. Literally, the term means difficult breathing and has been traced in English as far back as 1540. It is a disease of uncertain etiology, characterized by an increased responsiveness of the trachea and bronchi to various stimuli, many of which have been identified as allergens. The chief symptoms are marked wheezing and difficulty with expiration. The patient with asthma is subject to acute episodes of extreme **dyspnea,** principally due to prolonged and difficult exhalation of air. The smaller bronchi and bronchioles are narrowed and often occluded with excessive, tenacious mucus. The asthmatic patient has little difficulty with inspiration, but the narrowing and valve-like constriction causes a sensation of tightness that may be frightening and a wheezing that is loud and can be heard by others. This attack may subside within a few minutes or may continue sometimes for hours, or may lead to death. The chest may become distended by nature of the air-trapping, and the patient may become cyanotic and be desperately anxious. Immediate relief is usually obtained with the administration of epinephrine or aminophylline.

The cause of asthma is not clear. There is often a family history of allergy and an individual history of hypersensitivity. In addition, there is abundant evidence that psychologic factors play a role in some cases, and that asthmatic attacks can be precipitated by emotional factors.

ATELECTASIS

This word means collapse of the lung. The lung is a sponge filled with air. When compressed, it collapses. Before birth there is, of course, no air in the lungs, and they are therefore completely collapsed, a condition of **congenital atelectasis.** As soon as the newborn breathes after birth, the lungs become expanded with air. In medicolegal work, the absence of atelectasis is a proof that the child has lived after birth.

Apart from the congenital form, collapse of the lung may be produced in 2 entirely different ways: by compression of the lung or by obstruction of a bronchus. Compression of the lung may be caused by pleural effusion, by empyema, or by the presence of air under pressure in the pleural cavity (pneumothorax). Obstruction of a bronchus may be caused in a variety of ways. A foreign body such as a peanut, coin, or tooth may pass down the trachea and become lodged in a bronchus. No air can now enter that part of the lung supplied by the blocked bronchus; the air already there is absorbed into the blood, and the lung collapses. In debilitated children suffering from bronchitis, mucus may collect in the bronchi in such a large amount that obstruction and atelectasis re-

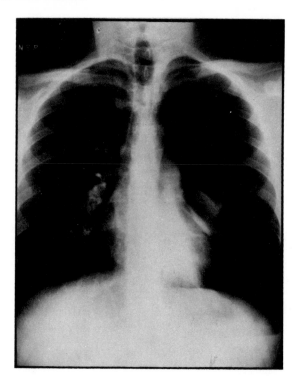

Fig. 15–23. This roentgenogram demonstrates a left-sided pneumothorax. The lung is completely collapsed on the left side and lies against the heart. Compare this with the right side, which is normal.

sult; owing to the debility, the mucus is not expelled by vigorous coughing. For the same reason, areas of collapse may develop after an abdominal operation, because mucus collects in the bronchi owing to the irritation of the anesthetic, and coughing is interfered with by the abdominal wound.

Pneumothorax

Pneumothorax is air in the pleural cavity. The air may come from the lung, usually as the result of rupture of an emphysematous bulla, occasionally of a tuberculous cavity on the surface. More rarely it may come from the outside, as in a perforating wound of the chest or a fracture of a rib. Whatever the cause of the pneumothorax, the air accumulates in the pleural cavity and compresses the lung, causing collapse in the same way as an accumulation of fluid may lead to collapse. The presence of air can easily be detected by the physician by the physical signs it produces and by the appearance in the roentgenogram (Fig.

15–23). Pneumothorax may be an emergency and requires rapid diagnosis and treatment, or suffocation will result.

ADULT RESPIRATORY DISTRESS SYNDROME

This is the name given to acute respiratory failure characterized by hypoxia with radiologic evidence of an extensive, bilateral infiltrate with an alveolar pattern. This life-threatening disorder has been found in many medical and surgical disorders, ranging from burns and aspiration of gastric contents to overdose of drugs and viral infections. It is seen most commonly in shock syndromes and has in fact been called "shock lung." The reason for the massive leakage of erythrocytes into the interstitial and alveolar spaces is unclear, but injury to the alveolar capillary tissue seems to be a common denominator. It does not seem to matter whether the injury is anoxemia, a chemical or toxic insult, or a physical injury such as high temperature, as in fire, the effect is the same, a marked respiratory impairment in the ability to oxygenate blood and to expand and ventilate the lung because of its increased turgor or stiffness. The hypoxemia may be fatal, and the treatment of this disorder is currently uncertain.

BRONCHIECTASIS

Bronchiectasis is a condition of dilatation of 1 or more of the smaller bronchi. It is similar to aneurysm of an artery, and, like an aneurysm, it is caused by weakening of the wall of the bronchus. This weakening has traditionally been attributed to infection. A single agent is seldom sufficient to produce the condition. It is most common in children after such viral infections as whooping cough or measles, in both of which the bronchial walls are inflamed, but it often occurs in young adults, and may persist into middle life. The most significant lesion is the destruction of the musculature and elastic tissue, for it is these that weaken the wall of the bronchus and allow the dilatation to occur. The bronchus dilates and forms a sac in which infection can occur. In time, a regular cesspool is formed, the wall of the bronchus is destroyed, and an abscess results.

The chief symptom of bronchiectasis is the coughing up at intervals of great quantities of purulent material that may be foul-smelling. In abscess, also, large quantities of pus are brought up and the breath may be foul. The disease may be confined to 1 or more segments, a point of great importance when it comes to a question of surgical removal of the lesion. (A segment is a section of lung parenchyma more or less completely separated from neighboring segments and supplied by a separate bronchus.)

RESPIRATORY FAILURE

The inability of the respiratory system to maintain normal arterial gas tensions of either oxygen or carbon dioxide, or both, may be caused by many or most of the pathologic processes outlined in this chapter. Today, the diagnosis of respiratory failure depends on laboratory examination of blood gases to determine the partial pressures of oxygen and carbon dioxide. Beyond the arbitrarily defined limits of arterial PO_2 of less than 60 mm Hg or PCO_2 of greater than 50 mm Hg while breathing room air, the situation is interpreted as respiratory failure that may be either acute or chronic.

The principal cause of the fall in arterial oxygen or the rise in arterial CO_2 is interference with the normal mechanisms of oxygen transfer or alveolar ventilation. This interference may be caused by inappropriately matched gas exchange and circulatory perfusion (ventilation-perfusion inequality) (Fig. 15–22). For example, when an alveolus is full of inflammatory exudate and air cannot fill the alveolus (as in acute bacterial pneumonia), the pulmonary capillary blood will return to the heart with a decreased capacity for carrying oxygen. In this instance, the alveolar oxygen tension is reduced, and this is reflected in the arterial oxygen level. Elevations in arterial carbon dioxide occur when the alveoli are poorly ventilated.

The physiologic effects of these disorders of oxygen and CO_2 transport are important, since hypoxia seriously interferes with the metabolism of all tissue, particularly that of the brain. The nature of the association between hemoglobin and oxygen dictates that, so long as the arterial oxygen level remains above 65 mm Hg, hemoglobin transportation will be effective. When the level falls below 60 mm Hg, there is a large decrease in the oxygen available to tissues. On the other hand, elevations of CO_2 are not so dangerous to tissues themselves, but rather have a decided effect on the central nervous system that results in a progressive loss of higher faculties, so that with CO_2 retention a person loses the ability to react or to think, and finally lapses into coma. This phenomenon is known as CO_2 narcosis and is well described, for example, by Charles Dickens in his account of the fat boy in the *Pickwick Papers.* The behavior of the fat boy was considered strange, perhaps drunken, because he was always falling asleep, even while eating. In his instance, CO_2 narcosis could be postulated because his obesity prevented his diaphragm from moving normally, and this impairment of a person's normal ventilatory excursions insidiously leads to carbon dioxide retention. Therefore the condition has been called the "Pickwickian syndrome."

A third effect of any disorder in gas exchange may be the change in arterial pH. Since blood has a limited buffering capacity, or a limited capacity particularly with respect to carbonic acid, any increase in PCO_2 will rapidly lead to acidosis. The most important obvious effects of such an acidosis are increased irritability of cardiac muscle, which may in turn lead to cardiac arrhythmias, or, on the other hand, to such changes as increased resistance in the pulmonary circulation. Fortunately, there are both respiratory and renal mechanisms that are brought into play to compensate for acidosis, whatever its cause.

One last word might be devoted to the accidental and often catastrophic event that follows inhalation, aspiration, or impaction of foreign material, particularly food, in the major airways. In the hospital, the accidental inhalation of gastric contents occurs once in a while in the unconscious, comatose patient. The acid gastric juices, which may contain enzymes as well as food particles, create a hemorrhagic pneumonia that, if it is not fatal, may destroy large areas of the lung. More commonly, particularly in persons who have been enjoying the fruits of Bacchus, large, incompletely mascerated particles of food, especially meat, may be aspirated, and the sudden convulsive actions of the unfortunate may be mistaken for an acute coronary occlusion (café coronary), whereas simple extraction maneuvers could clear the airway and save the person's life.

SYNOPSIS

The function of the lungs is to oxygenate blood, to excrete CO_2 and H_2O, and to act as a buffer. Its anatomy and physiology reflect these functions.

Infections cause the most common acute lung diseases. They may be local (abscess, tracheitis) or generalized (pneumonias), and they are caused by a wide variety of agents (virus, bacteria, fungi).

Tuberculosis is less common today, but it still is an important disease of the lung, because it destroys the pulmonary tissue and is treatable.

Bronchitis and emphysema are common chronic diseases and are related to air pollution (smoke, industrial pollutants).

Carcinoma of the lung is common in smokers and may only be recognized when it has either obstructed the bronchus or metastasized. Secondary tumors to the lung from other organs are found frequently.

Vascular disease of the lung may result in increasing pulmonary arteriolar resistance and cause heart failure. Pulmonary emboli are a frequent cause of death in postoperative, debilitated, or chronically ill patients.

Dyspnea has many causes and can best be understood in the context of all the pathologic processes involving both lung and systemic circulations.

Terms

Alveoli	*Consolidation*	*Pneumoconioses*
Bronchi	*Dyspnea*	*Mesothelioma*
Cilia	*Ghon complex*	*Pulmonary edema*
Pleura	*Hemoptysis*	*Pulmonary hypertension*
Surfactant	*Miliary tuberculosis*	*Atelectasis*
Pneumonia	*Fibrocaseous tuberculosis*	*Pneumothorax*
Resolution	*Emphysema*	*Bronchiectasis*

FURTHER READING

Bode, F. R., Paré, J. A. P., and Fraser, R. G.: Pulmonary diseases in the compromised host. Medicine, *53*:255, 1974.

Brewis, R. A. L.: Respiratory failure. Br. Med. J., *1*:898, 1978.

Comstock, G. W., et al.: The tuberculin skin test. Am. Rev. Respir. Dis., *104*:769, 1971.

Cosio, M., et al.: The relations between structural changes in small airways and pulmonary function tests. N. Engl. J. Med., *298*:1277, 1978.

Dalen, J.E., and Alpert, J.S.: Natural history of pulmonary embolism. Prog. Cardiovasc. Dis., *17*:259, 1975.

Dalen, J.E., et al.: Pulmonary embolism, pulmonary hemorrhage and pulmonary infarction. N. Engl. J. Med., *296*:1431, 1977.

Doll, R., and Hill, A. B.: Lung cancer and other causes of death in relation to smoking. Br. Med. J., *2*:5001, 1956.

Eller, W. C., and Haugen, R. K.: Food asphyxiation—restaurant rescue. N. Engl. J. Med., *289*:81, 1973.

Fekety, F. R., Caldwell, J., and Gump, D.: Bacteria, viruses and mycoplasmas in acute pneumonia in adults. Am. Rev. Respir. Dis., *104*:499, 1971.

Gewirtz, G., and Yalow, R. S.: Ectopic ACTH production in carcinoma of the lung. J. Clin. Invest., *53*:1022, 1974.

Gracey, D. R., Byrd, R. B., and Cugell, D. W.: The dilemma of the asymptomatic pulmonary nodule in the young and not so young adult. Chest, *60*:479, 1971.

Greco, F. A., and Oldham, R. K.: Current concepts in cancer: small-cell lung cancer. N. Engl. J. Med., *301*:355, 1979.

Lieberman, J.: Aryl hydrocarbon hydroxylase in bronchogenic carcinoma. N. Engl. J. Med., *298*:686, 1978.

Light, R. W., et al.: Pleural effusions: the diagnostic separation of transudates and exudates. Ann Intern. Med., *77*:507, 1972.

Macklem, P. T., Thurlbeck, W. M., and Fraser, R. G.: Chronic obstructive disease of small airways. Ann. Intern. Med., *74*:167, 1971.

Morse, James O., et al.: A community study of the relation of alpha$_1$-antitrypsin levels to obstructive lung diseases. N. Engl. J. Med., *292*:278, 1975.

Niewoehner, D. F., Kleinerman, J., and Rice, D. B.: Pathologic changes in the peripheral airways of young cigarette smokers. N. Engl. J. Med., *291*:755, 1974.

Reid, L.: *The Pathology of Emphysema.* London, Year Book Medical Publishers, 1967.

Sanford, J. P.: Legionnaires' disease—the first thousand days. N. Engl. J. Med., *300*:654, 1979.

Selikoff, I. J., et al.: Asbestosis and neoplasia (Editorial). Am. J. Med., *42*:487, 1967.

Stead, W. W., et al.: The clinical spectrum of primary tuberculosis in adults. Ann. Intern. Med., *68*:731, 1968.

Thurlbeck, W. M.: Small airways disease. Hum. Pathol., *4*:150, 1973.

West, J. B.: Causes of carbon dioxide retention in lung disease. N. Engl. J. Med., *284*:1232, 1971.

West, J. B.: *Respiratory Physiology—The Essentials.* Baltimore, Williams & Wilkins, 1974.

Upper Digestive Tract

16

Eating is touch carried to the bitter end.—ANON

The digestive or alimentary canal extends from the mouth, through which food enters the body, to the anus, through which the residue escapes (Fig. 16–1). Its function is twofold: (1) To convert the food into a digestible form in which it can be assimilated; (2) to absorb the food thus digested. Briefly, its functions are digestion and absorption. Digestion is begun in the mouth and continued in the stomach. Absorption is accomplished by the small intestine, although digestion also takes place in the upper portion of that tube. The digestive tract has been compared to a modern factory, for it is completely automated, and the owner's job merely consists of ordering bulk supplies and of disposing of the output. Table 16–1 illustrates the sites of digestion and absorption of the different components of food, namely, protein, carbohydrate, and fats.

We may, arbitrarily, divide the alimentary canal into an upper part—the mouth, esophagus, and stomach, and a lower part—the small and large intestine. The common diseases of the upper part are inflammation and tumors.

MOUTH

The principal structures of the mouth are the lips, tongue, salivary glands, tonsils, and teeth.

Cancer of the Lip. As the lips are covered by skin and gum, both of which are epithelial structures, the common tumor is carcinoma. Cancer of the lip is uncommon in women and extremely rare in the upper lip. It occurs principally in men past middle age, and begins as a thickening at the junction of the skin and mucous membrane (the red part of the lip) that may or may not be raised above the surface (Fig. 16–2). It is usually preceded by some chronic inflammatory lesion, such as an ulcer or crack, which may have been present for months or even years. The irritation produced by excessive smoking may be a factor. The most important single fact about cancer of the lip is that it is remarkably amenable to treatment. Surgical removal usually brings about a complete and lasting cure. The worst thing to do is to apply some form of caustic or irritant, with the idea of burning off the nodule. If the condition is untreated, it will gradually de-

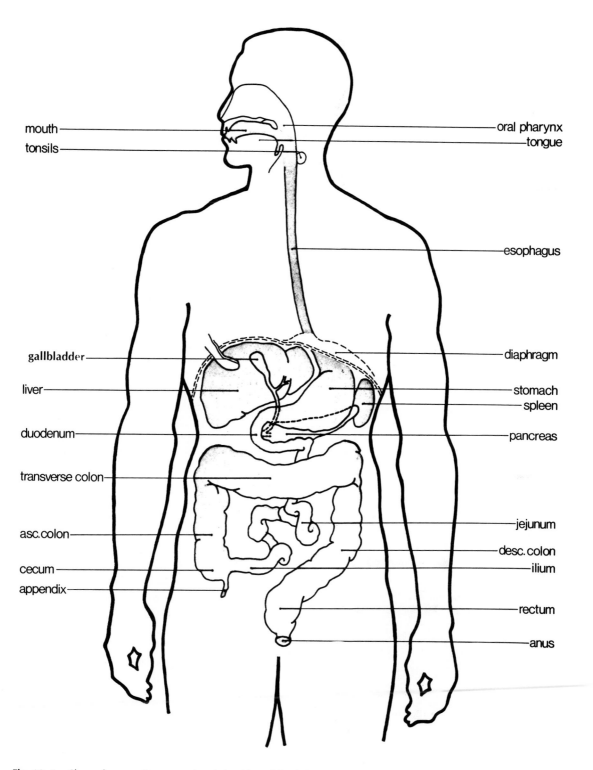

mouth

tonsils

oral pharynx

tongue

esophagus

gallbladder

liver

duodenum

transverse colon

asc.colon

cecum

appendix

diaphragm

stomach

spleen

pancreas

jejunum

desc. colon

ilium

rectum

anus

Fig. 16–1. Shown here are the anatomic relationships of the different parts of the digestive system and their approximate disposition within the body. The diagram might be referred to as disorders of different portions are discussed in this and the next chapter.

Table 16–1.   Sites of Digestion and Absorption of Food Components

FOOD EATEN	ORAL DIGEST. Ph≅7	GASTRIC DIGEST. Ph<7	INTESTINAL DIGESTION Ph>7		ABSORBED
protein	no action	┌pepsin └rennin → polypeptides	┌trypsin └chymotrypsin → polypeptides → dipeptides	┌carboxypeptidase ─aminopeptidase dipeptidase	amino acids
polysaccharides disaccharides	amylase	no action	amylase	┌maltase ─sucrase ─lactase	monosaccharides
fats	no action	┌lipase └fatty acids, glycerin	┌lipase ├bile salts		colloidal fats fatty acids, glycerin

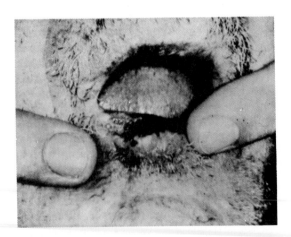

Fig. 16–2.   Cancer of lower lip. (Zegarelli et al.: *Diagnosis of Diseases of the Mouth and Jaws.* Philadelphia, Lea & Febiger.)

stroy the lip, and the tumor cells will be carried to the local lymph nodes under the jaw and in the neck, enlargement of which will form a large hard lump. When this occurs, the prospects of successful treatment are greatly lessened.

Cancer of the Tongue. As might be expected, the appearance of the lesion and the etiologic factors concerned are similar to those of cancer of the lip. Chronic irritation in the form of a jagged tooth or a badly fitting dental plate is an important factor. The tumor usually begins on the edge of the tongue, and is felt as a lump, which finally breaks down to form an ulcer. The tumor spreads much more rapidly than in the case of cancer of the lip, so that the presence of a lump in the tongue, however small, demands immediate attention. The prognosis is much worse than in cancer of the lip, particularly in cancer of the posterior part of the tongue, but radiation treatment has served greatly to lighten the gloom of the disease.

Cancer of the Mouth. Carcinoma may arise from the gum of the jaws and cheeks, from the palate, and from the throat. In the front of the mouth, the tumor is of the same character as cancer of the lip and tongue, and is again associated with chronic irritation. At the back of the mouth and in the throat, the tumor may present 2 special characteristics: (1) the local lesion may remain small and indeed undiscoverable for a long time, but the lymph nodes in the neck become greatly enlarged. (2) The tumor (mass in neck) may be radiosensitive, although it is seldom that a cure can be effected by this means.

Tonsillitis. The tonsils are masses of lymphoid tissue, 1 on each side of the throat. They are full of little recesses or crypts, and as the mouth is teeming with bacteria, it is natural that infection should be common. The infecting agent is frequently the streptococcus. As a result of the acute inflammation, the tonsils become swollen, narrowing the opening of the throat and causing great pain and difficulty in swallowing. Their surface may be covered with pus. One attack of tonsillitis predisposes to another, and a state of chronic infection may be established within the crypts. Acute or chronic sore throat, like tonsillitis, is due principally to streptococcal infection. Fortunately, the availability of antibiotics has decreased the need for tonsillectomy.

Salivary Glands. Diseases of the salivary glands are frequent and are important because of the resultant disfigurement, discomfort, and dysfunction. The most common disturbance of these glands is the inflammatory enlargement that occurs in the viral disease epidemic parotitis, mumps. Other inflammations may be due to bacterial infection of the ducts and gland, often related to ductal injury or obstruction. A more exotic inflammatory disease is the painless enlargement of 1 or more glands, histologic examination of which reveals only abundant lymphocytes. This inflammatory disease has been likened to other autoimmune diseases and is rare fortunately. It has been named after its discoverer, Mikulicz. Other infiltrations of the salivary glands may cause enlargement because of the presence of foreign material and functional atrophy because of mechanical interferences with the glandular structures.

However, with the exception of mumps, the most common cause of enlargement of the salivary glands is a benign growth called a mixed tumor. The parotid gland is often affected by this neoplasm, and over 80% of all salivary gland tumors are benign. The mixed tumor grows slowly and derives its name from its histologic appearance, which shows cartilage-like material in addition to the acinar structure, myoepithelial cells, and ducts. The slow growth of the benign tumors, which

are covered by a well-defined capsule, are a cosmetic hazard, but they also may compress the facial nerve, which lies between the deep and superficial lobes of the parotid gland.

Any rapid change in size, or pain associated with such a growth, heralds malignant change and is sufficient warning to have the tumor removed. The incidence of malignancy is low, but the eventual disfigurement and paralysis of the facial nerve with small operative risk warrants early surgical intervention.

TEETH

Structures. A tooth is composed of 4 structures: (1) enamel, (2) dentin, (3) pulp, and (4) cementum (Fig. 16–3). The enamel is the outer covering or crown of the tooth. It is calcified and extremely hard, so that it can stand the wear and tear of a long life and can enable a dog to crunch bones without itself becoming worn away. The enamel forms a perfect covering for the dentin, but, unfortunately, it is brittle and easily cracked. Moreover, fissures may form in the course of development, and through these fissures infection may reach the underlying dentin. The dentin forms the main bulk of the tooth. Like the enamel, it is calcified. The dentin is traversed by many minute channels, the dentinal tubules, which pass from the pulp and travel to the enamel. It

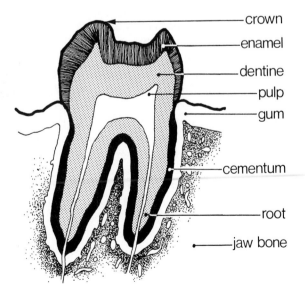

Fig. 16–3. Section through a tooth to show its structure.

is along these channels that infection may find its way, once it has reached the dentin. The pulp consists of soft, connective tissue filled with blood vessels and nerves.

Caries. One of the most widespread of diseases, caries or dental caries is found in the teeth of Egyptian mummies, so that it is no new affliction of mankind, and it is worldwide in its distribution, although certain races, such as Eskimos and some African natives, are remarkably exempt. It is principally a disease of childhood and adolescence; when that period is past, the threat of caries becomes much less. Both deciduous and permanent teeth are liable to the disease, but it is most likely to attack the permanent teeth on continued exposure to refined carbohydrates coupled with inadequate oral hygiene. The molars are most frequently affected.

There is no single cause of dental caries, but its essence is decalcification of the inorganic salts of which the tooth is composed. Anything that endangers the integrity of the enamel covering is liable to lead to caries. The factors may be exciting or predisposing. The exciting cause is bacterial infection with acid-producing organisms, which by enzyme action cause fermentation of refined carbohydrates retained as food debris in stagnant areas around the teeth with the elaboration of organic acids that attack the enamel. Of predisposing causes, faulty diet is all-important. Caries is essentially a disease of civilization, and it is the diet of civilization, particularly finely ground white flour, sugar, and starchy foods, that is the culprit.

The lesions of caries can be appreciated only when the structure of the tooth is understood. As in bone tuberculosis, caries is a gradual eating away of the tooth. All the elements of the tooth may be affected. The acids produced by the bacteria enter the enamel through cracks and defects and gradually dissolve the calcium of this hard substance. In time, the enamel is eroded away, exposing the dentin not only to the acids, but also to the bacteria themselves. Destruction of the dentin occurs much more rapidly and widely, so that a large cavity may be formed in the dentin, although there is only a small defect in the overlying enamel. The bacteria readily pass along the dentinal tubules and thus reach

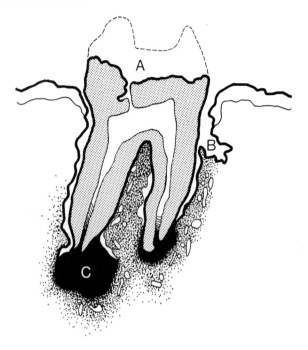

Fig. 16–4. Dental disease. *A,* Caries affecting the crown of the tooth and penetrating down to the pulp. *B,* peridontitis; shrinking of bone and gum away from tooth. *C,* root abscess.

the pulp, where they set up a true and often a violent inflammation. It is this inflammatory reaction in the pulp that is responsible for the pain of caries. The infection may pass down through the opening in the root of the tooth, through which the dental nerve enters the pulp, and may give rise to a root abscess (Fig. 16–4).

Other common conditions are periodontitis and gingivitis, but they will only be mentioned. Periodontitis, as the name indicates, is a disease of the surroundings of a tooth, not of the tooth itself. It is the greatest single cause of loss of teeth in the adult, for a gap is formed between the root of the tooth and the bone. Gingivitis is inflammation of the gingiva, the mucous membrane surrounding the neck of each tooth. The gums are swollen and inflamed and may bleed when the toothbrush is used too vigorously.

ESOPHAGUS

Considering its length and the variety of irritating fluids and solids that pass along it, the esophagus is remarkably free from disease. The only function of the esophagus is

A   B   C   D

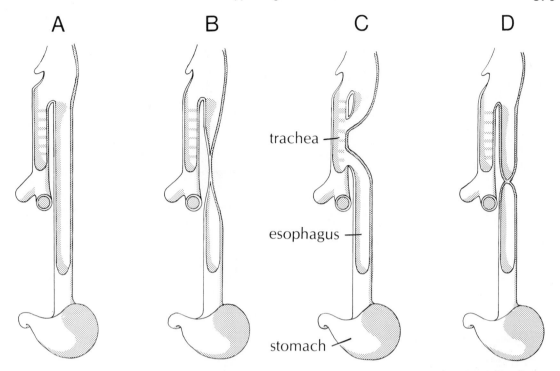

trachea —

esophagus —

stomach —

Fig. 16–5.   *A* illustrates a normal trachea and esophagus. In *B*, the upper esophagus is closed off and joined to the lower part only by a fibrous cord. *C* shows the proximal and distal portions of the esophagus opening onto the trachea. In *D*, the trachea is normal but the esophagus is divided by a stenosing web. *B*, *C*, and *D* are examples of congenital atresia of the esophagus (atresia meaning closure of a tubular organ). The symptoms, visible soon after birth, are excessive salivation, gagging, choking spells, cyanosis, and dyspnea. Surgery is the only treatment.

swallowing. We shall consider the lesions that interfere with this function.

Congenital Lesions. These often threaten the early days of life, because connections between the trachea and esophagus may lead to aspiration of foodstuffs and may thereby compromise both the respiratory and the digestive functions of the newborn (Fig. 16–5). Failure of development of the esophagus is well recognized, and a childhood injury to the esophagus by mechanical trauma or by chemical burns from accidental ingestion of caustic agents may lead to lifelong difficulties in swallowing. The act of swallowing, which we take for granted, is an extraordinary and well-integrated muscular activity, when you consider the variety of sizes and consistencies that travel our gullet, from graham crackers and peanut butter to oysters and horseradish.

Inflammatory Lesions. Chronic irritation or regurgitation of gastric acid may interfere with esophageal function and may lead to regurgitation of previously swallowed mate-

rials. One disease, a disorder of the esophagus that has a counterpart in the large bowel, is attributed to an imbalance in the autonomic innervation of the esophagus and leads to a grotesque dilatation, because the passage of foodstuffs into the stomach does not take place normally (Fig. 16–6). This huge dilatation, megaesophagus, fortunately is rare.

Another entity, particularly common in obese persons, is the occurrence of a hernia where the esophagus meets the stomach. After a large meal, while lying on the sofa, the stomach and its contents may slide into the chest because the distal esophagus is not properly anchored. This movement causes discomfort or pain and may be confused with pain arising from the heart. This entity is called a hiatus hernia.

Cancer of the Esophagus. The most serious and unpleasant disease of the esophagus is the malignant tumor that occurs most commonly in men of 50 years or more. The tumor

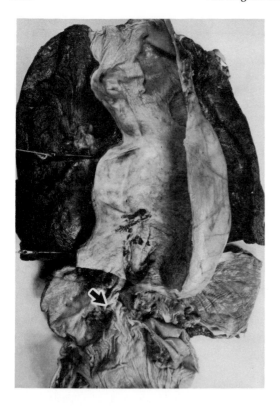

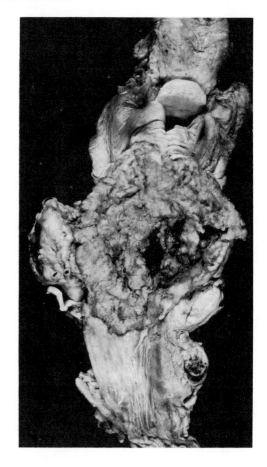

Fig. 16–6. In this greatly dilated esophagus, the entrance to the stomach (at arrow) is narrow. Food accumulates in this esophagus, which is dilated proximal to the obstruction. This gargantuan dilatation is called **megaesophagus** and fortunately is rare. (McGill University, Department of Pathology Museum.)

Fig. 16–7. The epiglottis is at the upper portion of the picture. The esophagus is replaced by a large, fungating, eroding **squamous carcinoma of the esophagus.** The esophagus in this instance has eroded into the trachea. This tumor sometimes occurs in middle-aged men and causes symptoms of difficulty in swallowing. (McGill University, Department of Pathology Museum.)

invades the muscular tube, so that difficulty in swallowing is the chief symptom. The common site is the middle, where the esophagus is crossed by the left bronchus. Another frequent site is the distal esophagus. No successful treatment exists for these squamous carcinomas, which interfere with swallowing (dysphagia) and many invade locally but seldom metastasize (Fig. 16–7). The prognosis is poor, with a mean survival time of less than 3 years. Although the surgical removal of the tumor is possible in some cases, no satisfactory substitute for the esophagus has been found, and most patients will be fed through a hole in their stomach.

STOMACH AND DUODENUM

The stomach serves several functions: it is a distensible muscular bag that can receive a seven-course meal and mix the dessert with the antipasto while waiting for a signal to proceed with further digestion, as the entry to the duodenum remains closed. It can mix all manner of foodstuffs with digestive juices and mucus (pepsin, rennin, and HCl) of a low pH (1.7), which begins the acid hydrolysis and proteolysis, key steps in all biochemical processes. The stomach also secretes a factor (intrinsic factor) responsible for the absorption of a vitamin essential to all cell maturation (vitamin B_{12}) (Fig. 16–8). As is well known, the stomach is exquisitely sensitive to mood, anxiety, rage, and all the expressions of personality.

The junction of the stomach with the esophagus is a sphincter, and the junction

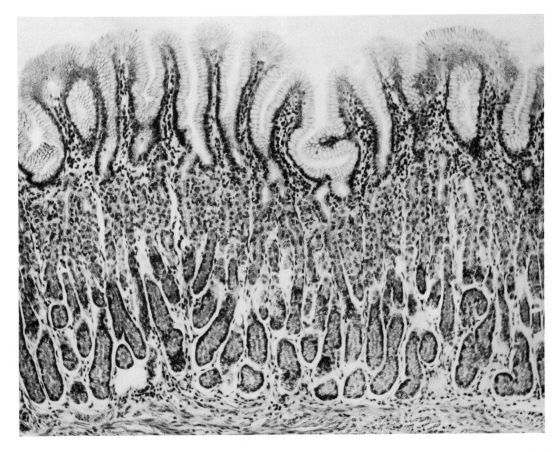

Fig. 16–8. This photomicrograph shows the **gastric mucosa.** The gastric glands at the bottom of the picture open into the pits and secrete hydrochloric acid and enzymes that are so important in the digestion of food. Four types of cells have been identified in these gastric glands. They secrete pepsin, hydrochloric acid, mucus, and 5-hydroxytryptamine. (From Bloom, W., and Fawcett, D. W.: *A Textbook of Histology,* 9th Ed. Philadelphia, W. B. Saunders, 1968.)

with the duodenum is another (the pylorus). In a few newborn children, the smooth muscle of the pylorus is hypertrophied, and a small olive-like mass can be felt in the infant's abdomen. This condition, which is suspected when the newborn repeatedly vomits, is referred to in patients of all ages as pylorospasm (Fig. 16–9). Occasionally, as in postoperative patients, or in instances of ulcer, inflammation, or tumor, the pylorus may remain contracted and the stomach will dilate, for which the simple remedy is to pass a tube (nasogastric) to decompress the organ and to retrieve the gas and gastric contents.

Perhaps, apart from inflammations due most frequently to excessive alcohol consumption, the most important disorders of the stomach are disorders of too much or too little secretion. Excessive amounts of pepsin

and hydrochloric acid are clearly related to the occurrence of ulcers in the stomach and duodenum, a disease that has been designated as the executive's "stress syndrome." Although the stimulus to excessive gastric acidity is still debated, recent insights into the various mechanisms responsible for secretion implicate at least 3 different routes by which the stomach is stimulated. The central nervous system (anxiety, tension, motion sickness) stimulates the stomach by the vagus nerve. Thus 1 of the more successful surgical treatments for ulcer has included transection of this nerve (vagotomy). Gastrin, a hormone, is a powerful secretagogue, and this substance may be secreted in excess amounts by the stomach, or even by a tumor. A third stimulus to secretion is histamine. How, exactly, histamine is involved in normal and

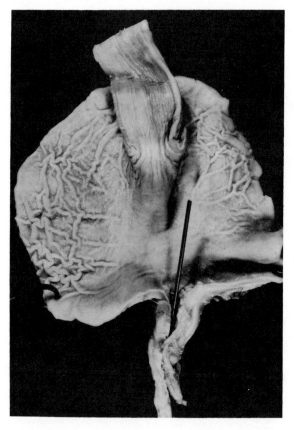

Fig. 16–9. This photograph shows the esophagus, stomach, and pylorus of an infant. At the probe the pylorus is markedly stenosed. This obstruction resulted in repeated vomiting and the untimely death of the infant. Today **pyloric stenosis** is recognized early and successfully treated in most instances. (McGill University, Department of Pathology Museum.)

abnormal secretions is debated. Empirically, however, histamine blockers (H_2) effectively reduce the amount and acidity of gastric secretion and thereby offer some relief to ulcer patients. Current management of ulcer patients is based on attempts to diagnose the underlying reasons for the ulcer before attempting surgical treatment or relying on pharmacologic agents alone. The current treatment is the use of cimetidine, an H_2 antagonist that seems to be particularly effective.

The other side of the coin is the stomach that secretes too little or no hydrochloric acid. This condition commonly occurs in the elderly, and whenever someone identifies a patient with little or no HCl (achlorhydria), there are 2 diseases that should come to mind.

The first is cancer of the stomach, because, for reasons that are not known, there is a high incidence of adenocarcinoma in the presence of achlorhydria. It is also of interest that patients with blood group type A have a much higher incidence of carcinoma of the stomach. The second disease is really not of the stomach, but of the bone marrow and hematopoietic system, since it seems that patients with achlorhydria frequently have a type of anemia in which the red blood cells do not mature normally (macrocytic anemia). This particular type of disease, which also affects the spinal cord and peripheral nerves, is due to the lack of a stomach secretion (intrinsic factor) and is called pernicious anemia. Thus the absence or presence of excessive HCl is a valuable diagnostic index, just as gastroscopy and radiology help to assess the morphology of the stomach.

Reference has just been made to the effect of nervous stimuli on gastric secretion. Food does not need actually to enter the stomach for the gastric glands to be stimulated. The mere presence of food in the mouth is sufficient for the stomach to respond in anticipation. This thesis was proved by the great Russian physiologist, Pavlov, who divided the esophagus in the neck of a dog, brought the end above the division out through the wound, and gave the dog as much to eat as he wished. The empty stomach poured out a plentiful supply of gastric juice, even though it received no food. The profound influence that psychic stimuli and stress have on the human stomach has been demonstrated by observations on patients in whom the interior of the stomach has been exposed to inspection over a long period as the result of a gunshot wound (Alexis Beaumont).

It must be appreciated that food in the stomach and bowel has not really entered the body and come into contact with the tissue for which it is intended. The food is merely in the alimentary canal, which runs through the body from the mouth to the anus. The large molecules of proteins, carbohydrates, and fats have to be broken down by the process of digestion before the food can be absorbed. The stomach and bowel represent the kitchen in which the food is prepared for use by the tissues. Neither water nor food is actually absorbed by the stomach itself. Both are taken up by the small intestine, and water by the large intestine.

The 3 common diseases of the stomach are gastritis, ulcer, and cancer.

Gastritis. When we consider the extraordinary assortment of substances, both fluid and solid, hot and cold, sweet and sour, alcoholic and aerated, to which the gastric mucosa is exposed, it is a wonder that we do not all have inflamed stomachs. Gastritis may be acute or chronic. In chronic gastritis, the signs of inflammation have faded into the past, leaving an atrophic mucosa. We shall confine our attention to the acute variety.

Acute gastritis may be caused by powerful surface irritants. The commonest of such irritants is alcohol. Acute gastritis must be present to some extent after every severe alcoholic bout, and this is largely responsible for the too familiar "morning-after" feeling. Chemical poisons swallowed accidentally by children or with suicidal intent by adults, dietary irritants, and bacterial and viral general infections may be accompanied by acute gastritis with dyspepsia. Food poisoning involves the intestine rather than the stomach. The mucous membrane is red, swollen, and infiltrated with inflammatory cells. If the acute attacks are repeated, as in the habitual alcoholic, the lesions become those of chronic gastritis, and eventually gastric atrophy results.

The most serious result of acute gastritis is bleeding. This may be minor and hidden in the gastric contents, or it may be revealed in the vomitus that often accompanies acute inflammation of the stomach. The vomiting of blood is called hematemesis and is an important sign, but its most frequent cause is acute gastritis, which is usually self-limited.

Peptic Ulcer. An ulcer of the stomach is called peptic, because the peptic or digestive juice plays an all-important part in its production (Fig. 16–10). A similar ulcer may occur in the duodenum next to the stomach, so that duodenal ulcer will be considered together with gastric ulcer under the common heading of peptic ulcer, since both are related to the hypersecretion of gastric products.

The cause of peptic ulcer can be stated in part, but only in part. When for any reason a

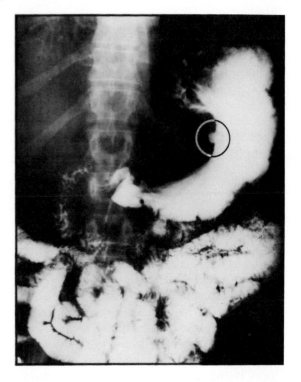

Fig. 16–10. A barium upper GI series shows a benign-appearing ulcer on the lesser curve of the stomach. The important aspects of this x-ray study are the projection of the ulcer into the wall of the stomach, and that the ulcer is on the lesser curvature.

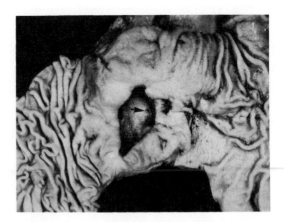

Fig. 16–11. This large, penetrating **peptic ulcer** is in the prepyloric area of the stomach. At the base of this ulcer is an artery (at arrow). The erosion of this artery led to massive gastrointestinal hemorrhage. The specimen demonstrates two classic complications of peptic ulcer—penetration and hemorrhage. (McGill University, Department of Pathology Museum.)

small area of gastric or duodenal mucosa is injured and becomes necrosed, the acid gastric juice digests the dead tissue, just as it would digest any piece of dead meat. In this way, a depression or hole is made that extends for a varying depth into the wall of the stomach or duodenum (Fig. 16–11). The chemical conditions are the same in the first part of the duodenum as in the stomach, for the acid gastric juice is poured into that part of the bowel when the pyloric sphincter relaxes. About 3 inches along the duodenum, the pancreatic and bile ducts open on the mucosa; as the juices from these ducts are strongly alkaline, the acidity of the gastric juice is neutralized. For this reason, peptic ulcer is usually confined to the first part of the duodenum (Fig. 16–12). The role of gastric juice in the production of peptic ulcer is easy to understand. However, we are still in the dark as to the cause of the initial necrosis of the mucous membrane. A bewildering variety of theories have been suggested, such as blood-borne bacterial infection, hyperacidity of the gastric juice, abnormal nervous impulses passing along the vagus nerve from the hypothalamic region of the brain to the stomach (vagotomy, i.e., division of the vagus nerve, may give spectacular therapeutic results), hormonal stimulation, and so on. In spite of all the

theories, peptic ulcer remains a mystery. The patient with peptic ulcer is usually high-strung, restless and irritable, prone to worry, and upset by strain. These characteristics are not the result of the ulcer; they are much more probably its cause and have to be considered by the physician who undertakes the treatment of a case.

The site of the ulcer is usually at the pyloric end of the stomach or along the upper border (lesser curvature). Treatment of an ordinary ulcer of the skin consists in putting the part at rest and in preventing irritation of the ulcer. However, in the case of a stomach ulcer, the organ is made to work every time a meal is taken. Hydrochloric acid acts as an acute irritant, so that the area of necrosis tends to be-

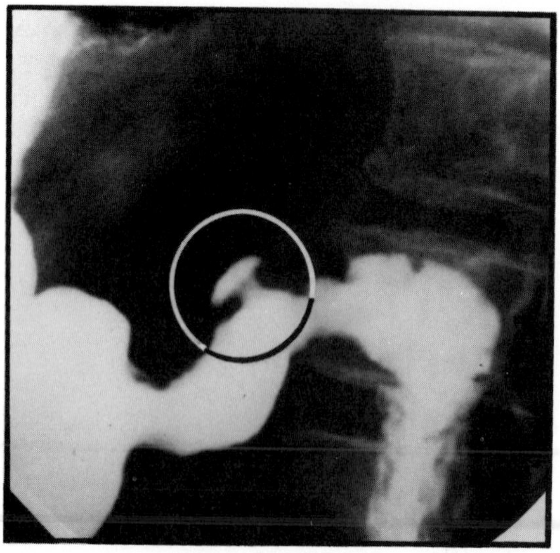

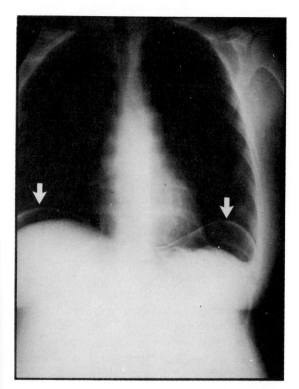

Fig. 16–13. This chest roentgenogram shows the presence of air under the diaphragm within the peritoneal cavity. A pneumoperitoneum (air in the peritoneal cavity) is seen with a penetrating wound of the abdomen, with a perforated stomach, as in an ulcer, or following an operation in which the wound has not been closed. The diagnostic sign is the presence of the increased contrast of air underneath the diaphragm at the arrows on both sides. If the patient is placed in another position, for instance on his back, the air will move as in a carpenter's level to the highest place, under the abdominal wall if the patient lies on his back, or along the posterior wall if the patient lies on his stomach.

Fig. 16–12. This barium swallow shows within the circle a collar button appearance typical of a benign duodenal ulcer. The edges of the ulcer are smooth.

come deeper. This necrotic tissue is in turn digested, and in time the hole may penetrate the whole thickness of the wall and may precipitate perforation into the abdominal cavity. One of the results of perforation is to permit the air that is normally in the stomach to escape into the peritoneal cavity. The presence of free air in the peritoneal cavity (Fig. 16–13), as seen in an upright x-ray examination, is an important clue to the diagnosis. Ulcers may be visualized on x-ray examination when the crater fills with barium outlining the mucosal penetration.

Fortunately, however, protective forces are at work that tend to prevent this catastrophe and to limit the spread of the ulcer. The continued irritation stimulates the formation of fibrous tissue in the floor of the ulcer, and this offers marked resistance to its spread. A chronic peptic ulcer is therefore a circumscribed area, usually not more than an inch in diameter, funnel-shaped, of varying depth, with a hard fibrous base. When the ulcer is still small, healing may take place, but when it is deep this is unlikely to occur. The abundant scar tissue at the base of the ulcer may contract to such a degree that obstruction of the pylorus is produced, or, if the ulcer is in the middle of the stomach, the contraction may divide that organ into 2 compartments.

Gastric ulcers are not so common as those in the duodenum, the former accounting for perhaps 20% of all peptic ulcers. Generally, persons with gastric ulcers are older (50 years) and male (3.5:1); sometimes they have no symptoms. The important aspect of gastric ulcers is the frequency of malignancy, but modern methods of fiberoptic gastroscopy and cytologic examination are increasing diagnostic accuracy to over 90%. Most benign ulcers show healing of up to 50% of their size after 2 weeks of medical therapy. Most heal completely after 12 weeks, but if they do not show healing, it is most likely that the ulcer is malignant.

CLINICAL PATTERN. The common symptom of peptic ulcer, whether gastric or duodenal, is **pain,** relieved by the taking of foods and alkalis. The pain may be a mild feeling of discomfort, or it may be severe. It bears a characteristic relation to food, being relieved by the taking of food for about an hour and then coming on again. The triple rhythm of pain-food-relief shows a remarkable regularity. An alkali such as sodium bicarbonate may relieve the pain to an even greater degree. The usual explanation given for the pain and its relief by food and alkalies is that the action of the hydrochloric acid irritates the raw surface of the ulcer, the acid being neutralized by food and alkali. Muscular contraction of the stomach wall may be even more important in producing pain than is the action of the acid. Inflammatory foci in the neighborhood of the ulcer cause contraction of the surrounding muscle and spasm of the pyloric sphincter. These factors increase the tension within the stomach and thus excite pain. Food and alkalies cause the stomach to relax for a time and thus relieve the pain. A large gastric ulcer sometimes produces no symptoms until it finally perforates, a situation for which no satisfactory explanation can be offered.

Hemorrhage is a frequent sign, varying from a slight oozing of blood to a copious flooding that may prove fatal. Severe hemorrhage is due to rupture of a large artery in the base of the ulcer. In gastric ulcer, there may be vomiting of blood, the vomitus being not red but "coffee grounds" in appearance, owing to the action of the gastric juice on the blood. The patient may not vomit, but may pass the blood in the stools, imparting to them a blackish color (tarry stools), a condition known as **melena.**

Fortunately, the occurrence of peptic ulcer seems to be declining, as has been shown from a study of British physicians. This group, aged from 35 to 64, showed an incidence of 3.1 cases of peptic ulcer per 1,000 in the years 1947 to 1951, and half this rate (1.7/1,000) in the same number of years from 1961 to 1965. It is of interest that peptic ulcers are more prevalent in monozygotic twins than in dizygotic twins, and there is a threefold increase of peptic ulcer among primary relatives. In addition, duodenal ulcers are more prevalent in persons with blood group O than in those with other blood groups, suggesting some heritable basis for this common, painful disorder, in which over 50% of patients have intractable pains and 30% have hemorrhage from their ulcers, which lead them often to seek surgical treatment for this disorder. It has been remarked that "surgical intervention is the substitution of one pathologic state for another, in the hope that the former is more acceptable than the latter." Surgical treatment for peptic ulceration was initiated by the great German surgeon Billroth in 1880, and has been used as a therapeutic modality with varying degrees of success ever since.

The **complications of peptic ulcer are hemorrhage, perforation, penetration** (into the pancreas, frequently), **fistula formation, and obstruction.** About one-third of all gastric ulcers perforate, and the overall mortality is about 10%, being higher in the older age group.

Cancer of the Stomach. This disease is much more common in men than in women. A remarkable (and unexplained) decline in gastric carcinoma in men has been taking place during the last 30 years. The usual age of occurrence is about 60 years, but it may occur much earlier. There is a curious epidemiologic pattern to stomach cancer: it is more frequent in the higher latitudes (Iceland, Finland), it is frequent in countries where smoked fish is commonly eaten, it is common in blood group A, and it is more frequent in relatives than in spouses.

The tumor is generally situated at the pyloric end of the stomach, but it may occur in any part of the organ. It may form a large mass projecting into the cavity of the stomach, or it may merely constitute a thickening of the wall in the pyloric region (Fig. 16–14). Gradually, however, this thickening leads to narrowing of the opening, until finally complete obstruction may be produced, causing marked dilatation of the rest of the stomach. The tumor in the stomach is best detected by means of radiologic examination. One pattern of infiltration of the wall of the stomach by cancer gives rise to an unusual appearance which has been called the "leather water bottle" stomach (Fig. 16–15A and B).

Spread of the tumor may occur by lymphatics or by the blood stream. Cancer cells are carried to the nearest abdominal lymph nodes by the lymphatics, but sometimes the lymph nodes in the supraclavicular fossa on the left side may be enlarged by tumor growth (Virchow's node). The cancer cells may be carried by the blood to the liver, brain, and other

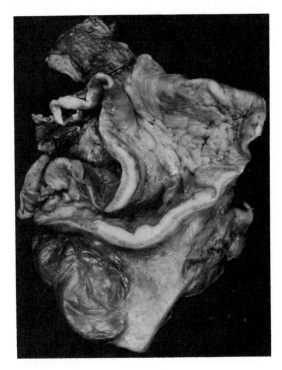

Fig. 16–14. This photograph shows the much-thickened wall of the stomach in a patient whose symptoms of loss of appetite and loss of weight had progressed for two years. This infiltrating tumor is called a **scirrhous carcinoma** of the stomach. (McGill University, Department of Pathology Museum.)

organs. When distant spread has occurred and metastases are formed, no treatment is of any avail. It is the early spread of carcinoma, often at a time when there are no warning symptoms, that makes the operative removal of the tumor often so disappointing. In this respect, the disease resembles bronchogenic carcinoma.

CLINICAL PATTERN. Unfortunately, pain is not an early symptom of cancer, either in the stomach or in other parts of the body, although it may be marked in the later stages, especially when pyloric obstruction has set in. Loss of appetite and a feeling of repletion before the meal is finished is much more characteristic, and should be regarded as a danger signal in a man in the cancer age who has previously had a healthy appetite, or who frequently states that up to that time he has been able to "digest nails." Absence of hydrochloric acid in the gastric contents obtained by the stomach tube is a sign of great importance. So

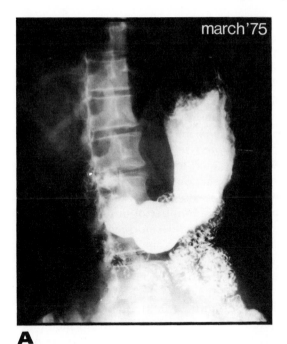
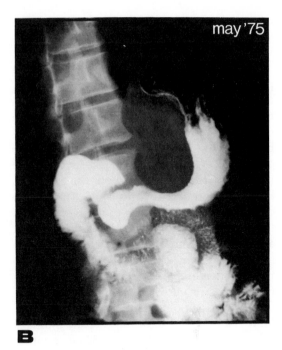

Fig. 16–15. *A* and *B*, These figures show barium meal studies given two months apart. The barium meal shows a much smaller stomach in May 1975, due to infiltration of the wall of the stomach by carcinoma. The decrease in the normal gastric volume and the rigid wall are classic signs of this particular type of cancer.

also is the presence of blood. This blood is most easily tested for by examination of the stools. It cannot be seen with the naked eye as it is too small in amount, but it is readily detected by a simple chemical test. Blood that can be detected by such a test alone is known as occult blood, because it is hidden from the eye. Anemia is a common symptom.

When pyloric obstruction has developed, vomiting from the dilated stomach may be a distressing symptom. The vomitus may have a coffee-grounds character owing to the presence of altered blood, as in the case of gastric ulcer. It will be noticed that nothing has been said about the presence of a lump or tumor that can be felt by the doctor. Such a mass can only be felt in the later stages, when it is too late to hope for cure of the patient.

Exfoliative cytology is another diagnostic aid. Gastric secretion rapidly digests any exfoliated cancer cells, and they soon become unrecognizable, so that a preliminary light diet and overnight fasting are essential. The minimum delay in examination of the aspirated material (special technician and laboratory facilities) is also of some importance. The

use of an abrasive balloon, which is inflated in the stomach, deflated before removal, and rubs off many tumor cells, has increased the number of positive results. Today, however, the single greatest advance in diagnosing the diseases of the stomach has come from the use of the flexible fiberoptic gastroscope, which permits visualization of the entire inside of the stomach without the need for an operation. Still, some cases are missed.

Gastric Analysis. The examination of the gastric contents gives 3 valuable pieces of information. (1) The emptying time of the stomach, i.e., whether or not there is obstruction at the pylorus that prevents the food from passing into the duodenum; (2) the presence or absence of hydrochloric acid (HCl), which is secreted by the normal stomach when food is taken; (3) the presence of blood and tumor cells. Various methods may be employed by the clinician, but the simplest is to give a standard test meal and to remove the stomach contents an hour later by means of the stomach tube. Sometimes a thin tube is left in the stomach for 2½ hours, samples being withdrawn by aspiration every half-hour. If the "fasting contents" are to be examined, the stomach tube is passed first thing in the morning before the patient has taken food.

In the normal stomach, there should be practically no fasting contents. Any considerable accumulation of fluid and food particles indicates pyloric obstruction, which may be caused by cancer at the pylorus or by the fibrotic contraction that accompanies a chronic gastric ulcer. Blood may be seen with the naked eye diffused throughout the contents. It may be red or brown in color. The brown color is due to conversion of the hemoglobin to acid hematin by the acid in the stomach, and it indicates that the blood has been in the stomach for some time. Blood in the stomach in any considerable amount is due to bleeding from a gastric ulcer or from cancer. A few streaks of fresh blood are of no significance, being caused by the passage of the stomach tube. For the same reason, delicate chemical tests for blood are of no value, as a trace of blood is likely to be present.

The free hydrochloric acid, which should normally be present after a test meal, is usually absent (achlorhydria) in both pernicious anemia and cancer of the stomach.

Whereas any of the disorders of the stomach and duodenum may be traced to a specific pathologic process (ulcer, tumor), they may share a common presenting feature such as hematemesis, or perforation with its accompanying physiologic complications. One additional disorder is obstruction, which, like hemorrhage or perforation, may require emergency treatment.

Whether the obstruction is mechanical, that is, some mass such as a benign or malignant tumor obstructing the pylorus, or caused by some physiologic or pharmacologic agent (acute gastric dilatation frequently occurs following surgical procedures), the effect on the patient may be the same. The patient may complain of a sense of fullness accompanied by epigastric pain and persistent vomiting of large volumes of fluid that may be bile-stained. The abdomen may be distended and hollow to percussion. Because of the vomiting and consequent fluid loss, the problems of the patient will become more acute rapidly as dehydration, alkalosis (due to loss of HCl), oliguria, and tachycardia become evident. The patient may then become hypotensive, and management may become more difficult as electrolyte imbalance (hypokalemia) complicates the problem. Because of the relative frequency and severity of this pattern, it is wise to be alert to early signs of acute upper intestinal tract obstruction, which can occur at any age in patients of any sex and may have any of a large number of underlying causes.

Gastrointestinal Hemorrhage. Gastrointestinal hemorrhage is a life-threatening emergency. It has a mortality of up to 30% and is often both difficult to manage and to diagnose. With the use of the fiberoptic scope, the site of bleeding can frequently be located more easily today than by ancient methods, such as having a patient swallow a string that was stained to see how far from the mouth the bleeding site might be! Over half the cases of gastrointestinal bleeding are due to peptic ulcer. Esophageal varices, gastric ulcer, gastritis (alcohol-induced), esophagitis, and rarely, systemic disease such as leukemia or a bleeding disorder may bring about the vomiting of blood. In at least 10% of patients, no specific source is found.

Important to the correct diagnosis are the careful noting of the patient's medical history (to identify aspirin or alcohol in particular), and a thorough physical examination (to discover signs of other disease such as cirrhosis). The immediate course is to stabilize the patient, to replace blood, and to attempt to visualize the site of bleeding. Endoscopy followed by radiology frequently solves the problem. It is characteristic of this emergency that rebleeding may occur; the final approach may have to be surgical, although even that does not guarantee that the bleeding will not recur. One final note is that the bleeding itself, particularly in the older patient, may lead to more serious illness such as myocardial infarction and renal tubular necrosis.

SYNOPSIS

The digestive system serves 3 purposes: to mix/digest, to absorb, and to store/excrete foodstuffs.

The stomach secretes pepsin and hydrochloric acid in response to cerebral stimuli (vagus nerve), hormones (gastrin), and histamine.

Peptic ulcerations occur in patients with gastric hyperacidity and hypersecretion and may lead to intractable pain, massive hemorrhage, perforation and peritonitis, or obstruction.

Achlorhydria is associated with gastric carcinoma and pernicious anemia.

Gastric carcinoma may be heralded by weight loss, pain, melena, anemia, or loss of appetite.

Terms

Mixed tumor

Esophagitis

Hiatus hernia

Gastritis

Hematemesis

Peptic ulcer

Melena

Achlorhydria

Pernicious anemia

FURTHER READING

Bynum, T. E., Hartsuck, J., and Jacobson, E. D.: Gastric ulcer. Gastroenterology, *62*:1052, 1972.

Cohen, S.: Motor disorders of the esophagus. N. Engl. J. Med., *301*:184, 1979.

Dodd, G. D.: Genetics and cancer of the gastrointestinal system. Radiology, *123*:263, 1977.

Fordtran, J. S.: Placebos, antacids and cimetidine for duodenal ulcer. N. Engl. J. Med., *298*:1081, 1978.

Griffiths, W. J., Newmann, D. A., and Welsh, J. D.: The visible vessel as an indicator of uncontrolled or recurrent gastrointestinal hemorrhage. N. Engl. J. Med., *300*:1411, 1979.

Himal, H. S.: Upper gastrointestinal hemorrhage. Can. J. Surg., *21*:192, 1978.

Isenberg, J. I., and Maxwell, V.: Intravenous infusion of amino acids stimulates gastric acid secretion in man. N. Engl. J. Med., *298*:27, 1978.

Katon, R. M., and Smith, F. W.: Panendoscopy in the early diagnosis of acute upper gastrointestinal bleeding. Gastroenterology, *65*:728, 1973.

Mendeloff, A. I.: Dietary fiber and human health. N. Engl. J. Med., *297*:811, 1977.

Menguy, R.: Pathophysiology of peptic ulcer. Am. J. Surg., *120*:282, 1970.

Rhodes, J.: Etiology of gastric ulcer. Gastroenterology, *63*:171, 1972.

Stabile, B. E., and Passaro, E.: Recurrent peptic ulcer. Gastroenterology, *70*:124, 1976.

Walsh, J. H., et al.: Gastrin. N. Engl. J. Med., *292*:1324, 1975.

Wolf, S.: *The Stomach*. New York, Oxford University Press, 1965.

Wynder, E. L., and Bross I. J.: A study of etiological factors in cancer of the esophagus. Cancer, *14*:389, 1961.

One finger in the throat and one in the rectum makes a good diagnostician.—OSLER

STRUCTURE AND FUNCTION

The lower digestive tract consists of 2 divisions,which differ in structure and function; they are called the small and the large intestine. The names apply to their diameter, not to their length; the small intestine is about 20 feet long and the large intestine about 5 feet long. The small intestine consists of a short upper section (12 inches), the duodenum, into which open the bile duct from the liver and gallbladder and the pancreatic duct; a longer lower section, the upper part of which is called the jejunum and the lower three-fifths, the ileum. The lower end of the ileum connects with the large intestine at the ileocecal valve, situated in the lower right part of the abdomen. The vermiform appendix opens into the large bowel just beyond it. The large intestine begins as a wide pouch, the cecum, and continues as the colon, which passes up into the right flank, across the abdomen beneath the liver and stomach, and down into the left flank, to become the sigmoid, an S-shaped portion, finishing as the rectum, which is about 5 inches long and opens onto the surface at the anus.

The small intestine is concerned with the digestion and absorption of the food, and its structure is designed to perform these 2 different functions. The mucous membrane lining this part of the bowel contains innumerable glands in the form of simple tubes, which secrete enzymes that act on food that has begun to be digested but is not yet absorbed (Fig. 17–1). The pancreas, a flat organ that lies transversely behind the stomach, synthesizes powerful secretions (lipase, amylase, chymotrypsinogen) that enter the bowel lumen at the same place as bile. By the emulsifying action of bile and the chemical action of enzymes on the foodstuffs in the upper bowel, digestion is enhanced and absorption can begin (Fig. 17–2).

The surface of the jejunum is arranged in small projections called villi, which look to the naked eye like velvet (Fig. 17–3). Each villus is composed of hundreds of thousands of intestinal absorptive cells that overlie the core of blood vessels and lymphatics (Fig. 17–4). Each absorptive cell itself is further modified to increase its surface area by the projection of microvilli on its surface, the brush border (Fig. 17–5). It has become apparent that these adaptations, which increase the surface area over fortyfold, facilitate absorption of the molecules that have been made available by digestive processes. It seems that different sugars, fats, and amino acids are absorbed preferentially at different levels in the small bowel.

The absorption at the surface of each cell is facilitated by the presence of extracellular enzymes that lie between the microvilli. All molecules that are absorbed pass into the intestinal cell and are then released into the extracellular space, the lymphatics, or the portal vein, whence they travel to the

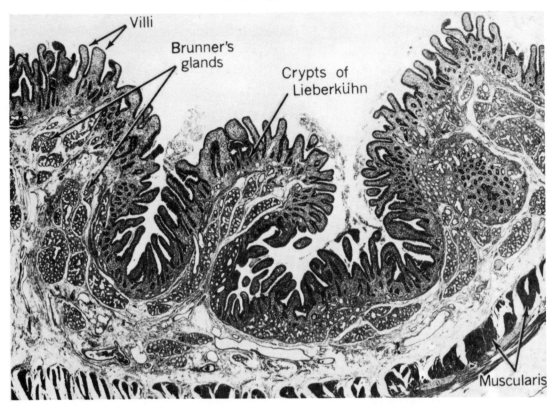

Fig. 17–1. This light microphotograph shows a section of the mucosa, submucosa, and muscularis of the duodenum. The villi are seen in the upper left as projections into the lumen of the bowel. The glands that secrete material into the lumen are in this portion of the bowel called Brunner's glands. (Courtesy of Dr. H. Mizoguchi.)

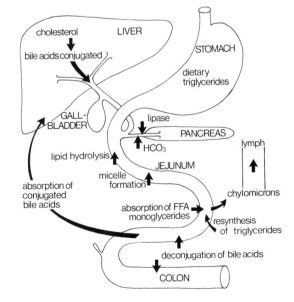

Fig. 17–2. This diagram shows a summary of fat digestion, fat absorption, and the enterohepatic circulation of bile acids in the digestive tract. It demonstrates the interrelationship of the liver, pancreas, jejunum, and circulation. A micelle is a water-soluble complex of emulsified lipid. FFA refers to free fatty acids. (Adapted from Hofmann, A. F.: The chemistry of intraluminal digestion. Mayo Clin. Proc., 48:618, 1973.)

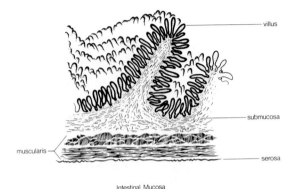

Intestinal Mucosa

Fig. 17–3. Intestinal mucosa. This drawing of the surface of the jejunum shows the velvet-like structure of the epithelial mucosa which is arranged in finger-like projections or villi. The function of this arrangement is to increase the absorptive area.

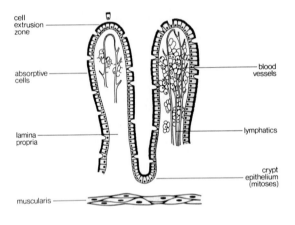

Villus of Intestinal Mucosa

Fig. 17–4. Villus of intestinal mucosa. This drawing shows the microscopic appearance of each villus. The epithelial cells, which cover the surface of the villus and absorb the sugars, fats, and amino acids, arise in the crypts. At the apex of each villus the cells are sloughed off. The core of each villus contains both lymphatic and blood vessels. Every molecule of substrate that is used for energy must pass across this epithelial barrier.

liver and are used or stored. As food passes down the small bowel, less and less of the absorbable materials remain, and contractions of smooth muscle in the wall of the bowel (peristalsis) facilitate the transport of materials from duodenum to ileum.

At the ileocecal valve, the structure and function of the intestine become different. At this point the residue contains water and indigestible materials. The principal role of the large intestine or colon is to absorb water and to store the materials (feces) until they are excreted. Most colonic uptake of water and salts occurs in the right colon, where up to 2 liters of fluid is absorbed every day. All but about 200 ml of this absorption occurs during the

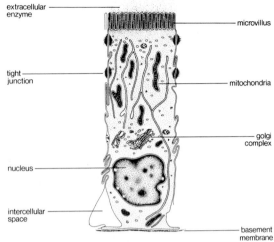

Intestinal Absorptive Cell

Fig. 17–5. Intestinal absorptive cell. This drawing shows the electron microscope appearance of a single intestinal absorptive cell. Note at the apex of this cell there are also projections to increase the surface area of the cell. This limiting membrane has the capacity to discriminate between D and L amino acids. Extracellular enzyme is held in place between the microvilli. (After Zetterqvist, H.: The ultrastructure of the columnar absorbing cells of the mouse jejunum. Ph. D. thesis, Karolinska Institute, Stockholm, 1956.)

passage of stool through the colon, where small amounts of sodium, potassium, chloride and bile acids are also absorbed. There normally are hundreds of millions of bacteria in the colon that aid in fermentation and degradation of the remaining foodstuffs. By-products include histamine and, depending on their substrate and the kinds of bacteria present, gases such as methane or sulfur-containing compounds, which have distinctive odors.

The colon can be considered to have several different parts; the diseases of these different parts frequently have different symptoms and signs. For instance, inflammation or tumors of the sigmoid and rectum may signal their presence by bright bleeding, obvious pain or lesions that may be felt by the examining finger or seen with a short sigmoidoscope. Examination of the terminal portion of the bowel should be mandatory in every middle-aged person because of the extraordinarily high incidence of easily diagnosed, curable cancer. Some degree of squeamishness and Victorian reluctance to look directly at the problem makes the proctoscopic examination an often-neglected opportunity to spot trouble. The old saying was, "if ı don't put your finger in it, you will put your ʋot in it later."

By contrast, tumors of the ileocecal valve may bleed silently for months until the patient has become severely anemic, with a hemoglobin of perhaps 6 instead of 13 grams.

DYSENTERY

This acute inflammation of the colon, colitis, is accompanied by frequent diarrhea and the passage of mucus, pus, and blood in the liquid stools. There are 2 kinds of dysentery due to entirely different causes, although with similar lesions and symptoms. These are amebic dysentery and bacillary dysentery.

Amebic Dysentery. This disease is caused by a unicellular organism, a protozoon, called *Entamoeba* or *Amoeba histolytica*. The parasite is swallowed in infected (uncooked) food or water, and when it reaches the lower part of the intestine (colon) it invades the wall of the bowel, causing the acute inflammation (colitis) known as dysentery. Amebic dysentery is a disease of the tropics, but it also occurs in temperate regions.

The chief symptom is profuse and painful diarrhea, the liquid stools containing slimy mucus, pus, and blood. Large numbers of amebas leave the body in the fecal discharge.

The characteristics of the ameba, together with the mode of infection, have already been discussed in connection with the protozoon parasites.

The lesions of both forms of dysentery are similar. Large and small ulcers are scattered along the length of the colon, and these are responsible for the pain, the diarrhea, and the mucus, pus, and blood in the stools. In the case of amebic dysentery, the amebas may be found to burrow deeply into the wall of the bowel, and they may invade the branches of the portal vein and be carried to the liver, in which they set up amebic abscesses of that organ. In spite of modern treatment with chemotherapy and antibiotics, it may not be possible to eradicate the infection in all cases, and some amebas may remain for a long time, even for years, protected by the bowel wall, and the patient may be subject to repeated attacks of dysentery.

Bacillary Dysentery. The Shigella group of bacilli, which are responsible for bacillary dysentery, are intestinal parasites peculiar to man. The characteristics of these bacteria and the mode of infection have already been described. The character of the lesions is similar to that of the lesions of amebic dysentery outlined in the foregoing paragraph.

ULCERATIVE COLITIS

Characterized by severe bloody diarrhea, up to 20 times per day, with alternating periods of worsening and improving, this is a disease of unknown etiology. The disease may last for many years. The diagnosis is made by excluding other causes of abdominal pain, weight loss, fever, and diarrhea. The lesions are nonspecific in that extensive ulceration of the mucosa of the colon and rectum does not suggest any particular pathogen. Frequently there is a hyperplastic growth of the damaged mucosa resulting in pseudo-polyps, but the muscular coats and draining lymph nodes are usually spared the disease.

Because circulating antibodies to the patient's own colonic cells have been demonstrated in some persons, an autoimmune etiology has been suggested. Hypersensitivity to milk, foods, or bacterial by-products has been implicated also as a pathogenic factor. Because hemorrhagic necrosis of the mucosa has been found in experimentally induced Arthus reactions, a vascular etiology has been proposed. In 1922, attention was drawn to the psychologic constitution of many patients with ulcerative colitis who, while appearing calm and serene, were really anxious and hostile. It has been said "the sorrow that has no vent in tears may make other organs weep." Recurrent attacks could often be related to overwork and worry. Attention to psychogenic factors continues to be relevant in the opinion of most physicians, while the patient's inflammatory disease is managed medically with anti-inflammatory agents (steroids) and, sometimes, surgically with colectomy.

The most important aspect of this disease is its characteristic pattern of exacerbation and remission coupled with our ignorance of its etiology.

REGIONAL ENTERITIS

This disease of the bowel is as mysterious as chronic ulcerative colitis and resembles it in many ways. The distribution of the lesions, however, is somewhat different. It was first described by Crohn of New York in 1932, so that it is commonly known as Crohn's disease. Here again, a psychogenic element is apparent. The patient is often frustrated for some reason or other, and emotional storms may precede the onset of the disease and the occurrence of relapses.

The lesions are limited to the small intestine in most cases, often to the terminal ileum, hence the name enteritis as opposed to colitis. The affected area is thick and rigid, like a hosepipe, owing to a progressive fibrosis and scarring. The great thickening of the wall results in marked narrowing of the lumen and in chronic obstruction, giving a characteristic "string sign" of the terminal ileum in the roentgenogram (Fig. 17–6). Although ulcers may be present, ulceration does not dominate the picture as it does in chronic ulcerative colitis. The bowel may become adherent to the abdominal wall, followed by slow perforation and the formation of a fistula. One of the most remarkable features is the patchiness of the lesions, areas of normal bowel referred to as "skip areas" alternating with areas of dense

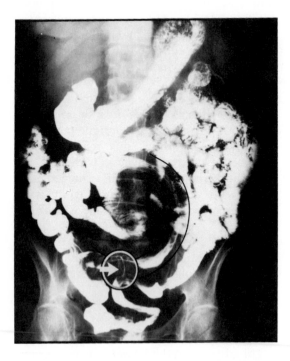

Fig. 17–6. This roentgenogram shows an upper GI series demonstrating the "string sign" of Crohn's disease. The terminal ileum is narrowed, its mucosa is destroyed, and there is separation of the bowel loops due to thickening of the bowel wall, and infiltration of the mesentery. A fistula between the sigmoid colon and the ileum can be seen at the arrow.

fibrosis, so that the appellation "regional" is well deserved.

Clinical Pattern. The outstanding features are a mass in the right iliac region, diarrhea, and fever. The disease may begin with an attack similar to appendicitis, but there is often blood in the stools due to bleeding from the mucous membrane, which is intensely congested in the early stage of the disease. The subacute and chronic forms are marked by recurring attacks of diarrhea with mucus in the stools, episodes of abdominal pain, symptoms of obstruction and sometimes vomiting. A peculiarly puzzling feature of Crohn's disease is the recurring nature of the attacks, with intervals of freedom. The condition is certainly an enigma.

There are those who feel that ulcerative colitis and regional enteritis are simply different forms of the same disease. Currently there are some hopes that a viral etiology will be proven, and it may be that, as in some other disorders, the genetic constitution (HLA antigens) of the person is important.

APPENDICITIS

The vermiform appendix is a small tube about 4 inches long and as thick as the tip of your little finger. It opens out of the cecum close to the spot where the small and large intestine join. If it has a function, it does not appear to be of any importance. The appendix is liable to the same diseases as the rest of the bowel, but the condition of importance from the point of view of both frequency and gravity is acute inflammation.

The causal factors are infection and obstruction, and it is becoming more and more apparent that the latter is the dominant factor. There is a sphincter-like mechanism at the base of the appendix that potentially makes it a closed loop. Obstruction can be due to the presence of a concretion at the proximal end, but probably more frequently to contraction of the sphincter or previous fibrosis at the proximal end. The acute attack has been likened to a knock at the door saying, "Let me out." As a result of the obstruction, the lumen becomes distended and the venous return is interfered with, so that the wall is poorly oxygenated and is then invaded by bacteria.

The infecting organisms appear to invade the mucosa from the lumen, the chief being streptococci and *Escherichia coli*. In exceptional cases, the infection may be carried by the blood stream from an acute tonsillitis or septic sore throat. Appendicitis is undoubtedly seen more in highly developed countries and in cities than in backward countries and rural districts. Acute appendicitis in children is becoming particularly frequent. Persons who live on a diet abundant in cellulose are immune to the disease, but when they adopt the diet of civilization, they lose that immunity. These and many other similar facts suggest that habits of life, and in particular modes of diet such as meat-eating, are important in predisposing someone to appendicitis.

There are all grades of acute appendicitis, from the most mild to the most severe, but for purposes of description, we shall take the severely inflamed organ that is removed just in time to prevent it from rupturing. Such an appendix is swollen and elongated, sometimes to an extraordinary degree, bright red in color, and covered by an acute inflammatory exudate (peritonitis). The inflammation is usually most marked toward the tip of the appendix. If gangrene (death of the tissue) has set in, usually at the tip, the gangrenous part will be green or black. As the process goes on, the wall of the appendix becomes thinned at 1 or more points and may rupture (perforation), so that the intestinal contents are poured out into the abdominal cavity and cause general peritonitis. A gangrenous appendix is certain to rupture unless it is removed.

The picture so far has been painted in the blackest colors—severe inflammation, gangrene, rupture, general peritonitis, death. Fortunately, such a sequence is the exception, not the rule. Most attacks of appendicitis are of a mild character and the patient recovers without operation. Unfortunately, no one can tell if a given case is going to result in spontaneous recovery or in gangrene. Rupture does not necessarily mean a fatal general peritonitis, for adhesions to surrounding structures tend to form before the rupture occurs. These adhesions limit the inflammatory process, so that the peritonitis remains local and an abscess is formed around the appendix. When this abscess is subsequently drained, it may be found that the appendix has been completely destroyed. This localization of the inflammation and infection is an excellent example of the beneficent effect of inflammation.

Clinical Pattern. The principal symptoms of a severe attack of appendicitis are pain and tenderness in the region of the appendix, nausea and vomiting, fever, and leukocytosis. The pain is at first of a general character, a "stomach-ache," but presently it settles in the right lower segment of the abdomen. Tenderness on pressure over the appendix is the most important single symptom. The pain and tenderness are caused by the great inflammatory swelling of the appendix with accompanying tension and pressure on the nerve endings. The pain goes on increasing in intensity until rupture occurs, when it is suddenly, completely, and most unfortunately relieved by the cessation of tension when the pus escapes. The relief is unfortunate because it may persuade the patient and the relatives, and even the nurse, that all is well, whereas the reverse is the case. The nausea and vomiting are reflex symptoms, since the same nerve (vagus nerve) supplies both the appendix and the stomach. Pain stimuli pass from the appendix to the brain and back again to the stomach, where they cause nausea and vomiting. The fever and leukocytosis are general symptoms due to absorption of bacterial toxins and the inflamed appendix. The leukocytosis is a valuable means of distinguishing between the appendicitis and simple colicky pains in that part of the abdomen unaccompanied by inflammation.

PERITONITIS

The peritoneum is the exquisitely thin layer of serous membrane that lines the abdominal cavity. It consists of 2 layers, 1 covering the inner surface of the abdominal wall, the other covering the stomach, intestines, and the other viscera. Between these layers lies the peritoneal cavity. Infection causing inflammation of the peritoneum generally comes from 1 of the hollow viscera covered by the membrane, but occasionally it is carried by the blood stream. The most common source of the infection is an acutely inflamed appendix, but rupture of a peptic ulcer in the stomach or duodenum or of a typhoid ulcer will flood the peritoneal cavity with infected material. The common microorganisms are streptococci and *Escherichia coli.*

Peritonitis may be local or general. Local peritonitis is inflammation limited to 1 region, e.g., the appendix and pelvic organs. The inflamed membrane, with its covering of fibrin, readily sticks to a neighboring part that is similarly inflamed. These adhesions are at first readily broken down and the parts separated, but they are invaluable in limiting the spread of the infection. This is particularly well seen in the case of appendicitis in which, if adhesions are formed before rupture occurs, a localized abscess in a walled-off space is the result, instead of a spreading fatal peritonitis. General peritonitis is the result of an infection that is not limited, but rather is spread throughout the peritoneal cavity. The surface covering the intestine is red and inflamed, and becomes covered with a sticky fibrinous exudate, which glues the coils of bowel together. A large amount of fluid may collect in the cavity and between the loops of bowel. This may be thick pus or thin watery fluid, depending on the organisms responsible for the infection.

The great danger of general peritonitis is intestinal obstruction. When the wall of the bowel (and the peritoneum forms the outer part of this wall) becomes inflamed, muscular movements are no longer able to pass along it, and the extremely serious condition of acute obstruction develops. This obstruction will kill the patient rather than the widespread infection, for reasons to be discussed in a subsequent section. The modern treatment of general peritonitis is largely directed toward the acute obstruction that accompanies it.

INTESTINAL DIVERTICULA

The diverticulum is a protrusion or herniation of the mucosa and submucosa through the muscular coat at some point of weakness. Diverticula of the intestine may occur in any part of the bowel, but the common sites are the duodenum and, more particularly, the sigmoid colon, which intervenes between the

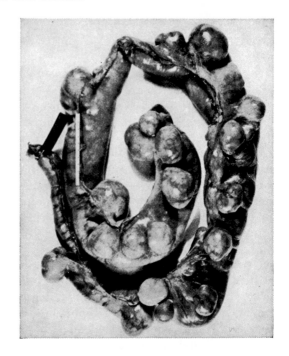

Fig. 17–7. Multiple diverticula of the small intestine. Death was due to infection and perforation of one large diverticulum. (Bell: *Textbook of Pathology.* Philadelphia, Lea & Febiger.)

descending colon and the rectum. It is here that these herniations may cause trouble. Diverticula may be present in great numbers, a condition known as diverticulosis. The usual size of each diverticulum is that of a large pea. In the sigmoid, the contents are naturally fecal and are sometimes in the form of concretions.

The condition of diverticulosis is unattended by symptoms, and is often discovered accidentally in the course of a barium series examination by the radiologist (Fig. 17–7). But if inflammation occurs in the diverticula, symptoms will be produced, just as they are in the appendix, which itself is a large diverticulum of the cecum. Acute diverticulitis, often associated with a hard concretion in the diverticulum, is similar to acute appendicitis, except that the symptoms are on the left side of the abdomen. Chronic diverticulitis is much more common, the characteristic feature being the formation of a large mass of chronic inflammatory tissue on the outside of the bowel, which may easily be mistaken for carcinoma in that region.

What is important about diverticulitis is that it may become complicated by peritonitis, which can be generalized or local; that pelvic abscesses may develop; that fistulas may occur; and that obstruction and bleeding may be life-threatening.

MALABSORPTION SYNDROMES

The persistence of diarrhea and the occurrence of abnormal bowel movements may be due to a disturbance of absorption, rather than to inflammation such as bacillary dysentery. Many disorders can result in stools that contain poorly digested foodstuffs, and these entities have been lumped together under the title malabsorption syndrome, since they have diarrhea in common. However, these disorders may have vastly different origins, as noted in Table 17–1.

One of the most interesting diseases causing the malabsorption syndrome is called adult sprue or gluten-induced enteropathy. A relatively large number of adults plagued by diarrhea and weight loss have their complaint traced to a hypersensitivity to the wheat protein, gluten. A small bowel biopsy shows atrophy of the villi in the jejunum that necessarily results in a decreased absorptive area. When placed on a trial diet, free from wheat gluten, the absorptive area is restored and their diarrhea disappears.

Table 17–1.   Classification of Malabsorption Syndromes

Inadequate digestion
  Following gastrectomy
  Pancreatic insufficiency
Reduced bile salts
  Liver disease
  Bile duct obstruction
  Abnormal intestinal pathways
Inadequate absorptive mechanisms
  Mechanical: intestinal resection or shunts
  Mucosal defects: genetic—enzyme deficiency
                inflammatory—tropical sprue
                infiltrative—amyloidosis
                allergic—celiac disease
  Obstructive disorders: lymphatic (intestinal lipodys-
                trophy or Whipple's disease)
                cardiovascular (congestive heart
                failure)
Endocrine and metabolic disorders
  Hyperthyroidism
  Diabetes mellitus

Of worldwide interest is the recent discovery that some persons lack the enzyme, lactase, which is necessary to digest milk. The genetically determined absence or decrease in lactase results in gaseous diarrhea and suggests that milk is an unsuitable food for such persons. However, more recent evidence has shown that, even in the absence of lactase, a considerable amount of nutritive value is still derived from the milk that is ingested. Clinical lists of the malabsorption syndrome include pancreatic diseases in which there is a loss of other digestive enzymes, but this problem may better be considered maldigestion.

Diseases that affect the liver and biliary tree result in reduced bile salts in the duodenum and are a major cause of malabsorption. In the absence of bile salts, fat cannot be absorbed. The stools are voluminous and frothy, and they float. Such a person with a gallstone in the common duct will have, in addition to other difficulties, malabsorption of fats that may result in a disorder of clotting; without adequate fat absorption, the vitamin essential to the coagulation process (vitamin K) is not absorbed, either.

Other diseases of a systemic nature such as lymphomas, and diabetes mellitus may result in the malabsorption syndrome by mechanical or metabolic means, and logically any obstruction to lymphatic or venous drainage may contribute to inadequate absorption.

NEOPLASIA

In the chapter on neoplasia, the thesis was advanced that there are degrees of abnormal differentiation leading to cancer. In the large bowel, one of the most common new growths is the polyp. Polyps frequently have a stalk and may be entirely asymptomatic, or they may obstruct or bleed and contribute to anemia. Most polyps represent hyperplasia. These growths are significant also because some are histologically malignant. A discussion of the debate as to whether all polyps are premalignant is unnecessary here, but it is important to know that there are families that transmit a trait as an autosomal dominant for multiple polyps of the colon. Such persons may have hundreds of polyps covering the surface of the bowel, and malignant transfor-

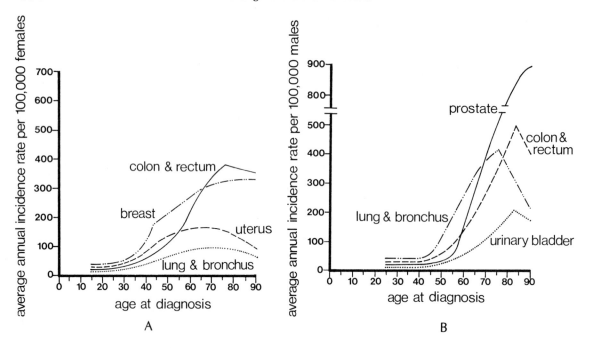

Fig. 17–8. *A,* This graph shows the average annual incidence per 100,000 women for carcinoma of the breast, uterus, lung and bronchus, and carcinoma of the colon and rectum. Note the rapid rise of carcinomas of the GI tract in ages 60 to 80. *B,* In men, carcinoma of the colon and rectum rises in a slightly older age group. (From Pitot, H. C.: *Fundamentals of Oncology.* New York, Marcel Dekker, Inc., 1978.)

mation is so frequent in members of these families that colectomy is routinely performed for this disorder.

Adenocarcinoma of the colon is among the most common carcinomas of man (Fig. 17–8). It is said that 70% of these cancers are within a few inches of the rectum and can therefore be detected by routine physical examination (Fig. 17–9). Fortunately, this tumor does not metastasize early and therefore the prognosis is good. In 1965, Gold and Freedman described an antigen present in the serum of patients with adenocarcinoma of the colon. Because this serum factor was identical to an antigen present in embryonic colon, this substance was called carcinoembryonic antigen (CEA). Its presence in patients with suspected or recurrent colonic malignancy has proved to be of diagnostic value.

Clinical Pattern. Any significant change in bowel habits, such as periods of diarrhea alternating with constipation, are warning signals that a tumor may be present. The presence of blood in the stool is another early

adenocarcinoma of sigmoid and anus

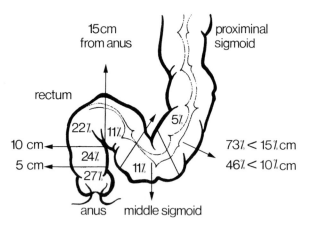

Fig. 17–9. This drawing illustrates the frequency of the sites of adenocarcinoma of the sigmoid colon and anus. The sigmoid colon and anus are divided into 5-cm, 10-cm, and 15-cm distances from the anal verge. The largest percentage of tumors of this area all lie within 15 cm and are thus detectable by proctoscopic or digital examination. (From Dionne, L.: Résultat du traitement chirurgical á visée curative des cancers recto-sigmoidiens. La Vie méd. au Can. fr., 8:149, 1979.)

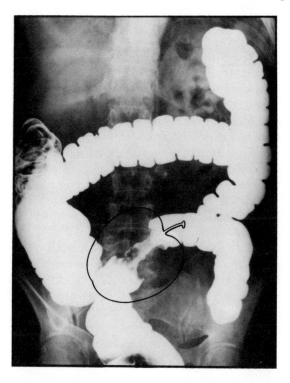

Fig. 17–10. This barium enema roentgenogram of the colon shows a constricting lesion that narrows the lumen and distorts the silhouette of barium. This lesion has been likened to the core of an apple and is shown within the outline of the apple. It is a common and often surgically resectable annular carcinoma.

warning signal. Radiologically, the carcinoma of the colon may be seen as a constricting lesion viewed as an "apple core" on barium enema (Fig. 17–10). Modern endoscopy with fiberoptic instruments permits both diagnosis and removal of suspicious lesions and greatly enhances the chance of early diagnosis. Carcinomas of the colon are treated surgically and the results are generally good.

Recently there has been much in the press about the theory that bulk in the diet promotes a rapid passage time, whereas the soft diet of western nations contains many potential carcinogens and promotes the incidence of cancer of the bowel. This debate will smoulder for several years until we glean data to confirm or deny the hypothesis. In the meantime it is sensible to vary your diet and to include as much fresh vegetable and fruit as you can afford.

OBSTRUCTIONS

The symptoms of intestinal obstruction vary, depending on the site and cause. With obstruction in the small bowel, vomiting may be the principal symptom; pain and distension are evidence of large bowel obstruction. However, some obstructions are relatively silent and the diagnosis as to the nature and cause of the disease may be hidden until the postmortem examination. Hernia, volvulus, and intussusception are all entities we can consider under this heading.

Hernia. The protrusion of a loop of bowel through an opening or weak point in the abdominal wall is called a hernia, although popularly it is often referred to as a "rupture." The most common sites for these protrusions are the groin (inguinal and femoral hernia) and the umbilicus. All these occurrences depend on an anatomic weakness; hernias do not occur from lifting or from hard work. The protrusion of a loop of bowel into a space where it does not belong may recur, and with time the opening may enlarge, or the bowel may become lodged in this new cavity and become irreducible. The danger arises when the venous return is compressed, the blood supply endangered, and necrosis of the bowel becomes imminent. This situation is called strangulation.

Because of the danger of perforation and peritonitis accompanying this acute intestinal obstruction, immediate surgical intervention is warranted. The surgeon's responsibility is to determine whether the bowel is viable, to return it to the peritoneal cavity, and to repair the opening so that herniation will not recur. It is of interest to note that the most common cause of intestinal obstruction is the presence of adhesions in the peritoneal cavity, and the most common cause of such adhesions is previous surgical exploration of the bowel.

Intussusception. A much more infrequent cause of bowel obstruction, intussusception occurs most often in children. Here, a segment of the bowel telescopes into another part, commonly at the ileocecal valve. Again, the hazards are gangrene, obstruction, rupture, and peritonitis. The preferred treatment today is to reduce the hernia with barium enema.

Volvulus. A twisting of the bowel on itself is another cause of obstruction.

Paralytic Ileus. Another name for a type of intestinal obstruction that occurs frequently after major surgery, anesthesia, or illness is paralytic ileus. The cause here is physiologic rather than mechanical: it is the absence of peristalsis, resulting in the accumulation of intestinal contents and gas, and dilatation, leading to pain and discomfort. Such obstruction is frequently relieved by the passage of a tube to drain the gas and contents.

Chronic Obstruction. This condition occurs frequently in the elderly or mentally incapable, who are often dehydrated or are unable to maintain a sufficient intake of foodstuffs, so that their feces becomes brittle, dry, and impacted. Tumors and old inflammatory disease may also constrict the lumen of the bowel.

DIARRHEA

In our survey of some of the principal diseases of the intestine, diarrhea has been noted as a frequent symptom. It may therefore be worthwhile briefly to review this important symptom. Diarrhea, the passage of stools that are too frequent and too soft, results when the fluid contents of the small intestine are hurried so rapidly through the large intestine that there is not sufficient time for the fluid to be absorbed. It is therefore to be expected that diarrhea will be most marked in an inflammatory disease of the large bowel such as dysentery. In this condition there is also a copious outpouring of mucus from the glands lining the colon that makes the stools still more liquid. Inflammation of the small intestine, especially when associated with ulcers, may also cause diarrhea.

Irritating foods tend to cause diarrhea. This may be because the food is particularly indigestible and coarse. The diarrhea may also be caused by food infections, bacteria-contaminated foods that have been allowed to decompose or "go bad."

Nervous diarrhea is well known, and is due to excessive nervous stimuli causing an undue amount of peristalsis. Some persons always have a looseness of the bowels when going for examinations and at other similar but equally inopportune moments.

FECES

In the course of digestion, the food passes from the stomach into the intestines, where it meets in the duodenum 2 powerful digestive agents, the bile and the pancreatic juice, both of which are necessary for the proper digestion of fat. In the small intestine, the food becomes completely fluid, because the solid masses of food are dissolved and because of the presence of the digestive fluids of the bowel. The food now passes slowly along the large intestine, where most of the water is absorbed, so that the stools or feces that leave the body are soft, well-formed, brown, cylindrical masses. If the bowel movements are accelerated to any marked degree, there is insufficient time for the water to be absorbed, so that the stools remain fluid (diarrhea). After the protein, carbohydrate, and fat have been absorbed, there remains indigestible material, chiefly cellular, from vegetable food, which acts as "roughage" and stimulates the motility of the bowel. The feces, however, are not just residues of food that have not been absorbed, but are composed in large part of material that has been excreted from the blood. For that reason, the bulk of the feces is not totally diminished during starvation. It is surprising to learn that bacteria make up more than 10% of the bulk of the feces.

Constipation is usually due to poor habits. The passage of feces into the rectum causes a desire to defecate, which should result in the complete emptying of the rectum. If this call is neglected or suppressed, the desire passes, and water is absorbed from the fecal mass, which becomes hard and dry. If this state of affairs is continued for long, the rectum, which is only 5 inches long and should normally be empty, contains feces all the time and comes to lose its sensitivity.

An examination of the feces will reveal many facts of importance with regard to the gastrointestinal canal, the process of digestion, and the many disorders that may affect it.

Form. The normal form and consistency of the stools depend on the extraction of water during their passage through the large intestine. If the time of this passage is shortened owing to the increased irritability of the bowel, such as occurs in dysentery, water is not absorbed, and the stools are therefore fluid in character. On the other hand, the feces may remain in the large bowel for an undue length of time, owing to chronic constipation. In this case, the stools take the form of small, hard, round masses, known as scybala. When the stools are narrow and ribbon-like, it is probable that there is some marked narrowing at the lower end of the large bowel, usually due to cancer of the rectum.

Mucus and pus are found in large amounts in acute dysentery and ulcerative colitis, often associated with blood. The mucus is produced by the cells lining the mucous membrane of the inflamed large bowel, just as mucus is discharged from an inflamed nose. The presence of pus is natural in an acute inflammation such as dysentery. The mucus can be seen with the naked eye as slimy streaks or shreds. Pus is best detected by means of the microscope.

The intestinal parasitic worms causing disease and the entamoeba of dysentery have already been described in Chapter 10.

Color. The normal color varies from yellow to brown. When the stool is large and pale, it contains undigested fat, the most common cause of which is obstruction to the flow of bile into the duodenum, either by a gallstone impacted in the bile duct or by a tumor. A chemical test for bile will give a negative result. In disease of the pancreas, the stool tends to be even more voluminous and greasy, owing to complete suppression of fat digestion on account of the absence of pancreatic juice.

The stools may be colored by blood. This blood may be bright red, dark, or black. Red blood comes from the lower part of the intestine. Streaks of bright blood, especially at the end of defecation, are probably due to bleeding piles. Bright blood may come from carcinoma of the rectum or of another part of the large intestine. During the third and fourth weeks of typhoid fever, the nurse must watch the stools carefully for bright blood, because a few specks or streaks may be the forerunner of a severe hemorrhage. Acute inflammation of the colon (colitis, dysentery) is often marked by the presence of blood in the fluid stools, associated usually with mucus and pus. Dark or black blood has been altered by digestion so that it comes from high up in the alimentary canal, usually the stomach or duodenum, the lesion being ulcer or cancer. If the bleeding from the ulcer or tumor is only slight, it will not be possible to detect the blood with the naked eye; it is hidden or occult. When these lesions are suspected, a specimen is sent to the laboratory to be tested chemically for occult blood. It is important that the patient be properly prepared before this examination by the omission of all red meat, meat soups, and meat extracts from his or her diet for at least 3 days. The inclusion of green vegetables in the diet does not interfere with most of the tests for occult blood. It must be remembered that the stools may be dark and tarry in appearance for reasons other than the presence of blood, especially the medicinal use of iron or bismuth.

SYNOPSIS

The lower digestive tract is divided by the ileocecal valve into the part that absorbs sugars, fatty acids, amino acids, iron, and essential substances (the small bowel: duodenum, jejunum, ileum) and the large bowel (colon), whose function is water absorption and storage.

Diarrhea is the most important symptom of bowel disease and its causes include infectious agents (amebic dysentery, typhoid fever, cholera), inflammatory diseases of unknown etiology (ulcerative colitis, regional ileitis), and diverse disorders of the bowel that range from rare infiltrates (amyloid) or tumors to obstruction of the bile ducts.

Complications of all inflammations of the bowel include obstruction, perforation, and peritonitis.

Impairment of the vascular supply, either arterial occlusions, emboli, or venous obstruction (thrombosis or torsion), will lead to gangrene of the bowel.

The malabsorption syndromes are caused by many disorders that result in weight loss, incomplete digestion of food, anemia, and diarrhea.

Tumors of the colon are the most common tumor in man and woman, and the majority of these are within 6 inches of the anus and are amenable to early diagnosis and treatment.

Terms

Duodenum	*Sigmoid*	*Malabsorption syndrome*
Jejunum	*Dysentery*	*Polyp*
Ileum	*Ulcerative colitis*	*Familial polyposis*
Appendix	*Crohn's disease*	*Hernia*
Villus	*Diverticulosis*	*Intussusception*
Brush border	*Diverticulitis*	*Volvulus*
Ileocecal valve	*Peritonitis*	*Ileus*
Colon	*Carcinoembryonic antigen*	

FURTHER READING

Editorial: Necrotising enterocolitis. Br. Med. J., *1*:132, 1978.

Almy, T. A., and Howell, D. A.: Diverticular disease of the colon. N. Engl. J. Med., *302*:324, 1980.

Barnes, B. A., et al.: Treatment of appendicitis at the Massachusetts General Hospital, 1937–1959. J.A.M.A., *180*:122, 1962.

Bayless, T. M., et al.: Lactose and milk intolerance: clinical implications. N. Engl. J. Med., *292*:1156, 1975.

Burkitt, D. P.: Some diseases characteristic of modern western civilization. Br. Med. J., *1*:273, 1973.

Dukes, C. E., and Bussey, H. J. P.: The spread of rectal cancer and its effect on prognosis. Br. J. Cancer, *12*:309, 1958.

Erbe, R. W.: Inherited gastrointestinal-polyposis syndromes. N. Engl. J. Med., *294*:1101, 1976.

Farmer, R. G., et al.: Clinical patterns in Crohn's disease: a statistical study of 615 cases. Gastroenterology, *68*:627, 1975.

Gold, P., and Freedman, S. O.: Specific antigenic similarity between malignant adult and normal fetal tissues of the human digestive system. J. Clin. Invest., *44*:1051, 1965.

Gorbach, S. L., et al.: Traveller's diarrhea and toxigenic *E. coli*. N. Engl. J. Med., *292*:933, 1975.

Hofmann, A. F.: The enterohepatic circulation of bile acids in man. Adv. Intern. Med., *21*:501, 1976.

Sacks, F. M., et al.: Plasma lipids and lipoproteins in vegetarians and controls. N. Engl. J. Med., *292*:1148, 1975.

Sleisenger, M. H.: Malabsorption syndrome. N. Engl. J. Med., *281*:1111, 1969.

Sleisenger, M. H., and Kim, Y. S.: Protein digestion and absorption. N. Engl. J. Med., *300*:659, 1979.

Stamland, J. R., et al.: Clinical presentations of diseases of the large bowel. Gastroenterology, *70*:22, 1976.

Yeomans, N. D.: Pathogenesis of coeliac sprue. Lancet, *2*:843, 1974.

Liver and Gallbladder

18

The liver is the lazaret of bile. —BYRON

LIVER

To the ancient Babylonians, the liver was the seat of the soul, whereas in ancient Greece it was considered the central organ of the body. The liver, tucked under the diaphragm, below the ribs on the right side of the abdomen, is the largest, warmest, and one of the most important organs in the body. Although it has remarkable regenerative powers, it also has an extraordinary reserve and can adapt to different loads of toxic substances or to nutritional excesses and deprivations. Without the liver we die quickly. One of the most interesting and puzzling things about the liver is that, although it performs many separate and distinct functions, as we shall shortly see, the cells of the liver are apparently identical and differ only in their position in the columns along which blood flows from the intestinal tract to the heart (Fig. 18–1). A diagram of the circulation of the liver is shown in Figure 18–2 and demonstrates that the liver, like the lung, receives blood from 2 sources. The minor component is blood from the hepatic artery, and the major (75%) is blood from the portal system, which derives its tributaries from the stomach, spleen, and small and large bowel.

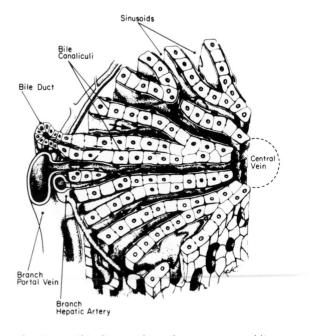

Fig. 18–1. This diagram shows the arrangement of liver cells in a hypothetical lobule, illustrating the different types of cells in the liver, namely the Kupffer cells and duct cells of the bile duct, and vascular cells. The liver cells are arranged in cords, as shown here. (From Bloom, W., and Fawcett, D.W.: *A Textbook of Histology.* Philadelphia, W. B. Saunders, 1968. After Ham.)

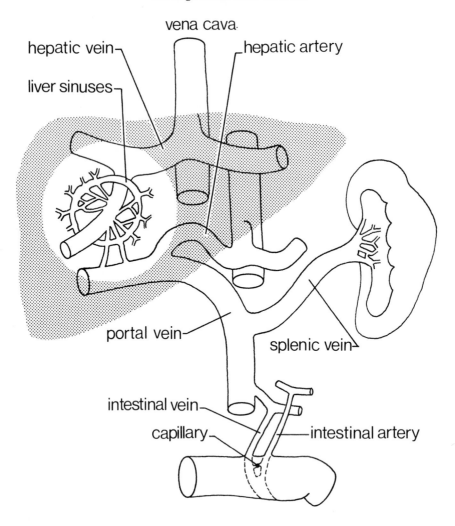

Fig. 18–2. This diagram of the circulation of the liver shows the portal vein, which is composed of veins draining from the intestine and spleen. The hepatic artery supplies blood to each liver lobule, and the blood then flows through the hepatic vein to the vena cava.

Although the liver is concerned with aspects of protein, carbohydrate, and lipid metabolism, it is possible to separate arbitrarily the many functions of the liver into 4 categories: synthesis, secretion, detoxification, and storage. Aberrations in most or all of these functions can be determined by laboratory tests and often form the basis for distinguishing 1 type of liver disease from another.

Synthetic Functions. Whereas the liver receives the elements of all digestive processes that arrive in the portal venous blood (a little like the groceries for the Christmas banquet arriving at the kitchen door), perhaps the most important products of the liver cell are the serum proteins. Serum proteins

(albumin, fibrinogen, prothrombin, to name 3) serve several specific functions, but collectively they contribute to the osmotic value of the serum of the intravascular fluid compartment and thereby enable the circulation to function, as reviewed earlier.

Albumin is the most important of these proteins; the liver is the only organ that makes it. About 10 grams of albumin are synthesized daily by a 70-kg man, but half this albumin will be lost in 2 weeks. A decrease in serum albumin (hypoalbuminemia) can result from increased excretion (glomerular disease), inadequate precursors (malnutrition), or decreased synthesis (liver disease). This decrease in serum albumin results in edema, ascites, or anasarca (the accumulation of fluid outside the vascular compartment).

Any acute or chronic injury to the liver may

result in decreased synthesis of important protein products of the liver, such as fibrinogen and prothrombin, which are blood clotting factors. Therefore, another serious result of liver damage may be small or large hemorrhages and impairment of the normal clotting mechanisms.

The liver also synthesizes a legion of enzymes, some of which appear in direct response to a need for them, such as alcohol dehydrogenase. A teetotaler will have little of this, whereas a souse will have a high specific activity of this inducible enzyme. When liver cells are injured by toxic agents (chemicals, viruses) or impaired blood supply (heart failure), enzymes may leak into the serum, just as necrotic heart muscle leaks both muscle-specific enzymes (CPK) and nonspecific cytoplasmic or mitochondrial enzymes, such as glutamic oxalacetic transaminase (SGOT) or lactic acid dehydrogenase (LDH). Elevations of transaminase and other isoenzymes (in the absence of necrosis of heart tissue) are good indications of damage to the liver.

The liver also synthesizes substances other than proteins. One important class are lipids, of which lipoproteins are the form that appear in the serum. The liver takes up free fatty acids from the portal circulation and esterifies them into triglycerides that may be stored or excreted (lipoproteins). Because the preferred form for the excretion of lipid is a complex of lipid with protein, the release and secretion of lipid depends also on the protein-synthesizing capabilities of the liver. If the liver's protein-synthesizing machinery has been poisoned, then the lipids that normally would be distributed accumulate in the liver cells, which results in a fatty, enlarged liver.

Secretory Function. The principal and most obvious product of the liver is bile. This colored fluid is derived from the hemoglobin of red blood cells that have reached the end of their normal life span. The obsolete red blood cells are broken down by cells of the reticuloendothelial system (Kupffer cells), and the iron (heme) that has been separated from the protein (globin) is converted into bilirubin via biliverdin. A small proportion of bilirubin comes from other heme proteins (cytochrome, myoglobin), and from the bone marrow. Liver cells take up bilirubin and conjugate it into a water-soluble derivative, using the microsomes of their cytoplasm to do the job. The principal product of this work is a bilirubin conjugated with sugars (bilirubin diglucuronide), a step that is required for bilirubin to pass into the bile. The liver cell is able to secrete this water-soluble material into the small space between 2 neighboring liver cells, the bile canaliculus, which, like the tributaries of a mountain stream that join to form a river, connects with the intrahepatic, extrahepatic, and common bile duct, terminating in the delta of the ampulla of Vater, where the bile enters the intestinal cavity and colors all the sediment a familiar muddy brown.

It is of interest that this conjugated bilirubin is not reabsorbed in the intestine, and the body is thereby permitted to excrete pigments for which it has no use. Bacteria of the large bowel have the capability, however, of converting conjugated bilirubin into urobilinogen, which can be reabsorbed and recycled, thereby conserving material if need be.

What is the function of bile? Bile contains bile salts and cholesterol as well as bilirubin. The salts in bile are surface-active substances that emulsify lipids and, by their action, permit lipids to be absorbed by the intestinal absorptive cell. In the absence of bile, fats and fat-soluble vitamins are not absorbed, and the body suffers the consequences of deficiency of vitamins D, K, and E and a lack of essential fatty acids (arachidonic, linoleic). The body has devised an ingenious mechanism for dealing with periods of famine and plenty by enabling large amounts of bile to be delivered to the intestine when a meal of seal blubber, cheesecake, or herring and sour cream has been ingested. The gallbladder is a reservoir that stores bile and can deliver relatively large amounts via the cystic and common duct on signal from the duodenum. Normally, small amounts of bile are constantly synthesized, secreted, and delivered to the intestine. It is one of Nature's devices to combine forces when possible. It is of note that the ducts from the pancreas enter the duodenum at the same site (ampulla of Vater) as the bile, and pancreatic enzymes, which are concerned with the hydrolysis of fats (lipases), are secreted at the same time into the duodenum as the emulsifier.

While we are on the subject of secretion of bile, it is appropriate to consider the problem of jaundice before going on to consider the other general functions of the liver (detoxification and storage).

Jaundice. "Jaundice," as William Osler said, "is the disease your friends diagnose." However, jaundice is not a disease. It is a sign of disease. Jaundice or icterus is a coloration of the skin, whites of the eyes, and urine; in fact, all the tissues of the body are stained by excess bile pigments that circulate in the serum. Normally, as we have seen, bile is secreted into the bowel and eliminated in the feces. Three general mechanisms can disrupt this pattern of flow and may cause bile to appear in the serum, thereby causing a complexion of a yellow, orange, or even green tinge, which we recognize as jaundice. Bilirubin may circulate either as free bilirubin or as conjugated (water-soluble) bilirubin, or as a mixture of both. In order to be conjugated, bilirubin must have been acted on by liver cells. To be detectable by a laboratory

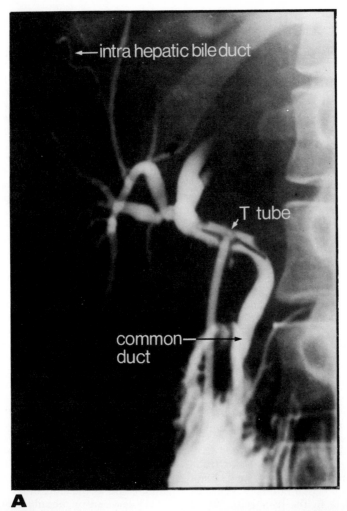

A

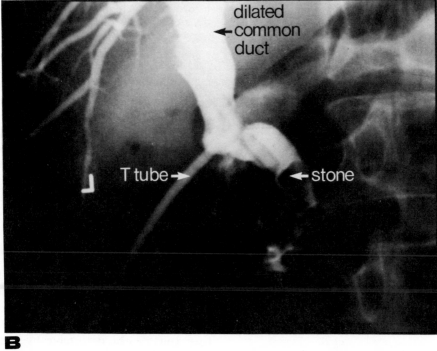

B

test, the total serum bilirubin should be in excess of 1.5 mg/100 ml, but it usually must reach 3.0 mg/100 ml before it is obvious to an observer. Jaundice (or an increase in serum bilirubin) has been divided into 3 groups.

The first of these types of jaundice is easy to understand and is called **obstructive**. Since bile normally flows from liver cells to canaliculi to ductules to ducts to the common duct and to the ampulla of Vater, an obstruction may occur at any of these levels and may cause a damming of flow and backup of bile. A tumor at or near the ampulla of Vater, a stone in the common duct, a misplaced suture, or scarring of the extrahepatic ducts may each prevent the normal passage of bile into the intestine. The accompanying roentgenograms (Fig. 18–3) show the appearance of both the normal, intra- and extrahepatic bile ducts and the dilated ducts that occur when obstruction has taken place. When this obstruction occurs, the secretion of bile from the liver continues. Since bile cannot traverse its normal route, it seeks another path, like the waters of a stream behind a beaver dam. The bile, which has already been through the liver cell (conjugated bilirubin), leaks into the serum, since it cannot follow its rightful tributary to the gut. This reflux of conjugated bilirubin into the serum causes staining of all tissues (and is clinically apparent when the serum bilirubin is greater than 3 mg/100 ml). The serum level of conjugated bilirubin can be determined by the van den Bergh reaction, a chemical test that can be used to distinguish between conjugated and unconjugated pigments. Conjugated bilirubin is said to be "direct-reacting." Because bile fails to reach the gut, the stools become pale and are not their normal brown (they are frequently referred to as clay-colored). The bile that circulates is cleared in the kidney, causing the urine to be much darker than normal, and in fact to foam. This is because bile is a surface-active agent. If the situation lasts for any length of time (a week or 2), there is impairment of fat digestion and absorption and interference with vitamin K absorption, which interferes with synthesis of prothrombin. The jaundice will progress and the liver cells themselves will become damaged. The pattern of jaundice, with an elevated direct-reacting bilirubin, pale stools, and bile in the urine, points to obstruction in the biliary excretory systems and suggests that surgical exploration for a stone or tumor is warranted. The longer the obstruction exists, the more likely it is that complications will arise, such as hepatocellular injury, infection of the ductal system, or other problems such as bleeding.

The second type of jaundice is called **hepatocellular**, because the elevated bilirubin is not conjugated with glucuronide. Unconjugated bilirubin levels cannot be measured directly. Total bilirubin and conjugated bilirubin levels are measured directly by means of the van den Bergh test, then the conjugated level is substracted from the total, yielding indirectly the unconjugated, or indirect-reacting, bilirubin level. This bilirubin, then, has not been acted on by the liver cells or secreted by them, usually because the liver cells have been damaged. Sometimes the circulatory system in the liver is no longer compartmentalizing the flow of pigments, and liberates bilirubin directly into the circulation. Thus an elevated serum unconjugated bilirubin can occur when many liver cells are destroyed or injured, as in infectious hepatitis (viral), or in acute toxic or vascular injury to the liver cells. It is important to recognize that if an obstruction continues, it may also injure the liver cells, resulting in an elevation of both the direct- and indirect-reacting bilirubin.

The search for the underlying cause of this type of jaundice is made more difficult when

Fig. 18–3. *A,* This x-ray study shows the appearance of the common bile duct and the intrahepatic bile duct, visualized by the presence of water-soluble iodinated contrast medium, which was inserted into the duct by means of a T tube following an operation. This x-ray study shows a normal, undilated, unobstructed biliary tree. *B,* Another postoperative cholangiogram shows the appearance of a markedly dilated intrahepatic biliary tree due to the presence of obstruction by a stone (arrow).

components of both obstruction and liver cell injury are present. The patient's prognosis is more guarded, because even the administration of general anesthesia, let alone the metabolic insult of a surgical operation, puts great stress on the liver.

The third type of jaundice is caused by the liberation of excessive amounts of bile pigments, that is, more than the liver can handle. This phenomenon occurs in all cases of massive hemolysis and is referred to as **hemolytic** jaundice. It appears most commonly during the first days after birth, when a transient or mild icterus should be no cause for alarm. Hemolytic jaundice is an unconjugated hyperbilirubinemia and can be expected in diseases in which hemolysis occurs (e.g., acquired or congenital hemolytic anemias), in bacterial infections, and occasionally in cases in which large areas of tissue are infarcted or bleeding. Traditionally, a mismatched transfusion is a cause of hemolysis.

With continuous excessive loads of bilirubin, as in the congenital hemolytic anemias (sickle cell disease), a complication may be the deposition of bilirubin in the form of stones that accumulate in the gallbladder, in the cystic duct, or even in the intrahepatic ducts. In this complication, 2 different types of bilirubin-overload intersect: the hemolytic jaundice (hemolytic anemia) may predispose a patient to a mechanical obstruction (stone), causing the obstructive type of jaundice!

Detoxification. The liver plays an important role in dealing with toxic and natural substances. Hormones, drugs, dietary pollutants—all are examples of substances that are excreted by the liver when they have been inactivated or converted to water-soluble materials. In order to do this job, the liver is capable of synthesizing new enzymes. Naturally, a diseased liver responds less effectively to demand than a normal one, and a dose of a drug that would be well tolerated in a normal person may be lethal in someone with severe liver disease. It has become clear that some drugs (for example, phenobarbital) may cause a change in the structure of liver cells that can even be visualized with the electron microscope. With regular doses, there is an increase in the smooth endoplasmic reticulum.

Storage. The famous experiments of Claude Bernard showed that the mammalian liver was a storehouse for glycogen, and thus provides a reservoir or physiologic buffer for the serum glucose. As serum glucose is used, additional supplies may be mobilized from the liver stores, and the constancy of the serum glucose level maintained. Other substances such as iron and lipids are also deposited in the hepatic bank account, although the normal turnover is rapid and the stored balance at any given time is small (just like the average bank account). With disease, with increased loads, or from decreased mobilization, materials may accumulate in liver cells. This accumulation leads to enlargement of the liver (hepatomegaly). Rarely, foreign materials (amyloid) may be deposited among the liver cells and may also increase the size of the liver. Moreover, in some rare hereditary disorders, such as those due to enzyme deficiencies, the liver may accumulate materials as in the glycogen storage diseases. Naturally, with acute destruction of the liver (hepatitis), there may be a failure of normal function. For example, a patient with acute hepatitis may be in coma because of an excessively low blood sugar, since the hepatic cells are capable neither of storing glycogen nor of releasing it.

Liver Function Tests. For each of these arbitrary functions of the liver (synthesis, secretion, detoxification, and storage) there are laboratory tests that can estimate the capability of the liver.

TESTS OF SYNTHETIC FUNCTION. The serum of albumin in the normal human being is about 4 to 5 gm/100 ml; the normal value of globulins is 2 to 3 gm/100 ml. Other proteins such as fibrinogen and prothrombin are not routinely measured directly. Any decrease in serum albumin in the absence of a demonstrated loss in the urine can be attributed to decreased synthesis. This implies a disordered function of the liver cells.

If a patient has a prolonged prothrombin time, the liver may be diseased; however, if the bile ducts are obstructed, a prolonged prothrombin time will also occur because vitamin K, essential for the synthesis of prothrombin, may not be available. A simple test to see whether this disorder can be reversed is to administer vitamin K to the patient. If, in the presence of exogenous vitamin K, the bleeding tendency reverses, it is clear that the liver cells themselves are capable of using this essential vitamin. Unfortunately, the longer mechanical obstruction lasts in any system, especially the liver, the more likely there is to be damage to the cells upstream of the obstruction.

Another group of tests for the integrity of the synthetic function of the liver are those for the presence of enzymes that are not normally present in the serum, or are present in low or trace amounts only. We have already mentioned the transaminases (SGOT and SGPT), which are only present in trace amounts in the serum (less than 40 units), but which are elevated in all types of liver disease (greater than 400 units). An isoenzyme of lactic acid dehydrogenase has been traced to hepatic cells and permits necrosis of liver to be distinguished from necrosis in the heart.

TESTS OF SECRETORY FUNCTION. As outlined previously, the functions of the liver include the secretion of bile and materials that have been detoxified: hormones, dyes (bromsulfophthalein), enzymes (alkaline phosphatase, 5′nucleotidase). In order to assess liver function, it is possible to use some tests that directly and/or indirectly measure the secretory function of the liver, other than the secretion of bile.

One test is to administer a dye, bromsulfophthalein (BSP), which is rapidly taken up, concentrated, conjugated, and secreted. A standard amount of dye (5 mg/kg body weight) is injected and a blood sample is withdrawn from another vein at a fixed time and analyzed for dye concentration. Normally, less than 5% of the dye remains in the serum 45 minutes after injection. Despite its nonspecificity, the test is of value in patients who do not have jaundice to assess the functional capability of the liver cells.

A second test, which complements the serum bilirubin assay, is that for serum alkaline phosphatase. This enzyme is present in the brush border of the intestine, in the kidney, in bones, and in the liver. Although its function is debated, it is well known empirically that extrahepatic biliary obstruction leads to great elevation in serum alkaline phosphatase. Perhaps hepatocellular disease leads to decreased synthesis of this enzyme,

but, in any case, in the presence of obstruction such as carcinoma of the head of the pancreas, or common duct stone, the alkaline phosphatase levels are many times normal. In order to distinguish elevations of alkaline phosphatase levels that occur in bone disease from those that occur in liver disease, another enzyme, 5′nucleotidase, may be measured.

TESTS OF STORAGE AND METABOLIC FUNCTION. In liver disease, not only may the storage and mobilization of glycogen be impaired, but the serum glucose levels, as assayed by a glucose tolerance test, may reflect damage to the liver. The glucose tolerance test may show a rapid rise of blood glucose to abnormally high levels and an abnormally slow return to normal. The most important finding is an unusually low serum glucose level. However, a glucose tolerance test in the presence of liver disease gives variable results and cannot be considered a specific indication of the kind or amount of damage to the liver.

OTHER TESTS OF HEPATIC FUNCTION. In addition to the tests outlined in the foregoing section, radiologic examination of the liver is frequently useful. A plain film of the abdomen may demonstrate calcified structures within the liver or biliary tract, and the presence of fluid (ascites) in the peritoneal cavity often points to hepatic disease. Radiopaque substances taken by mouth (oral cholecystog-

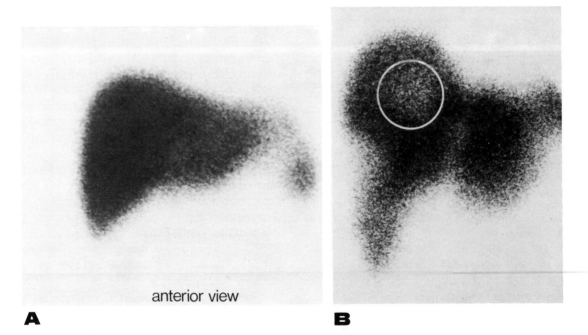

anterior view

A   **B**

Fig. 18–4. *A,* This roentgenogram shows a scan of a liver 15 minutes after the intravenous injection of technitium sulfur-colloid. The uniform distribution and uptake shows the outline of a normal liver. *B,* In this instance, within the circle, there is an area of decreased uptake of the technitium sulfur-colloid. Such an absence of normal liver is compatible with the diagnosis of tumor, abscess, or cysts. The technitium is normally taken up by Kupffer's cells of the reticuloendothelial system.

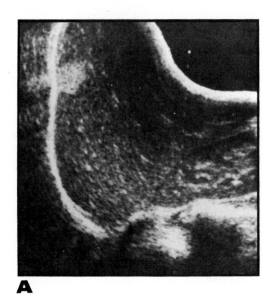
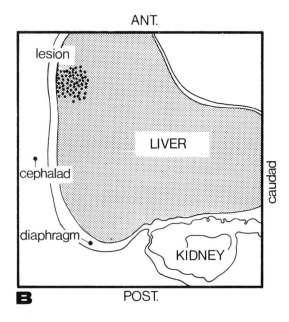

Fig. 18–5. *A* and *B,* This ultrasound scan, using the B-mode, shows a 2-cm area in the superior aspect of the liver. This lesion is labeled in the accompanying diagram. The presence of an echogenic mass is consistent with a solid growth such as a metastasis from cancer of the colon to the liver. (The dense white line at the left of the picture is the position of the diaphragm.)

raphy) or injected intravenously (IV cholecystography) or directly into the liver (transhepatic cholangiography) often outline the biliary tree, indicating an obstruction or an anatomic abnormality, guiding the surgeon to the diagnosis and treatment. Other more recent techniques take advantage of the liver's synthetic, storage, and secretory functions. When radioactively labeled substances are administered, they may be taken up by the liver and may reveal nonfunctional areas (cysts) or space-occupying lesions that may represent tumor (Figs. 18–4 and 18–5).

In the absence of any bleeding disorder, a needle biopsy of the liver can be done, yielding a small piece of tissue from which a histologic diagnosis may be made. With this background of structure, function, and possible tests of the liver's integrity, we may progress to consider the circulation of the liver before discussing important and common diseases.

Hepatic and Portal Circulation. Each liver cell is bathed in blood derived from the venous return from the intestine. This blood naturally has a lower oxygen content than arterial blood and higher content of substrates derived from the absorptive processes.

The flow of blood through the liver is estimated at 1.5 liters per minute, and the blood flows from the portal triads along the columns of cells to drain into the central veins. Thus,

each liver cell is exposed to a gradient of portal blood with varying amount of oxygen and substrate, depending on whether the liver cell is first in line (portal zone) or last at the banquet table (central zone). Should the venous pressure in the systemic circulation be raised owing, for example, to heart failure (old myocardial infarct), then there will be stasis in the venous circulation that can be reflected as far downstream as the liver. This passive congestion may result in a slow attrition of the liver cells around the central veins of each lobule, because they are the last to receive any oxygenated blood and the last to receive any amino acids, glucose, or fatty acids. The anatomic result of longstanding congestion is a loss of functional capability that may lead to abnormalities in test dye retention, serum, bilirubin, enzyme elevations, and even in decreased synthesis of albumin. Anatomically, the liver may be smooth and enlarged. The patient complains of a dull ache in the right upper quadrant, and, if you press on the liver, a wave may be seen in the jugular veins. This chronic passive congestion of the liver is a common disorder (Fig. 18–6), and the older pathologists talk about the "nutmeg liver" because the stasis and congestion of blood in

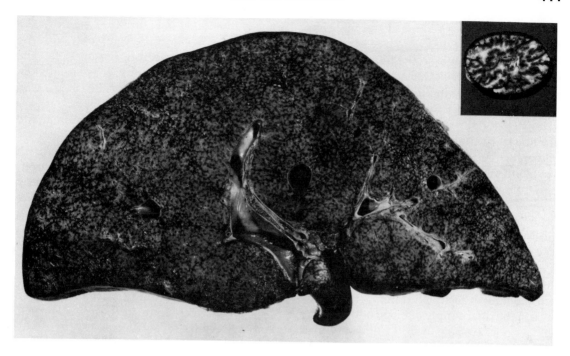

Fig. 18–6.   This gross photograph of a liver from a patient with chronic, congestive heart failure, shows the marked mottling that is typical of this condition. Its resemblance to the *inset,* a photograph of a section through a nutmeg, has caused generations of students to wonder what a nutmeg looked like. A classic cause for chronic, passive congestion in the liver is old myocardial infarctions or chronic valvular heart disease, such as mitral stenosis. (McGill University, Department of Pathology Museum.)

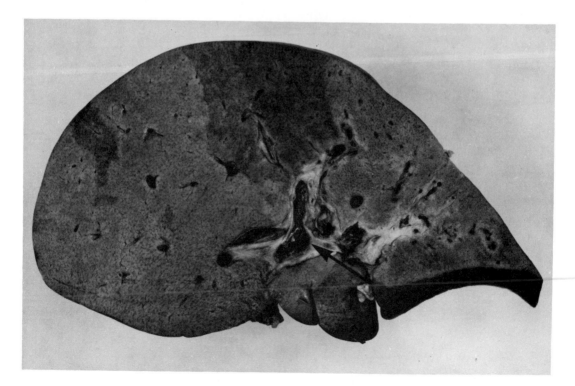

Fig. 18–7.   Section through the liver showing an area of discoloration at the top of the liver. The portal vein is thrombosed at the arrow, and this has caused the **infarction** despite the fact that the liver has a dual circulation. (McGill University, Department of Pathology Museum.)

the liver resemble a sectioned nutmeg (Fig. 18–6, *inset*).

Disease upstream or in the liver may affect the intrahepatic circulation and the portal venous system below the liver. Chronic injury to the liver with scarring (cirrhosis) may lead to elevated portal venous pressure and even to thrombosis of the portal veins. Fortunately, collateral circulations may be available to return blood to the heart, but complications can arise from the use of this collateral pathway, as we shall see. The hepatic vein may also become occluded, and all the predisposing causes of thrombosis discussed earlier may be relevant in considering this uncommon circumstance.

In the liver, as in any organ, infarction may occur, but it is relatively rare, perhaps because of the dual supply of blood and because the liver cells are able to shift from aerobic to anaerobic glycolysis. The rare infarct in the liver is illustrated in Figure 18–7, and the discolored local area can be compared with the diffuse congestion seen in Figure 18–6. The most common antecedent to these infarcts in the liver, which have been called infarcts of Zahn, are episodes of profound shock associated with blood loss as in major trauma, and in surgical and obstetric accidents.

Acute Necrosis of the Liver. A more frequent occurrence than simple ischemic infarction, necrosis of the liver is most often caused by specific viral infections (hepatitis, yellow fever), by poisons that have a profound effect on the liver, such as carbon tetrachloride (CCl_4) and phosphorus (rat poison), or by special instances of unknown etiology, such as toxemia of pregnancy (eclampsia) and shock. An example of the massive injury to the liver that can occur in these instances is shown in Figure 18–8. Naturally such a widespread and extensive hepatic injury as shown

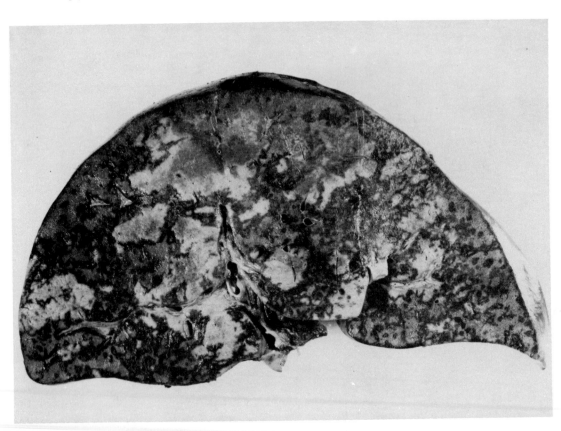

Fig. 18–8. This gross photograph of a section of the liver shows large, irregular, pale areas surrounded by red borders. This appearance is typical of widespread **necrosis**. Such an injury, as shown here, is so severe as to cause death, despite the remarkable regenerative capacity of the liver. This is from a case of **eclampsia**. (McGill University, Department of Pathology Museum.)

in this figure may result in death. Because of the remarkable regenerative capacity of the liver, owing to the active recruitment of the pluripotential liver cells to mitosis and subsequent resumption of the organ's many functions, if the patient can be kept alive until the liver has had time to recover from such a massive injury, regeneration may restore many of the functions of this essential organ. However, following such an extensive injury, it is likely that scars will develop that will leave a permanent mark on the liver, both anatomically and physiologically. Broad bands of scar may remain to testify to the near-fatal episode of hepatic necrosis, and the portal circulation may be disordered because of the collapse of the hepatic architecture, leaving the patient with venous shunts that bypass the usual detoxifying and filtration mechanisms represented by the normal portal system. Fortunately, acute, massive, hepatic necrosis is relatively rare, as compared with the diseases we shall now consider.

Infectious Diseases of the Liver. From the worldwide point of view, infections of the liver are extremely common. Earlier we have considered schistosomiasis, yellow fever,

echinococcal cysts, and amebiasis, all of which are serious and often fatal diseases of the liver (Fig. 18–9). In North America, when considering infections of the liver, we usually think first of viral hepatitis and bacterial infections of the bile ducts; the latter are a frequent complication of obstruction to the biliary tree. Abscesses, both bacterial and fungal, and tuberculous infections of the liver are becoming much less common than in the preantibiotic era. A solitary abscess is shown in Figure 18–10 that might have given only a mild sense of discomfort to the patient, but it might also have provided a general feeling of ill-being together with a fever. The etiology of the abscess could have been related to septicemia or endocarditis, and might have occurred in someone who was debilitated by intercurrent systemic disease such as diabetes mellitus. The diffuse abscesses of the biliary tree (Fig. 18–11) are equally difficult to diagnose clinically and are more frequent, being a complication of stones and cholecystitis. In this instance, jaundice as well as a hectic fever may point to the correct diagnosis of cholangitis with abscess formation, especially if the patient was known to have chronic inflamma-

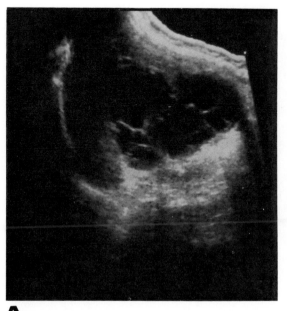

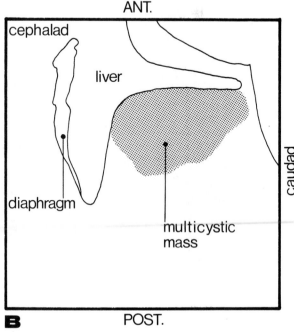

A

B

Fig. 18–9. *A,* This ultrasound scan of the liver shows a large, multicystic mass, as illustrated in *B.* This is typical of a hydatid cyst.

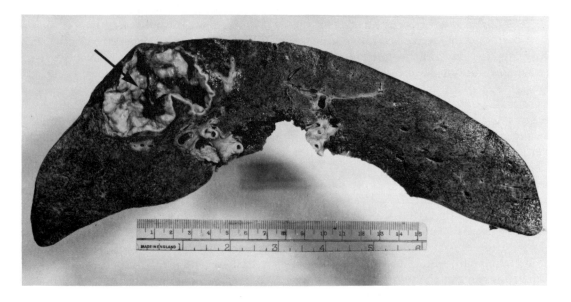

Fig. 18–10.   Arrow points to walled cavity, which was an **abscess**. The remainder of the liver is normal. Such an abscess could be caused by either gram-positive or gram-negative bacteria, or by amebas, coming from the blood or gastrointestinal tract. (McGill University, Department of Pathology Museum.)

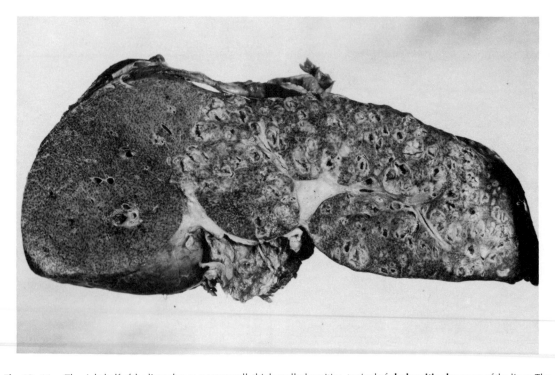

Fig. 18–11.   The right half of the liver shows many small, thick-walled cavities, typical of **cholangitic abscesses** of the liver. The remaining portion of the liver is normal. This type of infection commonly arises from motile bacteria in the partly obstructed biliary tree. (McGill University, Department of Pathology Museum.)

tion of the gallbladder. Rarely, diffuse abscesses throughout the liver may arise when bacterial infections (commonly *E. coli*) from the appendix ascend to the tributaries of the portal vein and reach the liver by that route (pylephlebitis).

Currently, the most intriguing infectious disease of the liver is viral hepatitis. The term hepatitis is often misleading, since one frequently expects the suffix -itis to imply inflammation in the conventional sense, that is, inflammatory cells followed by the vascular phase of congestion and exudate. In the liver, however, the injury caused both by specific agents, such as the viruses of hepatitis, and by toxic agents, is necrosis of hepatic cells. As suggested earlier, when the injury is slight and transient, the dead cells are removed quickly and are replaced by new liver cells, but when the injury is severe and prolonged, there is usually proliferation of fibroblasts and bile ducts, collections of macrophages, and the deposition of large amounts of collagen. These phenomena are the hallmarks of the chronic liver disease cirrhosis, but we are getting ahead of ourselves.

The term hepatitis covers a multitude of disorders. Any reader is bound to become confused by the many uses of the word in the literature. It is a little like blue jeans, which have been stretched to cover every shape and have been used on every social occasion. The key to successful usage of the term hepatitis is to use it with some qualifying adjective, such as acute, viral, or chronic. For example, we are now recognizing an entity that was regarded entirely differently 25 years ago. The term chronic hepatitis has been defined as "inflammation of the liver continuing for at least 3 to 6 months," and has been divided into several subsets that need not concern us here except to indicate that the causes of the inflammation may be different (viral, immunologic).

VIRAL HEPATITIS. **Fulminant viral hepatitis** is a serious disease with an appalling mortality rate. Survival is only 10 to 20% among those who develop liver failure serious enough to lapse into coma. Characteristically, it is estimated that only 1 of 10 persons afflicted with viral hepatitis develops liver damage sufficiently severe to become identified clinically because of jaundice or other evidence of hepatic dysfunction. The typical signs and symptoms of viral hepatitis are a nonspecific malaise, loss of appetite, fever, headache, nausea, and abdominal discomfort, all of which may be followed by jaundice. On examination, the liver may be tender and enlarged, and laboratory tests may show evidence of hyperbilirubinemia, elevated transaminases, and other signs of disordered liver function, depending on the severity and extent of the hepatocellular necrosis. Whereas most cases are self-limited and run a benign course without complication, a few cases have a rapid course and result in the patient's death within as short a time as 10 days, with deep jaundice, prolonged prothrombin time, and hepatic coma. In a few patients, the course of the disease is prolonged and may involve relapse with recurrent or persistent malaise and enzymatic evidence of continuing hepatocellular damage. As we shall discuss, a few patients develop the late complications of cirrhosis of the postnecrotic type.

For several decades it has been possible to identify 2 types of viral hepatitis (Types A and B). Type A, with a short incubation period (2 to 6 weeks) and a peak incidence in the winter and spring, is more common in young people and has an abrupt onset with a short course and few complications. It is usually associated with oral-fecal contamination. The mortality is slight (less than 0.1%). The etiologic agent is identified as hepatitis virus A. An example of a hepatitis epidemic is shown in Figure 18–12.

The second type of viral hepatitis, caused by hepatitis B, used to be called serum hepatitis because its occurrence could often be traced to transfusion, to contamination of syringes, or to other blood sources. The presence of virus may raise antibodies as early as 6 days after infection, there is no seasonal or age predilection, and unlike type A, the course may be long and insidious, frequently with complications and a mortality rate of 1 to 10%. It now seems that both types of viruses are excreted in the feces, and that both types of viral hepatitis can be spread by person-to-person contact or by contaminated materials (Fig. 18–13).

Both diseases may have a flu-like pro-

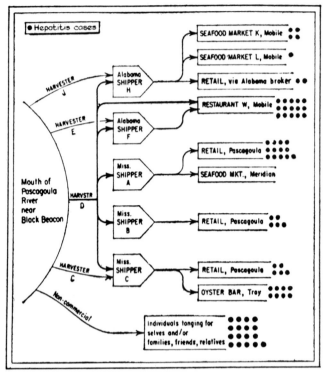

Chart adapted from Public Health Service report shows distributors of oysters linked to 70 hepatitis cases.

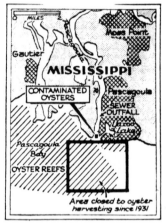

Area where contaminated oysters were harvested.

Fig. 18–12.   This chart shows the distribution of oysters from the mouth of the Mississippi River and the 70 cases of hepatitis that resulted. (From *The New York Times*, November, 19, 1961.)

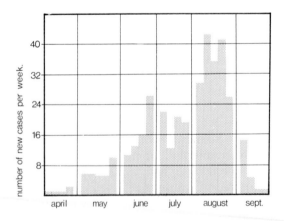

Fig. 18–13.   This figure shows the weekly clinical case rate of hepatitis in an institution for the mentally retarded during the period of an infectious hepatitis epidemic in 1972. (From Matthew, E. B., et al.: A major epidemic of infectious hepatitis in an institution for the mentally retarded. Am. J. Epidemiol., 98:203, 1973.)

drome, with malaise, fatigue, headache, and nausea. Arthritis, itching, urticaria, and thrombophlebitis have all been associated with hepatitis, but jaundice is the outstanding clinical feature. The symptoms of the prodromal phase usually decrease as jaundice becomes more apparent, and may last as long as 8 weeks. Abnormal liver function tests, together with specific serologic identification, confirm the diagnosis.

Biopsy may often help to determine the severity of the disease and may shed some light on the possible outcome of a particular case.

The economic importance of viral hepatitis cannot be overstated when the numbers of annual clinical cases are considered. In southern and eastern Europe, it is estimated that there are between 200 and 300 new cases of

Table 18–1.   Prevalence of Antibody to Hepatitis B Surface Antigen (Anti-HB's) in the Population Surveyed for HAV Infections

COUNTRY	NO. TESTED	NO. ANTI-HB's POSITIVE	% POSITIVE (CRUDE)	% POSITIVE AGE-STANDARDIZED*
U.S.A.	1,000	108	10.8	12.1
Switzerland	98	3	3.1	2.9
Belgium	133	7	5.3	4.6
Yugoslavia	97	33	34.0	32.8
Israel	112	17	15.2	17.4
Taiwan	123	96	78.0	72.8
Senegal	96	60	62.5	55.6

* Direct method; rates for Taiwan and Senegal were standardized to the 1974 Taiwan population distribution; rates for the remaining countries were standardized to the 1970 United States population distribution.

(From Szmuness, W., et al.: The prevalence of antibody to hepatitis A antigen in various parts of the world: a pilot study. Am. J. Epidemiol., *106:*392, 1977.)

acute viral hepatitis per 100,000 population per year. The number of new cases in the United States is estimated at between 9 and 43, a testimony to different standards of hygiene more than anything else, but even this figure is high. In the United States, for all patients tested, at least 10% have antibodies against hepatitis B antigen, whereas in Taiwan, for example, 78% have presumably been exposed to the virus (Table 18–1). The figures are even higher for antibodies against hepatitis A antigen (Fig. 18–14).

Viral hepatitis (hepatitis B) has been the focus of attention recently, with the recognition of the importance of Australia antigen as a diagnostic tool to identify carriers and persons who have had previous infections. Blumberg was awarded the Nobel prize in 1976 for his identification of an antigen specifically related to serum hepatitis. He had hypothesized that patients receiving multiple transfusions would receive proteins of a phenotype different from their own and would therefore produce antibodies to them. While pursuing this line of reason, he discovered an antigen from an Australian aborigine that was commonly present in the blood of leukemic patients. Further study soon established a closer relationship between this antigen and patients with serum hepatitis. The Australia antigen is now recognized as the surface antigen of the double-shelled hepatitis B virus (Fig. 18–15). One million carriers of the virus are estimated to live in the United States alone, and

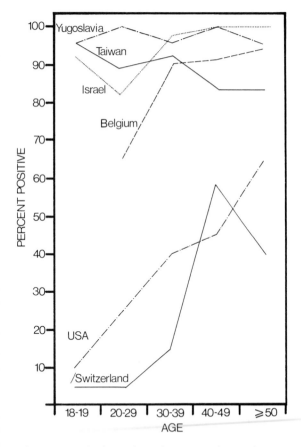

Fig. 18–14. This figure shows the age-specific prevalences of antibody to hepatitis A antigen in population samples from 6 countries. This antibody is a sensitive and specific indicator of previous hepatitis infections. The prevalence of the presence of antibody does provide valuable information about the presence of viral heptatitis A. (From Szmuness, W., et al.: The prevalence of antibody to hepatitis A antigen in various parts of the world: a pilot study. Am. J. Epidemiol., *106:*392, 1977.)

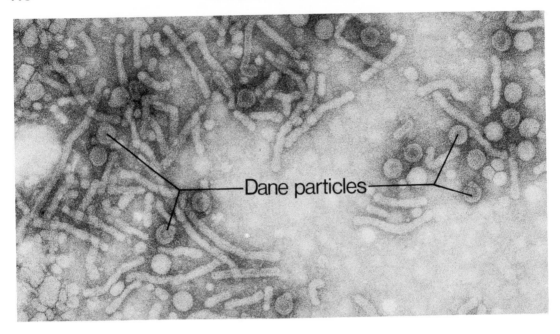

Fig. 18–15. This electron photomicrograph shows the Dane particle (hepatitis B virus) as indicated. In the serum of patients with hepatitis there are also incomplete particles and particles that are antigenic. These appear as the other material in this photograph. ×150,000 (Courtesy of Dr. S. N. Huang.)

100,000,000 in the world. It is of serious import that this virus is not only associated with viral hepatitis, but also with hepatocarcinoma, a primary carcinoma of the liver.

Because of the evidence of the widespread distribution of this virus, and because it may be transmitted not only by blood and blood products, but also orally, the virus is a public health problem of great concern. Since we now can identify the Australia antigen, we can identify carriers and sequester contaminated blood, which might have been used therapeutically. The classic routes of infections, such as tattooing needles, drug-abuse syringes, and the careless handling of human blood and excreta, will still expose numbers of people to hepatitis, but with the identification of hepatitis-associated antigen, we can anticipate the development of a vaccine for at least this type of viral liver disease.

HEPATITIS DUE TO OTHER CAUSES. There are a few patients with enlarged, tender livers, who show accompanying laboratory disorders of elevated transaminases without jaundice. Often these persons have arthritis. The disorder is found most commonly in young women. This liver disease is of uncertain etiology, and some have claimed that the hepatic damage has an autoimmune basis. The disease is designated chronic hepatitis in some, and when evidence of connective tissue disease is present, it has also been called lupoid hepatitis.

We can also identify hepatic disease occurring in small numbers of persons who have been taking drugs such as phenothiazines (tranquilizers), or antibiotics (isoniazid), or anesthetics (halothane). This disease may take the form of acute necrosis, or of a subacute injury. Patients who take steroids such as methyltestosterone may also develop jaundice, which has been found to be due to cholestasis.

Fatty Liver. Another major classification of liver disorders is that in which most or a major portion of the liver is filled with fat in the form of triglyceride droplets. Acute fatty liver may reflect many different insults to this organ, which has only a limited repertoire of responses to insult. Excessive caloric intake, usually in the form of ethanol is the most common cause of a large, greasy, yellow liver unable to function normally because most cells have their cytoplasmic organelles displaced by the accumulated lipid droplets.

Other important causes of fat in the liver are

hepatotoxins (CCl_4, PO_4), and systemic metabolic disorders such as uncontrolled diabetes mellitus and toxemia of pregnancy. The most serious of these disorders is the chronic fatty liver seen in alcoholics, who persist in taking large amounts of ethanol, which by itself is an agent that depresses glycogen synthesis and inhibits normal hepatic cell metabolism, and which provides as well a caloric fuel without some of the essential cofactors (vitamins) normally found in the diet. The fatty liver in acute alcoholism may progress, with continuing alcohol abuse, to chronic hepatitis, in which there is evidence of necrosis, leukocytic infiltration, Mallory's alcoholic hyaline bodies, and disorganization of the parenchyma. Chronic hepatitis will frequently result, eventually, in cirrhosis.

Cirrhosis. Most of the disorders we have been discussing are acute diseases of the liver. Now we shall consider a group of disorders collected under the term cirrhosis, a chronic disease of the liver. One may identify several anatomic types of cirrhosis, each of which has a differing etiology. A reasonable definition for cirrhosis is **"a diffuse structural disorganization characterized by necrosis,** **with nodular regeneration of liver parenchyma and fibrosis"** (Fig. 18–16). Cirrhosis inevitably produces disordered hepatic function. We should consider the respective roles played by the anatomic aberrations. First, however, it may be wise to outline some of the symptoms, signs, and physiologic abnormalities of a typical case of cirrhosis, regardless of origin.

The patient with early cirrhosis may be asymptomatic and unaware of the disorder, but physical signs such as hepatomegaly, peripheral edema, ascites, vascular hemangiomas (spider nevi), gynecomastia, and testicular atrophy may bear testimony to the diagnosis. With progression of the disease, anasarca, splenomegaly, and other evidence of portal hypertension and a collateral circulation (hemorrhoids, esophageal varices, and collateral veins about the umbilicus) may appear. Finally, the complications of cirrhosis are full blown, and massive bleeding into the gastrointestinal tract from ruptured esophageal varices, hemorrhage, hepatic coma, and hepatic cell carcinoma may leave no doubt as to the underlying disorder.

Cirrhosis represents a morphologic re-

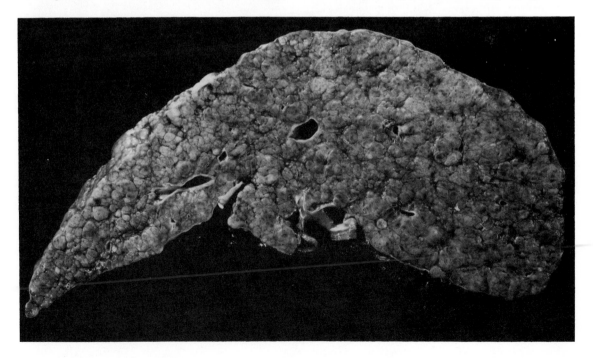

Fig. 18–16. Liver with diffuse nodularity that is typical of **cirrhosis.** Small and irregular nodules of liver are separated by bands of scar. Within these areas of regeneration, necrosis may progress and sometimes carcinoma arises. (McGill University, Department of Pathology Museum.)

sponse to continuing injury to the liver. Regardless of the etiology of the cirrhosis, one may generalize that the cirrhosis is a reflection of the type, location, and duration of the injury to the liver. If the injury has been a chronic inflammation of the bile ducts, the scarring will be principally in the region of the bile ducts, namely the portal area (biliary cirrhosis). If the injury has not been limited to a specific anatomic segment of the lobule, but has involved large areas of the liver, as in viral hepatitis, the scarring may consist of broad bands of collagen coursing throughout the organ (postnecrotic cirrhosis). The extent of the scarring depends on the extent and severity of the injury.

What happens when large numbers of liver cells are injured on a long-term basis? The loss of liver cells may produce ascites (due to hypoalbuminemia), jaundice (due to loss of secretory function and disturbance of excre-

tory pathways), and hepatic coma (loss of urea synthesis and shunting). The structural disorganization and collapse distort the vascular pattern of the liver, so that the portal blood may pass directly to the vena cava without being exposed to cords of liver cells. This shunting of blood then exposes the brain to blood that contains ammonia absorbed from the colon, but is not detoxified by the liver. This shunting is believed to be a reason for the disordered central nervous system function that is such a serious complication of cirrhosis (hepatic encephalopathy). The fibrosis and nodular regeneration compress the sinusoidal spaces and the venous and portal tributaries, resulting in elevated sinusoidal and portal pressure (portal hypertension). Stasis in the circulation may even lead to portal vein thrombosis (Fig. 18–17). The lymphatic drainage is also affected and contributes additionally to the development of as-

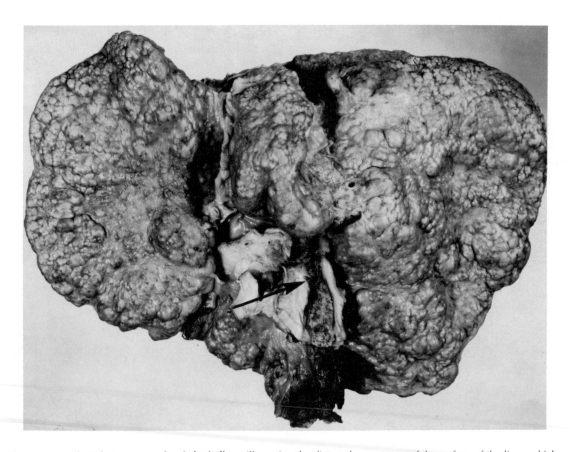

Fig. 18–17. The inferior aspect of a **cirrhotic liver**, illustrating the distorted appearance of the surface of the liver, which sometimes can be palpated through the abdominal wall. At the arrow, the portal vein is thrombosed. (McGill University, Department of Pathology Museum.)

cites. The continued stimulus to regeneration in the liver may be an important factor in the development of still another complication of cirrhosis, hepatocarcinoma. In North America, this disease arises rarely in the non-cirrhotic liver, but is seen more commonly in cases of cirrhosis.

Although one may classify the types of cirrhosis on anatomic or etiologic bases, contemporary usage confuses these taxonomic schemes and groups cirrhosis into 5 general classes:

1. Cirrhosis due to dietary factors such as alcohol (Laennec's, portal, alcoholic).

2. Cirrhosis following massive necrosis such as viral hepatitis (postnecrotic).

3. Cirrhosis associated with pigment deposition (hemochromatosis).

4. Cirrhosis associated with disease of the bile ducts (primary and secondary biliary cirrhosis).

5. Miscellaneous cirrhoses.

Cirrhosis following congestive heart failure

does not really conform to the criteria that require regenerative nodules to be present, and it is not considered by us to be a legitimate type of cirrhosis.

For our purposes, it does not seem necessary to delve into the specific reasons for separating 1 type of cirrhosis from another, or to describe the morphologic features of each type. It does seem important to recapitulate the significance, in physiologic terms, of the disordered structures. When the liver is injured and necrosis occurs, the pattern of collapse, regeneration, and new collagen formation takes place on a continuing basis; when inflammation of the bile ducts continues, or repeated episodes of alcohol excess occur, or hepatitis virus is not cleared from the liver, this organ is then unable to synthesize normal amounts of protein. In addition, the pressures in the intrahepatic and portal circulations gradually rise, and a collateral circulation is recruited. This venous system is less well protected from the daily abrasions of life, and bleeding from unsupported veins may occur, precipitating a hemorrhage. Such a hemorrhage may plunge the patient with cirrhosis into shock and initiate new episodes of hepatic cell necrosis because of ischemia, thereby accelerating the **process of necrosis, collapse, fibrosis, and regeneration**.

Historically, the fate of most patients with cirrhosis was to die of infection, commonly of pneumonia, with gastrointestinal hemorrhage, hepatic coma, or hepatic cell carcinoma as less frequent complications. Today, hepatic coma is the most frequent and most common cause of death, as infections and hemorrhages are managed more successfully by modern methods (Fig. 18–18).

The cause of hepatic coma is frequently debated, and no absolute answer is available to explain this fateful disorder. Explanations range from toxic effects of ammonia absorbed from the gut to the failure of metabolism of insulin by poorly functioning hepatocytes. In fact, insulin-glucagon therapy has been used with some success in the therapy of acute hepatic failure, and a low-protein diet is the rule for all cirrhotics.

Because of the intractable nature of advanced cirrhosis, liver transplants have been attempted.

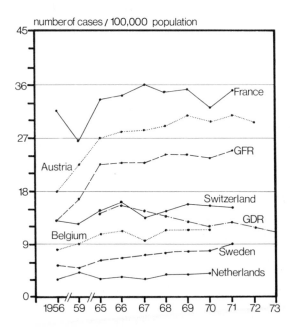

Fig. 18–18. This graph shows the relative incidence of chronic liver disease in different countries from 1956 to 1973. It is of interest that countries with high alcohol consumption show the highest incidence, although this graph does not distinguish among specific types of chronic liver disease. (From Jorke, D., and Rheinhardt, M.: Epidemiology of chronic liver diseases. Acta Hepatogastroenterol. (Stuttg.), 24:220, 1977.)

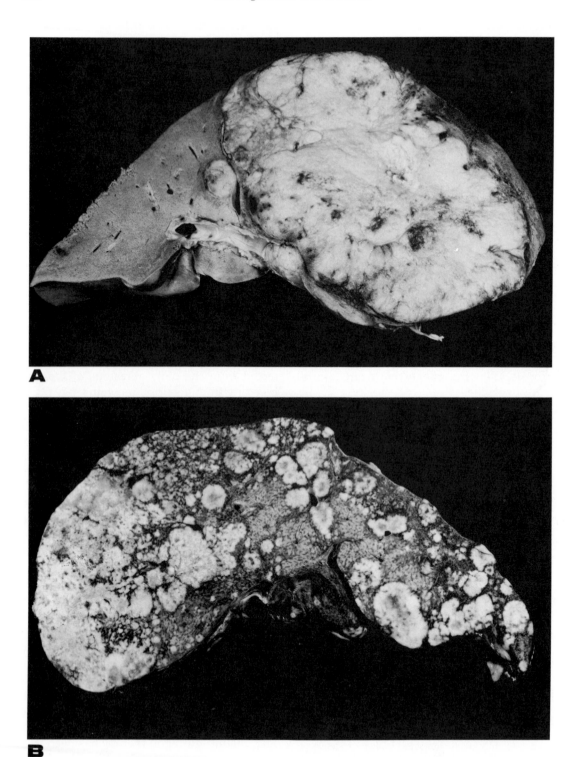

Fig. 18–19. *A,* More than half of this liver has been replaced by a **carcinoma**, which arose in the stomach and metastasized to the liver. One can see compression of the remaining liver parenchyma at the border of the white tumor. *B,* **Multiple metastases** to the liver are scattered randomly throughout the organ. The whitish, cauliflower-appearing material compresses the liver parenchyma. This carcinoma arose in the breast. (McGill University, Department of Pathology Museum.)

Tumors of the Liver and Bile Ducts. The most common malignant tumor of the liver is metastatic tumor, most frequently arising from the lung, colon, pancreas, breast, or gallbladder (Fig. 18–19). These tumors reach the liver by hematogenous, lymphatic, or direct extension, frequently are silent, and often do not impair liver function in any recognizable way. When the metastases replace most of the liver parenchyma, as happens occasionally, signs of hepatic failure may become apparent. Even small tumors that involve the liver may give rise to signs and symptoms if they occupy such strategic points as the portal vein or bile ducts, giving rise to ascites or jaundice. The rapid increase in size of the liver, the presence of palpable nodules, and the occurrence of bloody ascitic fluid all point to the diagnosis of malignant tumor in the liver. Hepatography by liver scan has unfortunately not proved to be as reliable as hoped for, and liver biopsy seems to be the best method to prove the diagnosis of malignancy.

In Africa and Asia, hepatic cell carcinoma is a much more common tumor than in North America and accounts for up to 30% of all malignant disease. This has been attributed to dietary habits and to the presence of car-cinogens in foodstuffs or beverages. In North America, 75% of carcinoma of the liver arises in patients with cirrhosis. Carcinoma arising in the bile ducts is also associated with cirrhosis and its first sign may be jaundice.

Benign tumors arising in the liver (hemangiomas) are common incidental findings and are seen frequently at autopsy (Fig. 18–20). Recently, a peculiar vascular tumor, an angiosarcoma, has been found in workers exposed to vinylchloride. This is another example of environmental hazards of which we were not previously aware.

Primary carcinoma of the liver, properly called hepatic cell carcinoma, but often referred to as hepatoma, is frequent in the world population. It is unusual in North America, except in patients with cirrhosis.

Hemochromatosis. Although this rare disease need not be placed in the chapter on the liver, it seems reasonable to discuss it here, as the liver is 1 of the principal targets affected by this disorder of iron metabolism, and frequently the disordered liver functions and cirrhosis are diagnosed by biopsy as being due to some type of iron storage disease. It occurs 10 times as frequently in men as in women, usually after the age of 40, and is a

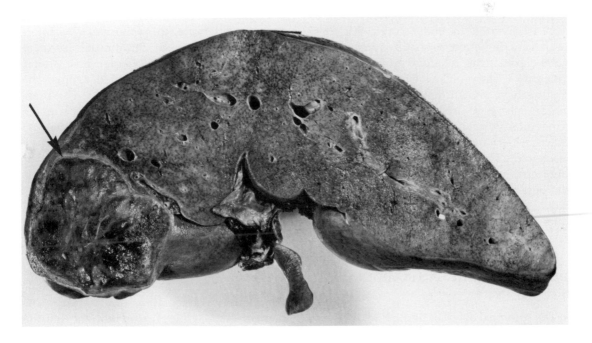

Fig. 18–20.   Shown here is the most common tumor of the liver, a benign tumor of blood vessels, a **hemangioma**. It is circumscribed by a capsule at the arrow. (McGill University, Department of Pathology Museum.)

classic cause of an enlarged liver and liver failure. The diagnosis is made by tissue demonstration of liver damage and of grossly increased body iron stores. The diagnosis is established when other causes for the same pattern are excluded. Hemochromatosis is not a disease of the liver alone and is sometimes diagnosed because of diabetes mellitus in a person who has an unusually darkened skin, hence the term "bronzed diabetes." Histologically, every organ can be demonstrated to contain excessive amounts of iron, from the pituitary, the pancreas, and the liver to the skin. Even the heart may be involved. These deposits of iron impair normal function of the respective organs and produce fibrosis in the liver and pancreas in particular. There is an extraordinarily high incidence of carcinoma of the liver in persons with hemochromatotic liver disease.

The causes of hemochromatosis are continually debated. It is clear that in South Africa, owing to native custom, a diet excessively rich in iron is the principal reason for the extraordinary incidence of cirrhosis and carcinoma of the liver in the Bantu. In all instances of the disease, alcohol seems to be a significant factor in increasing the iron load. Clearly, there are many persons who have a defect in red blood cell synthesis and in whom iron is diverted to body stores. All these causes are thought of as acquired instances of hemochromatosis. A second group of persons gives no history of any exogenous source. Studies have shown that their siblings have abnormally high iron levels, suggesting a congenital defect, perhaps in the intestinal mucosa, perhaps in the pancreas itself, that leads to the iron overload. It is an interesting but rare disorder in North America for which the best treatment seems to hark back to the days of Robin Hood, because bleeding, and thus depleting the body of iron, gives the best results.

DISORDERS OF THE GALLBLADDER AND BILE DUCTS

The principal diseases of the bile ducts and gallbladder are obstructions and infections. We shall consider the gallbladder and its diseases first.

The gallbladder is a small sac with a muscular wall and an epithelial lining that lies on the undersurface of the right lobe of the liver. It contains normally about 100 ml of bile, and its distal surface projects just to the free margin of the liver, so that if it is distended or inflamed, it may be palpated. In fact, a physician's name (Murphy) is associated with the presence of a palpably enlarged gallbladder. Bile flows continuously into the gallbladder from the liver by way of the cystic duct, but bile is only expelled from this small sac when a meal containing fat enters the duodenum. Bile in the gallbladder is concentrated by absorption of water. The epithelium of the gallbladder lining is a delicate series of folds filled with capillaries, much like the mucosa of the small intestine. When the gallbladder has been repeatedly inflamed due to chemical, mechanical, or infectious irritation, the ability to concentrate bile is impaired. The gallbladder wall may become markedly thickened and incapable either of responding to the stimuli to secrete or of enlarging in the face of partial obstruction.

Visualization of the gallbladder by radiographic means in the person who has experienced discomfort after a fatty meal or pain in the right upper quadrant is done by the administration of an organic iodine-containing compound, usually by mouth. This radiopaque material is selectively concentrated in the normally functioning gallbladder as water is resorbed and bile stored. If the gallbladder does not fill and cannot be visualized after repeated attempts, this failure can be interpreted as evidence of chronic disease or of obstruction. If the gallbladder fills, stones may sometimes be silhouetted against the radiopaque material (Fig. 18–21). The presence of small stones may then explain the reason for the discomfort and may suggest to the physician that the gallbladder could be surgically removed on an elective basis, or that an attempt to dissolve the stones may be undertaken.

Acute Cholecystitis. This most common disease of the gallbladder occurs most frequently in conjunction with obstruction at the neck of the gallbladder or in the cystic duct due to small stones. In much the same way as the appendix reacts to obstruction, the gallbladder becomes edematous and acutely inflamed. For a while, it was thought that the inflammation could be caused by some infectious agent (bacteria), but today it is generally held that the process is due to chemical injury.

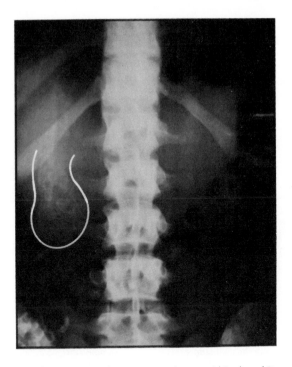

Fig. 18–21. This roentgenogram shows, within the white line, the appearance of the gallbladder filled with numerous translucent stones. The gallbladder itself contains contrast from the orally administered dye.

The edema and inflammation may impair venous return and may result in infarction or gangrene of the gallbladder. Naturally, as the small sac with its highly concentrated surface-active bile salts becomes necrotic, a great danger is rupture. The result of rupture is an abdominal catastrophe. Bile peritonitis is often fatal, since it rapidly leads to shock.

The outstanding features of both acute and chronic inflammation of the gallbladder are pain in the right upper quadrant (which sometimes masquerades as a peptic ulcer, pancreatitis, or even a myocardial infarction) and nausea and muscle guarding.

Clearly gallstones, or cholelithiasis, play a key role in the development and recurrence of cholecystitis; in fact, the diagnostic terms are used most often in conjunction. Biliary calculi, or gallstones, may be formed at any place in the biliary tree, but are most often found in the gallbladder. From many studies, estimates have been made of the frequency of gallstones in the general population, and some autopsy series give figures as high as 1 in every 5 cases. It has been estimated that

18,000,000 persons have gallstones in North America.

Gallstones are more frequent in women than in men. The old adage is that one should suspect gallstones in anyone who is "female, fat, fecund, fair, flatulent, and forty."

Recently there has been more and more evidence from studies on selected populations that heredity affects the generation of gallstones, and we have come to talk of "lithogenic" bile in certain populations such as the Pima Indians of Arizona, in whom gallstones occur in as many as 70% of adult women. A recent study shows that this highly saturated bile appears with puberty and is correlated with obesity and high levels of estrogens (Fig. 18–22).

The types of gallstones formed depend on many factors, such as heredity and certain body changes (infections, pregnancy). The most common stones are composed of a mixture of cholesterol, bilirubin, and calcium. Other types are pure cholesterol and calcium-bilirubin stones, each constituting about 10% of the stones analyzed. Frequently, gallstones are multiple; they range in size from the head of a pin to a hen's egg. As it is often the little dogs that make the most noise, the same is true of gallstones. The small ones (gravel) may pass into the cystic duct and lodge there or in the common duct and cause

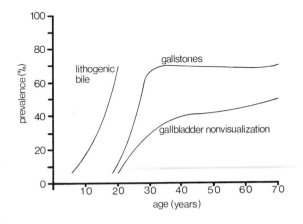

Fig. 18–22. This chart shows the prevalence of gallstones correlated with age in a population that has highly saturated bile. The first curve shows the high incidence of lithogenic bile (60% at age 10) in this population; the second curve shows that 75% have gallstones by 25 years of age. (From Bennion, L. J., et al.: Development of lithogenic bile during puberty in Pima Indians. N. Engl. J. Med., *300*:873, 1979.)

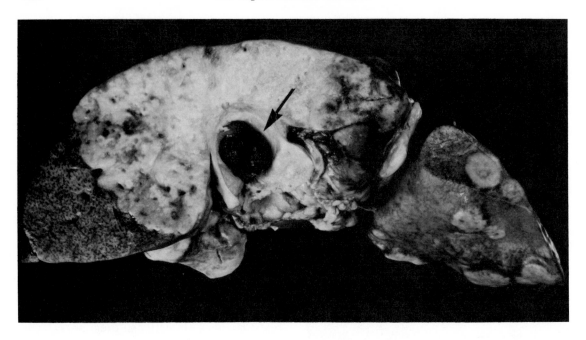

Fig. 18–23. **Two gallstones** are shown lying in a case of **carcinoma of the gallbladder** (at arrow). Surrounding this thickened wall is firm, white tumor, extending into and replacing the liver parenchyma. In the small lobe at the right of the photograph are umbilicated metastatic nodules of carcinoma. (McGill University, Department of Pathology Museum.)

exquisite pain and/or obstruction. Gallstones are often asymptomatic and may only be discovered by accident. Because of the complications of gallstones, the presence of a solitary, silent stone in an elderly patient raises important questions about the role of elective surgery. The complications of obstruction, leading to distension of the common bile duct and the intrahepatic ducts and predisposing a person to infection (cholangitis), are much more serious in the elderly, debilitated patient. Occasionally, large stones may erode from the gallbladder and create a fistula into the large bowel, where they may cause obstruction (ileus).

In addition to these complications, there is a much higher incidence of carcinoma of the gallbladder in patients who have had gallstones for many years, to the point where gallstones are considered a predisposing cause for carcinoma of the gallbladder (Fig. 18–23). Gallstones were present in 75% of all cases of carcinoma of the gallbladder in 1 study.

Table 18–2 illustrates various complications that may be caused by the presence of lithogenic bile. First, it predisposes a patient to gallstones, either in the gallbladder or in common duct. Whenever stones occur in the common duct, a number of complications

Table 18–2.   Complications of Gallstones

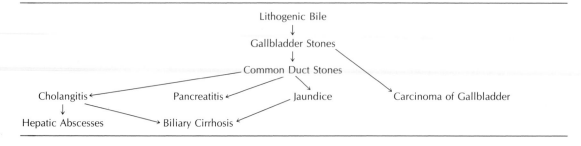

may arise: cholangitis, pancreatitis, jaundice, biliary cirrhosis. Stones in the gallbladder predispose a person to carcinoma of that organ.

All this leads to the view that this small storage bladder is not essential to health and, when there are indications, it should be removed. In every hospital, however, there should be a tissue committee that reviews all such procedures to be sure that the reason for removal was true disease, not "acute remunerative cholecystitis."

SYNOPSIS

The liver, supplied by blood from the portal veins and hepatic artery, synthesizes proteins, secretes bile, detoxifies drugs, and stores glycogen, among other functions.

Jaundice is a sign of disease. The causes of hyperbilirubinemia may be hepatocellular injury, obstruction to the bile ducts, or hemolysis.

Necrosis of liver cells is a common response to many types of injury. Acute hepatic failure may be due to viral infections, to poisons, to congestion, to ischemia, or to particular diseases such as toxemia of pregnancy.

Infections of the liver may be caused by flukes, protozoa, fungi, bacteria, and viruses, and may result in local abscess or diffuse injury, which may be either acute or chronic.

Viral hepatitis is an important public health problem in North America.

Cirrhosis is a chronic, diffuse, structural disorganization of the liver, characterized by necrosis, fibrosis, and nodular regeneration of hepatic cells.

The complications of cirrhosis are ascites, splenomegaly, gastrointestinal bleeding, hepatic coma, and occasionally portal vein thrombosis and hepatic cell carcinoma.

Carcinoma of the liver is relatively rare in North America but arises commonly in patients with cirrhosis. It is a common disease in Asia and Africa.

The principal diseases of the gallbladder and bile ducts are obstruction and infections. Cholelithiasis and cholecystitis are virtually synonymous.

Terms

Portal circulation	*Hepatomegaly*	*Hepatic coma*
Hypoalbuminemia	*Cholangiogram*	*Hepatocarcinoma*
Bilirubin	*Hepatitis*	*Cholecystitis*
Jaundice	*Cirrhosis*	*Cholelithiasis*

FURTHER READING

Bainton, D., et al.: Gallbladder disease: prevalence in a South Wales industrial town. N. Engl. J. Med., *294*:1147, 1976.

Beaumont, C., et al.: Serum ferritin as a possible marker of the hemochromatosis allele. N. Engl. J. Med., *301*:169, 1979.

Bennion, L.J., et al.: Development of lithogenic bile during puberty in Pima Indians. N. Engl. J. Med., *300*:873, 1979.

Boyer, J. L.: New concepts of mechanisms of hepatocyte bile formation. Physiol. Rev., *60*:303, 1980.

Braverman, D.Z., Johnson, M.L., and Kern, F., Jr.: Effects of pregnancy and contraceptive steroids on gallbladder function. N. Engl. J. Med., *302*:362, 1980.

Dane, D.S., et al.: Virus-like particles in serum of patients with Australia-antigen-associated hepatitis. Lancet, *1*:695, 1970.

Isselbacher, K.J., and Greenberger, N.J.: Metabolic effects of alcohol on the liver. N. Engl. J. Med., *270*:402, 1964.

Klatskin, G.: Hepatic tumours: possible relationship to use of oral contraceptives. Gastroenterology, *73*:386, 1977.

Krugman, S., et al.: Viral hepatitis, type B. Studies on natural history and prevention re-examined. N. Engl. J. Med., *300*:101, 1979.

Lee, Y.: Liver scanning in patients with malignancy: rationale, results and limitations. Cancer Treatment Rep., *62*:1183, 1978.

Lieber, C.S.: Pathogenesis and early diagnosis of alcoholic liver injury. N. Engl. J. Med., 298:888, 1978.

Jorke, D., and Reinhardt, M.: Epidemiology of chronic liver diseases. Acta Hepatgastroenterol. (Stuttg.), 24:220, 1977.

Piehler, J.M., and Crichlow, R.W.: Primary carcinoma of the gallbladder. Surg. Gynecol. Obstet., 147:929, 1978.

Rimland, D., et al.: Hepatitis B outbreak traced to an oral surgeon. N. Engl. J. Med., 296:953, 1977.

Robinson, S.H.: The origins of bilirubin. N. Engl. J. Med., 279:146, 1968.

Sherlock, S.: Diseases of the Liver and Biliary System, 5th Ed. London, Blackwell, 1975.

Starzl, T.E.: Liver transplantation. Johns Hopkins Med. J., 143:73, 1978.

Stone, W.D., et al.: The natural history of cirrhosis. Q. J. Med., 37:119, 1968.

Sveger, T.: Liver disease in alpha$_1$-antitrypsin deficiency detected by screening of 200,000 infants. N. Engl. J. Med., 294:1316, 1976.

Szmuness, W., et al.: The prevalence of antibody to hepatitis A antigen in various parts of the world: a pilot study. Am. J. Epidemiol., 106:392, 1977.

Warren, K.S.: The relevance of schistosomiasis. N. Engl. J. Med., 303:203, 1980.

Zuckerman, A.J.: Hepatitis B vaccines. Nature, 267:578, 1977.

Medical science is a contradiction in terms.—LOEB

STRUCTURE AND FUNCTION

The pancreas, known in animals as the "sweetbread," is an elongate flat organ that crosses the left side of the abdomen behind the stomach. It is the most powerful digestive gland in the body, and has been called the salivary gland of the abdomen, because not only does it resemble the salivary glands in structure, being composed of tubular acini, but it pours its secretion into the digestive canal by a duct. The pancreatic duct opens into the duodenum at the same point as the common bile duct enters the bowel; indeed the 2 ducts usually have a common opening, the importance of which will soon become evident. The pancreas is partly exocrine, producing 3 digestive enzymes, and partly endocrine, releasing at least 2 hormones into the blood. One of the enzymes prepares carbohydrates for absorption, whereas the hormones regulate the metabolism for carbohydrates once absorbed.

Exocrine Function. The pancreatic secretions produced by the acini contain several powerful digestive enzymes, 1 for the digestion of proteins, 1 for carbohydrates, and 1 for fats. (1) Trypsin, like the pepsin of gastric juice, acts on the proteins, but it carries the process a step further. (2) Amylase breaks large molecules of starch into smaller molecules of maltose, which are converted into still smaller molecules of glucose in the intestinal juice. The glucose is absorbed and carried by the portal vein to the liver, where it is stored as glycogen, to be reconverted into glucose as needed. (3) Lipase splits ingested fats into fatty acids and glycerol with the aid of bile.

Endocrine Function. The endocrine part of the pancreas is not visible to the naked eye; it is represented by tiny groups of cells called the islets of Langerhans, after the man who first described them in 1869, never guessing their function. The islets are scattered among the acinar tissue throughout the length of the pancreas. Their cells are of 2 general types and contain granules that stain differently, so that they are known as A or alpha and B or beta cells. The alpha cells stain red and the beta cells blue. The beta cells, which secrete insulin, comprise 60 to 90% of the cells. The

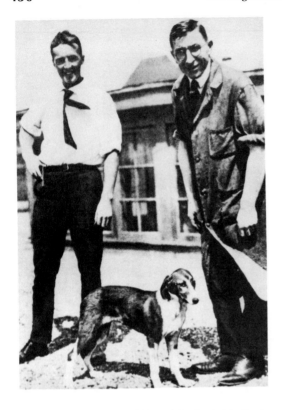

Fig. 19–1. Charles Best (left) and Sir Frederick Banting (right) with their experimental animal seen in the late 1920's.

alpha cells produce glucagon, the other internal secretion. A third group of cells has been found to produce another hormone (somatomedin), which is discussed in the endocrine chapter.

Insulin, secreted by the beta cells, is absorbed directly into the blood that passes through the pancreas. Were it to enter the pancreatic duct, insulin would immediately be destroyed by the pancreatic enzymes. It has been known since 1889 that removal of the entire pancreas in animals was followed by fatal diabetes, but we had to wait until 1922 for the demonstration, by Banting and his coworkers in Toronto, that an extract of islets of Langerhans would control the diabetes produced by pancreatectomy (Fig. 19–1). They named the substance insulin because it came from the islets (Latin *insula*, island). The function of insulin is to regulate carbohydrate metabolism; when insufficient insulin is produced, diabetes develops. Insulin acts: (1) by making the storage of sugar possible, especially in the liver and muscles; (2) by enabling the tissues to burn sugar. When the blood sugar in the portal vein carrying blood from the pancreas to the liver is above normal (hyperglycemia), insulin is released into the vein.

Glucagon is the alpha cell hormone. It may be regarded as the opposite twin of insulin, for it is released into the portal vein when the blood sugar is below normal. It brings about the breakdown of liver glycogen into glucose, so that there is a prompt rise in the glucose content of the blood leaving the liver.

Tests of Pancreatic Function. These depend on an estimation of 1 or more of the 3 main digestive enzymes in the blood. The lipase and amylase levels in the serum give invaluable information. Lipase estimation takes longer, but serum amylase can be measured within an hour, so that it is the method of choice in acute pancreatitis, which may constitute an abdominal emergency that has to be differentiated from acute appendicitis, perforated peptic ulcer, and biliary colic. These tests are of little help in chronic pancreatitis. Tests for endocrine dysfunction will be considered in connection with diabetes.

The 3 most important diseases of the pancreas are acute hemorrhagic pancreatitis, diabetes mellitus, and cancer, although others will be mentioned briefly.

PANCREATITIS

As with all organs, inflammatory conditions of the pancreas are an important source of pain, discomfort, and dysfunction. There are 2 general classes of inflammatory disease in the pancreas. We shall dismiss from our consideration the chronic inflammatory conditions, which require much space and time, and instead refer the reader to a textbook of medicine or surgery. Suffice it to say that chronic pancreatitis is seen most commonly in alcohol abusers; it may occur in individuals with disease of the biliary tract, particularly where there are gallstones, and after abdominal injuries such as trauma. We shall consider here only acute pancreatitis.

Perhaps mumps virus is the most common cause of acute inflammation of the pancreas. If the other salivary glands are afflicted, the diagnosis is not difficult, and as with most viral diseases, the course is self-limited. There is little we can do except to adhere to the traditional practice of "watchful waiting."

There is another acute disease of the pancreas that is fortunately rare, but is so serious as to be life-threatening, with a mortality rate of 50% or greater. It is often seen around Christmas or the New Year, at times of gastronomic and alcoholic celebration, and is known as acute hemorrhagic pancreatitis.

The entity is an acute abdominal catastrophe and may be confused with a ruptured peptic ulcer or even with a dissecting aneurysm, because of the intense pain, coupled with shock and a rigid abdomen with guarding and tenderness. Steady, penetrating pain in the upper abdomen, which may be referred to the back and may be relieved by the patient's assuming the fetal position with the knees drawn up and the trunk folded, is typical of acute pancreatic disease. The physical signs are typical of shock, and the laboratory data will show leukocytosis, perhaps hemoconcentration, and occasionally jaundice, if the duct is compromised. A fall in the serum calcium points to fat necrosis and helps to establish the diagnosis, but the pathognomonic finding is an elevated serum amylase, which rises within a few hours of the onset of the disease. Any level above 500 Somogyi units suggests the diagnosis of acute pancreatitis.

What is the mechanism of this disease, what are the predisposing causes, and what are the complications or eventual outcome? The disease is believed to depend on the activation of pancreatic enzymes, which are normally excreted through the ducts into the duodenum. In cases in which it is anatomically possible for bile to reflux into the pancreatic ducts, this is believed to be the mecha-

nism. Although the secreting pressure of the pancreas exceeds that of the bile ducts, and although not all ducts have a common orifice, it has been shown that a mixture of bile and pancreatic juices can produce pancreatitis.

It is well recognized that biliary tract disease, particularly the presence of stones, predisposes a person to acute hemorrhagic pancreatitis. One postulate is that a stone may obstruct the ampulla of Vater and may rechannel the bile into the pancreas, but this has not been observed in all cases. Rich and Duff found squamous metaplasia in pancreatic ducts and suggested that this led to a degree of pancreatic obstruction that set the stage for autodigestion. Alcohol in quantity, a strong stimulus to secretion, is associated with other gastrointestinal diseases, as well as with the occurrence of pancreatitis. Suffice it to say that we do not know the precise etiology of pancreatitis, but we can invoke several hypotheses, all of which require the activation of pancreatic enzymes, which then digest not only the tissues of the pancreas itself, but also neighboring structures, including blood vessels. These vessels may then rupture and bleed vigorously into the retroperitoneal space and may lead to shock. The proteolytic and lipolytic pancreatic enzymes have been

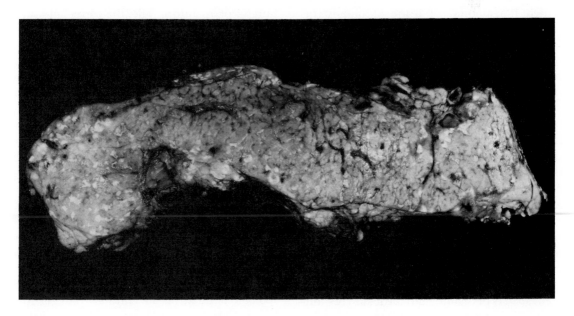

Fig. 19–2. Mottled areas of whitish material are distributed randomly throughout the pancreas. These white areas represent fat necrosis and are areas where inflammation has taken place in acute pancreatitis. (McGill University, Department of Pathology Museum.)

implicated in the destruction of the tissues that leads to fat necrosis and destruction of the pancreas itself (Fig. 19–2).

The sequel to this acute episode depends on the degree of damage. If the injury is slight (small amounts of enzymes—small areas of destruction), edema and slight sudden discomfort may be the only indication that anything was wrong, whereas a severe episode may lead to death. In between, various degrees of disability may result from loss of the exocrine and endocrine pancreas. Naturally, severe damage to the exocrine pancreas may leave the patient a digestive cripple; his or her stool may show abundant fat that cannot be absorbed and meat fibers that are not digested because of the lack of enzymes. The patient may have hyperglycemia because of damage to the islets of Langerhans, and cysts and infection in the necrotic area are always feared as results of the acute episode. Fortunately, the most severe type of pancreatitis is rare.

DIABETES MELLITUS

Diabetes means a "running through;" mellitus means "sweet" (literally, honeyed). The word diabetes is also used as an abbreviation for another disease, diabetes insipidus, in which the amount of urine is greatly increased, but contains no sugar and is therefore insipid or tasteless. The nomenclature obviously dates from the time, happily now past, when tasting the urine was a recognized part of urinalysis.

As diabetes insipidus is rare, diabetes mellitis is usually known simply as diabetes. The increases in both volume and frequency of urine and its sugar content might suggest that this was a disease of the kidneys. This is not so; the kidneys may be normal. It is a metabolic disorder, as a result of which the carbohydrate of the food is not used by the tissues. Paradoxically, the diabetic may have adequate fuel, but may shiver, metaphorically speaking, because he cannot ignite the furnace. The cause of the disorder is a deficient supply of insulin, and the lesion responsible is in the islets of Langerhans in the pancreas.

We do know, however, that insulin in some way serves as a spark that enables the glucose carried to the tissue cells, particularly the muscles, to unite with the oxygen there and to be burned and thereby produce energy. Glucose is to the body as gasoline is to the internal combustion engine. Every time the heart beats or we move a muscle, we use glucose, and, just as a spark is necessary to fire the gasoline in the engine, so insulin is necessary to burn the glucose. Insulin also enables the glucose carried from the intestine to the liver to be converted into glycogen. When insulin is lacking, it is evident that glucose will neither be changed into glycogen in the liver nor be burned by the muscles, so that it will accumulate in the blood in large amounts. When the blood reaches the kidneys, the glucose will flow out into the urine. A diagnosis of diabetes can be made by testing either the urine or the blood for sugar, remembering that some is always present in the blood. The normal fasting blood sugar level is 60 to 100 mg per 100 ml, but in diabetes it may reach 300 mg or higher.

There is an even greater danger than the failure to burn carbohydrates, namely, a failure to burn fats. For the proper combustion of fat, a certain proportion of carbohydrates must be burned at the same time. In the carburetor of an automobile, the correct mixture must be present, or else the engine will "smoke" and will misfire. So also in the tissues, if the correct fat-glucose mixture is not present, it will "smoke" during combustion, the smoke representing toxic acid substances that result from incomplete combustion of the fat. These substances are known as ketone bodies, and the clinical condition is known as acidosis or ketosis. We may say, then, that diabetes is initially a derangement of carbohydrate metabolism, but that this disorder leads to a perverted fat metabolism, which, if unchecked, will result in death.

It is estimated that 200,000,000 persons in the world have diabetes. In Sweden, in each of the 5 years from 1970 to 1975, there was a mean yearly incidence of 19.6 cases per 100,000 population in children, suggesting that the country could expect 330 new cases annually, with some clustering of cases in

January and in the autumn, and peaks at 7 and 12 years of age. The disease is of worldwide distribution, but there are some countries that report a higher frequency than others. In the United States, it is estimated that the frequency is 1.3 diabetics per 1,000 in the population up to age 17, 17 between 25 and 44 years, 43 in the age group from 45 to 64, and 79 over 65 years of age. These numbers will continue to increase as the population grows older. Successful management of the disease prolongs life, and more diabetics live long enough to procreate.

Diabetes is 2.5 times more frequent in relatives than in the general population, and 85% of diabetics have been obese at some time. We do not know the fundamental cause of diabetes; the lesions in the islets are hardly striking, and may indeed be difficult, and sometimes impossible, to detect. There is increasing evidence that in the maturity-onset diabetic, the pancreas produces normal quantities of insulin and the problem is a reduced sensitivity of fat and muscle cells to the effects of insulin.

There are many steps involved in the action of insulin: its biosynthesis, liberation, circulation, uptake and activation, binding, and its effect on intermediary metabolism. There are just as many loci in which lesions that result ultimately in elevated blood glucose can occur. We have stated that the most obvious metabolic cause of diabetes is the lack of insulin, without specifying whether this is a lack of synthesis of insulin or of an abnormal insulin molecule, or whether it is a failure to secrete the synthesized molecule.

Clearly we may have another lesion, namely resistance to insulin. This resistance has been recognized in clinically overt diabetics who respond poorly to insulin in standard doses, but who may respond to greater than normal doses. Defects in insulin receptors have been recognized recently, anti-insulin antibodies are frequently found, and accelerated rates of insulin breakdown are often discovered; these biochemical disorders can lead to diabetes.

Perhaps it it better to consider for a moment what is meant by diabetes mellitus by considering the **diabetic syndrome**. Diabetes may be defined as a metabolic disorder characterized by hyperglycemia.

Because of the body's inability to use glucose, there is starvation in the midst of plenty, and the mobilization of body fat and protein occurs, leading to acidosis. With the occurrence of hyperglycemia and the loss in the urine of glucose in large amounts, there is an obligatory water loss that leads to dehydration and consequent thirst, increased drinking of water, and more urination, as a vicious cycle continues. If the central nervous system does not receive adequate glucose, coma may ensue (Fig. 19–3). In the chronic condition, there is the classic development of changes in small blood vessels throughout the body, particularly in the retina and kidney (see Fig. 14–6). These changes can be visualized with the ophthalmoscope or in the kidney biopsy, and they result in premature visual difficulties (even blindness in some persons) and in abnormal permeability to proteins in the glomeruli, which may precipitate the nephrotic syndrome. Since it is now recognized that the basement membrane around small blood vessels is unusually thickened in diabetic patients, even biopsy is sometimes performed for diagnosis. Because of these lesions, we have come to think of diabetes as a systemic disease, rather than simply a disorder of insulin production.

The relationship between the vascular lesions and the availability of insulin is not understood, and it may be that they are not causally related, but are simply associated genetically determined defects.

It is convenient to classify diabetes into 4 stages, implying that there may be progression from 1 to another (although this is an hypothesis). The stages range from the theoretic to the obvious, ending with the clinical, overt, or "decompensated" diabetes about which we have been speaking. In testing for the **potential diabetic**, we can identify the asymptomatic person whose fasting blood sugar is normal, but whose blood glucose tolerance curve shows an abnormally slow return to normal levels. A glucose tolerance curve is the serum glucose level taken at specific times after a challenge dose of glucose (Fig. 19–4), and this delayed return to normal

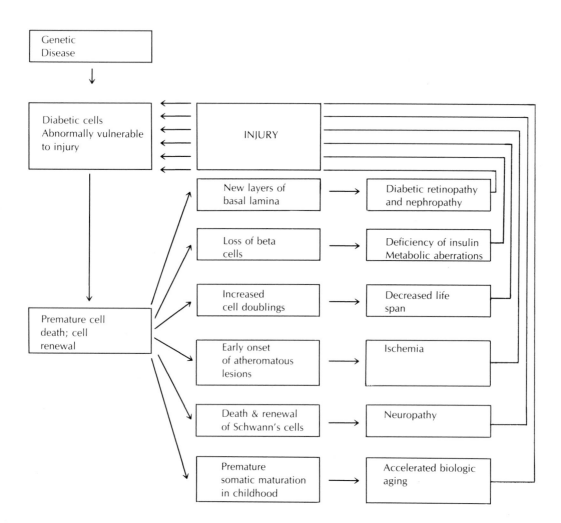

Fig. 19–3. Hypothetical flow of events in diabetes mellitus. Diabetic cells, which by the nature of a genetically transmitted defect, are more vulnerable to injury, die prematurely as a result of ordinary wear and tear. The accelerated cell turnover gives rise to (a) formation of new layers of basal lamina (the hallmark of diabetic microangiopathy), (b) loss of beta cell mass—the problem is compounded by a limited capacity of pancreas to replenish beta cells, (c) increased use of cell doublings *in vivo* and, consequently, decreased *in vitro* replicative life span, (d) lesions of atherosclerosis caused either by increased opportunity for expression of smooth muscle cell transformation or proliferation in response to release from feedback inhibition, (e) death and regeneration of Schwann's cells associated with intermittent symptoms of neuropathy, and, conceivably, (f) accelerated maturation and aging of diabetic individuals. The vascular problem, metabolic aberrations related to insulin deficiency and neuropathy, all provide additional opportunity for injurious events and probably further increase the speed and frequency of accelerated cell turnover. (From Vracko, R., and Benditt, E.P.: Manifestations of diabetes mellitus—their possible relationships to an underlying cell defect. Am. J. Pathol., *75*:204, 1974.)

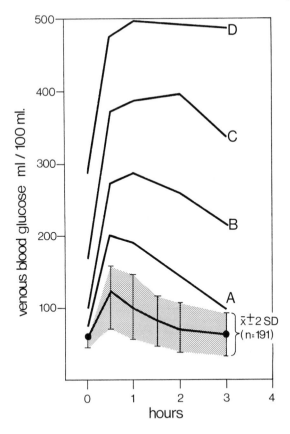

Fig. 19–4.   This figure shows glucose tolerance curves for 191 normal controls (shaded area) and for 4 diabetic patients (A to D). (From Cahill, G.F., Jr.: Diabetes mellitus. In *Cecil Textbook of Medicine,* 15th Ed. Edited by P. B. Beeson, W. McDermott, and J. B. Wyngaarden. Philadelphia, W. B. Saunders, 1979.)

shows an inappropriate handling of glucose. **Latent diabetes** is the term used for those persons whose random blood sugar levels are normal and whose glucose tolerance curves are normal, but who have been identified, when under stress of pregnancy or serious illness or when they were obese, as diabetic. This concept is useful, as the disease may become clinically evident again. Finally, the term **prediabetes** has been introduced to describe those who can be considered to be at risk to develop diabetes, for example, a twin of a diabetic, or the child of diabetic parents. It is a concept rather than a diagnosis, because all testing shows normal metabolism of carbohydrate.

Etiology. Heredity is undoubtedly a most important factor in the development of diabetes. The genetics of diabetes are confusing

at best. First, we recognize several different types of diabetes: in the child (juvenile), in the obese middle-aged adult (late onset), and the diabetes that can be detected only by rigorous testing (latent). Of course, there is as well diabetes due to other disorders of the pancreas (pancreatitis) and diabetes as a part of another syndrome (Cushing's disease). The difficulties in perceiving the patterns of diabetes are compounded by recent studies on twins that reverse the traditional view that juvenile diabetes is hereditary, and adult onset is acquired. In a study of 106 pairs of twins with insulin-dependent diabetes, almost half have only 1 member with diabetes. Dr. Pyke recalls the tragedy of a pair of female twins, of which the nondiabetic won a beauty contest at age 20, and has a happy marriage with 3 children; her sister, meanwhile, developed retinopathy, became nearly blind, developed glomerular disease, and died in her early 30's from the complications of her disease. For her whole life, she had only to look at her sister to see how life would have been without diabetes. A further study of a group of adult-onset diabetics, on the other hand, has shown that there is a high concordance or frequency of diabetes in the identical twin of the adult-onset diabetic, implying a genetic predisposition for this particular form of the disease. These data reverse the widely held concept that juvenile diabetes is hereditary, and adult-onset acquired.

Different hypotheses to explain the confusing patterns have been put forward, but none is satisfactory. At this time, the most comfortable hypotheses are that diabetes is a multifactorial disease in which both heredity and environment play a significant role. Evidence that (1) there is a strong association between the HLA antigen groups, B8 and BW15, and juvenile diabetes, and that (2) infections with viruses such as Coxsackie and mumps in such persons are often followed by diabetes in children, points out the fallacy of an either (heredity) /or (precipitating factor) explanation for diabetes. Without treatment, the downhill progress is much more rapid the younger the patient is, and the untreated child will not usually survive for more than a year.

There are many other possible causes of

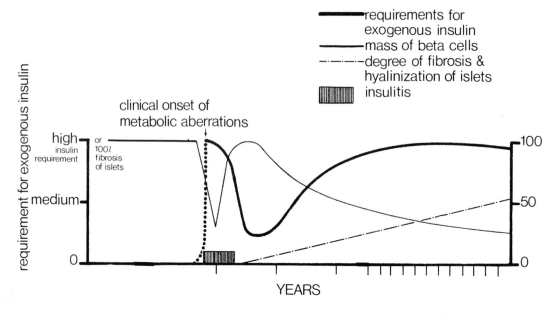

Fig. 19–5. This diagram shows the time relationships between inflammation of the islets of Langerhans and the development of diabetes. (From Vracko, R., and Benditt, E.P.: Manifestations of diabetes mellitus—their possible relationships to an underlying cell defect. Am. J. Pathol., 75:204, 1974.)

diabetes mellitus, in addition to a deficiency of insulin. For example, we now know there are instances in which the presence of antibodies to insulin makes the available insulin ineffective. In some cases, the target cells of insulin are refractory to the presence of this hormone, and in others there is a pituitary-dependent insulin antagonist present. However, the generalities with which we can work are: (1) there is some decrease in the total mass of B cells in the islets (Fig. 19–5); (2) there is some decrease in extractable insulin in the majority of diabetic patients, but not in all; (3) there is a widespread tendency to differentiate 2 major clinical types of diabetes; and (4) etiologic factors other than insulin deficiency may play a role in early stages of diabetes.

Clinical Pattern. As shown in Table 19–1, the chief signs and symptoms of untreated diabetes are polyuria (excessive urination), glycosuria (sugar in the urine), high blood sugar, excessive thirst and hunger, marked weakness, and loss of weight. Other symptoms due to the incomplete combustion of fats are manifestations of acidosis, e.g., air hunger, coma, and ketone bodies in the urine. Still other accompaniments to the dis-

ease are itching, boils, gallstones, arteriosclerosis, and gangrene of the limbs. Nowadays, as the result of insulin treatment, most patients do not die of diabetes itself, but of complications and infections. Many of these symptoms have been alliterated by generations of students, and diabetes has been referred to as the "P" disease: pruritus, polyuria, polyphagia, polydipsia, and Opie, the last being the name of a great pathologist who studied the pancreas.

The glycosuria is due to the excess blood sugar in the urine, since there is a maximum that the tubules of the kidney will absorb. The large amount of sugar dissolved in the urine raises the latter's specific gravity or density, so that it becomes 1.030 or 1.040 in place of the normal of around 1.020. Sugar acts on the kidneys as an osmotic diuretic, hence the polyuria. On account of the large amount of water, the urine is characteristically pale in color. The tissues are dehydrated, which causes thirst. Because of the unavailability of glucose, there is hunger, weakness, and loss of weight. The diabetic patient draws on protein and fat reserves for nourishment and fuel. Itching, in many instances, can be traced to infections, particularly fungal infections of

Table 19–1. Pathophysiology of Diabetes Mellitus

	SOURCE	PROCESS	END RESULT
	Increased blood sugar	Sugar overflows into urine ⟶	Glycosuria
		Water loss to preserve osmotic balance ⟶	Polyuria, Thirst
DECREASED INSULIN	Decreased usable glucose	Incomplete fat combustion ⟶	Ketoacidosis ↓
		Brain starvation ⟶	Coma
	Excess glucose in tissues ⟶	Provides excellent bacterial culture medium ⟶	Infections
?	Increased serum cholesterol ⟶	? Atherosclerosis ⟶ ⟶	Gallstones, Ulcers, Gangrene, Myocardial infarcts
?	?	Small vessel disease ⟶	Kidney damage, Retinopathy, Blindness
?	?	?	Peripheral neuropathy

the genitourinary tract, but its real cause is unknown. The boils and carbuncles are also thought to arise because of the excellent culture medium provided by the excess glucose in all tissues.

Acidosis is a chief danger to life. Often, air hunger (deep respirations) signals the onset of diabetic coma, owing perhaps to the combination of acidosis, ketone bodies, and inadequate blood glucose for the central nervous system. For unknown reasons, the serum cholesterol is elevated, which predisposes a person to gallstone formation and also favors the acceleration of atherosclerosis. Characteristically, diabetics suffer from premature atherosclerosis and occlusion of blood vessels, particularly of their extremities. Gangrene of the toes and legs and ulcers that do not heal may be the first sign of diabetes in an older person. Neuropathy, numbness, tingling, and loss of motor skills are also typical for the diabetic patient.

The treatment of the disease is directed first to the lack of insulin and second to the ad-ditional complications. The effect that "well-controlled" diabetes has on the progression of such complications as arteriosclerosis is disputed, but it is clear that thousands of patient-years have been added by good management of diabetes. The wonder of modern medicine is nowhere better seen than in the treatment of this disease, from which so many patients used to die in diabetic coma.

CARCINOMA OF THE PANCREAS

Carcinoma of the pancreas is rising rapidly in incidence in the western world and now ranks fourth among the important cancers. The prognosis of this tumor is poor indeed, with only a 2% survival rate for 5 years. Contemporary treatments such as radical surgery carry high operative mortality (20%), and chemotherapy does not seem to be much better.

Most carcinomas of the pancreas arise as epithelial tumors (adenocarcinoma) of the ductal epithelium and make their presence known by obstruction and local invasion. The pancreas is richly supplied with nerves; therefore, pain is a prominent feature of cancer of the pancreas, whether it arises in the head, the body, or the tail of that organ.

If the tumor arises in the body or tail, the prognosis is even worse than usual, because the symptoms that allow patient and doctor to suspect cancer in this centrally placed organ are so vague that the tumor has ample time to advance to a stage at which it is inoperable and will respond poorly to radiation or to chemotherapy. These tumors metastasize to regional nodes and to the liver. The only good thing that can be said about the disease is that it occurs relatively late in life, the peak incidence being in the fifth decade. Unfortunately, life expectancy after such a tumor has been diagnosed seldom exceeds a year.

What are the possible explanations for this rise in incidence? There is a clear-cut association with cigarette smoking, and the medium age for pancreas cancer is 15 years earlier in smokers. Cancer of the pancreas also appears frequently in patients with diabetes mellitus. One thought is that the continued stimulus of the modern diet, rich in fat and protein, may lead to hyperplasia of the pancreas, which eventually becomes neoplasia. Of course, there is always the possibility of some unidentified carcinogen in modern processed food that is the offending agent.

Cancer of the head of the pancreas, which accounts for more than half of tumors of the pancreas, behaves in a less secretive way because of its proximity to the common bile duct (Fig. 19–6). These tumors may make their presence known by jaundice, in addition to the nonspecific symptoms of weight loss, pain, anorexia, and nausea, which can be attributed equally well to biliary, hepatic, or gastric causes. There is a time-honored association between pancreatic tumors and thrombophlebitis, which may herald the

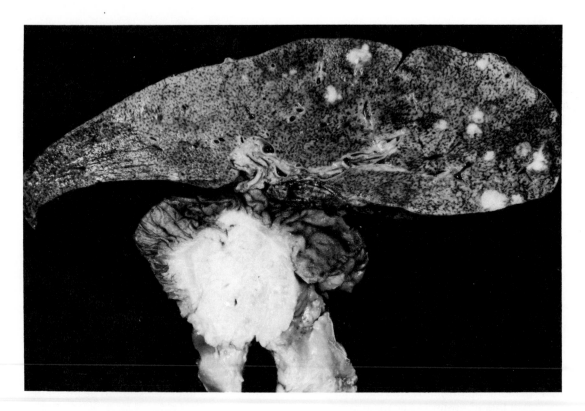

Fig. 19–6. Gross specimen of the liver, duodenum, and pancreas. The firm, white appearance in the bottom center of the photograph is typical of carcinoma. Scattered throughout the lobe of the liver are whitish nodules which are metastatic tumor from the primary, pancreatic carcinoma to the liver. This type of carcinoma frequently is associated with jaundice. (McGill University, Department of Pathology Museum.)

search for a tumor in the pancreas, but this is certainly not a universal finding, and its explanation is unclear.

Symptoms of adenocarcinoma of the head of the pancreas may be pain, or painless jaundice in a middle-aged patient without any clear-cut etiologic, environmental, or antecedent relationship of which we are aware. The patient's jaundice may be principally of the direct type and his stools may be clay-colored, since bile is unable to pass into the duodenum because of the narrowed bile duct. As in the case of destruction of the pancreas by inflammation or obstruction of the pancreatic ducts from other causes, there will also be maldigestion when the pancreatic secretions do not reach the duodenum. Naturally, it is important, whenever one encounters these symptoms, to be certain that the pain, jaundice, and evidence of obstruction are truly due to a cancer, and not to a more treatable disorder such as a stone, or polyp, or inflammation, that has a much better prognosis and can often be remedied. Laparotomy and tissue diagnosis are important in such cases.

Islet Cell Tumors. Another tumor of the pancreas is that of the endocrine portion of the islet cells. These tumors form an uncommon but interesting group because, although they are benign adenomas, often not more than 1 cm in diameter, they may result in the death of the patient unless a correct diagnosis is made. When that is done, the condition can usually be cured promptly. As there are 2 types of islet cells, alpha and beta, so there are 2 varieties of adenoma.

BETA CELL TUMOR. The tumor is usually a small adenoma, 1 or 2 cm in diameter, and is more readily felt than seen by the surgeon at operation, being really a gigantic islet that is easily enucleated. Occasionally, there is a general enlargement of the islets, and, still more rarely, carcinoma with metastases.

The symptoms are those of hyperinsulinism or insulin shock, with correspondingly low blood sugar owing to overactivity of the islet tissue in the adenoma. There may be attacks of weakness and unconsciousness when the interval after a meal is too long. In severe attacks, the patient may pass into a stupor, which may be followed by convulsions. The attack is at once aborted by the administration of sugar. It will be seen that the condition is the reverse of diabetes. The occupational hazard for airplane pilots, engine and taxi drivers, window cleaners, and the like is all too obvious, and the beneficial effect of enucleation of the adenoma is almost unbelievable to the despairing patient.

ALPHA CELL TUMOR. In 1955, Zollinger and Ellison of Ohio State University reported 2 cases of curious association of (1) recurring peptic ulcers, (2) marked gastric hypersecretion and hyperacidity, and (3) an islet cell tumor that did not produce insulin. This combination is now known as the Zollinger-Ellison syndrome, and the tumor is recognized as an alpha cell adenoma which secretes the hormone gastrin, hence the tumor may be referred to as a gastrinoma. Severe watery diarrhea may be a feature. Other cases of this syndrome have been reported in instances in which there was only hyperplasia of the islets, and, rarely, the syndrome has been reported in cases of carcinoma of the islets. The diagnosis is now made by determining the serum gastrin levels in patients with the symptom complex. Management with cimetidine has proved useful in some cases, but resection of the tumor, if possible, is desirable.

CYSTIC FIBROSIS

This condition, called fibrocystic disease of the pancreas, was not recognized 50 years ago, yet it is now identified as a cause of death in children. It is a familial disease of young children, the genetic defect being transmitted as an autosomal recessive gene, resembling diabetes in this respect. In a family in which both parents carry the recessive gene, there is a 25% chance in every pregnancy that the baby will develop the disease. The condition is rare in the Negro. The defect causes an increased viscosity of mucous secretions involving perhaps all the mucous glands of the body, but more especially the pancreas, lungs, and liver. It is also known as mucoviscidosis. Six or 7 years after the onset of the first symptoms, 90% of the afflicted children used to be dead, but modern understanding of the disease has materially improved the outlook. The cause and physiologic or biochemical lesion are unknown.

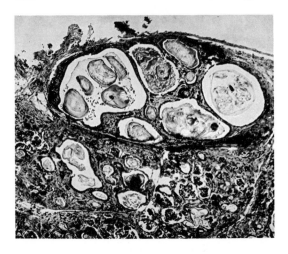

Fig. 19–7. Cystic fibrosis of the pancreas. (Boyd, W.: *Textbook of Pathology*, Philadelphia, Lea & Febiger.)

In the pancreas, the small and large ducts and also the acini are dilated and converted into small cysts filled with inspissated mucus that prevent pancreatic secretions from entering the duodenum (Fig. 19–7). The child therefore fails to gain weight, although he or she develops a healthy appetite. The normal fecal matter of the newborn consists of a mixture of mucus and bile known as meconium. In mucoviscidosis, the intestinal mucus may be so sticky that it forms a plug that blocks the lumen of the bowel and leads to obstruction and even rupture of the ileum, a condition known as meconium ileus. This is a cause of death. If the child survives, the distended pancreatic acini become replaced by fibrous tissue, so that the term cystic fibrosis is well deserved.

In the lung, the mucous glands of the trachea and bronchi are filled with inspissated mucus, which blocks the air passages and leads to atelectasis and emphysema. A few years elapse before the development of marked pulmonary symptoms such as cough, wheezing, shortness of breath, and recurring staphylococcal infections, which may readily produce a fatal bronchopneumonia.

In the liver, evidence of obstruction of the bile ducts is still later to develop. If the patient lives long enough, the result may be cirrhosis with portal hypertension, but this complication is exceptional.

It is evident that, despite its name, cystic fibrosis is not fundamentally a disease of the pancreas, but is one in which this organ is frequently, although not necessarily, involved. Pulmonary involvement dominates the clinical picture of cystic fibrosis and determines its outcome. The deficient pancreatic enzymes can be supplied daily, although at a cost that may well be imagined. With the aid of antibiotics, the threat of staphylococcal pneumonia may be held off, so that the child may have time to grow up.

A simple and reliable test depends on the involvement of the sweat glands in nearly every case. There is excessive perspiration with a corresponding loss of sodium, potassium, and chloride, so that the patients are unduly susceptible to heat exhaustion in hot weather. The test indicates the presence of excessive chloride on the skin. The "sweat test" has shown that adults as well as children may show the hereditary defect and may manifest mild forms of the disease.

SYNOPSIS

The pancreas secretes digestive enzymes (lipase, amylase, and chymotrypsinogen) into the duodenum through the ducts that join the common bile duct at the ampulla of Vater. It also secretes hormones into the blood, glucagon and insulin.

The exocrine function of the pancreas may be destroyed by inflammation, cancer, or surgery, or by obstruction of the ducts.

Pancreatitis may be acute, chronic, or hemorrhagic.

Tumors of the pancreas may involve the organ's head, body, or tail, or they may arise in the endocrine portion. Each type may develop a different clinical pattern.

Diabetes mellitus is systemic disease of uncertain etiology. The diabetic syndrome of polyuria, polyphagia, and polydipsia should include accelerated atherosclerosis, acidosis, neuropathy, and coma.

Terms

Diabetes mellitus	*Glucagon*	*Pancreatitis*
Insulin	*Amylase*	*Cystic fibrosis*

FURTHER READING

Editorial: Death from acute pancreatitis. Lancet, *2*:632, 1977.

Editorial: Carcinoma of the pancreas. Br. Med. J., *2*:1497. 1977.

Creutzfeldt, W., and Schmidt, H.: Aetiology and pathogenesis of pancreatitis: current concepts. Scand. J. Gastroenterol. (Suppl.), *6*:47, 1970.

Cudworth, A.G., and Festenstein, M.B.: HLA genetic heterogeneity in diabetes mellitus. Br. Med. Bull., *34*:285, 1978.

Davis P.B., and Di Sant'Agnese, P.A.: A review. Cystic fibrosis at forty—quo vadis? Pediatr. Res., *14*:83, 1980.

Deveney, C.W., Deveney, K.S., and Way, L.W.: The Zollinger-Ellison syndrome—23 years later. Ann. Surg., *188*:384, 1978.

Diamond, D., and Fisher, B.: Pancreatic cancer. Surg. Clin. North Am., *55*:363, 1975.

Flier, J.S., Kahn, R., and Roth, J.: Receptors, antireceptor, antibodies and mechanisms of insulin resistance. N. Engl. J. Med., *300*:413, 1979.

Gabbay, K.H.: The insulinopathies, N. Engl. J. Med., *302*:165, 1980.

Hermann, R.E., and Cooperman, A.M.: Current concepts in cancer: cancer of the pancreas. N. Engl. J. Med., *301*:482, 1979.

Salt, W.B., and Schenker, S.: Amylase; its clinical significance. A review of the literature. Medicine (Baltimore), *55*:269, 1976.

Sarles, H.: Chronic calcifying pancreatitis—chronic alcoholic pancreatitis. Gastroenterology, *66*:604, 1974.

Solow, H., Hidalgo, R., and Singal, D.P.: Juvenile onset diabetes: HLA-A, -B, -C, and -DR alloantigens. Diabetes, *28*:1, 1979.

Strum, W.B., and Spiro, H.M.: Chronic pancreatitis. Ann. Intern. Med., *74*:264, 1971.

Vracko, R., and Benditt, E.P.: Manifestations of diabetes mellitus—their possible relationships to an underlying cell defect. Am. J. Pathol., *75*:204, 1974.

Warren, S., LeCompte, P.M., and Legg, M.A.: *The Pathology of Diabetes Mellitus*, 4th Ed. Philadelphia, Lea & Febiger, 1968.

Winegrad, A.I., and Greene, D.A.: The complications of diabetes mellitus. N. Engl. J. Med., *298*:1250, 1978.

The Kidney and Male Genital Tract

20

The three most important things a man has are his private parts, his money and his religious opinions.—S. BUTLER

The genitourinary system includes the kidneys, ureters, urinary bladder, urethra, and the genitalia and accessory glands. In this chapter we consider the urinary system first and then the male genital tract. The excretion of urine is common to both males and females, whereas the female genitalia deserve a separate chapter.

URINARY SYSTEM

Structure and Function

The urinary system removes waste products from the blood (filtered at a rate of 1.2 liters per minute), particularly those waste substances containing nitrogen, e.g., urea. Excretion is accomplished by means of filtration and reabsorption in the kidneys. The normal glomerular filtration rate is about 120 milliliters per minute or 180 liters per day, but the urine output is less than 1% (1.5 liters for men, 1 liter for women). The urine so formed passes from each kidney in the corre-sponding ureter to the bladder (Fig. 20–1), and thence through the urethra to the exterior. The urinary bladder differs from the

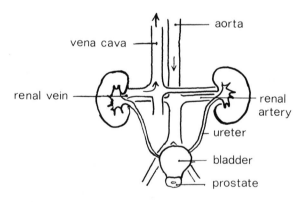

Fig. 20–1. The anatomic relationships of the kidney. Its arterial blood supply, the renal arteries, break up into progressively smaller blood vessels until the afferent arteriole is reached. The renal veins, which drain blood back to the heart, are important because increased pressure or thrombosis may cause renal disease. The kidney shows to the naked eye a cortex and medulla and collecting system, the pelvis, which terminates in the ureter. The left and right ureters join the urinary bladder, which opens to the exterior through the urethra.

gallbladder in that it is only a reservoir and does not absorb or significantly concentrate the fluid that it contains. Absorption and concentration do take place in the kidney to a marked degree; an early sign of renal disease is loss of this concentrating power.

The mechanism for filtration is elegant. Each kidney, with an average weight of around 150 grams, is composed of over 1,000,000 units or nephrons (Fig. 20–2), all of which are minute filters and resorbers (Fig. 20–3). The nephron is a complex tube, partly coiled (convoluted tubule) and partly straight (collecting tubule), the upper end of which is formed by a spherical structure, Bowman's capsule. The lower end opens into the chamber or pelvis of the kidney, from which the urine passes to the bladder. In the glomerulus, which is the filter, a small artery, the afferent arteriole of the glomerulus, breaks up into a little cluster of capillary loops that project like a bunch of grapes into the dilated upper end of the tubule. As the blood passes through the loops, water and solids in solution diffuse into the space around the capillaries and pass down the convoluted tubule, where secretion and reabsorption of the protein and electrolytes take place. The urine then passes into the collecting tubules, where the contents are concentrated as water is resorbed, and finally into the pelvis of the kidney. Table 20–1 outlines the function of different portions of the nephron.

The process of filtration or secretion of urine depends partly on the pressure under which the blood is forced through the glomerular capillaries. If the blood pressure falls markedly, the secretion

Table 20–1. Functions of the Nephron

SEGMENT OF NEPHRON	FUNCTION
Glomerulus	PRODUCES ultrafiltrate of PLASMA (120 ml/min)
Proximal Tubule	REABSORBS 66% of filtered Na, Cl, H_2O
	REABSORBS HCO_3, glucose, K, P, amino acids, uric acid, and some proteins
Loop of Henle	REABSORBS NaCl
Distal Tubule	REABSORBS Na, Cl, H_2O
	SECRETES H^+, K^+, NH_4
Collecting Duct	REABSORBS Na, Cl, H_2O
	SECRETES H, NH_4, K

of urine diminishes or stops. Although water, urea, and salts pass from the blood through the walls of the glomerular capillaries into the tubules, the albumin and other large molecules of the blood plasma are not allowed to escape (Fig. 20–4). The presence of albumin in the urine indicates disease of the glomeruli; the presence of sugar is nearly always due to the elevated blood sugar level characteristic of diabetes.

It is evident that in the formation of the urine there are 2 opposite factors at work, glomerular filtration and tubular reabsorption. Were it not for reabsorption in the tubules, the body would soon be drained of its fluid, for only 1% of the fluid that passes through the glomeruli appears as urine. The normal amount of urine passed is about 1,000 ml per day, but this will vary with, for example, the amount of water drunk or the amount lost in perspiration, as well as with body size.

One important indication that all is not well with the kidneys is any serious departure from this average, particularly in the direction of too little (oliguria). However, frequency of urination, that is, an increase in the number of voidings in any given time, is a common sign of some urinary tract disorder. Under unusual circumstances, this frequency is determined by factors other than a person's physiology (Fig. 20–5). The accompanying chart shows how the clinician might evaluate a problem involving frequency of urination (Table 20–2). As illustrated by this table, frequency (frequent urination, usually with some pain, i.e., dysuria) is a common symptom of urinary tract disease. Obstructions may be due to stones, strictures, tumors, or other causes, as shown in the left-hand columns of Table 20–2.

Large volumes of urine may be due to diabetes insipidus (either the loss of antidiuretic hormone due to pituitary surgery, for example, or tubular unresponsiveness to ADH), or to the presence of osmotically active substances in the urine, such as occurs in diabetes mellitus (glucose), in glomerulonephritis (albumin), or in therapeutic treatment (mannitol).

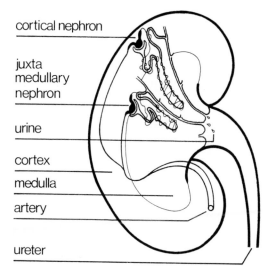

cortical nephron

juxta medullary nephron

urine

cortex

medulla

artery

ureter

Fig. 20–2. This figure shows the relationship of the nephron to the cortex of the kidney. Note the 2 different types of nephrons, those that arise in the cortex and those that arise in the corticomedullary junction.

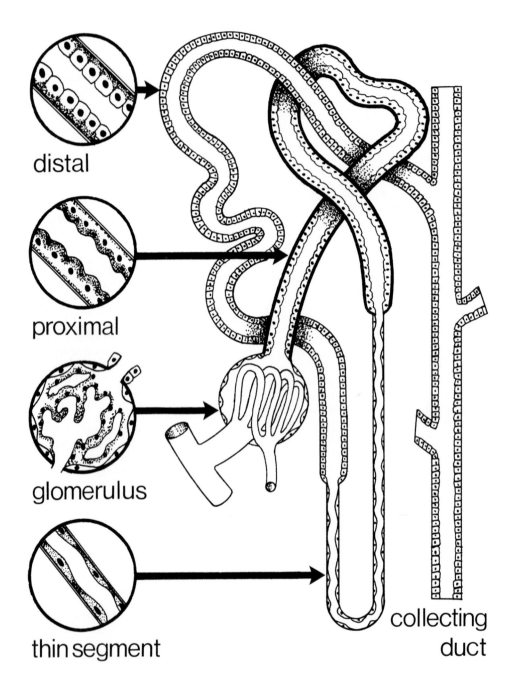

distal

proximal

glomerulus

thin segment

collecting duct

Fig. 20–3. The nephron is the fundamental unit of the kidney. Shown here is the glomerulus and the respective parts of the tubular epithelium, the proximal and distal convoluted tubules that proceed to the collecting ducts.

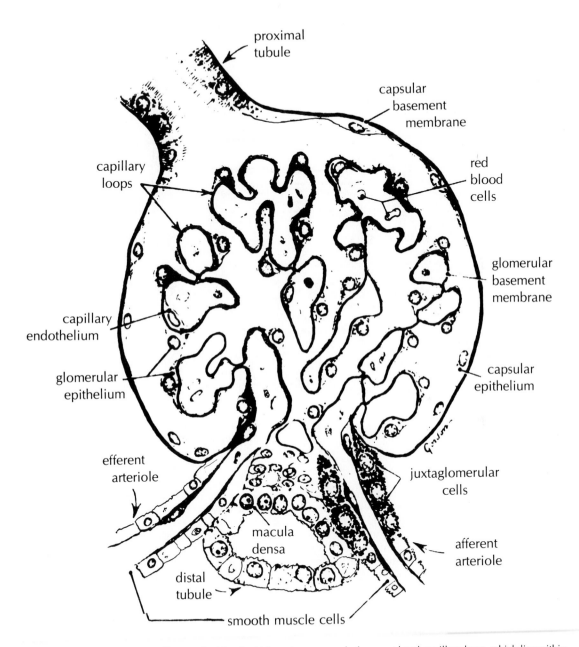

Fig. 20–4. The glomerulus, or filtration bed for the kidney, is composed of a convoluted capillary loop, which lies within Bowman's space. Outside the cells of the capillary are epithelial cells. Between the capillary and the epithelial cell is a complex basement membrane, which frequently reflects inflammatory injury to the glomerulus. (From Ham, A. W.: *Histology,* 7th Ed. Philadelphia and Toronto, J. B. Lippincott, 1974.)

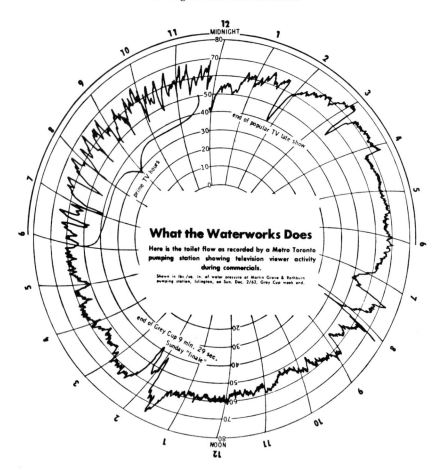

Fig. 20–5. This figure illustrates the effect of television viewing on synchronizing urinary output in Toronto. The fall in water pressure shown in each hour is directly related to the number of gallons poured into Lake Ontario. (From Daily Pressure Chart from Martin Grove Pumping Station, 1962. Toronto, Metropolitan Works Department.)

Although we have spoken of the kidneys as excretory organs, it is known that the regulation of the acid-base balance of the body fluids and the maintenance of the normal concentrations of electrolytes are functions of equal importance. This regulation, as readers will recognize, represents the preservation of the internal environment. The acid-base balance is preserved by the formation of carbonic acid by the epithelium of the convoluted tubules and by the reversal of the proportion of acid and alkaline phosphates with the exchange of hydrogen for sodium ions. As the result of these interchanges, the alkaline serum of the blood that is excreted by the glomeruli becomes the acidic urine that enters the bladder.

The concentrations of solutes and substances in the urine contribute to its specific gravity. Depending on the dilution of urine or the dehydration of the person, the specific gravity of urine from normal kidneys varies between 1.015 and 1.025. If the glomeruli are inflamed and albumin is present in the filtrate, the specific gravity will be greater than normal, as is the case of the diabetic patient's urine, which may contain significant amounts of glucose. If the nephrons have been injured by disease, their ability to secrete and to resorb will be impaired; therefore, the specific gravity of the urine may be fixed at a low value and the kidney cannot respond to such a physiologic challenge as the need to conserve water by excreting a concentrated urine.

We may classify kidney diseases according to the anatomic structures involved (glomerular, vascular, interstitial, or tubular disease), or we may classify them according to origin (hereditary, neoplastic, infectious, inflammatory), but neither taxonomy is entirely satisfactory. For purposes of this chapter, we consider them arbitrarily in order of frequency, that is, the more common diseases first.

We start our consideration with the most

Table 20–2. Assessment of Urinary Frequency

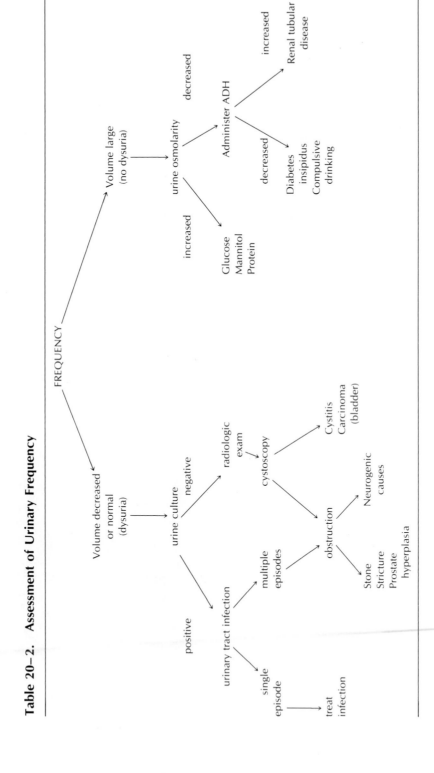

common and treatable type of kidney diseases, those caused by infectious agents.

Pyelonephritis and Infectious Disease

The word pyelonephritis means inflammation of the kidney and the renal pelvis, the emphasis on the pelvis indicating that the infection is often ascending. The inflammation is different from that of glomerulonephritis, for it is primarily an inflammation of the interstitial tissue rather than of the parenchyma (glomeruli and tubules) of the kidney; it is patchy in distribution. One may use special terms to describe infections in and around the kidney, such as acute pyelonephritis, renal abscess, pyelitis, etc., as illustrated in Figure 20–6.

Urinary tract infections are common, and as many as 1 out of 4 sexually active women have pyelonephritis at some time; for men the incidence is much lower, perhaps one-tenth as frequent.

The diagnosis is generally made and confirmed by examination of uncontaminated urine (clean catch) in which the colony count is greater than 100,000 bacteria per ml, with observable bacteria in the sediment.

The inflammation is caused by pyogenic bacteria, particularly *E. coli*, streptococci, and staphylococci. The colon bacilli ascend from the bladder in infections of the kidney, which are especially apt to occur in women and children. In men it is a common complication of enlarged prostate. The infecting organisms may also reach the kidney by the blood stream (hematogenous route).

The kidneys are seldom equally affected, and often only 1 is involved. Numerous small abscesses are scattered throughout the kidney (Fig. 20–7). These abscesses may open into the renal pelvis, so that a characteristic symptom is the presence of a large amount of pus in the urine, which is called pyuria. The progress of the disease varies, and it may end in 2 different ways:

1. The suppuration may extend; more and more renal tissue is destroyed, and the small abscesses fuse and form large ones that communicate with the renal pelvis. The clinical picture is that of hectic, septic infection. If the patient lives long enough, 1 or both kidneys may become converted into large bags of pus. As so much kidney tissue is destroyed, the patient will show symptoms of renal failure and may die of uremia, if he has not already died of septic infection.

2. In other persons, the inflammatory process is much less violent, and in many of the inflamed areas healing occurs, followed by scar formation. The infection continues in other areas, until these also become scarred.

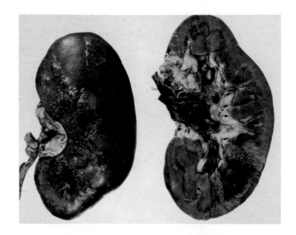

Fig. 20–7. This photograph of a kidney shows the cortical surface at the left, with numerous small whitish areas surrounded by a hemorrhagic zone. On the right, the pelvis is opened and its mucosal surface shows a shaggy, hemorrhagic appearance. This kidney shows abscesses and inflammation of the pelvis, the diagnostic term **pyelonephritis** being appropriate. *E. coli* is a common cause of such infection. (McGill University, Department of Pathology Museum.)

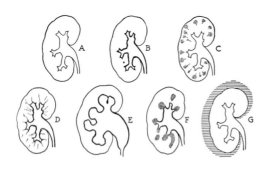

A-Normal ; B - Pyelitis; C - Cortical abscesses; D-Diffuse pyelonephritis; E- Infected hydronephrosis ; F- Pyonephrosis; G- Perinephric abscess.

Fig. 20–6. This drawing shows schematically the disposition of infection in various anatomic areas of the kidney. *A*, Normal; *B*, pyelitis; *C*, cortical abscesses; *D*, diffuse pyelonephritis; *E*, infected hydronephrosis; *F*, pyonephrosis; *G*, perinephric abscess. (From Christopher, F.: *A Textbook of Surgery*. Philadelphia and London, W. B. Saunders.)

In this way the kidney is gradually destroyed, but it is now a mass of scar tissue instead of a bag of pus. The scar tissue contracts, so that the kidney becomes shrunken in size and has a granular surface. In other words, the picture of granular contracted kidney is similar to that of chronic glomerulonephritis. If both kidneys are involved, the patient shows evidence of renal failure and dies of uremia.

Fortunately, both outcomes are rare today, when antibiotics are readily available.

Hypertension may develop in the chronic stage of pyelonephritis. Even though only 1 kidney is involved, there may still be hypertension. The involvement of a single kidney has suggested the possibility of curing the hypertension by removing the diseased kidney. This procedure has been done on a number of occasions, but the results have been disappointing. Although there is temporary benefit, sooner or later, and usually sooner, the hypertension returns. There is also the danger that the remaining kidney may be affected, in which case the state of the patient will be worse than before.

Pyelonephritis is the commonest type of kidney disease. It occurs particularly frequently in school-age female children and is attributed to both poor hygiene (a soiled perineum) and a short urethra. It is clear, however, that pyelonephritis can be successfully treated, as can any infectious disease, and the widespread and abundant use of antibiotics has reduced the severity and has improved the prognosis of the disease.

Recurrent episodes of pyuria (pus in the urine), fever, and flank pain should always raise the question of some underlying cause that predisposes a person to recurrent infections in the kidney. It is well established that any partial obstruction to the flow of urine makes it easier for infections to gain a foothold (another example of the dictum: obstruction leads to stasis and stasis predisposes to infection).

The most important contributing factors to pyelonephritis are instrumentation or catheterization, which is frequently necessary in the aged or in persons with tumors, spinal cord CNS injuries, obstructions, such as stones or tumors, or even pregnancy and infections elsewhere in the body (Fig. 20–8).

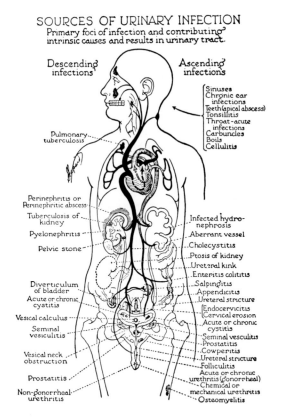

Fig. 20–8. This schematic drawing shows sources of infection that may arrive at the kidney. Frequently a predisposing cause is partial obstruction in the genitourinary tract. Additionally, infections elsewhere in the body may cause pyelonephritis because of the transient septicemia. (From Christopher, F.: *A Textbook of Surgery.* Philadelphia and London, W. B. Saunders.)

In order to establish the diagnosis of pyelonephritis, microscopic examination of the urine is all-important. In the acute stage, the urine is loaded with polymorphonuclear leukocytes, so that the diagnosis is easy. In the chronic stage, there may be only an occasional pus cell, and the bacteriologic examination becomes particularly important. True bacterial infection must not be confused with contamination due to the use of a catheter for obtaining a specimen of urine. The distal 1 or 2 centimeters of the urethra, both male and female, contain numbers of bacteria, so that the tip of the catheter inevitably becomes infected, and the bacteria thus collected grow readily in the urine. It is far better to use a midstream specimen, rejecting the first and the last parts. This procedure is followed by high dilution with sterile saline solution, prompt inoculation of culture plates, and a count of the resulting colonies. Significant bacteriuria is present when there are 100,000 bacteria or more per milliliter of urine.

There are specific infections of the kidney that can be considered under the same heading. Perhaps the most significant is tuberculosis. Its importance arises from the difficulty in making the diagnosis on one hand, and from the extreme destruction of the kidney that it can cause on the other. Microscopic hematuria, the presence of a few round cells in the urine, and a history of low-grade fever and weight loss will suggest the diagnosis, which can only be established by isolating the tubercle bacillus from the urine, not an easy task. Because the response of the host to the tubercle bacillus is often slow and indolent, the infection may smolder for months and years until all that remains of the kidney is a thin line of tissue surrounding a tennis-ball sized mass of caseous necrosis, known as the "putty kidney" (Fig. 20–9). Fortunately, the diagnosis is often made in time and the disease rarely involves both kidneys to the same degree simultaneously. Modern antibiotic therapy for tuberculosis is successful, and contemporary surgery for removal of a useless and destroyed kidney has less risk than ever.

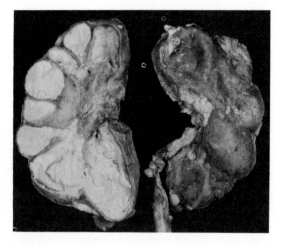

Fig. 20–9. This photograph shows the cortical surface on the right and the sectioned surface of the kidney on the left. The cortex and medulla cannot be perceived due to their destruction and replacement by the cheesy white material, which has given this **tuberculous** kidney the name of a "putty kidney." (McGill University, Department of Pathology Museum.)

Naturally, the tubercle bacillus had to come from somewhere, and in most instances there is pulmonary tuberculosis as well. Renal tuberculosis may also spread to the urinary bladder.

Vascular Diseases

Perhaps the second most common cause of impaired kidney function has its origin in disease of the blood vessels, more specifically the arterial and arteriolar supply to the kidneys. Various names have been used for these vascular diseases, ranging from nephrosclerosis, which simply means hardening of the kidney, to arteriosclerotic renal disease, or arteriosclerotic nephritis. Because the kidney has an immense reserve capacity, as do most of our organs, it is not until more than 75% of the kidney structure has been destroyed that we have any symptoms of dysfunction, but with careful testing, lesser degrees of physiologic loss can be detected. As we age, one of the targets of time is our vascular tree, and it is common to find branches of small arteries significantly narrowed, as in the coronary arteries, the cerebral vessels, and the kidneys.

Naturally, this narrowing may be partial or complete and may have varying effects. As with other vessels, if the occlusion is sudden and the area it supplies relatively large, the infarct may be symptomatic (Fig. 20–10). On the other hand, if the narrowing is gradual, atrophy of the area will occur slowly and, if the vessel is small, the loss in function will go undetected. However, if enough small vessels are narrowed over decades, a large percentage of the nephrons will be lost, and there can be a loss in function detectable by a rising blood urea nitrogen level (BUN) and by decreases in creatinine clearance.

This relationship of loss of renal function to loss of anatomically and physiologically functional nephrons is shown in the accompanying graph (Fig. 20–11), in which it can be seen that the rise in creatinine as an important measure of renal failure occurs only after 80% of the kidney tissue is damaged, which is late in the progress of any disease.

We have been describing arteriosclerosis and arteriolosclerosis of the kidneys, and we

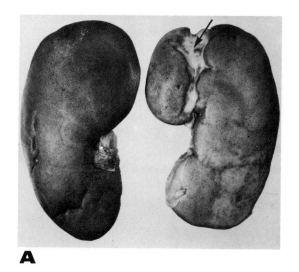

A

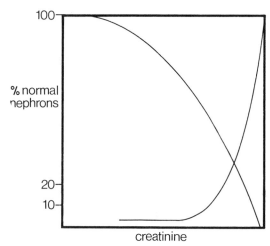

Fig. 20–11.   This diagram shows the percentage of normal nephrons that must be lost before the serum creatinine level begins to rise significantly.

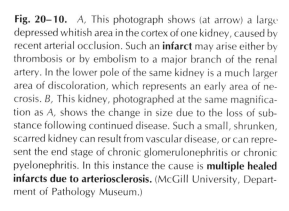

B

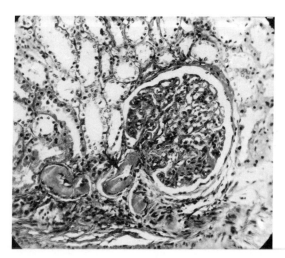

Fig. 20–10.   *A,* This photograph shows (at arrow) a large depressed whitish area in the cortex of one kidney, caused by recent arterial occlusion. Such an **infarct** may arise either by thrombosis or by embolism to a major branch of the renal artery. In the lower pole of the same kidney is a much larger area of discoloration, which represents an early area of necrosis. *B,* This kidney, photographed at the same magnification as *A,* shows the change in size due to the loss of substance following continued disease. Such a small, shrunken, scarred kidney can result from vascular disease, or can represent the end stage of chronic glomerulonephritis or chronic pyelonephritis. In this instance the cause is **multiple healed infarcts due to arteriosclerosis.** (McGill University, Department of Pathology Museum.)

Fig. 20–12.   This light photomicrograph of a glomerulus shows the afferent arteriole (at arrow). It is a markedly thick-walled and hyalinized vessel. This is typical of **arteriolosclerosis** in the kidney, often a concomitant of hypertension. (McGill University, Department of Pathology Museum.)

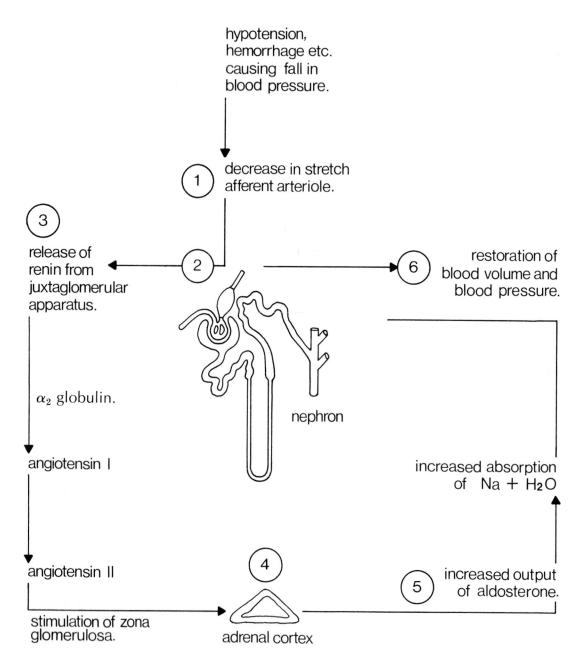

hypotension,
hemorrhage etc.
causing fall in
blood pressure.

(1) decrease in stretch
afferent arteriole.

(3)

release of
renin from
juxtaglomerular
apparatus.

(2)

(6) restoration of
blood volume and
blood pressure.

α_2 globulin.

nephron

angiotensin I

increased absorption
of Na + H_2O

angiotensin II

(4)

(5) increased output
of aldosterone.

stimulation of zona
glomerulosa.

adrenal cortex

Fig. 20–13. This drawing illustrates the relationship of several factors in the development of hypertension. A decrease in the stimuli to the afferent arteriole may result in the release of renin from the juxtaglomerular apparatus which may produce stimulation of the zona glomerulosa of the adrenal, resulting in increased reabsorption of sodium. Equivalently, angiotensin may cause an increase in the peripheral resistance alone due to vasoconstriction of the peripheral arterioles.

consider it to be an extension of the normal aging process (Fig. 20–12). There is another, less readily explainable, cause of arteriolosclerosis. From decades of observation in hundreds of cases, it is clear that narrowing of small arterioles in the kidney follows a raised systemic blood pressure. In other words, people with hypertension (regardless of its etiology) demonstrate reactive changes in their peripheral arterioles, and, significantly, these changes may be severe in the kidneys.

It has been shown experimentally that an elevation in blood pressure can cause hyperplasia of the arteriolar smooth muscle and even an increase in the size of the endothelial cells, so that they narrow the lumen. This phenomenon is seen most dramatically in a syndrome called malignant hypertension (severe rapidly progressive hypertension, retinal hemorrhages with papilledema, and renal failure), a disease of uncertain etiology in which the arterioles not only become narrowed, but also undergo a peculiar fibrinoid necrosis and are prone to thrombosis and

hemorrhage (arteriolonecrosis) (Fig. 20–13). These lesions are seen particularly clearly in the kidney, but they can occur in all parts of the body, especially the brain. In malignant hypertension, rapidly progressive renal failure follows the small vessel disease in the kidneys.

The corollary of these observations is the discovery by Dr. Goldblatt, many years ago, that partial occlusion of a renal artery leads to hypertension. The mechanism by which this "Goldblatt effect" is achieved is as follows: surrounding each afferent arteriole in each glomerulus is a mechanoreceptor composed of a group of granule-containing cells. These granules contain renin, which may be released into the blood stream by the stimulus of a decrease in blood pressure or by hypoxia. This release apparatus serves as a mechanism to maintain the blood pressure because renin, once it is released, acts on angiotensin, a serum globulin produced in the liver. This in turn is converted to another substance (angiotensin II), which has powerful pressor ef-

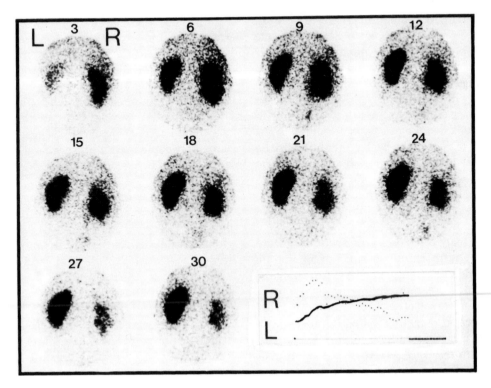

Fig. 20–14. The diagnosis of renovascular hypertension may be aided by the use of radio-Hippuran. This series of films taken every 3 minutes demonstrate normal function on the right but delayed uptake and excretion on the left, with no evidence of an obstructed or dilated collecting system. The curves at the bottom illustrate normal uptake and excretion in the right kidney (dotted line) and delayed uptake and secretion in the left (solid line), mirroring the information provided by the sequential films.

fects on smooth muscle, causing arterioles everywhere to constrict, thereby increasing the peripheral resistance and raising the diastolic pressure.

So we have an intimate relation between arterial and arteriolar diseases and hypertension (Fig. 20–14). We have also seen how hypertension can cause vascular diseases, especially in the kidney, by narrowing small blood vessels, which in turn leads to a loss of nephrons by ischemic atrophy. On the other hand, we have heard how disease of large vessels (Goldblatt lesion) or small vessels can initiate hypertension, starting a vicious cycle of vessel disease → hypertension → small vessel disease. Thus, hypertension may both cause and result from arteriolosclerosis!

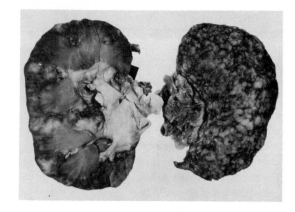

Fig. 20–15. This kidney is typical of **end-stage glomerulonephritis.** Compare this photograph with Figure 20–10, an end-stage kidney caused by vascular disease. With sufficient destruction of renal parenchyma due to any chronic renal disease, the uremic syndrome appears. (McGill University, Department of Pathology Museum.)

Glomerulonephritis

The clinical picture of headache, puffy eyes, pain in the lumbar region, and small amounts of dark urine of increased specific gravity is quickly recognized as the pattern of acute glomerulonephritis. This disease is an acute proliferative inflammation of the glomeruli for which no infectious agent is immediately responsible. We believe glomerulonephritis occurs as an allergic inflammatory response.

The headache is attributed to the accompanying hypertension, the puffy eyes to edema consequent to the loss of albumin in the urine (a result of the leaky inflamed capillaries), the pain in the back is attributed to the turgid swollen kidneys, and the oliguria (smaller than normal amount of urine, e.g., less than 400 ml/24 hrs) to the damage to the nephron and to the congestion in the capillary bed.

The disease often occurs as a sequel to acute infection with certain strains of hemolytic streptococci in the upper respiratory tract or in the middle ear and following scarlet fever after an interval of 2 weeks or more. This latent period, together with the absence of bacteria and the peculiar proliferative type of lesion, strongly suggests that sensitization of the tissue is an essential feature and that the inflammation is immunologic in character, owing to an antigen-antibody reaction in the glomeruli, perhaps the most vulnerable part of the whole renal vascular system. The structural element of the glomerulus that is involved in antigen-antibody reaction is the basement membrane, which becomes significantly thickened and, with fluorescent microscopy, can be shown to be the site of antigen-antibody complexes.

It is important to recognize that most cases of acute glomerulonephritis resolve completely and the kidney returns to normal; however, a few persons are left with kidneys that are anatomically scarred and physiologically incompetent (Fig. 20–15). These patients actually become uremic and are candidates for permanent dialysis or for kidney transplantation.

New methods of study by biopsy and by fluorescent and electron microscopy have permitted us to recognize several varieties of glomerulonephritis: those with minimal lesions, those with focal lesions, and those in which there are different types of structural changes in the basement membrane. However, it is beyond the scope of this chapter to discuss the specific pathologic classification of glomerulonephritis. The common feature is a glomerular lesion that renders the glomerular capillary unusually permeable to large molecules and even to erythrocytes, resulting in an abnormal urinary sediment and secondary tubular dysfunction. These characteristics distinguish this group of kidney diseases from the previous groups, the infectious and the vascular.

Acute Renal Failure

Distinct from, but related to, the 3 principal entities we have just considered is the situation in which there is an acute episode of renal failure not directly attributable to infection, inflammation, or conventional vascular disease. Although there may be a precipitate onset of oliguria (less than 400 ml urine/24 hrs) or anuria accompanying the inflammation of kidney disease, there are some other causes of renal failure that can be collected under this heading and should be mentioned briefly.

For many years, it has been recognized that in the case of a patient severely injured by trauma, as in a car accident, or after severe burns, there is oliguria or anuria in the 24 to 48 hours following the injury. Examination of the kidneys in these cases shows that the proximal convoluted tubules have become necrotic. We now know that this is attributable to the shock following the injury. This lesion, whether it is caused by trauma, by burns, or by septicemia, has been called acute tubular necrosis and, fortunately, is reversible in a large percentage of cases, since the tubule cells are capable of regenerating and of repopulating the length of the nephron that has been rendered ischemic and necrotic. The principal causes of acute tubular necrosis at Montreal's Royal Victoria Hospital in 1978 were equally divided between septic conditions (28%) and shock due to cardiogenic causes (26%). Drugs, chemicals, and pigments (hemoglobin, bile) accounted for the balance.

An identical lesion can be produced by such poisons as mercury or carbon tetrachloride, which may be accidentally or intentionally taken. In this situation, the toxic material acts directly on the tubular epithelium. One result of this injury is the obstruction of the tubular lumen because of the necrotic debris, and this obstruction is a reason for the decrease in urine excretion.

Again, in situations in which a mismatched transfusion has taken place, there may be the excretion of hemolyzed red blood cells, which precipitate and obstruct the kidney tubules just as in some cases of overwhelming jaundice, bile pigments may accumulate in the tubules and directly injure the cells and obstruct the outflow of urine.

The kidneys may reflect this injury grossly by appearing larger than normal, pale, and swollen. Microscopic amounts of substances such as hemoglobin or bilirubin may be present. The urine, if any can be obtained, will show casts of the offending material or of tubular cells that are being shed.

Acute tubular necrosis is an entity with a much better prognosis today because of the life-support techniques, such as dialysis, which were not widely available 30 years ago.

Figure 20–16 shows graphically the course of a patient's urine production and the retention of blood urea during episodes of renal failure, transplantation, and final renal failure, to illustrate the complex nature of the disease and its treatment.

Nephrotic Syndrome

Between this acute phase of kidney injury and the chronic phase of renal failure, there is a frequent extension of injury that is called the nephrotic syndrome. The term is a misnomer and should be discarded, but age does not seem to wither nor time decay its usage.

The term nephrotic syndrome is applied to the patients who demonstrate: generalized **edema** (anasarca), massive **proteinuria** (more than 4 gm protein/24 hrs), **hypoalbuminemia** (less than 2.5 gm/100 ml) and **hyperlipidemia**. These abnormalities are all traditionally related to the inflammatory glomerular lesion; however, in about one-fifth of the cases, renal vein occlusion or the deposition of such material as amyloid may be the cause. The mechanism by which these abnormalities exert their effect is explained in the following way.

The loss of albumin into Bowman's space and its consequent excretion (albuminuria) depletes the serum (hypoalbuminemia). The decreased serum protein level renders the Starling hypothesis unworkable, and the interstitial fluid fails to return to the vascular compartment at the venous end of the capillary, thus leading to diffuse edema. The explanation of hyperlipidemia is not so clear. It

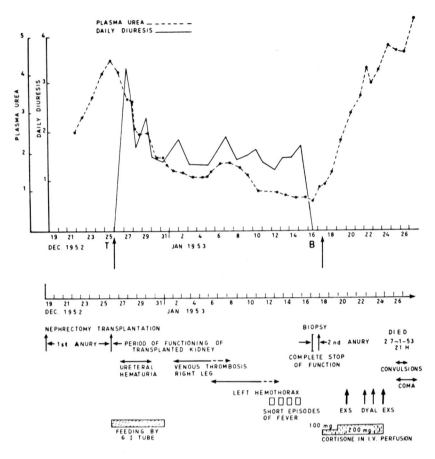

Fig. 20–16. This graph demonstrates several functions of the kidney. Note blood urea nitrogen and urine production (diuresis) during the period from December to the end of January in the 1950s. This particular patient had a renal transplant which ultimately failed to function. (From Michon, L., et al.: Une tentative de transplantation renale chez l'homme: aspects medicaux et biologiques. Presse Med., 61:1419, 1953.)

has been suggested that, in the race to synthesize new albumin, the liver coincidentally synthesizes lipids, or alternatively, since albumin is a serum carrier for lipids, in hypoalbuminemia there is not enough albumin to transport lipids normally. It is sufficient here to refer the interested reader to more complete accounts of this interesting but uncommon disorder.

Uremia

The final common pathway for all renal diseases is the condition known as uremia. It is estimated that 10,000 Americans develop renal failure each year, that 40,000 people are treated by means of dialysis, and that another 27,000 have received transplants. The cost of

all treatment is enormous; the cost of the first year of a transplant is estimated at $25,000, an amount equal to the annual cost of dialysis in hospital. The total cost of these current cases in the United States is 5% of the Gross National Product or $1,000,000,000 a year in 1979, and it may double by 1981.

Because the symptoms occur as the kidney reaches the limit of its function, uremia can be viewed best in the light of disorders of normal renal physiology. We have discussed the kidney's role in excretion of waste products, water balance, acid-base regulation, and regulation of electrolytes. The kidney also synthesizes erythropoietin, a hormone that helps to regulate production of red blood cells. When a significant amount of kidney tissue has been destroyed by infection, by vascular disease, or by glomerulonephritis, there will be a diminished ability to excrete nitrogen-containing compounds. This leads to an increase in the number of molecules of urea, uric acid, ammonia, and creatine, which circulate in the blood. These molecules may have specific action on the central nervous system (CNS), promoting such symptoms as irritability, insomnia or stupor, and loss of appetite. One of the major mysteries of uremia is the cause of the **central nervous system derangements**, which are certainly as serious as the more treatable chemical disorders and are often more debilitating to the patient. Current explanations suggest that there is no single factor, such as creatinine, or small molecule such as urea, but that probably the physiologic response to a reduced glomerular filtration rate calls out a variety of hormones in an effort to restore homeostasis. The best known of these middle-sized molecules is parathyroid hormone, and there is some evidence that the CNS-depressing effects may be traced to such hormones.

The destruction of the kidney also decreases the patient's buffering capability, and with retention of anion excess, he becomes **acidotic**. At the same time, the kidney fails to excrete adequate amounts of potassium, sodium, and phosphates. The elevated serum phosphate level is met with a reduction in serum calcium, which in turn leads to the muscle twitching commonly seen in uremic patients. The retention of the sodium leads to increased water retention, and patients usually become edematous. Most important, perhaps, is the elevated serum potassium level that frequently occurs. This condition is life-threatening because hyperkalemia (high serum potassium) has a direct effect on cardiac muscle contractility. Sudden death in uremia is often due to cardiac arrhythmia traceable to abnormal serum electrolytes.

The **anemia** that occurs so often in uremic patients and is so serious has been attributed to the microscopic blood loss that occurs in many types of kidney disease. There is some evidence that the loss of erythropoietin due to destruction of kidney tissue may be significant in the etiology of this anemia, or perhaps the acidosis depresses the production of these red blood cells.

Kidney Stones

A urinary calculus is a stone that forms in the urinary tract. The common site of formation of the stone is the kidney, but it may form in the bladder. Stones in the kidney originate in the renal pelvis most frequently. Stone in bladder may begin in the bladder, but more often it starts in the kidney (Fig. 20–17) and passes down into the bladder, where the stone continues to grow.

The causes of stone are attributed classically to infections, to irritation, and to disease of the parathyroid glands (hyperfunction). In the kidney, in addition to infection, a high concentration of crystalline salts in the urine probably plays a part, for a urinary stone is composed of such inorganic materials as uric acid, oxalates, and calcium phosphate. Some stones consist entirely of one of these materials, but usually there is a mixture of 2 or more. Diet may be a factor in some cases, for stones are common in some parts of India, where a large proportion of the population lives on a vitamin-poor diet. Vitamin A is perhaps the

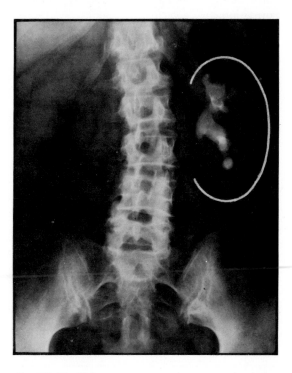

Fig. 20–17. This roentgenogram shows a renal calculus (kidney stone) on the patient's left side. The white mark outlines the kidney. Incidentally, there is scoliosis of the vertebral spine.

most important of the vitamins in this respect. A small tumor of the parathyroid glands may cause stone formation. These glands, which are 4 in number and lie in contact with the thyroid gland in the neck, are important regulators of calcium metabolism. When they become overactive, owing to the development of an innocent tumor, too much calcium phosphate is removed from the bones, carried by the blood to the kidneys, and deposited there. Risk factors for stone formation are shown in Table 20–3, and the percentage of these factors that contribute to stone formation are shown in Table 20–4.

The significance of kidney stones is twofold. First, the presence of stone may cause extreme pain and may obstruct or partially obstruct some part of the "waterworks." This obstruction, as we have outlined before, predisposes a person to stasis and infection. Although the pain may be alleviated when the stone is removed or passed, the underlying cause of the stone raises the second and more

Table 20–3. Risk Factors for Kidney Stone Formation

Family history
Dehydration
Medications
  Vitamins A, D, and C
  Acetazolamide
Urinary pH
Diet
Hyperoxaluria
Hyperuricosuria
Hypercalcemia

Table 20–4. Causes of Stone Formation

Idiopathic hypercalciuria	20.7%
Marginal hypercalciuria	11.5%
Hyperuricosuria	14%
Hypercalciuria and	
hyperuricosuria	11.7%
Primary hyperparathyroidism	5.2%
No disorder	20.2%
Other disorders	16.2%

(From Coe, F. L.: Treated and untreated recurrent calcium nephrolithiasis in patients with idiopathic hypercalciuria, hyperuricosuria, or no metabolic disorder. Ann. Intern. Med., 87:404, 1977.)

important question. Why did the stone occur in the first place? As outlined, whenever a stone is identified in the genitourinary system, it is desirable to identify the possible physiologic disturbance that permitted the condition to develop. Stones are fortunately rare, and such diseases as gout and cystinosis are treatable today, whereas 25 years ago, the recurrence of stones was a dreaded and inevitable consequence of those diseases.

Malignant Tumors of the Urinary Tract

Although tumors of the kidneys are sufficiently common to keep us aware of their existence, they are sometimes amenable to surgical treatment and can often be identified early enough to be cured. Hematuria is the most common early sign of a tumor, and the occurrence of a palpable mass in the region of the kidney suggests a new growth (Fig. 20–18). Because of their tendency to invade and to metastasize, kidney tumors offer a serious threat. Tumors of the genitourinary system are classified in different ways; it is sufficient here to name the hypernephroma or clear cell tumor, which is the most common tumor of adults, and the Wilms tumor, the most common tumor of children. Tumors of the pelvis, urethra, and bladder also occur, and hematuria may be the first signal of their presence.

Long-continued fever is a remarkable feature in some cases of kidney tumors. Removal of the affected kidney is often curative, provided metastases have not occurred.

Wilms Tumor. This neoplasm, first described by Wilms, has a peak incidence at 15 months of age and usually occurs during the first 3 years of life. It has a constant geographic occurrence and an incidence of 6 per 100,000 children under 15 years of age.

The tumor often appears as an abdominal mass, sometimes nearly filling the child's abdomen. Surgical removal results in a cure rate of 80% when the tumor is removed under 1 year of age. Fever occurs in 50% of cases, and distant metastases are a common complication.

Recently, this germinal tumor has been recognized to occur in children with the syndrome of mental retardation, other genitouri-

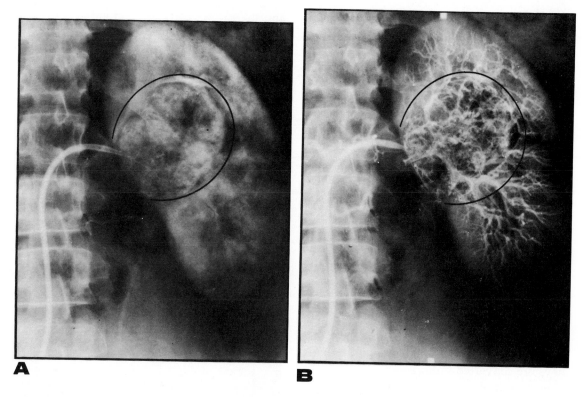

Fig. 20-18. *A,* This selective arteriogram shows an increased vascularity in the upper pole of the kidney. The injection material is present in the catheter on the left. The area of neovascularity is outlined in black. *B,* A later film from the same arteriogram shows, within the black outline, the abnormal area of small blood vessels. This is interpreted as a renal tumor.

nary abnormalities, and the absence of the iris of the eye. This pattern has been credited to the deletion of a small portion on the short arm of chromosome 11, thus relating the tumor whose origin has been much debated to a chromosomal abnormality.

Carcinoma of the Bladder. The chief tumor of the bladder is carcinoma, and it is often a low grade of malignancy. In the last 50 years, epithelial bladder tumors have been found much more frequently among old persons than before. Although the tumors used to be much more common in men than in women, this pattern too is changing. Carcinoma of the bladder is also slightly more common than it used to be, but this increase can be attributed to the rise in the number of biopsies, largely owing to better techniques for visualization and operation.

The tumor usually projects into the bladder in a papillary form. Sometimes it assumes a villous form, the growth consisting of delicate fern-like processes that unfold like a piece of seaweed when the bladder is filled with water and is viewed with the cystoscope. Each of these processes contains a thin-walled blood vessel, which is readily injured when the bladder contracts during urination, so that hemorrhage is common. The outstanding symptom is therefore blood in the urine, usually unaccompanied by pain (painless hematuria). Such tumors may be removed by surgery only to recur repeatedly; in fact, it may be necessary to remove the whole bladder and to transplant the ureters into a loop of ileum.

ETIOLOGY. A number of substances are known to be carcinogenic for the bladder. Workers in aniline dye factories are liable to develop the disease, the material being inhaled, and then carried to the bladder by the blood. The sharp-pointed ova of *Schistosoma haematobium* or bilharzia can stimulate the development of cancer of the bladder. That condition has its highest incidence in Egypt, where bilharzia infection is prevalent. The latest discovery is that cigarette smoking in excess is associated with the disease, carcinogenic metabolites being excreted in the urine.

TREATMENT. This consists in opening the bladder and in treating the tumor either by radium or by surgical removal. If an early diagnosis is made with the aid of the cystoscope, an instrument passed into the bladder by means of which a view of the interior can be obtained, the prognosis is good in many cases.

Congenital Cystic Kidney

Known also as polycystic kidney, this condition is a congenital defect of the kidney, an error in development. About 30% of cases are symptomatic in infants, the majority stillborn. In the remaining cases, symptoms are noted in early adult and middle life. The condition is nearly always bilateral. The kidneys are converted into a series of cysts, and may be enormously enlarged (Fig. 20–19). The contents of the cysts are watery, but hemorrhage may occur from intervening vessels, so that, should the cyst rupture into the renal pelvis, there will be hematuria. Hardly any renal tissue may be left, so that the occurrence of hypertension, renal insufficiency,

and uremia is easily understood. There is a strong hereditary tendency. Small cysts in other organs, more particularly the liver and the pancreas, are an indication of a general disturbance in development.

Summary

A reflection on the variety of syndromes that occur in kidney disease of different types indicates the wide spectrum of complaints that can be traced to these organs. We have seen that flank pain, chills, and fever—signs of infection—can often be traced to acute abscess or pyelonephritis in 1 or both kidneys. At another extreme, nonspecific signs of

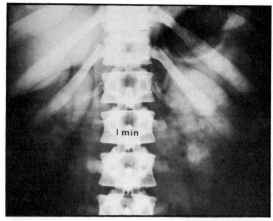

A

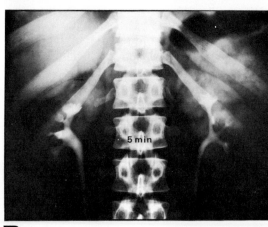

B

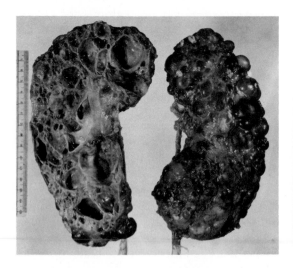

Fig. 20–19. This photograph of a **congenital cystic kidney** shows the absence of any normal renal parenchyma. It is no wonder that the uremic syndrome eventually occurs with this progressive, slow destruction of the kidney. (McGill University, Department of Pathology Museum.)

Fig. 20–20. *A,* This film shows a normal intravenous pyelogram after 1 minute. The kidneys are normal in position, size, shape, and contour. This is called the renal phase. *B,* This is the 5 minute film, which shows the excretion of dye into the pelvis and ureters. Again, this is a normal film.

Table 20–5.   Rehabilitation Rate for Dialysis Patients and Cadaver Kidney Recipients

	HEMODIALYSIS	TRANSPLANTATION
Total patients	359 (100%)	272 (100%)
Complete rehabilitation	179 (50%)	205 (75%)
Partial rehabilitation	79 (22%)	14 (5%)
No rehabilitation	101 (28%)	53 (20%)

(From Kreis, H.: Selection of hemodialysis versus cadaveric transplantation. Kidney Int. [Suppl.], *13*:S–91, 1978.)

loss of appetite, weakness, and muscle twitching are traceable to the uremic syndrome, a terminal phase in any renal disease. In between, signs such as hematuria, oliguria, edema, proteinuria, or palpably enlarged kidneys can herald such diverse entities as glomerulonephritis, tubular necrosis, stones, tumors, or congenital cystic disease of the kidney.

The correct diagnosis is arrived at when careful history-taking and physical and laboratory examinations have been carried out, and when such special studies as are warranted, e.g., pyelograms (Fig. 20–20), arteriography, and biopsy may have been undertaken. The most heartening thought, however, is the recent success in managing serious kidney disease by a combination of dialysis and transplant. Table 20–5 and Figure 20–21 illustrate the rehabilitation rates for dialysis and transplant patients, and also show the improvement during 3 periods of patient and cadaver kidney transplants. More than in any other organ system, modern medical and surgical advances offer the patient with severe renal failure hope for a reasonable life.

Examination of the Urine

Urinalysis serves to show the presence of disease in the kidneys and in the bladder. It also indicates the presence of diabetes, although this disease is not connected in any way with a disorder of renal function. In a complete urinalysis, the following points are noted: color, reaction, specific gravity, a chemical examination for albumin and sugar, and a microscopic examination for blood, pus, and casts.

Color. The normal color of the urine is yellow or amber. The intensity of the color depends on the amount of water the urine contains. If the patient is drinking a large amount of water, the urine is di-

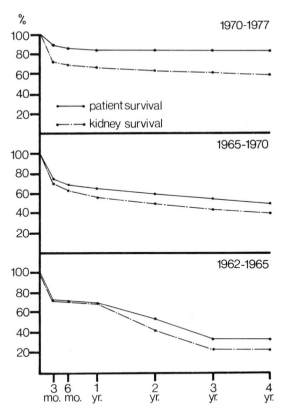

Fig. 20–21. These graphs show the improvement in survival from the time of operation of patients who received transplanted cadaver kidneys between June 1962 and January 1977. The graphs illustrate both the survival rates of the patients and the success of the kidney transplants. (From Kreis, H.: Selection of hemodialysis versus cadaveric transplantation. Kidney Int., *13*, [Suppl.] *8*:S-91, 1978.)

lute and pale. On the other hand, if much water is lost by perspiration in hot weather or as the result of fever, the urine becomes darker. In diabetes, there is a marked increase in the output of water, so that the urine is correspondingly pale. The same is true of chronic nephritis, in which the kidneys lose their normal power of concentrating the urine. A smoky red or brown color is usually due to the presence of large amounts of blood.

pH. Although the blood is alkaline in reaction, the normal reaction of the urine is acidic. In infections of the bladder, the reaction tends to be alkaline, owing to the action of bacteria. It is important to remember that if the specimen of urine is allowed to stand for many hours in a warm room, the normal acidic reaction may be changed to alkaline because of the action of contaminating bacteria. The urine should therefore be fresh and sent at once to the laboratory. Decomposing urine has a characteristic ammoniacal smell (to be noted in some urinals), owing to the production of ammonia from the urea in the urine.

Specific Gravity. The concentration or specific gravity of the urine depends on the amount of solids (waste products of the tissues) held in solution. When the urine is secreted by the glomeruli, it is of low concentration, but during its passage along the convoluted tubules a large amount of water is absorbed; this normal process is known as the concentrating power of the kidney. Extensive kidney disease, particularly chronic nephritis, results in destruction of many of the renal tubules, with corresponding interference with the concentrating power. This loss of the normal concentrating power of the kidneys is most valuable as evidence of the presence of chronic diffuse renal disease. For this reason, the estimation of the specific gravity of the urine is a procedure of the greatest importance.

The specific gravity of pure water is 1.000. The specific gravity of normal urine varies from 1.010 to 1.025, but it may be even higher as the result of loss of water through profuse perspiration, diarrhea, or other means. In health there should be a variation of at least 10 points in the course of 24 hours, the first specimen in the morning being always the most concentrated. A high fixed specific gravity (1.030 to 1.040) suggests the presence of sugar (i.e., diabetes) or protein.

Albumin. When albumin is present in the urine (albuminuria), it comes from the blood and is an indication of inflammation in the glomeruli, as a result of which the permeability of the capillaries is increased.

Sugar. In nearly all cases, the presence of sugar in the urine (glycosuria) indicates diabetes mellitus. The rare exceptions need not be discussed here. The kidneys are normal, but the blood sugar is so high that some of it leaks out into the urine. As the sugar is dissolved in the urine, the specific gravity is considerably above normal, i.e., 1.040 or higher.

Diacetic Acid and Acetone. In the discussion of diabetes, reference was made to the presence in the urine of diacetic acid and acetone, known as ketone bodies and indicative of acidosis, a grave complication of diabetes. When sugar is found in the urine, it is therefore essential to test for the presence of ketone bodies.

Blood. If there is much blood in the urine, the former imparts to the latter a dark brown or smoky character. If the quantity of blood is small, there may be no apparent change, and microscopic examination of a centrifuged specimen for red cells is necessary. Blood in the urine (hematuria) with rare exceptions indicates disease of the kidney, ureter, or bladder. The disease may be inflammation (acute or chronic nephritis), tuberculosis, stone, or tumor. Painless hematuria without any other symptoms suggests a malignant tumor of the kidney or bladder. When associated with pain, hematuria suggests a stone in the kidney or bladder, or tuberculosis of these organs.

Pus. Pyuria or pus in the urine gives a cloudy or turbid appearance. Microscopically, large numbers of pus cells (polymorphonuclear leukocytes) are readily recognized. Pus in the urine may be caused by suppuration in the kidney, inflammation of the bladder (cystitis), and tuberculosis or stone in the kidney or bladder. In the male, pus may come from the urethra, and in the female, from the vagina. If pus is found in female urine, a second specimen should be obtained from the bladder by means of a catheter.

When tuberculosis of the kidney is suspected, a search must be made for tubercle bacilli. These may be found in the centrifuged deposit. If not, a guinea pig may be inoculated with a small quantity of urine, or a culture may be made on special media. In both cases, unfortunately, several weeks may elapse before a definite result can be obtained.

Casts. A urinary cast is a cast or mold of the renal tubules formed by a collection of precipitated albumin. Red and white blood cells and epithelial cells from the lining of the kidney are often incorporated with the cast. Casts, which are oblong in shape, tend to disappear when the urine has been kept for some time; the specimen should therefore be fresh. The importance of casts is that they form an important feature of urinary findings in the various forms of nephritis. A few casts, spoken of in case reports as "an occasional cast," may, however, be present in the absence of definite disease. When the urine is found to contain albumin, it must always be examined for casts.

Crystals of various kinds are often found in the urine, but as they are of no special pathologic significance, they will not be described here.

The accompanying Table 20–6 summarizes findings in normal urine and in different diseases.

MALE GENITAL TRACT

Prostate

The prostate is a gland about the size of a horse chestnut situated at the neck of the bladder and surrounding the urethra. It really belongs to the male reproductive system, but, when diseased, it produces symptoms associated with the urinary system on account of its position at the outlet of the bladder. Three diseases of the male accessory gland, the prostate, deserve mention in this brief section: prostatitis, benign hyperplasia, and carcinoma.

Prostatitis. As in other organs that are hidden in the body, inflammation may frequently occur, but the predisposing causes and etiologic agents are not always discovered or understood. Whenever there is inflammation in a glandular structure that elim-

Table 20–6. Observations in the Normal Urine and in Different Kidney Diseases

NATURE OF RENAL LESION	PROTEIN EXCRETION G/24 HR	R.B.C. MILL/24 HR	EPITHELIAL & W.B.C. MILL/24 HR	ABNORMAL CELLS	CASTS MILL/24 HR	BLOOD CASTS	R.B.C. CASTS	FATTY CASTS	BROAD CASTS	WAXY CASTS	OTHER CASTS
Normal	male 0 to 0.060 female 0 to 0.090	0 to 0.130	0 to 0.650	—	0 to 0.002	—	—	—	—	—	—
Glomerulitis	0.5 to 5.0	1 to 1,000	1 to 400	—	0.1 to 0.5	+	+	—	—	—	+
Tubular necrosis	5.0 to 40.0	1 to 100	20 to 1,000	oval fat bodies	0.1 to 2.0	—	—	+	—	—	+
Malignant arteriolitis	2.0 to 10.0	1 to 100	1 to 200	—	0.1 to 1.0	—	+	+	—	—	+
Renal failure	2.0 to 7.0	1 to 10	1 to 50	—	0.5 to 4.0	—	—	—	+	+	+
Infection	0.5 to 7.0	0 to 1	20 to 2,000	pus cells	0 to 0.1	—	—	—	—	—	—
Neoplasm	0	0 to 1,000	0	tumor cells	0	—	—	—	—	—	—

inates its secretions by a duct, or a system of ducts, and when the controls over secretion include nervous stimulation, hormones, and a variety of other agents, there are legitimate theories as to the importance of each factor in causing the inflammation (consider the theories of the etiology of pancreatitis).

Inflammation of the prostate can commonly arise as a result of infection by bacteria from neighboring structures such as the urethra (gonococcus) or bladder (E. coli). Often, a history of exposure to venereal disease or of urinary tract infection can be elicited, and the prostate secretions can be stained and cultured to show the offending organism. Treatment with appropriate antibiotics usually limits the disease, although the prostate does not always respond rapidly to chemotherapy because of the difficulties some drugs have in reaching the site of inflammation. Naturally, an abscess in the prostate is anatomically a different matter from a boil of the buttock. The prostate is a favorite site for occult or hidden infections to smolder, causing fever of obscure origin and a long-term feeling of ill health.

Another frequent cause of prostatitis is the occurrence of acute, sterile inflammation in young or middle-aged men who have indulged in high living with lots of alcohol, coffee, spiced foods, cigars, and little sleep, as is common at a convention or on a holiday. The symptoms of urgency, frequency, and retention of urine lead one to suspect cystitis and/or prostatitis. The absence of discharge, fever, and flank pain, combined with the history of fatigue and dietary excess, point to this diagnosis. It is not clear why the prostate should be the target for such inflammation (as sometimes involves the pancreas in similar situations) but it is well known to urologists that this small gland is a kind of Achilles heel.

Hyperplasia in the Prostate. When the gland becomes enlarged, and can be felt through the rectum as being increased in size, the cause of this is an increase in the number of glandular cells and stroma. Enlargement of the prostate is common in men over 60 years of age, but, fortunately, it only produces symptoms in about 8% of these cases. The disease is hardly ever seen in early life. The cause of the enlargement is probably some disturbance of the hormones from the sex glands that is likely to occur as the period of reproductive activity declines. It is really a hyperplasia or overgrowth rather than a hypertrophy or enlargement. It is comparable to the condition of the breast known as chronic mastitis or cystic hyperplasia, which is described in Chapter 21.

The effects of prostatic enlargement are partial obstruction to the outflow of urine and an inability to empty the bladder completely (Fig. 20–22). The residual urine retained in the bladder tends to become infected. Two great dangers that threaten the man suffering from enlargement of the prostate are (1) urinary retention with back-pressure on the ureters and kidneys, and (2) infection that ascends from the bladder to the kidneys. The results will be distension of the bladder, cystitis, dilation of the ureters, hydronephrosis (Fig. 20–23), and pyonephrosis. Death may be due either to sepsis or to renal failure.

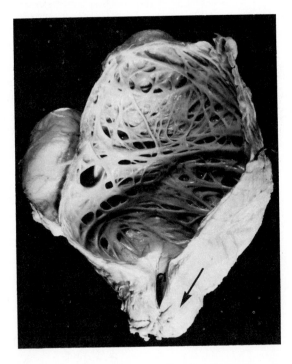

Fig. 20–22. The **prostate,** a small walnut-sized organ, can be recognized at the arrow. Most of the photograph shows the interior wall of the urinary bladder, which is markedly trabeculated. This is the result of the partial obstruction at the level of the prostate. A prominent posterior lobe is apparent at a. Benign prostatic hyperplasia is a common disease in men over 60. (McGill University, Department of Pathology Museum.)

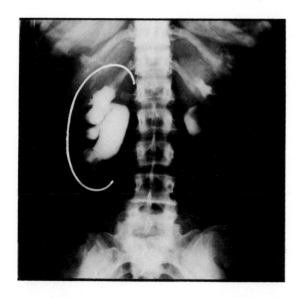

Fig. 20–23. This roentgenogram shows the collection of dye in the kidney, displaying an extraordinary amount of material. This illustrates right-sided hydronephrosis due to obstruction in the ureter.

Treatment has entirely changed the outlook for the man in declining years whose last days used to be made pitiable by prostatic enlargement. The enlarged gland can be removed by various surgical measures. One of these days, it may be possible to control the enlargement by the use of hormones and thereby to render operation unnecessary.

Cancer of the Prostate. Carcinoma of the prostate is common, unfortunately. An old saying is that 70% of men over 70 have cancer of the prostate. Of course, this may be only a histologic diagnosis of a microscopic lesion.

However, the problem is real enough. Each year there are 42,000 new cases of prostatic carcinoma in the United States, with 17,000 deaths, which makes the disease the second leading cause of cancer deaths among men. The incidence has continued to rise to a present figure of 21 per 100,000 population, and is accounted for by improvements in screening and in accuracy of diagnosis.

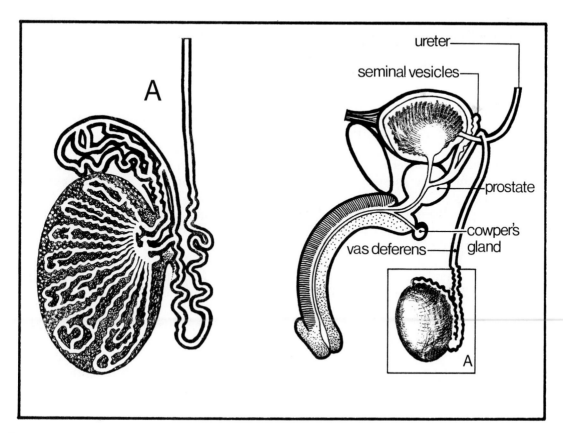

Fig. 20–24. *Left,* This diagram shows the anatomy of the testicle and epididymis. *Right,* The urinary bladder and external genitalia are shown schematically. (Redrawn from Christopher, F.: *A Textbook of Surgery,* 5th Ed., Philadelphia and London, W. B. Saunders.)

The prostate becomes enlarged and hard and may cause symptoms of urinary obstruction. The tumor infiltrates the surrounding structures early and extensively, and, on that account, surgical treatment is far from satisfactory. The blood vessels and lymphatics are also invaded at an early date, and metastases are formed in various organs, particularly in the bones. When an elderly man is found to be suffering from bone pain, carcinoma of the prostate should always be suspected.

However, new light and new hope have been shed on the subject of carcinoma of the prostate by the demonstration that the male hormone of the testicle exerts an important influence on the growth of the prostate (Fig. 20–24). Castration (removal of both testicles) before puberty prevents development of the prostate, and castration in adult life causes regression of the normal gland. These factors have been applied to the problem of the control of cancer of the prostate with remarkable results, for castration often leads to shrinking of the tumor and to relief of the severe bone pains caused by metastases in the skeleton, particularly in the spine. The administration of stilbestrol, the synthetic form of the female sex hormone, also affords marked relief, probably because of interference with the male hormone. This form of therapy has largely replaced castration. Sometimes the 2 are combined.

A valuable means of determining the improvement produced by these methods of treatment is afforded by estimating the acid phosphatase in the blood. Acid phosphatase is an enzyme produced by the prostate. The amount in the serum is greatly increased when cancer of the prostate develops, and especially when secondary tumors are formed in the bones. Under these circumstances there is a marked rise in the level of the blood acid phosphatase, a rise that disappears if the treatment is successful. The word "success" is used in a relative sense only, for it is not claimed that cancer of the prostate can be cured by these means.

Testis and Epididymis

One word before considering the diseases of the testis. Jules Verne described a marvel-

Table 20–7.   Sperm Journey

Seminiferous tubule	30 to 80 cm
Straight tubule	0.2 cm
Rete testis	1.0 cm
Efferent ductule	4 to 6 cm
Common lower vas	15 to 20 cm
Epididymis	400 to 600 cm
Vas deferens	40 to 45 cm
Ejaculatory duct	1.9 cm
Urethra	20 cm
Uterus	2.5 cm
Uterine tube	7.1 cm
	7.84 m

ous journey in *Around in the World in 80 Days*, which is known to many, but the sperm of man makes what seems to us to be an equally incredible journey, as shown in the accompanying Table 20–7. Surely, to take a voyage of 7.84 meters within the real distance of something significantly less than a foot requires remarkable engineering.

Although there is much reference in idle conversation to the "male menopause," there is no biologic evidence for any such phenomenon. There are abundant recorded instances of gentlemen in their 80's who have sired progeny, and histologic examination of testes often demonstrate spermatogonia in nonagenarians. It seems that the male menopause is more a frame of mind or an attitude; it has been called the time when a man's attention turns to his teeth rather than to his testes.

The epididymis is the convoluted excretory duct of the testis and, although it lies separate from, although attached to, the testis, it may be considered with the latter in connection with disease.

Epididymitis. By far the most common cause of inflammation of the epididymis is the gonococcus, which may reach the male urethra during an acute attack of gonorrhea. The epididymis becomes enlarged, hard, and tender. Minute abscesses are formed, but there is no extensive breaking down of tissue, such as might be expected. The inflammation is acute and subsides quickly, but often leaves fibrous scars that obliterate the seminiferous tubules. When the condition is bilateral, complete sterility may result.

Orchitis. The 2 common causes of inflammation of the testis (orchitis) are injury and mumps. Traumatic orchitis, caused by a blow, is often followed by acute inflammatory edema of the organ. Mumps orchitis is usually unilateral, and is rarely seen before the age of puberty, being most common in young men. It may follow or may precede the enlargement of the parotid gland or involvement of the pancreas, which is characteristic of mumps.

Tuberculosis. This disease usually starts in the lower pole of the epididymis (Fig. 20–25). Tuberculous nodules are formed throughout that organ, and caseation may occur later, with ulceration through the skin. Infection may spread to the testis and along the spermatic cord, which is felt to be thickened and nodular. If the disease is progressive, there may be successive involvement of the prostate, the other epididymis, the bladder, and finally the kidneys.

Tumors. In the testis, tumors are fairly common. There are 2 principal groups, named seminoma and teratoma. The seminoma appears to arise from the seminiferous tubules of the testis, whereas the teratoma is believed to arise from a primitive germ cell, and consists of a variety of structures. Both tumors are highly malignant

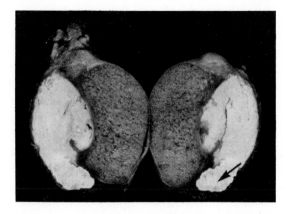

Fig. 20–25. This section of a testicle shows a large area of white material, which is caseous necrosis caused by the tubercle bacillus. Tuberculosis usually starts at the lower pole of the epididymis (at arrow) and involves the whole epididymis. (McGill University, Department of Pathology Museum.)

and tend to spread both by the lymphatics and along the blood stream. Fortunately, the seminoma is radiosensitive, and early diagnosis combined with irradiation has resulted in many cures. Other rare tumors are found in the testis, but these do not need to be considered here.

SYNOPSIS

The kidneys filter blood and excrete urine; they act as excretory organs for catabolic waste products, as water conserving organs, as electrolyte monitors, as buffering agents, and as stimulators of the bone marrow.

Infectious diseases (pyelonephritis and abscesses) are the most common and important of all kidney diseases. Partial obstruction leads to stasis and is an important predisposing cause to kidney infections.

Renal vascular diseases may be of large or small vessels and may be either the cause or result of hypertension.

Glomerular diseases are of immune etiology and may result in proteinuria and the nephrotic syndrome.

Acute renal failure may have diverse etiologies and should be differentiated from other causes of little urine output.

Chronic renal failure (uremia) may be caused by any renal disease, but usually more than 80% of the kidney is diseased anatomically. The symptoms and signs are diverse and are sometimes difficult to recognize.

Examination of the urine is the most important laboratory approach to kidney disease.

Three diseases of the prostate, prostatitis, hyperplasia, and cancer, occur frequently.

Terms

Nephrosis	*Arteriolosclerotic nephritis*	*Nephrotic syndrome*
Glomerulus	*Arteriolonecrosis*	*Uremia*
Pyelonephritis	*Gomerulonephritis*	*Hematuria*
Arteriosclerotic nephritis	*Acute tubular necrosis*	*Hypernephroma*

FURTHER READING

Editorial: What causes toxicity in uraemia? Br. Med. J., 2:143, 1977.

Bakir, A. A., and Dunea, G.: Current trends in the treatment of uraemia: a view from the United States. Br. Med. J., 1:914, 1979.

Brenner, B. M., and Humes, H. D.: Mechanics of glomerular ultrafiltration. N. Engl. J. Med., 297:148, 1977.

Broadus, A. E., and Thier, S. O.: Metabolic basis of renal-stone disease. N. Engl. J. Med., 300:839, 1979.

Campbell, J. D., and Campbell, A. R.: A patient's perspective of end-stage renal disease. N. Engl. J. Med., 299:386, 1978.

Coe, F. L., Keck, J., and Norton, E. R.: The natural history of calcium urolithiasis. J.A.M.A., 238:1519, 1977.

Dixon, F. J., Feldman, J. D., and Vasquez, J. J.: Experimental glomerulonephritis. J. Exp. Med., 113:899, 1961.

Fawcett, D. W.: The cell biology of gametogenesis in the male. Perspect. Biol. Med., 22:S56, 1979.

Freeman, R. B.: Does bacteriuria lead to renal failure? Clin. Nephrol., 1:61, 1973.

Guttmann, R. D.: Renal transplantation. N. Engl. J. Med., 301:975, 1979.

Heptinstall, R. H.: *Pathology of the Kidney.* Boston, Little, Brown, 1966.

Jamison, R. L., and Maffly, R. H.: The urinary concentrating mechanism. N. Engl. J. Med., 295:1059, 1976.

Klein, L. A.: Prostatic carcinoma. N. Engl. J. Med., 300:824, 1979.

Leaf, A., and Cotran, R.: *Renal Pathophysiology.* New York, Oxford University Press, 1976.

Levinsky, N. G.: Pathophysiology and acute renal failure. N. Engl. J. Med., 296:1453, 1977.

Mauer, S. M., et al.: Development of diabetic vascular lesions in normal kidneys transplanted into patients with diabetes mellitus. N. Engl. J. Med., 295:916, 1976.

Merrill, J. P.: Glomerulonephritis. N. Engl. J. Med., 290:257, 1974.

Ober, W.: Boswell's gonorrhea. Bull. N. Y. Acad. Med., 45:587, 1969.

Smith, L. H., Van Den Berg, C. J., and Wilson, D. M.: Nutrition and urolithiasis. N. Engl. J. Med., 298:87, 1978.

Female Reproductive System (Including Breast)

21

Natural man has only two primal passions: to get and to beget.—OSLER

FEMALE REPRODUCTIVE SYSTEM

Anatomy

The female genital system includes the external genitalia or vulva, vagina, uterus, fallopian tubes, and ovaries (Fig. 21–1).

The external genitalia or vulva include the mons pubis, the labia majora and minora, the clitoris, the openings of the urethra and vagina, and the perineum. These structures are covered by stratified squamous epithelium and may contain skin appendages such as hair and sebaceous glands.

The vagina or birth canal connects the opening of the uterus with the vulva, and is the usual mode of exit of menstrual fluids and the products of conception. The vagina is lined by stratified squamous epithelium and contains 2 layers of smooth muscle in its wall.

The cervix is the neck of the uterus. Its funnel shape connects the uterine cavity with the upper vagina. The portion of the cervix that extends into the vagina (exocervix) is covered by squamous epithelium. The endocervical canal is lined by mucus-secreting columnar epithelium. The wall of the cervix contains dense connective tissue and some smooth muscle.

The uterine corpus or body is a pear-shaped organ, about the size of a large spoon, that sits on the lower pelvis between the bladder and the rectum. It provides a proper environment for the growth and development of a fetus. It is lined by the endometrium, which changes remarkably during the course of a menstrual cycle (Fig. 21–2). The myometrium (uterine wall) is a thick layer of muscle. The outer surface (serosa) is covered by the smooth pelvic peritoneum. The uterus grows tremen-

469

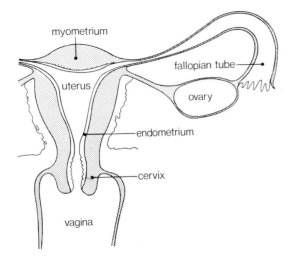

Fig. 21–1. This drawing shows the relationships of ovary, fallopian tube, and uterus. The muscular wall of the uterus is called the myometrium, the lining is called the endometrium, and the junction and entrance to the uterus is called the cervix. The vagina is shown at the bottom.

dously in shape and in volume during pregnancy, and then returns almost to its original size like a deflated balloon within 6 weeks after the birth of an infant.

The fallopian tubes extend from the upper corners of the uterine cavity to the ovaries. They are suspended by folds of the broad ligament and tend to fall back behind the uterus. Each tube is 8 to 12 cm long. The portion near the uterus (the isthmus) is narrow. The diameter increases gradually toward the fimbriated (fringed) end, next to the ovary. The function of the fallopian tubes is to receive mature ova from the ovary, to provide the site where fertilization occurs, and to transport the fertilized ovum to the uterine cavity, where it will implant and continue its growth.

The ovaries are 2 almond-sized organs on the pelvis at the fimbriated end of each fallopian tube. They are attached to the broad ligament, and also to the posterior wall of the uterus. The ovary releases mature ova and steroid hormones, mainly estrogen and progesterone.

Menstrual Cycle

The average menstrual cycle lasts for 28 days and is divided into the follicular or proliferative phase, ovulation, and the luteal or secretory phase.

During the follicular (proliferative) phase, follicles on the ovary begin to grow under the influence of FSH (follicle-stimulating hormone, released from the anterior pituitary on orders from the hypothalamus) (Fig. 21–3). The hypothalamus issues its orders for the release of FSH when it senses

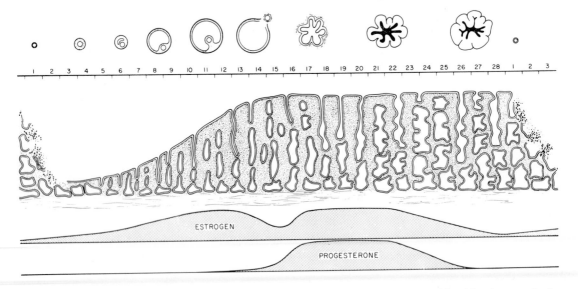

Fig. 21–2. This drawing shows the size and appearance of the endometrial epithelium in the middle of the picture, at the days of the menstrual cycle shown as numbers at the top. The appearance of the ovum and corpus luteum is shown above the top line, and the relative levels of the 2 hormones, estrogen and progesterone, are indicated at the bottom of the figure. (From Bloom, W., and Fawcett, D. W.: *A Textbook of Histology,* 10th Ed. Philadelphia, W. B. Saunders, 1975.)

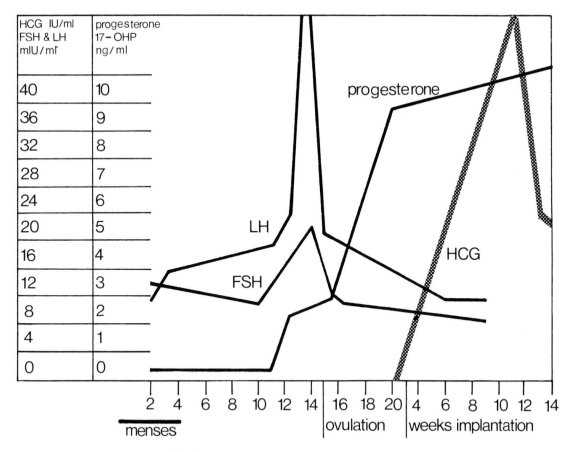

HCG IU/ml FSH & LH mIU/ml	progesterone 17-OHP ng/ml
40	10
36	9
32	8
28	7
24	6
20	5
16	4
12	3
8	2
4	1
0	0

Fig. 21–3. This chart shows the relative amounts of the differing hormones, luteinizing hormone (LH), follicle-stimulating hormone (FSH), progesterone, and human chorionic gonadotropin (HCG) during the menstrual cycle. (From Speroff, L., Glass, R. H., and Kase, N. G.: *Clinical Gynecologic Endocrinology and Infertility,* 2nd Ed. Baltimore, Williams & Wilkins, 1978.)

the declining level of estrogen in the blood, which has occurred at the end of the previous menstrual cycle and during the days of endometrial shedding or menstruation. As follicles grow, they produce estrogen, which acts on its target organs to induce growth. The main target organ is the endometrium. Endometrium responds to estrogen by growth of epithelium, by reformation of its connec-tive tissue, and by growth of the small spiral arterioles that supply it with blood. Although several follicles begin to grow under the influence of FSH, usually only 1 becomes fully mature.

At approximately the fourteenth day of the cycle, a sudden increase in estrogen and FSH stimulates the hypothalamus to release a surge of luteinizing hormone (LH) from the anterior pituitary. LH

Table 21–1. Risk-Benefit Ratio of Contraceptives

METHOD	FAILURE RATE OR EFFECTIVENESS	MAJOR SIDE EFFECTS	MINOR SIDE EFFECTS	APPROXIMATE COST $
Female sterilization	1 in 200–1 in 1000	post-tubal syndrome	none	850
Male sterilization	1 in 1000	possible atherosclerosis	none	175
Oral contraceptives	0.5 per 100 woman years	thrombophlebitis, pulmonary embolus, cerebral thrombosis	pseudopregnancy	75/yr
Intrauterine devices	2–3 per 100 woman years	uterine perforation, pelvic infections	uterine bleeding and cramping	75/yr
Barrier methods	3–20 per 100 woman years	none	allergic reaction, nuisance to use	30/yr

(From Droegemueller, W., and Bressler, R.: Effectiveness and risks of contraception. Annu. Rev. Med., *31*:329, 1980.)

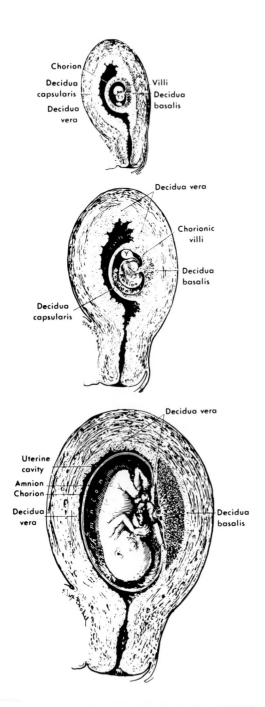

Chorion
Decidua capsularis
Decidua vera
Villi
Decidua basalis

Decidua vera
Chorionic villi
Decidua basalis
Decidua capsularis

Decidua vera
Uterine cavity
Amnion
Chorion
Decidua vera
Decidua basalis

Fig. 21–4. These drawings show the appearance of the different components of the implanted, fertilized egg in the wall of the uterus. These are shown at different stages of growth. The fetus lies within the amniotic cavity in the bottom figure. (From Bloom, W., and Fawcett, D. W.: *A Textbook of Histology*, 10th Ed. Philadelphia, W. B. Saunders, 1975.)

travels to the ovary and releases a mature ovum into the fallopian tube. This is called **ovulation**. It is signalled by a rise in body temperature that can be detected by daily measurement. The follicle that contained the maturing ovum is transformed into a corpus luteum by the action of LH. The corpus luteum produces large amounts of progesterone that cause the endometrium to undergo changes that characterize the secretory phase of the cycle.

The ovum should be fertilized within 48 hours of its release from the ovary (Table 21–1). If this does not occur, the ovum disintegrates, the corpus luteum wanes and collapses, hormone production declines, and the endometrium breaks down and is shed. When the hypothalamus senses the low level of estrogen in the blood, it begins again to order the anterior pituitary to release FSH, which starts a new cycle of follicular growth in the ovary.

If the ovum is fertilized, it spends 2 to 3 days passing through the tube, where it begins to divide (Fig. 21–4). When it reaches the endometrial cavity, it spends another 2 to 3 days dividing before it implants itself in the endometrium on the wall of the uterus. By this time, the secretory activities of the endometrial glands are at a peak and are able to provide a wealth of nutrients, which the tiny conceptus needs. Already, the conceptus has divided itself into a portion that will form the embryo and a portion that will form the placenta (the trophoblast cells). The trophoblast cells begin to produce human chorionic gonadotrophin (HCG), which is released into the mother's blood, travels to the ovary, and causes the corpus luteum to continue full production of progesterone. This process insures that the endometrium will not break down and shed, and that the endometrial gland will continue to secrete nutrients for the embryo until the placenta has developed sufficiently to take nutrients directly from the mother's blood. This development is fully established by 17 days after fertilization. The entire sequence of the menstrual cycle, fertilization, and implantation, is an amazing achievement of neatly synchronized events.

There is considerable evidence that the time of conception after ovulation affects the gender of the offspring. Studies on 2 populations of women have confirmed that the proportion of male babies is higher in the offspring of women who have sexual intercourse 2 days after ovulation. The proportion is lower on or near the day of ovulation than on the previous day or so.

Vulva

Inflammations

The vulva may be the site of many skin diseases that occur elsewhere on the body.

The most common inflammations in this area are contact dermatitis from use of soaps, deodorant sprays, or dyes in clothing; fungal infections, particulary candida; herpes simplex type II; and condyloma acuminatum.

Candidal vulvitis often occurs with a concomitant candidal vaginitis, and is particularly frequent in women with diabetes mellitus. Other predisposing conditions include pregnancy, use of oral contraceptives, and recent treatment with broad-spectrum antibiotics. The vulvar skin itches intensely and is red, edematous, weeping, and may show small, white patches on the labial folds. The diagnosis can be established by microscopic examination of skin scrapings, vaginal secretions, or by culture. Prompt relief is obtained when appropriate medication is given.

Herpes simplex type II causes painful, vesicular lesions on the vulva and vagina that ulcerate to form small craters filled with necrotic gray-white material surrounded by a red rim. The diagnosis can be confirmed by cytologic examination of scrapings from the crater base. Specific treatment for this painful condition does not exist at present. Symptomatic improvement may be obtained by soaking the lesions in povidone-iodine or in Burow's solution.

Condyloma acuminatum is a warty, papillary growth caused by the papillomavirus. They occur on the labia, perineum, perianal skin, vagina, or cervix, and are usually several millimeters in diameter. They grow larger and may become flat and confluent under the influences of pregnancy or oral contraceptive use. Treatment is by chemical destruction with podophyllin, cryosurgery, or cautery.

Other inflammations of the vulva are syphilis, chancroid, granuloma inguinale, and lymphogranuloma venereum (LGV).

Cysts

The most common cystic lesion affecting this region is the Bartholin's gland cyst or abscess. Bartholin's glands are located in the deep tissues on each side of the vaginal opening. They frequently become infected with gonococci, *E. coli,* or anaerobic bacteria, with formation of an abscess. Clinically, the patient has an enlarged, tender, red, fluctuant mass at the base of the labia majora on 1 side that may make sitting or walking difficult. Treatment is by incision and drainage of the infected material and by administration of antibiotics. Sometimes, the duct that normally drains these glands becomes obstructed, leading to retention of the gland secretions. In this case, a Bartholin's gland cyst develops. These are usually nontender, unilateral swellings at the base of the labia majora brought to the physician's attention when the patient notices a lump. The treatment for these cysts is surgical.

Dystrophy

In some women, the vulvar skin may undergo changes of atrophy or hyperplasia. These changes usually occur in older women and often present clinically as intense itching. The skin may appear thin, shrunken, or thickened, with red, pink, white, scaling, or weeping patches. Microscopically, one sees variable patterns of atrophy of hyperplasia of the skin structures. These changes are called vulvar dystrophy and are benign. They are treated medically.

It is important to realize that it is not possible to distinguish between the types of dystrophy (i.e., atrophic or hyperplastic), or between these benign conditions and early cancer (carcinoma *in situ*), without a small biopsy. Only then can the correct medical therapy or need for further surgery be determined.

Carcinoma

Cancer of the vulva is the fourth most common cancer of the female genital tract. It usually affects elderly women (over age 60). Histologically, the majority are squamous cell carcinomas.

The patient may notice a small lump or sore on the vulva that begins to itch or to ulcerate and bleed. Often she is embarrassed or afraid to seek medical advice and will treat the lesion with assorted creams and other preparations for many months. By the time the patient comes to the physician's attention, the lesion is often greater than 2 cm in size and it may have caused extensive destruction of the vulvar skin and spread to the lymph nodes of the groin.

Unfortunately, there is also an element of delay by the physician in establishing the diagnosis. In early cancers, the skin changes may not be so obvious. The skin may appear similar to that described for vulvar dystrophy, and itching may be a prominent complaint. The physician may treat the patient with various lotions or creams, and only after some months have passed without improvement will a biopsy be done. By this time, an early, *in situ* cancer may have become invasive, with the danger of lymph node metastases and a decreased chance of successful surgical treatment.

The treatment of invasive cancer of the vulva is by radical surgery in which all the vulvar skin, subcutaneous fat, and lymph nodes of the groin are removed and submitted for microscopic analysis. The five-year survival rate depends on the size of the lesion at the time of surgery, and on the presence or absence of lymph node metastases. It ranges from more than 80% for a lesion under 2 cm in size with negative lymph nodes, to 15 to 30% for a large lesion (greater than 3 cm) with positive lymph nodes. The importance of early diagnosis is obvious.

Vagina

Inflammations

The most common causes of vaginitis are candida, trichomonas, *Hemophilus vaginalis,* and infections. Inflammation with discharge often occurs after insertion of a foreign body—such as a forgotten tampon, or an object inserted by a child.

In candidal vaginitis, the vagina appears red and edematous. The discharge may be thick, white, and may resemble cheese curds, or it may be thin with small, white patches stuck to the mucosa. Diagnosis and treatment are as described in the section on the vulva.

Trichomonas vaginalis is a single-celled protozoan which commonly causes vaginal discharge and itching. The discharge may be heavy and watery, or it may appear greenish and frothy. Diagnosis is established by demonstration of the organism on a wet smear of the vaginal secretions. Treatment is with metronidazole (an antifungal agent). The vaginitis may recur if the woman's sexual partner is not treated, because the organism survives well in the male genital tract and is transmitted during sexual intercourse.

Hemophilus vaginalis causes a grayish discharge with a disagreeable odor. It gives little inflammation of the underlying tissue, in contrast to candida and trichomonas. The diagnosis may be suspected by finding so-called "clue cells" in the vaginal secretions (epithelial cells filled with bacteria). Treatment is with antibiotics.

The thin vaginal mucosa of postmenopausal women is prone to infection by various bacteria from the gastrointestinal tract. Treatment with intravaginal antibiotics and estrogen creams kills the offending bacteria and promotes growth of a thicker, more resistant vaginal mucosa.

Cysts

Sometimes, cysts develop from embryologic remnants located deep in the side walls of the vagina. These growths are called Gartner's duct cysts and may be small or large. They may be asymptomatic, or the patient may notice a bulging mass in the vagina. The treatment is by surgical excision. These cysts are benign.

Intrauterine DES Exposure

During the 1940's and 1950's, patients with certain pregnancy complications, such as threatened abortion, were treated with diethyl stilbestrol (DES), a synthetic estrogen compound. In the early 1970's, it became apparent that some of the daughters of these patients were developing cancers of the vagina and cervix during their teenage and young adult years. Cancer of the vagina is almost unheard of in young women, and these cancers were of a particularly rare type: clear cell adenocarcinoma. A frantic attempt to find other offspring of these DES-treated mothers began, so that the former could be examined and treated if a cancer was found.

Since the first reports on this subject appeared, it has been learned that, although there are many young women who had been exposed to DES prenatally, particularly in the United States, the vaginal and cervical cancers occur in only about 1 to 2% of them. There are only 300 cases reported worldwide. Careful examination of these women has revealed that many have developmental abnormalities of the vagina and cervix. Some of these abnormalities are areas of persistent columnar epithelium and gland formation, called vaginal adenosis (the vagina and exocervix are normally covered by squamous epithelium), partial or complete blockage of the vagina by excess tissue (vaginal septa), and an abnormal shape of the cervix. These abnormalities may be detected by careful pelvic examination, including Pap smears and colposcopy.

The colposcope is a stereoscopic magnifying instrument that looks like a pair of binoculars on a stand. It magnifies from 2 to 50 times. Through it, the external surfaces of the vagina and cervix can be carefully studied. Abnormalities such as adenosis, dysplasia, carcinoma *in situ*, and invasive cancer show specific changes in the contours of the epithelium that are too small to be seen without the aid of this magnifying instrument. Its chief benefit is to help the physician to determine the location of abnormal areas, which should be examined by biopsy.

It is not known whether these women will have an increased risk of developing other cancers at the sites of adenosis as they grow older, so it is important that these patients be identified and undergo regular follow-up examinations.

The male offspring of DES-treated mothers may also show certain genital tract abnormalities (epididymal cysts and small testes), and some of these young men have low sperm counts.

Cervix

The cervix or neck of the uterus is divided into the exocervix which is covered by squamous epithelium, and the endocervix, a canal lined by mucus-secreting columnar epithelium, folded into deep clefts (called "glands" by convention, although they are not true glands).

The meeting place of these 2 types of epithelium may be located on the anatomic exocervix, exactly at the mouth of the cervix (external os), or up in the endocervical canal. This meeting place is called the squamocolumnar junction and it varies in location throughout a woman's life: it is on the exocervix during childhood and puberty; then it gradually retreats to approximately the external os during the reproductive period, and is finally located up inside the endocervical canal in the postmenopausal age group.

The exocervix is readily available for examination by general inspection, more detailed inspection using the colposcope, and microscopic examination of the cells that it sheds (i.e., Pap smear). It can also be easily examined by biopsy as an office procedure, without the need for anesthesia, and the tissue examined microscopically.

The gradual replacement of columnar epithelium by squamous epithelium that causes this apparent migration of the squamocolumnar junction is called squamous metaplasia. Metaplasia occurs in response to the various hormonal and local environmental conditions present during the different phases of a woman's reproductive life. The process is especially active at puberty and during pregnancy. Although metaplasia itself is an orderly process, the areas undergoing this change risk the development of disorderly patterns of cell maturation, namely, dysplasia and anaplasia (carcinoma).

Ectropion is the name given to areas of columnar epithelium located on the anatomic exocervix. This appears to the naked eye as a red, granular area surrounding the external os. Although these areas used to be called "erosions," we know now that ectropion is the normal finding during childhood, puberty, and early reproductive life, and that it is neither an ulceration nor an erosion. Ectropion is often extensive in women who have been exposed to DES, and it covers all of the anatomic exocervix and extends onto the vaginal walls in some cases.

Inflammatory Conditions

The endocervical glands may become infected by a variety of agents. These are bacterial (e.g., gonorrhea), fungal (e.g., candida), spirochete (e.g., syphilis), protozoan (e.g., *Trichomonas vaginalis*), or viral (e.g., herpes simplex type II).

The cervix appears boggy, red, and inflamed. A characteristic type of lesion or discharge may be present, which aids the physician in making the diagnosis.

A common finding is a small, yellow cyst protruding from the surface. This growth is called a nabothian cyst, and results when an endocervical gland becomes obstructed and material collects behind the obstruction. This obstruction may be caused by inflammation or by active metaplasia in the area.

Polyps

Endocervical polyps result from a localized overgrowth of endocervical glands. The polyps vary in size and often will protrude from the external os (opening), where they appear as a soft, red, raspberry-like mass, attached by a stalk. They are composed of delicate blood vessels and of fibrous tissue covered by endocervical glands. Because the vessels are fragile, these polyps frequently cause abnormal bleeding, i.e., bleeding between menstrual periods, postcoital bleeding, or postmenopausal bleeding. Endocervical polyps rarely contain cancer.

Dysplasia (Cervical Intraepithelial Neoplasia)

Dysplasia is an abnormal growth pattern in which some of the epithelial cells have features of malignancy. In the normal maturation sequence of squamous epithelium, the most common immature cells (basal cells) occupy a single layer just above the basement membrane, which separates the surface epithelium from the connective tissue (stroma) of the cervix. In dysplasia, some of these basal cells take on malignant criteria and begin to occupy more of the thickness of the surface epithelium than just a single layer.

Although exact definitions of dysplasia have not been set down, the condition is usually graded as mild, moderate, or severe, depending on how much of the epithelial thickness is replaced by abnormal cells. In the mildest forms, up to about 25% of the epithelium is made up of abnormal cells. In severe dysplasia, only a thin rim of non-malignant, nondysplastic cells are left at the surface. When the entire epithelial thickness is replaced by these cytologically malignant cells, it is called *carcinoma in situ* (CIS). At this point, the disease has still not broken through the basement membrane, i.e., it is still confined to the epithelium.

The newer terminology for this spectrum of lesions is **cervical intraepithelial neoplasia**, and it is graded I, II, and III, corresponding to mild (CIN I), moderate (CIN II), and severe dysplasia, plus *carcinoma in situ* (CIN III). This terminology helps to emphasize that these lesions do form a continuous spectrum and that the process is, in fact, a type of neoplasia. Severe dysplasia and CIS are grouped together because the dividing line between the 2 is often fine, and because CIS is still a disease confined to the epithelium, i.e., it is not invasive.

The significance of cervical intraepithelial neoplasia (CIN) is that, if left alone, a certain percentage will progress to CIS, and eventually to invasive carcinoma. The higher the degree of dysplasia at the time of diagnosis, the greater the chance of progression to a more severe lesion if left untreated.

CIN is diagnosed initially by an abnormal Pap smear—the cervix usually appears normal to general inspection. The abnormal cells tend to be less cohesive than normal squamous cells, and are readily removed when a Pap smear is performed. Further examination of the cervix is recommended with the colposcope, with which it is possible to see abnormalities of color, surface contour, and vascular pattern too small to be noticed with the naked eye. These abnormal patterns are then examined by biopsy so that an exact diagnosis can be made and appropriate treatment can be given to destroy the abnormal cells. The exact type of treatment depends on the degree of the abnormality and on the patient's desire to keep her uterus. After definitive therapy, it is important for the patient to be followed closely by regular examination and cytology, because she is at increased risk for developing other areas of CIN.

Microinvasive Carcinoma

This is a special category of invasive cervical carcinoma in which small groups of malignant cells break through the basement membrane into the cervical stroma, but penetrate less than 3 mm below the point of the rupture in the basement membrane. These patients are usually treated by simple hysterectomy, but a small proportion of them (less than 5%) will have micrometastases to regional lymph nodes.

Invasive Carcinoma

Invasive squamous carcinoma of the cervix was the most common female genital tract malignancy until recent times. In the past 25 years, Pap smear examinations have permitted detection of the disease in early, potentially curable, stages. The middle-aged woman who suddenly visits her physician because of abnormal vaginal bleeding, not having been examined since the birth of her last child 20 years before, and who is found to have a far advanced cervical cancer, has largely become a thing of the past.

The average age of patients with invasive cervical carcinoma is 45, versus age 35 for those with CIS, and under 35 for CIN. There is good epidemiologic evidence to support the belief that this spectrum of disease is related to sexual intercourse, i.e., early age of beginning sexual activity, multiple sexual partners, and prior infection with agents known to be sexually transmitted, notably herpes simplex type II.

The usual presenting symptom is abnormal vaginal bleeding, particularly postcoital bleeding. Inspection of the cervix shows an obvious lesion that may be cauliflower-like and friable, or deeply ulcerated. A portion of the cervix, or its entirety, may be replaced by the tumor. Microscopically, one sees nests and cords of malignant squamous cells infiltrating the cervical stroma. The major routes of spread are to the vaginal mucosa, to the pelvic and para-aortic lymph nodes, and by growth directly into the soft tissues around the uterus with further extension out to the pelvic side walls. As the tumor grows, it may entrap the ureters as they pass close to the cervix, or it may invade the bladder and rectum. It may also spread to distant sites. The usual cause of death is entrapment and blockage of the ureters by tumor, causing uremia and death over a period of months.

The treatment and prognosis for survival depend on the stage of the disease at the time of diagnosis. Staging includes a careful pelvic exam, radiologic investigations, and sigmoidoscopy and cystoscopy to determine the extent of disease (see Table 21–2). The primary treatment is radiation therapy. Radical hysterectomy with pelvic lymph node dissection is a formidable operation reserved for the younger patient with a small, localized lesion.

Five-year survival figures range from 90% for stage I lesions to about 40% for stage II, and under 15% for stage IV.

Endometrium

The endometrium is unique in that each month it undergoes a complex series of structural changes in response to hormonal signals from the ovary, in order to receive and to nourish a fertilized ovum, and is broken down and shed if conception has not occurred.

The sequence of endometrial changes during a menstrual cycle has been described in detail, so that it is possible to determine which day of the cycle a sample of endometrium represents by noting its appearance.

The first part of the cycle is called the menstrual phase. In a twenty-eight-day cycle, this represents days 1 to 5. It is characterized by breakdown of the endometrial glands and stroma from the previous cycle, accompanied by a variable amount of bleeding from the small, spiral arterioles. Days 6 to 13 make up the proliferative phase, which is characterized by regrowth of the endometrial glands and stroma. Day 14 is the day of ovulation, although histologic evidence of this event can only be detected at day 16, when large, clear vacuoles appear on all the glands just below the cell nuclei. Days 14 to 28 are characterized by proliferation of the epithelium, and growth of the spiral arterioles. By the time the next menstruation occurs, the endometrium has grown to be about 5 mm thick.

Table 21–2. Clinical Stages in Carcinoma of the Cervix

Stage I.	Carcinoma strictly confined to the cervix (extension to the uterus should be disregarded).
Stage Ia.	Microinvasive carcinoma (early stromal invasion).
Stage II.	The carcinoma extends beyond the cervix but has not extended onto the pelvic wall. The carcinoma involves the vagina, but not the lower third.
Stage III.	The carcinoma has extended onto the pelvic wall. On rectal examination there is no cancer-free space between the tumor and the pelvic wall. The tumor involves the lower third of the vagina.
	All cases with a hydronephrosis or nonfunctioning kidney.
Stage IV.	The carcinoma has extended beyond the true pelvis or has clinically involved the mucosa of the bladder or rectum.

(Adapted from DiSaia, P. J., et al.: Definitions of different clinical stages in carcinoma of the cervix uteri. In *Synopsis of Gynecologic Oncology*. New York, John Wiley and Sons, 1975.)

The endometrial pattern depends on the proper sequence of hormonal stimuli from the ovary. The ovary, in turn, cannot put forth the proper stimuli unless it receives accurate signals from the anterior pituitary. The anterior pituitary receives its orders from the hypothalamus, which receives stimuli from higher centers in the brain, such as the cerebral cortex, thalamus, and limbic system. We can see that any disturbance along this complex pathway may result in an abnormal endometrial response. The patient will then experience what is for her an abnormal menstrual period—too scanty, too heavy, delayed in onset, or skipped altogether. These abnormal bleeding episodes are not caused by a specific structural abnormality of the endometrium, but reflect a derangement in the hypothalamic-pituitary-ovarian control system. The derangement may exist for a single cycle only, or it may be the dominant feature of all the woman's menstrual cycles. This derangement is called **dysfunctional uterine bleeding** (DUB).

DUB is most common in the teenage years just after the onset of menses and in the several years just before menses stop (perimenopausal age group). This common disorder can also occur at any other time in between those 2 age groups. The young woman who leaves her family to attend college or to take a job in another city, and who then begins to have menstrual problems, is the classic example of DUB. Because DUB is a reflection of alteration in the normal, orderly transfer of hormonal signals between the parts of the reproductive control system, it is a frequent finding in women who are infertile because of absent or infrequent ovulation.

Contraceptive pills have a characteristic effect on the endometrium. Intrauterine devices (IUD) also produce a characteristic picture. There is indentation of the endometrial surface and inflammatory changes (acute and chronic) at the places where the intrauterine device touches the endometrial surface. Sometimes, areas of ulceration or of squamous metaplasia may occur.

Inflammation

Acute inflammation of the endometrium occurs most commonly following abortion or delivery, especially when fragments of the placenta remain in the uterus, when the delivery has followed a long labor with multiple vaginal examinations, or when cesarian section was required. A mild degree of acute inflammation is frequent following insertion of an intrauterine device.

Microscopically, one sees collections of polymorphonuclear leukocytes (microabscesses) that destroy the gland architecture and are scattered throughout the epithelium.

Chronic endometritis is found in association with retained products of conception, pelvic inflammatory disease (see section on fallopian tubes), and the presence of an IUD. A mixed chronic inflammatory infiltrate of lymphocytes, histiocytes, and plasma cells is found in the epithelium. Since plasma cells are never found in a normal endometrial tissue, the presence of even 1 is sufficient for the diagnosis. These patients usually have menstrual irregularities and may have pain.

Antibiotics are successful in treating both acute and chronic endometritis after the retained products of conception or the IUD have been removed.

Hyperplasia

When the endometrium has been subjected to prolonged stimulation by estrogen, unopposed by the effects of progesterone, it becomes hyperplastic.

The unopposed estrogen stimulation may be the result of noncyclic activity of the hypothalamic-pituitary-ovarian axis, which causes anovulation and a lack of progesterone production by the ovary; the use of estrogen-containing drugs commonly given to perimenopausal age women to control symptoms such as hot flushes; or the conversion of certain steroid compounds made in the ovary and adrenal to estrogens by the body's fat tissue.

When hyperplasia is neither severe nor grossly atypical, it can be removed by endometrial curettage and prevented from recurring by eliminating the sources of excess estrogen. When severe and atypical, hysterectomy is usually recommended. Although the number of women with hyperplasia that progresses to adenocarcinoma is only 5 to 10%, the chances increase when the hyperplasia has been untreated for a long time, or when it is severe and atypical.

Polyps

Endometrial polyps result from small areas of endometrial hyperplasia. They are usually located near the top of the endometrial cavity. These glands do not usually respond to hormonal stimuli. Endometrial polyps may become large and are a common cause of postmenopausal bleeding. They may ulcerate, become infarcted, or protrude through the external cervical os. Sometimes, adenocarcinoma develops in a polyp.

Carcinoma

Adenocarcinoma of the endometrium has now become the most common invasive cancer of the female genital tract (Fig. 21–5). It usually occurs in postmenopausal women (over age 50). The typical patient is described as an obese, diabetic, hypertensive woman who has never had children. She often has a family history of endometrial carcinoma.

Recent studies have indicated that women taking estrogens for relief of menopausal symptoms have an increased risk (4 to 8 times)

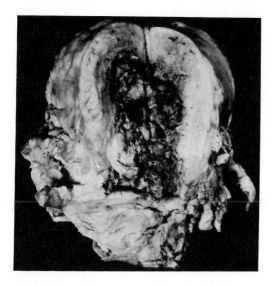

Fig. 21–5. This uterus shows an irregular outer surface, a thick wall, and a fungating necrotic mass occupying the endometrical cavity. (McGill University, Department of Pathology Museum.)

of developing carcinoma of the endometrium. Because the use of these drugs is so widespread today, and because the Pap smear is not a reliable detector of endometrial carcinoma, aspiration biopsies of the endometrium are frequently performed to follow these patients. This biopsy is an office procedure done on an annual or semiannual basis. If any abnormality is seen in the biopsy, or if the patient develops postmenopausal bleeding, a full curettage is done.

When curettage is performed on any patient suspected of having carcinoma of the endometrium, the specimen should be separated into 2 parts (fractional D & C). The endocervical specimen is examined separately from the tissue of the body of the uterus, so that it can be determined whether a carcinoma is confined only to the body (stage I), or whether it has spread to involve the cervix as well (stage II). Treatment and prognosis for survival are vastly different in the 2 stages.

The pathologist has a responsibility to grade the tumor as I, II, III (corresponding to well-differentiated, moderately well-differentiated, and poorly differentiated carcinoma), depending on how well the tumor can duplicate the glandular pattern of endometrial tissue, and to determine (on a hysterectomy specimen) the depth to which the tumor has penetrated the myometrium.

The common routes of spread of this tumor are downward growth to involve the cervix, paracervical lymphatics, and vagina, penetration into and finally through the myometrium, with implantation of tumor on the pelvic and abdominal organs, spread to pelvic and para-aortic lymph nodes, and distant metastases, especially to the lung.

The tumor is staged as shown in Table 21–3. Treatment is by simple hysterectomy and bilateral salpingo-oophorectomy for early lesions, or preoperative irradiation followed by total hysterectomy or salpingo-oophorectomy. Postoperative radiation may be given if it is found that the tumor is more poorly differentiated or more widespread than originally thought.

A good prognosis with a five-year survival of more than 90% is found with a stage I, well-differentiated lesion that does not pene-

Table 21–3. Clinical Stages of Carcinoma of the Corpus Uteri

Stage I.	The carcinoma is confined to the uterus.
	The Stage I cases should be subgrouped with regard to the histologic type of the adenocarcinoma, as follows:
	Grade 1. Highly differentiated adenomatous carcinomas.
	Grade 2. Differentiated adenomatous carcinomas with partly solid areas.
	Grade 3. Predominantly solid or entirely undifferentiated carcinomas.
Stage II.	The carcinoma has involved the uterus and the cervix.
Stage III.	The carcinoma has extended outside the uterus, but not outside the true pelvis.
Stage IV.	The carcinoma has extended outside the true pelvis or has obviously involved the mucosa of the bladder or rectum.

(Adapted from DiSaia, P. J., et al.: Definitions of different clinical stages in carcinoma of the corpus uteri. In *Synopsis of Gynecologic Oncology*. New York, John Wiley and Sons, 1975.)

trate the myometrium. The five-year survival rate drops to about 50% for stage II, 25% for stage III, and less than 10% for stage IV tumors.

Endometriosis

Endometriosis is the presence of normal-appearing endometrium in sites other than their normal location inside the uterus. The most common locations are the ovaries and tubes, pelvic peritoneum (especially the posterior surface of the uterus and cul de sac), other pelvic organs such as large bowel, and soft tissues, for example, abdominal scars, episiotomy scars, and the umbilicus. Occasionally such distant sites as the lung and pleura may be involved.

Inspection of the organs involved shows hemorrhagic or dark brown nodules surrounded by dense fibrous scars and adhesions. In the ovary, large cysts may be formed that are filled with old, dark brown blood (chocolate cysts). These cysts sometimes become large enough to destroy most of the normal ovarian tissue.

Microscopically, one must find typical endometrium to make a diagnosis. Usually there is also surrounding fibrosis and evidence of old hemorrhage in the area.

Several theories have been put forth to explain how the endometrial tissue appears in such unusual locations. Some of these are: reflux of endometrial fragments backward through the tubes during menstruation with implantation in the pelvis, metaplastic transformation of multipotential cells on the abdomen and pelvis, implantation of endometrial fragments during surgery or delivery, and blood or lymphatic spread to distant places.

The patients are usually in their late 20's or early 30's. The presenting complaints depend on the organs involved. The more common symptoms include pelvic pain, dysmenorrhea, and infertility, whereas more unusual implantation sites may lead to monthly episodes of bloody sputum production or partial bowel obstruction.

Myometrium

The 2 common conditions affecting the uterine muscle mass are adenomyosis and leiomyomas.

Adenomyosis is the presence of normal-appearing endometrial glands and stroma deep in the muscle wall of the uterus. The uterus may appear grossly normal or round and globular in shape, with tiny areas of hemorrhage surrounded by bands of smooth muscle.

The patient is usually a middle-aged woman complaining of pelvic pain, abnormal menstrual bleeding, and dysmenorrhea. This condition is usually not associated with endometriosis. Treatment is by hysterectomy.

Leiomyomas are benign smooth muscle tumors that are present in at least 20% of all women. They have been misnamed fibroids or fibroid tumors, although they are composed of interlacing bundles of smooth muscle and not of fibrous tissue. Leiomyomas may be either small or large, and a patient may have 1 or many. They vary on location from submucous (which distort the endometrial cavity and often produce menorrhagia), to intramural (the most common), to subserous (or just beneath the outer surface of the uterus).

Leiomyomas are frequently asymptomatic. However, they may become large enough to distort the shape of the uterus completely. When symptoms do occur, they consist of pelvic pressure, frequent urination because of compression of the bladder, constipation due to rectal pressure, abnormal bleeding, or infertility. The patient may also notice a mass in her lower abdomen. Leiomyomas tend to grow under the influence of estrogens.

The cut surface of these tumors is characteristic. They are white, solid, rubbery, and have a whorled pattern. Sometimes they contain small areas of hemorrhage or of cystic degeneration. They may be densely calcified. Rarely, the tumors may be malignant (leiomyosarcoma).

The treatment depends on the size of the uterus and on the patient's symptoms. Small, asymptomatic tumors may be left alone, whereas larger, symptom-producing ones will often require hysterectomy.

Fallopian Tube

The major conditions that affect the fallopian tube are acute and chronic salpingitis (pelvic inflammatory disease) and ectopic pregnancy.

Acute salpingitis is most often the result of infection with the gonococcus, which is thought to travel along the mucosa from its portal of entry at the endocervical glands to the fallopian tubes. Other organisms, such as streptococcus, E. coli, and anaerobes, can also cause acute salpingitis. Acute salpingitis may result from an unsterile abortion or delivery, or it may follow the insertion of an IUD. Salpingitis is usually bilateral, but in cases associated with an IUD, it is often unilateral.

The fallopian tube appears red and swollen, may be covered with exudate, and is often leaking pus from the fimbriated end. The patient has a fever, lower abdominal pain, nausea, and vomiting. There is often severe pain on pelvic examination. Treatment is with high-dose antibiotics and bed rest.

Chronic salpingitis frequently follows 1 or several episodes of acute salpingitis. The delicate mucosal folds may be damaged or destroyed by the inflammatory process, and adhesions frequently occur both in and around the fallopian tube, causing it to bind to neighboring structures. Often, the fimbriated end of the tube becomes occluded by adhesions and the tube fills with fluid (hydrosalpinx). Repeated flare-ups of salpingitis are common. When a hydrosalpinx becomes infected, the fallopian tube may become filled with pus and greatly distorted in shape and size. If the ovary is also involved, this mass is called a tubo-ovarian abscess. Rupture of such an abscess is a serious emergency that requires high-dose intravenous antibiotics and surgical drainage. Although mild flare-ups of salpingitis may be treated with antibiotics, the long-term complications of this condition, chronic pelvic pain, infertility, and ectopic pregnancy, frequently require surgery.

Tuberculosis as the cause of salpingitis is uncommon and may manifest as infertility. It is usually brought to the fallopian tube by hematogenous spread from a tuberculous focus in the lung.

Ectopic pregnancy is described under the disorders of pregnancy.

Ovary

The ovary is a small but complicated organ with 2 functions:

1. To release a mature egg at a specific time of the menstrual cycle.
2. To receive signals from the anterior pituitary (by means of the gonadotrophins FSH and LH), to interpret the signals, and to translate them into the production of steroid hormones (mainly estrogen and progesterone), which are then released into the blood and cause characteristic changes in the other female reproductive organs.

It is easier to understand the abnormalities of ovarian structure and function if we divide the ovary into 5 compartments:

1. the surface epithelium
2. the germ cells
3. the follicles
4. the stroma or interstitial tissue
5. the hilus and medulla.

Surface Epithelium. The ovary is covered by a single layer of cells, the same cells that form the linings of the fallopian tube, the endometrium, and the endocervical canal. The most common types of ovarian tumors develop from these surface epithelial cells, which will change as they grow from their usual cuboidal shape to resemble endometrial- or endocervical-type cells.

Germ Cells. The mature germ cell is called the ovum and is released at ovulation. The germ cells come to the ovary from the yolk sac during early embryologic life and populate the cortex (located just beneath the surface epithelial cells).

Follicles. After each germ cell arrives in the ovarian cortex, it is surrounded by a double layer of specialized cells that are important in the production of estrogen and progesterone. This unit of germ cell surrounded by a special double cell layer is called a follicle. The inner ring of cells is called the granulosa cell layer. This is surrounded by an outer layer, called the theca cells. During development of the follicle on days 1 to 14 of the menstrual cycle, these cells (especially the theca cells) are actively producing estrogen. When the egg is released at ovulation, the granulosa and theca cells remain behind on the ovary. The granulosa cells, lining the cavity in which the ovum matured, become bright yellow, plump, and full of vacuolated cytoplasm. This change is called luteinization and the cavity is called a corpus luteum (CL). It is here that progesterone, which causes the secretory changes in the endometrium, is made. If fertilization of the ovum does not occur, the CL regresses, hormone production wanes, and a small, white scar, the corpus albicans, is left. The ovary repeats this cycle in response to FSH and LH signals from the anterior pituitary.

Stroma (Interstitial Tissue). The ovarian follicles sit in a bed of dark, spindle-shaped cells, called the stroma. During early embryologic life, the primitive gonad is bipotential. It will develop into a definite male or female gonad only after certain influences push it in one direction or the other. The ovarian stroma retains some of this bipotential ability. It produces a full range of steroid hormones, including androgenic and estrogenic compounds. When tumors develop from these cells, they may also produce these hormones, leading to rare, but clinically striking, pictures.

Hilus and Medulla. This is the innermost region of the ovary, and it contains the ovarian vessels and nerves as well as small groups of special luteinized hilus cells.

Functional Cysts

The ovary forms small cystic structures (i.e., the follicle and corpus luteum) during a normal menstrual cycle. Sometimes, these cysts become much larger than usual. They can cause symptoms such as pain or pressure on the bladder, or they may be discovered at a routine pelvic examination. Characteristically, their size changes quickly and they may be 4 to 5 cm in size when first examined, only to disappear completely within a few weeks.

Because they are related to the normal small cystic structures (follicle and CL) in the ovary, these growths are called functional cysts.

The most common types are the follicle cyst, which is an exaggerated development of a normal follicle, and the CL cyst, an overdilatation of a normal CL. The CL cyst may be filled with hemorrhagic fluid and may occasionally rupture and cause serious intraperitoneal bleeding. Both kinds of cysts frequently cause some abnormality in the menstrual period.

Polycystic Ovaries

A common cause of female infertility is anovulation. Many infertile women have polycystic ovaries or Stein-Leventhal syndrome. These patients have absent or infrequent ovulations, and they suffer from oligomenorrhea, amenorrhea or DUB, infertility, and often some signs of virilization, such as increased facial hair and acne.

The ovaries are usually bilaterally enlarged with a smooth surface capsule. The cut surface shows multiple small cysts just below the thickened external capsule, an absence of corpora lutea, few corpora albicantia, and hyperplasia of the ovarian stroma.

The hypothalamus of these women fails to send its signals to the anterior pituitary. The proper amounts of FSH and LH are not released in time to promote the normal maturation sequence in an ovarian follicle and to cause ovulation to occur. The primary treatment is by drugs to induce ovulation.

Neoplastic Cysts

The neoplastic cysts and tumors of the ovary are described according to their compartment of origin. The ovarian neoplasms may be totally cystic, totally solid, or a mixture of both. The benign types usually affect 1 ovary, whereas the malignant ones are more often bilateral. These neoplasia cause symptoms such as pressure in the pelvis, frequent urination, rectal pressure, increasing abdominal size (if large), or they may be asymptomatic.

Tumors from the Surface Epithelium. These tumors may be lined by serous-type tall columnar epithelium similar to that on the fallopian tube, or by mucus-producing columnar cells similar to those of the endocervix.

The serous tumors are the most frequent kind of ovarian tumors. Up to 50% are bilateral.

The serous carcinoma is the most common type of ovarian cancer. These tumors are often both cystic and solid, large, and adherent to other pelvic structures. The cut surface shows areas of hemorrhage and necrosis. Papillary projections may be seen on the inner and outer surfaces. Microscopically, they range from well-differentiated adenocarcinomas with delicate frond-like projections to poorly differentiated cancers in which no attempts at gland formation are seen.

The mucinous tumors are more often unilateral. The benign ones are unilocular, smooth-lined cysts filled with a thick, mucoid fluid. They are lined by a single layer of mucus-producing columnar cells. Benign mucinous tumors often grow large before detection, filling the entire pelvis and abdomen.

Mucinous carcinomas are multilocular, cystic, and solid tumors. They may be well or poorly differentiated. They may rupture and fill the pelvis with thick mucus-containing tumor cells, which implant on the surfaces of bowel, omentum, or liver. This condition is called pseudomyxoma peritonei and is rare.

Other malignant ovarian tumors arising from surface epithelial cells are endometroid carcinoma (which resembles endometrial cells), and clear cell adenocarcinoma. Some of these tumors are so poorly differentiated that it is impossible to classify them.

Carcinoma of the ovary is rare in patients under 40. Because these tumors are often asymptomatic in the early stages, patients tend to have widespread disease by the time a diagnosis is made. These cancers invade their capsule and sow tumor cells all around the pelvis and abdomen. These cells grow into tumor nodules that eventually encase the pelvic organs, small bowel, omentum, stomach, and liver. Ascites and pleural effusions are common. The usual presenting symptoms are abdominal swelling, abdominal discomfort, or vague pain, and nonspecific gastrointestinal symptoms such as bloating, nausea, anorexia, or heartburn. Sometimes, abnormal vaginal bleeding alerts the patient. Rarely, the first symptoms may be shortness of breath due to a malignant pleural effusion.

The treatment consists of surgery, to remove the uterus, tubes, ovaries, and as much tumor bulk as possible, followed by chemotherapy or radiation. Recently, improved survival rates have been obtained by the use of multiple-drug chemotherapy. Survival depends on the stage of the tumor, on the degree of differentiation of the cells, and on the amount of residual tumor left behind after surgery.

Germ Cell Tumors. Tumors derived from the germ cells of the ovary are rare. (They usually occur in children or in young adults.) Except for the benign cystic teratoma or dermoid cyst, they are malignant. They are microscopically the same as the germ cell tumors that arise on the testis.

These tumors are divided into the dysgerminoma, endodermal sinus tumor, embryonal carcinoma, teratomas, and choriocarcinoma.

The benign cystic teratoma or dermoid cyst is the most common germ cell tumor. It contains mature tissues derived from all 3 germ cell layers—ectoderm, endoderm, and mesoderm. Grossly, this is a smooth cystic tumor that contains an unforgettable, greasy mixture of keratin, sebaceous material, and hair. Occasionally, teeth are found and, if present, give a diagnostic x-ray picture. Microscopically, many tissues such as skin, cartilage, bone, nerve, brain, and thyroid are seen.

Tumors of the Gonadal Stroma. These tumors are rare, but remarkable because they may produce hormones that cause characteristic clinical manifestations.

The granulosa cell tumor is composed of granulosa cells alone or mixed with theca cells. These are the same cells that form the lining of the ovarian follicle, and many of these tumors produce estrogens. They can cause precocious puberty when present in a child, or postmenopausal bleeding in an elderly woman, because the estrogen produced by the tumor stimulates the endometrium. Microscopically, the tumor cells arrange themselves in small rosettes around a central area filled with pink material. This grouping is called a Call-Exner body and helps to identify this type of tumor.

The Sertoli-Leydig cell tumor contains cells resembling those seen in the testis. It should be remembered that in the embryo, the primitive gonad is bipotential. These tumors are thought to arise from cells of the ovarian stroma that suddenly begin to differentiate along the lines of a testicle. When these tumors are steroid-forming, they make androgenic hormones, which cause a striking degree of masculinization in the patient—including acne, growth of facial and chest hair, clitoromegaly, and deepening of the voice. These tumors are extremely rare.

The fibroma is a non-hormone-producing tumor, which arises from stromal cells that grow into fibroblast-like cells. Small fibromas are not uncommon and consist of whorls of spindle cells arranged in bundles. They rarely may be associated with ascites and hydrothorax, called Meig's syndrome. These tumors are benign; once removed, the ascites and hydrothorax disappear.

Metastatic Tumors

This type of tumor frequently involves the ovary. The most common primary sites are the breast, the colon, and the stomach.

Metastatic tumors are bilateral in 50 to 60% of cases and are often asymptomatic. Microscopically, the general architecture of the ovary is preserved, but tumor cells are seen infiltrating in nests or cords between the ovarian structures.

A special type of metastatic ovarian tumor is the Krukenberg tumor, in which the ovary contains metastatic signet-ring adenocarcinoma cells within a strikingly hyperplastic ovarian stroma. These tumors are usually bilateral, hard, and solid. The classic Krukenberg tumor was described in association with a signet-ring adenocarcinoma of the stomach, but metastatic colon carcinoma can also produce this tumor.

Placenta

The placenta is a temporary organ that accomplishes the transfer of nutrients and oxygen to the fetus and the passage of metabolic waste products back to the mother for excretion. It is composed of numerous arborizing villi through which fetal blood circulates. The placenta attaches itself to the wall of the uterus, and these villi penetrate into the maternal endometrium (called decidua in pregnancy). The decidua at the site of implantation contains many sinuses into which maternal blood flows. The villi are bathed in the blood of these sinuses, and the exchange of nutrients, oxygen, CO_2, and waste products occurs at this point. Although the blood of the mother and the fetus pass close to each other, they usually do not mix.

Except at the implantation site, the placenta is surrounded by a double layer of membranes—the inner amnion and the outer chorion (Fig. 21–6). Inside the membranes, the

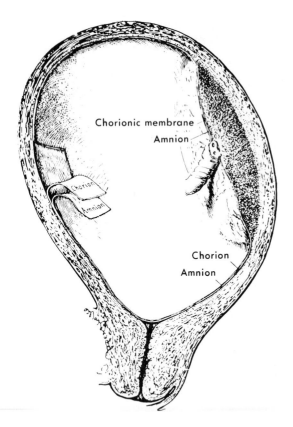

Fig. 21–6. This drawing shows the different layers of the envelope containing the fetus, namely the amnion, the chorion, and the umbilical cord. It demonstrates the placenta at the upper right. (From Bloom, W., and Fawcett, D. W.: *A Textbook of Histology*, 10th Ed. Philadelphia, W. B. Saunders, 1975.)

fetus floats on a bath of amniotic fluid. (The fetus is attached to the placenta by the umbilical cord, which ranges from 35 to 120 cm in length, and usually contains 2 arteries and 1 vein.) It has now become commonplace to remove a sample of amniotic fluid using a needle inserted through the mother's abdominal wall (amniocentesis). By this means, chemical analysis of the fluid can determine fetal lung maturity, can detect certain congenital abnormalities, or can follow the course of Rh-induced hemolytic disease. Fetal cells in the fluid can be cultured and examined for evidence of chromosomal abnormalities such as Down's syndrome, certain inborn errors of metabolism, and determination of the fetal sex.

Abnormalities of the Cord

The umbilical cord contains only 1 artery and 1 vein in about 1% of cases (about 7% of twins). Up to 25% of infants with a two-vessel cord have other congenital anomalies. The cord may occasionally contain a true knot, but this usually does not tighten enough to cut off the blood supply to the fetus.

Abnormalities of the Placenta

The placenta may contain an accessory lobe, connected to the main placenta by blood vessels. Accessory lobes are important chiefly because they may be left behind in the uterus after delivery and may cause a postpartum hemorrhage.

Placenta previa is insertion of the placenta near or covering the cervical canal. It usually causes bleeding in the latter part of pregnancy.

Placenta accreta is an abnormal adherence of the placenta to the uterine wall. At the implantation site, there is thin or absent decidua, so that the placental villi are directly in contact with the myometrium. In more severe degrees of this abnormality, the villi invade the myometrium (placenta increta), or perforate the uterus (placenta percreta). In these rare situations, the placenta does not separate from the uterine wall after the baby is born, heavy bleeding results, and immediate hysterectomy is usually necessary.

Sometimes a portion of the placenta separates from the implantation site prematurely. This is called **placental abruption** and may be severe enough to cause fetal death. Usually the size of the abruption is small (less than 20% of the surface of the placenta). Inspection may show a depressed area on the maternal surface of the placenta filled with clotted blood.

Abnormally large placentas are found with severe Rh incompatibility (erythroblastosis fetalis), syphilis, cytomegalic inclusion disease, toxoplasmosis, and polyhydramnios. Abnormally small placentas are seen with prematurity, severe maternal diabetes, hypertension, or renal disease, some fetal chromosome abnormalities, and rubella.

Twins

The placenta should be carefully examined in cases of twin pregnancy possibly to determine whether the twins resulted from a cleavage of the ovum within the first days after fertilization (monozygotic or identical twins) or from the simultaneous fertilization of 2 separate ova (dizygotic, nonidentical, or fraternal twins).

The possibilities are shown in Fig. 21–7.

Ectopic Pregnancy

The fertilized ovum may implant outside of the endometrial cavity. Such a condition is called ectopic pregnancy. The implantation

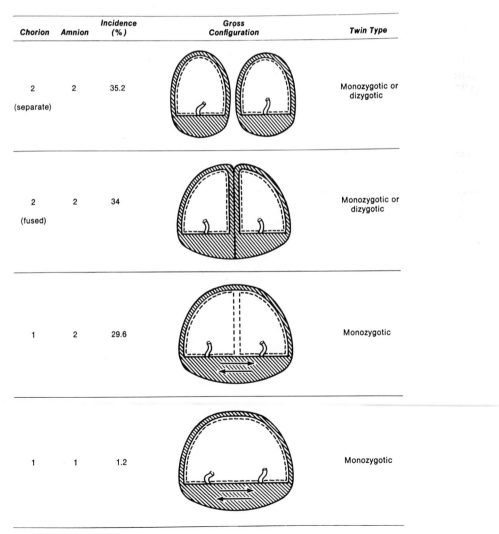

Chorion	Amnion	Incidence (%)	Gross Configuration	Twin Type
2 (separate)	2	35.2		Monozygotic or dizygotic
2 (fused)	2	34		Monozygotic or dizygotic
1	2	29.6		Monozygotic
1	1	1.2		Monozygotic

Fig. 21–7. This drawing shows the possible varieties in the appearance of the placenta in twins. (From Benirschke, K., and Driscoll, S. G.: *The Pathology of the Human Placenta.* New York, Springer-Verlag, 1967.)

occurs in the fallopian tube (most cases), on the ovary, cervix, or in the abdominal cavity (rare).

The etiology of tubal implantation is usually delayed or obstructed passage of the ovum through the tube because of adhesions from previous salpingitis, endometriosis, or previous surgery on the fallopian tube. The ovum implants and penetrates the wall of the fallopian tube, which will either rupture or attempt to abort the pregnancy through its fimbriated end. Both situations cause serious intra-abdominal hemorrhage.

Clinically, the patients often have severe lower abdominal pain, menstrual abnormalities, a tender mass on 1 side of the uterus, fainting, or shock from loss of blood. The patient may not even be aware that she is pregnant. The pregnancy test is frequently negative. Ectopic pregnancy must be distin-

guished from salpingitis, a ruptured or twisted ovarian cyst, appendicitis, and threatened abortion. An uncertain diagnosis is confirmed by laparoscopy, which requires the insertion of a viewing scope through a small incision just below the umbilicus. If an ectopic pregnancy is found, the affected tube must be excised.

Abortion

An abortion is the termination of pregnancy before fetal viability, either spontaneously or electively. The risk of abortion at different ages is shown in Figure 21–8, which also illustrates the risk of other forms of contraceptive control. Viability is usually set at 500 gm (about 20 weeks gestation) even though infants weighing less than 1,000 gm at birth usually do not survive.

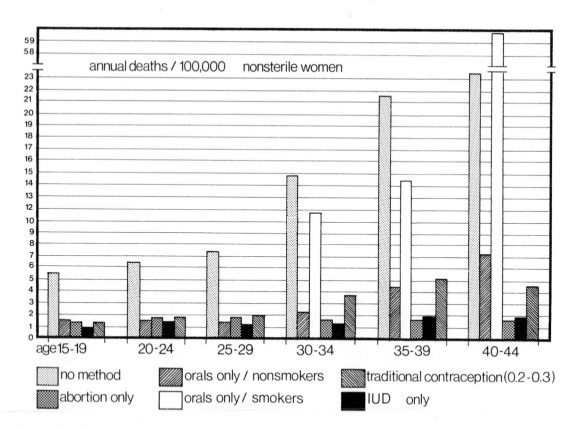

Fig. 21–8. This figure shows the annual number of deaths per 100,000 fertile women at different ages on different contraceptive regimens, and with different smoking histories. The graphs show that the number of deaths in the 15 to 19-year-old age group is highest in those who are on no contraceptive regimen, whereas the death rate in the 40 to 44-year-old age group is 60/100,000 for women who smoke and take oral contraceptives. (Adapted from Kase, N.: The ovaries. In *Cecil Textbook of Medicine,* 15th Ed. Edited by P. B. Beeson, W. McDermott, and J. B. Wyngaarden. Philadelphia, W. B. Saunders, 1979.)

Spontaneous abortions are said to occur in about 20% of all conceptions. The incidence may be higher than this, because some conceptions abort before the pregnancy is diagnosed. Most spontaneous abortions occur in the first trimester (first 14 weeks) of pregnancy, and reflect chromosomal or developmental abnormalities in the fetus that are incompatible with life (blighted ovum). If a careful search of the aborted material is performed, one usually finds only an empty gestational sac, or a sac containing a malformed portion of fetal tissue.

Spontaneous abortions are clinically categorized as threatened, incomplete, or missed. In threatened abortion, there is vaginal bleeding and cramping, but the cervix remains closed and no tissue is passed. **Incomplete abortion** occurs when the cervix opens and the patient spontaneously passes some of the products of conception. However, some pieces of placental tissue remain behind on the uterus and must be removed by curettage. In **missed abortion**, the fetus dies, but for some reason is retained in the uterus for 6 weeks or longer. The products of conception may abort spontaneously after several weeks, but curettage is often required to remove them. Microscopically, a missed abortion usually shows degenerated, hyalinized villi with chronic inflammation. Fetal parts are usually not seen.

Septic abortion occurs when there has been contamination of the uterine cavity by bacteria with acute inflammation of the products of conception and decidua. Before safe, elective abortions were widely available, sepsis was common after attempted illegal abortions, which were frequently done under unsterile conditions. Septic abortion may be life-threatening to the mother. It requires aggressive antibiotic therapy and prompt evacuation of the uterus.

Trophoblastic Disease

Trophoblast is the name given to the cells that form the placenta. These are the light-staining cytotrophoblast and the smaller, dark-staining syncytiotrophoblast. These cells are characterized by rapid growth and by their tendency to invade the maternal endometrium and myometrium as part of the normal course of pregnancy. Trophoblastic tissue also manufactures human chorionic gonadotropin hormone (HCG). Detection of this hormone in urine or in blood forms the basis of tests for pregnancy. HCG also provides a "marker" by which the physician may follow the course of patients who have recently been treated for 1 of the 3 types of trophoblastic disease. In these situations, a falling or absent titer of HCG in the blood indicates eradication of the abnormal trophoblastic tissue.

Hydatidiform Mole

Hydatidiform mole is an abnormal product of conception in which there is usually no fetus. The uterus is filled with cystically dilated chorionic villi that look like a bunch of grapes (Fig. 21–9). It is felt that hydatidiform mole may represent the missed abortion of a blighted ovum. The villi then continue to absorb fluid and become swollen. Microscopically, one finds edematous villi that contain no fetal blood vessels, and degrees of overgrowth of the trophoblastic tissue ranging from mild to marked.

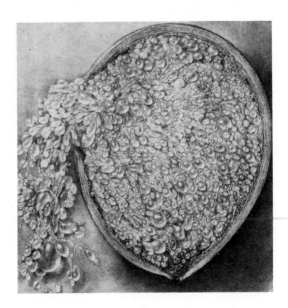

Fig. 21–9. This drawing shows the appearance of an hydatidiform mole. The grape-like clusters of edematous villi without fetal blood vessels appear as tiny grape-like cysts. (From Eastman, N. J.: Williams Obstetrics, 10th Ed. New York, Appleton-Century-Crofts, 1950.)

Hydatidiform mole occurs in about 1 in 2,000 pregnancies in North America, but the incidence rises to about 1 in 300 in parts of the Far East. The reason for this geographic difference is unknown.

Molar pregnancy is more common in older women. The patient has vaginal bleeding early in pregnancy. The uterus is often found to be larger than expected for the length of the pregnancy. No fetal heart tones can be found, and a characteristic pattern is seen on ultrasound. The HCG titer remains elevated, instead of showing the expected decline after the first trimester.

A molar pregnancy usually aborts spontaneously early in the second trimester. Sometimes, however, this does not occur, and suction curettage must be done. The patient is followed closely with serial measurements of the HCG blood titer. After complete evacuation of a molar pregnancy, the titer should be normal within 8 weeks. Follow-up is continued for 6 to 12 months because, although more than 80% of patients require no further treatment after evacuation of the mole, about 16% develop invasive mole and 2 to 3% have choriocarcinoma.

Invasive Mole

An invasive mole is one in which molar tissue is found deep in the myometrial wall. It appears grossly as a circumscribed, hemorrhagic nodule deep in the uterine wall. Microscopically, one sees the edematous mole villi surrounded by overgrown trophoblastic tissue mixed with hemorrhage. An invasive mole can be thought of as a molar pregnancy with placenta increta.

It is impossible to diagnose invasive mole from uterine curettings. The diagnosis can be established if the uterus is received after hysterectomy, or, more commonly, by an HCG titer that remains elevated after evacuation of a molar pregnancy by curettage.

Invasive mole responds quickly to treatment by chemotherapy, with prompt return of the HCG titer to normal.

Choriocarcinoma

Choriocarcinoma is a malignant tumor of the trophoblast. In choriocarcinoma, the trophoblast grows wildly, without production of villi. This tumor deeply invades the myometrium and rapidly spreads to distant organs. The most common sites of metastasis are lungs, vagina, brain, and liver.

Aside from the 2 to 3% of patients, mentioned previously, with hydatidiform mole who develop choriocarcinoma, the disease can also rarely occur following a normal term delivery and after spontaneous abortion of a nonmolar pregnancy.

If patients with choriocarcinoma are considered as a group, 50% have had a prior hydatidiform mole, 25% give a history of spontaneous abortion, and 25% have had a normal term delivery.

Foci of choriocarcinoma are located deep in the myometrial wall, surrounded by hemorrhage and cavitation of the tissue.

Microscopically, one sees sheets of cytotrophoblast and syncytiotrophoblast cells growing together uncontrolledly in a plexiform, double-layer arrangement. Chorionic villi are almost never present.

The diagnosis is usually not made on the basis of uterine curettings, but because of persistently elevated HCG titers and evidence of distant metastases.

Before the discovery in 1956 that choriocarcinoma is sensitive to methotrexate, death from widespread disease occurred in under a year. Now, aggressive chemotherapy with methotrexate and actinomycin D have greatly improved this dismal prognosis.

BREAST

Diseases of the breast are frequent, and breast biopsy is a common surgical procedure. The differential diagnosis in these cases is essentially "cancer or not cancer." When a woman hears the word "cancer," it is breast carcinoma with mastectomy that comes to her mind.

In the section to follow, the most common breast conditions are described.

Anatomy

The breast is a special type of secretory gland derived from the skin. It is made up of about 12 lobes arranged around a central nipple. The lobes are composed of lobules, or clusters of epithelial cells arranged in gland formations. These gland spaces are drained by a system of ducts that join to form a main excretory duct for each lobe. The main excretory ducts radiate out from the central nipple like the spokes of a wheel. Just beneath the nipple, they dilate into lactiferous sinuses, which act as small reservoirs. The ducts of the breast are lined by cuboidal to low columnar epithelial cells, sometimes arranged in 2 layers. Each duct is also surrounded by a layer of myoepithelial cells that contracts the ducts and expels the milk when suckling occurs (Fig. 21–10).

The lobules and ducts of the breast are supported and held in place by connective tissue, called the stroma. The contour of the breast is filled out by fat tissue. It is largely the amount of fat that determines the size of the breast.

During pregnancy, maternal hormones cross the placenta and stimulate the fetal breast tissues. After delivery, the baby may show mild enlargement of the breasts with secretion of small amounts of milk (witch's milk). This condition disappears after a few days.

Up to the time of puberty, the breast structure is similar in males and females. At puberty, hormones produced by the ovaries stimulate an increase in breast size and development of the pigmented areola around the nipple. Estrogen causes the ducts of the breast to elongate and to branch out. Progesterone is thought to act mainly on the lobules and promotes gland formation.

The breast is sensitive to estrogen and progesterone. It responds to the hormonal fluctuations of the menstrual cycle by growth and regression of its epithelial and stromal components. Many women notice increases in breast size and tenderness just before each menstrual period.

Pregnancy provides the major stimulus for growth and complete development of the breast

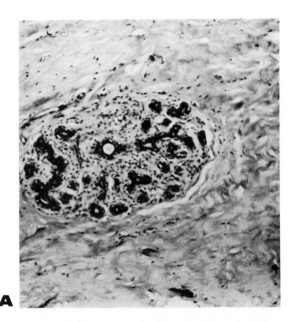

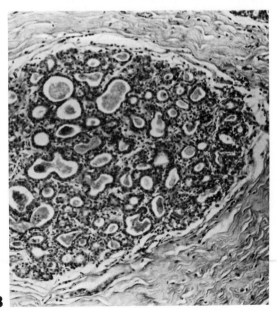

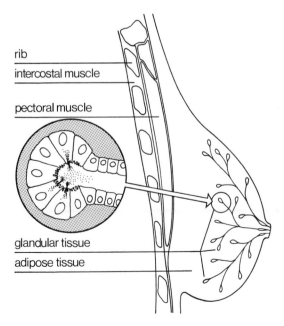

Fig. 21–10. This drawing shows the appearance of the tissues of a normal breast, illustrating the relationship of the lobular architecture to the ducts and to the nipple.

rib
intercostal muscle
pectoral muscle
glandular tissue
adipose tissue

Fig. 21–11. *A,* This histologic section shows the glandular tissue of **normal breast** surrounded by a large area of connective tissue. The dark cells surround a small cavity in this resting state. *B,* This section is from a **lactating breast.** Here a lobule of secretory epithelium secretes milk into the cavities of each acinus. Compare the relative amount of cell per square unit of surface area in the resting and lactating breasts.

(Fig. 21–11). In addition to elevated levels of estrogen and progesterone, prolactin from the anterior pituitary and special hormones from the placenta (placental lactogen) are present in large amounts. During the early months of pregnancy, further growth of ducts, and particularly lobules, occurs. The breasts become larger and firmer. During the latter part of pregnancy, secretion of nonmilk colostrum begins. Following delivery of the baby, the influence of prolactin is dominant. This hormone causes the lobular epithelial cells to produce milk, which is then secreted into small ducts. When suckling occurs, the posterior pituitary is stimulated to release oxytocin. Oxytocin causes the milk to be propelled along the duct system and to be ejected out of the nipple to the infant. Suckling also stimulates the anterior pituitary to continue prolactin secretion, so that the production of milk will be maintained. Thus, suckling the infant insures a continuous milk supply by releasing the hormones that cause milk production (prolactin) and milk ejection (oxytocin) from the pituitary gland.

Breast milk is a unique blend of proteins, lactose, and fatty acids. It also contains immunoglobulins that guard the newborn against certain types of infections. The exact "formula" of breast milk has never been duplicated in the laboratory. Because its mixture of proteins, sugar, and fatty acids is specifically designed to nourish human infants, is easy to digest, and does not cause allergies, breast milk is the best possible food for newborn babies.

When breast-feeding is stopped (or if the woman did not breast-feed after delivery), the secretory lobules and ducts regress and become less prominent. The breast is again composed mainly of connective tissue, stroma, and fat.

After menopause, the lack of hormonal stimulation by estrogen and progesterone causes a gradual atrophy of the lobules, ducts, and stroma. The breasts become smaller and flattened.

Developmental Conditions

Sometimes an imbalance of hormones causes 1 or both breasts to become overly large. This phenomenon occurs in the adolescent age group and is called virginal hypertrophy. The hypertrophy is mainly due to increased fibrous tissue. The breast ducts show hyperplasia of their epithelial cells. The hypertrophy is permanent and reconstructive surgery is necessary to restore the breast or breasts to their normal size.

Gynecomastia is the name given to hypertrophy of the male breast. It is due to hormonal imbalance in which a relative increase in estrogen as compared to testosterone occurs. Gynecomastia is found in adolescents,

and in old age, in patients with cirrhosis of the liver, testicular atrophy, decreased gonadotropin levels (i.e., Klinefelter's syndrome), and in some men receiving estrogen as part of the treatment for carcinoma of the prostate.

The breast ducts become elongated and branching. The surrounding connective tissue undergoes a pale bluish change, and inflammatory cells are present about the ducts. Pronounced gynecomastia must be treated surgically.

Inflammatory Conditions

The most common inflammation of the breast is puerperal mastitis, a bacterial infection occurring in the first few weeks after giving birth. The organisms involved are usually *Staphylococcus aureus* or streptococci. These bacteria invade the breast tissue through cracks or fissures in the nipple, which are common in the early weeks of breast-feeding. The breast appears red, swollen, hot, and tender. The woman may develop chills, fever, and malaise. Treatment consists of antibiotics, local application of heat, and frequent emptying of the affected breast. With prompt treatment, formation of a breast abscess can usually be avoided.

Fibrocystic Disease

Fibrocystic disease or cystic mastitis is a spectrum of benign breast abnormalities that occur because the breast tissue becomes out of phase with the ovarian hormone cycle.

Instead of an orderly pattern of growth and regression, any of the breast elements (the lobules, ducts, myoepithelial cells, intralobular stroma, or general connective tissue) overgrow. The exact pattern produced depends on which of these elements is dominant. Thus one may see multiple dilated ducts or cysts, growth of duct structures on an area forming a mass (adenoma), or increased fibrosis around and between lobules. It is usual to see more than 1 pattern in different areas of the breast.

Fibrocystic disease is common and affects women in the middle and late reproductive years. It may affect 1 or both breasts. The patient usually notices discomfort in the breast and may feel a lump. The physician may palpate a discrete lump or notice only a poorly defined "thickening." If a cyst is present, aspiration and cytologic examination of the fluid may be helpful in establishing the diagnosis. Mammography or xerography (both x-ray techniques) may better define the abnormal area. However, the ONLY way to establish the diagnosis definitely and to rule out cancer is by excision biopsy and histologic examination of the tissue. It is not always possible to distinguish a lump of fibrocystic disease from a small lump of carcinoma using only palpation or x-ray studies (Figs. 21–12 and 21–13). All breast lumps should be suspected of being cancer until proven otherwise, and only excision biopsy with careful tissue examination can give the answer.

Neoplasms

Fibroadenoma

The fibroadenoma is a benign breast tumor formed by an overgrowth of connective tissue and haphazardly branching ducts. It is found in young women and may grow rapidly during prenancy.

The fibroadenoma is a well-defined nodule that often has a surrounding capsule. Typically, it can easily be "shelled out" at the time of surgery. It is rubbery, white, moist, and lobulated. The cut surface shows a delicate, fissured pattern. Fibroadenomas may undergo cystic degeneration, become hyalinized, or calcify when old. Excision is curative.

Papilloma

A papilloma is a small nodule of duct epithelium covering a fibrovascular core. It usually grows on a large duct lumen or cyst cavity, where it looks like a raspberry attached to the wall. Because of its location, the papilloma frequently causes a cloudy or bloody nipple discharge that brings the patient to the physician.

Although most intraductal papillomas are benign, some may become malignant, and these lesions should be excised.

Carcinoma

Carcinoma of the breast is the most common cancer in women. About 70,000 new cases are diagnosed, and 30,000 patients die from breast cancer each year in the United States. It is estimated that 1 of 15 North American women will develop breast cancer in her lifetime. The disease also occurs rarely in men.

Breast cancer is more frequent in women who have never been pregnant, in sisters and daughters of breast cancer patients, and in patients who have previously had certain types of benign breast disease—particularly the types of fibrocystic diseases where the

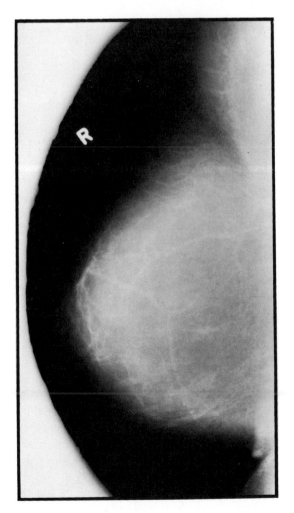

Fig. 21–12. This mammogram shows the normal appearance of blood vessels and tissue.

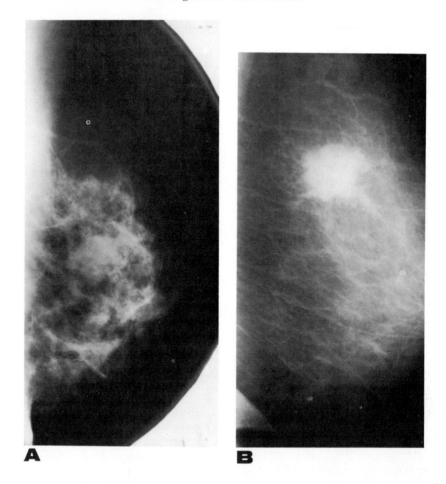

Fig. 21–13.   Mammogram *A* shows dysplasia, a diffuse abnormality, otherwise called fibrocystic disease. *B* shows a carcinoma of the breast.

duct epithelium shows hyperplasia or atypia. Women who have had a carcinoma in 1 breast are at risk for developing carcinoma in the other breast. This risk is estimated at about 1% per year.

Pregnancy before age 30, frequent pregnancies, and early menopause seem to decrease the risk of breast cancer. Use of oral contraceptive pills has not been found to increase the risk.

Many breast cancers are sensitive to estrogen and grow more rapidly under its influence. It is possible to determine which tumors are estrogen-dependent and to use this information to help plan subsequent therapy.

The etiology of breast cancer is not known, although theories incriminating hormonal factors and viruses are popular (see Chap. 11).

The disease is most common after age 45, but it can also occur in younger women. It is usually discovered by the patient herself (or her mate) as a firm lump in the upper outer quadrant or central portion of the breast.

The typical patient has a single, hard, nonmobile lump. If the lump is located in the central part of the breast, the nipple may be deformed or inverted (Fig. 21–15). The tumor may be fixed to the overlying skin, causing retraction or ulceration (if advanced) (Fig. 21–14). The lump may be fixed to the pectoral muscle lying beneath the breast. Sometimes the skin over a breast cancer resembles the skin of an orange (peau d'orange), owing to infiltration of the connective tissue by tumor.

The tissue is firm and cuts with the same gritty consistency as that of an unripe pear.

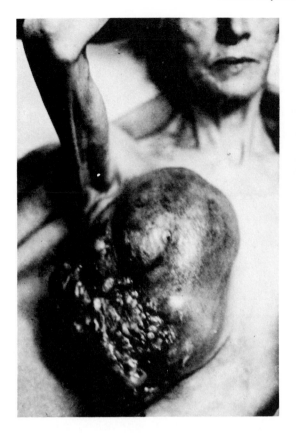

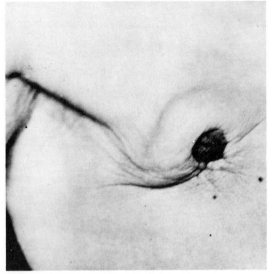

Fig. 21–15. This photograph of an elderly patient with **adenocarcinoma** of the right breast shows the indrawing of the nipple and dimpling of the skin. (The Evans Collection, Osler Library, McGill University.)

Fig. 21–14. Gross deformity of the breast with ulceration due to **adenocarcinoma** is shown in this photograph taken 75 years ago. It is uncommon for patients today to let a cancer develop to this degree. (The Evans Collection, Osler Library, McGill University.)

The cut surface shows an ill-defined opaque mass surrounded by radiating translucent lines of connective tissue containing yellow-white dots and streaks (Fig. 21–16). The tumor is depressed below the cut surface. Its infiltrating nature and the pronounced fibrous tissue response around the tumor cells give it the name "scirrhous" carcinoma.

Other gross appearances of breast cancer are less common and include the soft, large, hemorrhagic medullary carcinoma, papillary carcinoma, and comedocarcinoma (a cancer-filled duct containing a central necrotic area). Paget's disease of the breast is a variant of infiltrating duct carcinoma in which the skin of the nipple and areola shows a red, weeping, scaly appearance. Microscopically, the epidermis contains large vacuolated, so-called Paget's cells. These are not cancer cells,

however. A ductal carcinoma is found in the deeper breast tissue under the nipple.

Most cancers of the breast are adenocarcinomas arising from the epithelial cells of the ducts. Cancer may also arise from the breast lobules (lobular carcinoma), or, rarely, from the connective tissue (sarcomas).

The major route of metastasis is to the lymph nodes, particularly of the axilla. It is estimated that more than 50% of patients have axillary node metastases at the time of initial surgery. The skin lymphatics may be involved, or the disease may spread across to the opposite breast. Tumor cells in the blood grow most commonly in the lungs and pleura (more than 50% of cases), and in the liver, bones, brain, adrenal glands, and ovaries.

The standard treatment for breast carcinoma used to be radical mastectomy, in which the breast, pectoral muscle, and axillary contents were removed. More recently, the modified radical mastectomy (includes breast and axillary lymph nodes) has been used. Other possibilities include excision of the lump, with or without x-ray therapy or chemotherapy. Patients with estrogen-dependent tumors and known metastases are

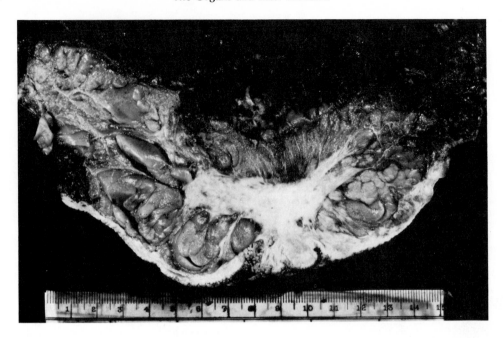

Fig. 21–16.   This section of a surgically removed breast shows the firm, whitish tissue in the center, which is **adenocarcinoma.** (McGill University, Department of Pathology Museum.)

often treated with hormonal manipulations (removal of the ovaries or adrenals, administration of testosterone). The exact method of treatment depends on the type and size of the lesion, on the presence of known metastases, and on the preference of the surgeon. Clinical studies are currently in progress in an attempt to determine the best approach to this disease. That the overall five-year survival rate (about 55%) has not changed significantly in the past 40 years reflects the need for continuing research in this area.

SYNOPSIS

Bleeding from the uterus in excessive amounts or at unusual times should always be investigated.

Carcinoma of the cervix is common and can be diagnosed early by either smear or biopsy. Carcinoma of the endometrium is less common and occurs at an older age.

Infections of the female genitourinary tract occur most commonly in the urinary bladder (cystitis), fallopian tubes (salpingitis), and occasionally in the endometrium (endometritis). Puerperal sepsis used to be much more significant as a life-threatening disease than it is today.

Benign tumors of the female genitourinary tract include leiomyomas of the uterus and cysts of the ovary of different designations.

Malignant tumors of importance are carcinoma of the cervix and adenocarcinoma of the endometrium. Tumors of the ovary are less common.

Mammary dysplasia is the commonest disease of the female breast. Biopsy is the surest way to confirm the diagnosis.

Carcinoma of the breast is a common important lesion with a tendency to early local metastases and generalized metastases. All single nodules of the breast should be regarded as malignant until proven otherwise.

Terms

Menorrhagia	*Endometriosis*	*Salpingitis*
Metrorrhagia	*Chorionepithelioma*	*Dermoid cyst*
Amenorrhea	*Choriocarcinoma*	*Teratoma*
Leiomyoma	*Hydatidiform mole*	*Mammary dysplasia*
Endometrium	*Carcinoma of cervix*	*Fibroadenoma*
Endometritis	*Carcinoma of endometrium*	*Adenocarcinoma of the breast*

FURTHER READING

Editorial: Genital herpes and cervical carcinoma. Br. Med. J., *1*:807, 1978.

Anderson, W. A. D., and Kissane, J. M. (Eds.): *Pathology,* 7th Ed. St. Louis, C. V. Mosby, 1977, Vol. II.

Blaustein, A. (Ed.): *Pathology of the Female Genital Tract.* New York, Springer-Verlag, 1977.

Bottoms, S. F., et al.: The increase in the cesarean birth rate. N. Engl. J. Med., *302*:559, 1980.

Coulson, W. S. (Ed.): *Surgical Pathology.* Philadelphia, Lippincott, 1978, Vol. I.

Crile, G., Jr.: The case for local excision of breast cancer in selected cases. Lancet, *1*:549, 1972.

Currie, A. R. (Ed.): *Endocrine Aspects of Breast Cancer.* Edinburgh, Livingstone, 1958.

DiSaia, P. J., Morrow, C. P., and Townsend, D. E.: *Synopsis of Gynecologic Oncology.* New York, John Wiley & Sons, 1975.

Friedrich, E. G.: *Valvular Disease. Major Problems in Obstetrics and Gynecology.* Philadelphia, W. B. Saunders, 1976, Vol. 9.

Goldfarb, J. M., and Little, A. B.: Abnormal vaginal bleeding. N. Engl. J. Med., *302*:666, 1980.

Goldzielier, J. W., and Dozier, T. S.: Oral contraceptives and thromboembolism: a reassessment. Am. J. Obstet. Gynecol., *123*:878, 1975.

Haagensen, C. D.: *Diseases of the Breast,* 2nd Ed. Philadelphia, W. B. Saunders, 1971.

Harlap, S.: Gender of infants conceived on different days of the menstrual cycle. N. Engl. J. Med., *300*:1445, 1979.

Henderson, I. C., and Canellos, G. P.: Cancer of the breast: The past decade. N. Engl. J. Med., *302*:17, 1980.

Herbst, A. L. (Ed.): Intrauterine exposure to diethyl stilbestrol in the human. American College of Obstetricians and Gynecologists, Proceedings of Symposium on DES, 1977.

Koss, L. G.: Dysplasia—a real concept or a misnomer? Obstet. Gynecol., *51*:374, 1978.

LiVolsi, V. A., et al.: Fibrocystic breast disease in oral-contraceptive users: histopathological evaluation of epithelial atypia. N. Engl. J. Med., *299*:381, 1978.

Mack, T. M., et al.: Estrogens and endometrial carcinoma in a retirement community. N. Engl. J. Med., *294*:1262, 1976.

McDivitt, R. W., Stewart, F. W., and Berg, J. W.: Tumors of the breast. Bethesda, Md., AFIP Fascicle #2, Second Series, 1968.

Pytkowicz Streissguth, A., et al.: Teratogenic effects of alcohol in humans and laboratory animals. Science, *209*:353, 1980.

Smith, D. C., et al.: Association of exogenous estrogen and endometrial carcinoma. N. Engl. J. Med., *293*:1164, 1975.

Spencer, J. D., Millis, R. R., and Hayward, J. L.: Contraceptive steroids and breast cancer. Br. Med. J., *1*:1024, 1978.

Speroff, L., Glass, R. H., and Kase, N. G.: *Clinical Gynecologic Endocrinology and Infertility,* 2nd Ed. Baltimore, Williams & Wilkins, 1978.

Weiss, N. S., Szekely, D. R., and Austin, D. F.: Increasing incidence of endometrial cancer in the United States. N. Engl. J. Med., *294*:1259, 1976.

Ziel, H. G., and Finkle, W. D.: Increased risk of endometrial carcinoma among users of conjugated estrogens. N. Engl. J. Med., *293*:1167, 1975.

Endocrine System

22

Science has promised us truth—it never has promised us either peace or happiness.—LeBon

The body has 2 major communication networks that enable its many parts to operate in a coordinated, efficient manner. One of these is the nervous system, in which messages are passed from neuron to neuron, as a network of wires connects all the telephones of a city. Communication depends on the integrity of these neurons, and if the wires were cut, communication would cease just as in our telephone system.

The other major communication network is the subject of this chapter, namely, the endocrine system. Endocrine communication is not like telephone communication; it generally does not depend on wires. It is more like radio communication, of which the essential elements are transmitter, signal, and receivers. The signal is not transmitted by wires to a specific destination, rather it is carried through the blood all over the body, just as any radio in the general area will receive a radio message. Thus endocrine signals may come into contact with cells throughout the body; however, some cells, like radio receivers tuned to the right frequency, are particularly sensitive to and dependent on the signals, and these are referred to as the "target organ." For example, the pituitary secretes adrenocorticotropic hormone (ACTH) into

the blood, which carries the hormone all over the body. However, the cells of the adrenal cortex appear to be the only ones to respond to this signal, as far as we know.

Endocrine organs are commonly referred to as glands, a term that connotes secretion of a substance. Endocrine glands secrete their products into the blood (as opposed to exocrine glands, which secrete onto a surface, e.g., sweat glands).

The products of endocrine glands are called **hormones,** and these are the chemical signals we have mentioned. Hormones are chemical substances of different kinds: steroids (cortisone), proteins (growth hormones), peptides (antidiuretic hormone), amino acids (thyroxine), or amines (epinephrine). They range from large to small molecules and have chemical structures of varying complexity. The term hormone (which means to set in motion) was introduced at the turn of the century from the work of Bayliss and Starling, who demonstrated that there were substances that could initiate secretion in a distant organ.

The endocrine system includes all endocrine glands and their products, the hormones. Thus this system is composed of anatomically and histologically distinct parts, possessing many individual functions. However, the system as a whole is regarded as having a regulatory function. It is the system that, on orders from above, regulates and coordinates many of the functions of the organism.

Historically, we came to understand the function of the endocrine organs largely through the effects of their destruction. Disorders of the endocrine system are the result of lesions in the transmitting organ (and occasionally in the target receptor; Fig. 22–1). Whereas a lesion in the wires of the nervous system may have disastrous results, this kind of signal disruption is not possible in the endocrine system, for reasons described. However, lesions in the endocrine transmitters may have lethal ramifications. This situation may be compared with that of an army general whose radio transmitter breaks, which causes all troops, who depend on his orders, to run completely amok. The troops may simply not act, or they may act in such an unregulated fashion that the war is lost. War cannot be successfully waged unless the actions of the individual troops are coordinated; so it is with the functioning of the body.

There are 3 important principles of endocrine disease that should be kept in mind:

1. Endocrine disease can arise from a malfunction of control mechanism (a breakdown in the transmitter).

2. Such a malfunction may lead to insufficient, excessive, or inappropriate emission of signal. Any of these alternatives leads to disordered function. For example, when the anterior pituitary is destroyed by necrosis, all the target organs, whose functioning depends on pituitary hormones, become atrophied. Conversely, when a tumor of the eosinophilic cells of the anterior pituitary produces excess growth hormone, an afflicted child may grow up to be a great basketball player, with a height of 7 or 8 feet. Finally, a diseased endocrine gland may secrete more or less or the right amount of hormone, but at the wrong times. Acromegaly, which is a syndrome caused by excessive secretion of the growth hormone, is an example of this last type of disorder.

3. Although most hormones may demonstrate their effects on a single target area most obviously, since hormones are chemical mes-

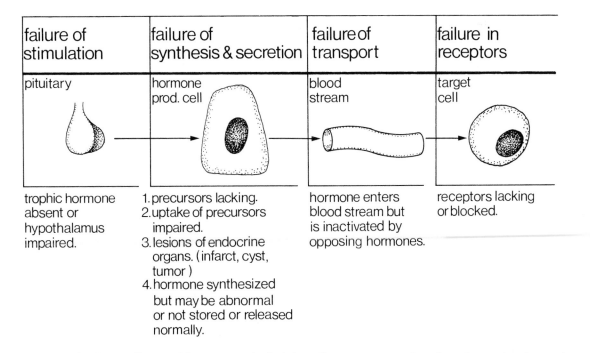

failure of stimulation	failure of synthesis & secretion	failure of transport	failure in receptors
pituitary	hormone prod. cell	blood stream	target cell
trophic hormone absent or hypothalamus impaired.	1. precursors lacking. 2. uptake of precursors impaired. 3. lesions of endocrine organs. (infarct, cyst, tumor) 4. hormone synthesized but may be abnormal or not stored or released normally.	hormone enters blood stream but is inactivated by opposing hormones.	receptors lacking or blocked.

Fig. 22–1.   This diagram illustrates different reasons for the failure of hormone action. Failure of stimulation, of synthesis and secretion, of transport, and in receptors are all easy to understand conceptually, but each may be difficult to prove in an individual patient.

Table 22–1. Endocrine Glands, Hormones, and Their Effects

ENDOCRINE GLAND	HORMONE	EFFECT
HYPOTHALAMUS	Thyrotropin releasing factor (TRF)	Stimulates the anterior pituitary to secrete thyrotropic hormone (TSH).
ANTERIOR PITUITARY	Thyrotropic hormone (thyroid stimulating hormone, TSH)	Stimulates thyroxine formation and release from the thyroid gland.
	Adrenocorticotropic hormone (corticotropin, ACTH)	Stimulates the adrenal cortex to secrete cortisone.
	Follicle-stimulating hormone (FSH)	♂: Stimulates development of germinal epithelium in testes and, therefore, spermatogenesis as well.
		♀: Induces maturation of ovarian follicle.
	Interstitial cell-stimulating hormone (ICSH, luteinizing hormone, LH)	♂: Stimulates interstitial cells of testes to produce testosterone.
		♀: Develops corpus luteum.
	Prolactin	♂: No known action.
		♀: Maintains activity in fully developed corpus luteum and stimulates milk secretion.
POSTERIOR PITUITARY*	Oxytocin	Stimulates pregnant uterus to contract.
	Vasopressin (antidiuretic hormone ADH)	Promotes reabsorption of water from distal tubule in the kidney.
THYROID	Thyroxine (T_4) Triiodothyronine (T_3)	Increases metabolism in most tissues of the body.
PARAFOLLICULAR CELLS OF THYROID	Calcitonin	Inhibits reabsorption of calcium from bone (lowers serum calcium level).
PARATHYROID	Parathormone	Mobilizes calcium and phosphorus from bone (increases serum calcium level).
ADRENAL CORTEX	Aldosterone	Stimulates sodium and chloride reabsorption in the kidney. Promotes potassium excretion.
	Cortisone	Regulates carbohydrate metabolism (and is used clinically to suppress inflammation).
	Androgens	Promote masculinization.
ADRENAL MEDULLA	Epinephrine and Norepinephrine	Neurotransmission. Preparation for "flight or fight."
PANCREAS: B CELLS	Insulin	Lowers blood glucose. Mobilizes glycogen from liver.
TESTIS	Testosterone	Develops male secondary characteristics.
OVARY	Estrogen	Develops female secondary characteristics. Helps to regulate menstruation.
CORPUS LUTEUM	Progesterone	Prepares uterus for implantation of fertilized ovum during "luteal" phase of menstrual cycle.

*Hormones secreted by the posterior pituitary are not in fact produced there. They are formed in the hypothalamus, in nerve cells that have long axons extending down into the posterior pituitary (hence the synonym: neurohypophysis). The pituitary stores and secretes these hormones.

sengers that circulate to all tissues and cells, the absence or excess of their effects may be seen in all tissues, if we know how to perceive them. To be more specific, whereas endocrine disorders such as hyperthyroidism may be viewed as a disturbance of the control mechanisms of thyroid hormone production, the effects of excessive thyroxine can be detected not only in skeletal and cardiac muscle, but also in biochemical and submicroscopic lesions in the liver, as well as in the general behavior of the patient. Conversely, the destruction of the thyroid gland causes many symptoms that are manifest in the attitude of the torpid patient himself or herself.

Thus endocrine diseases may be best viewed as **multisystem disorders**, that is, their effects cut across anatomic boundaries and create disorders of function in many different parts of the body. They are not confined to 1 system alone.

In this chapter, we first consider the pituitary, its relationship to the hypothalamus and its target organs, then the adrenal, thyroid, and parathyroid glands, and, finally, the islets of Langerhans (see Table 22–1). The testes and ovary have already been considered in chapters on the male and female genitourinary systems, respectively.

PITUITARY

This small organ, about the size of a cherry pit, is hidden deep in the skull. It develops from an outpouching of the oral cavity during embryonic life and comes to rest dead center at the base of the brain, attached to it by the most slender stalk (Fig. 22–2). This stalk carries nerves from the hypothalamus to the posterior part, but only blood vessels to the anterior portion. The blood supply of the anterior pituitary is curious because, unlike any other in the body (usually a simple extension of the arterial blood supply, with the standard arrangement of capillaries and veins), it consists entirely of venous blood from the hypothalamus (the anterior pituitary receives no arterial blood), so the blood to the pituitary has already been circulated to a part of the brain.

This venous blood divides into a second capillary network that arborizes around the

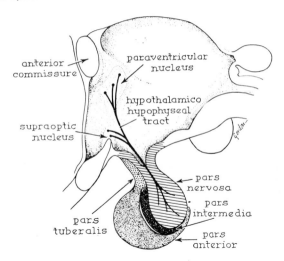

Fig. 22–2. This drawing shows the relationship of the pituitary to the hypothalamus. The tracts joining the hypothalamus to the pituitary are illustrated in the black, dark lines. The anterior pituitary is shown in the stipple, the pars intermedia in the dark shading, and the pars nervosa or posterior pituitary by the cross-hatching. (From Ham, A. W.: *Histology*, 7th Ed. Philadelphia and Toronto, J. B. Lippincott, 1974.)

cells of the anterior pituitary. The arrangement is elegantly suited to the transport of chemical messengers arising in the brain itself, for this is how the pituitary receives its signals. It is not by a system of wires, but by a hydraulic waterway. It is now clear that the anterior pituitary produces its hormonal products intermittently, in spurts that are greatly dependent on the functioning of the central nervous system. Figure 22–3 shows the rhythmic and pulsatile secretion of a variety of hormones from the anterior pituitary, each of which is modulated, if not governed, by stimuli from the hypothalamus through the mechanism of releasing hormones.

The hypothalamus itself receives signals from the afferent or incoming pathways such as sight, smell, temperature, even hunger, and especially rage and fright. Its connection to the pituitary thus makes it possible for the experience of the world to be interpreted and reacted to, preparing the individual by grading and stimulating or by inhibiting the hormone production from the pituitary by its own products, those small polypeptides known as releasing or inhibitory hormones. These polypeptides are secreted into the vascular system just described, and are received

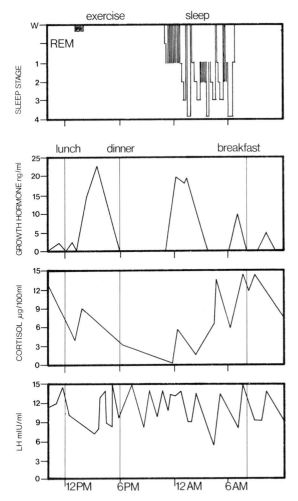

Fig. 22–3. This set of graphs illustrates human activities during a full 24-hour day. The top graph illustrates the levels of growth hormone at different times, illustrating the intermittent nature of the secretion of growth hormone and its relationship to exercise and sleep. Meals, exercise, and sleep are illustrated in the second graph. Cortisol has a diurnal cycle with two peaks, and luteinizing hormone is secreted discontinuously in small amounts throughout the 24-hour period. (From Federman, D. D.: Endocrinology. In *Scientific American Medicine.* Edited by E. Rubenstein and D. D. Federman. New York, Scientific American Illustrated Library, 1979, Vol. I.)

and reacted to by anterior pituitary cells. Hormonal products of the anterior pituitary cells are quickly circulated in the blood stream to all parts of the body, where they may signal for more testosterone, more thyroxine, or more cortisone, for example.

A second and important aspect of the blood supply to the anterior pituitary is that the cells are also exposed to direct chemical messen-

gers from the rest of the body, so that signals of hypoglycemia, high serum sodium levels, and the feedback hormones from the peripheral endocrine organs are all constantly perfusing these cells. These signals are received simultaneously, together with those from the hypothalamus. This arrangement permits a finely graded tuning that makes the life of an air traffic controller at a major international airport seem simple by comparison.

The secretion of the releasing hormones from the hypothalamus depends in turn on biologic rhythm such as the sleep-waking cycle, but it may be modified by anxiety, stress, exercise, and diet.

As we have said, the **anterior lobe** secretes hormones in response to releasing and inhibitory factors of the hypothalamus and in response to the hormones produced by the glands that they stimulate. This form of regulation can be likened to a thermostat and furnace. On a warm day, the heat, the product of the furnace, signals to the thermostat to turn off the furnace, just as a high blood level of thyroxine turns off the thyroid. Similarly, when the temperature falls, the thermostat turns on the furnace, and, despite changes in the weather, the house remains at a given temperature. However, the thermostat can be regulated just as the hypothalamus regulates, and at times resets, the pituitary. The principal hormones of the anterior pituitary are:

Growth hormone (GH), as its name implies, regulates growth; therefore, its target is the whole body. An animal that has undergone hypophysectomy (removal of the pituitary) cannot grow unless growth hormone is replaced. The secretion of growth hormone is usually regulated through somatomedin, a substance made in the liver. A tropic hormone that might govern the release of growth hormone has been postulated, but not identified. Instead, many other signals, such as exercise, amino acids, hypoglycemia, sleep, all promote its secretion. Growth hormone also helps to protect the body from hypoglycemia during fasting. The secretion of this hormone is triggered by hypoglycemia and is increased in response to a rise in amino acids (particularly arginine) or following either stress or the administration of alpha-adrenergic stimuli (such as L-DOPA). Growth hormone is secreted shortly after sleep starts, even during the day. Its secretion is suppressed by a newly discovered substance called somatostatin. Growth hormone has a short half-life in the peripheral blood of about half an hour. The amount of circulating growth hormone is constantly fluctuating in the normal individual. GH and insulin combine to provide tissues with a continuously available source of fuel. This function of GH explains why patients with hypopituitarism are subject to severe hypoglycemia after a small injection of insulin, which could be easily tolerated by a patient with an intact pituitary. When the function of a patient's anterior pituitary is uncertain, insulin or arginine is administered to see whether the gland can secrete growth hormone normally.

Gonadotropic follicle-stimulating hormone (FSH) and **luteinizing hormone** or Interstitial Cell-Stimulating Hormone (LH, ICSH) are necessary both for the proper development of the male and female reproductive organs and for the menstrual cycle, since the hormones stimulate the ovaries to monthly activity, which in turn produces hormones responsible for the changes in the uterus that result in menstruation. One of the first signs of pituitary disease in the female is cessation of the normal menstrual function.

Thyrotropin (TSH) signals for the release of thyroxine from the thyroid gland and is essential for normal well-being. Thyrotropic hormone occasionally occurs in excess, and the normal serum values are a sensitive indicator of the integrity of the feedback mechanism between the liberation of thyroxine and the availability or inhibition of TSH.

Prolactin stimulates the production of milk in the female animal. Its effectiveness depends on the previous effect of adrenal hormones on breast tissue. Suckling initiates the release of prolactin. Prolactin is a large peptide hormone that has many functions in lower animals, but apparently only 1 in man. It shows physiologic variations, as does growth hormone, in association with sleep, stress, and other stimuli. The secretion of prolactin seems to be regulated by an inhibitory factor, secreted from the hypothalamus. Prolactin secretion rises progressively during pregnancy, reaching its maximum at term, coincident with the delivery of the fetus.

Adrenocorticotropin (ACTH) is the hormone that indicates to the adrenal cortex that it should produce a number of hormones. Hyperproduction of ACTH is the most common cause of Cushing's syndrome, which we discuss later in this chapter.

Melanocyte-stimulating hormone. In lower animals, this hormone is produced in the intermediate lobe of the pituitary, and it stimulates melanocytes (pigment-producing cells). In man, it is produced in the anterior lobe and has some melanocyte-stimulating properties.

The posterior lobe, called the neurohypophysis, produces 2 hormones: oxytocin and vasopressin (antidiuretic hormone).

Oxytocin derives its name from its ability to cause contraction of smooth muscle, principally in the uterus (Greek *oxys*, swift, and *tokos*, birth). This hormone is used clinically to induce uterine contractions during ineffective labor, and to cause tonic constriction of the uterus following delivery to control postpartum bleeding. Oxytocin also seems to have an effect on the mammary gland and aids in the ejection of milk.

Antidiuretic hormone (ADH), or vasopressin, increases the rate of reabsorption of water and electrolytes by the renal tubules, so that it reduces the output of urine. It thus performs the important function of guarding the organism against excessive water loss. In the absence of antidiuretic hormone, continued loss of fluid and accompanying thirst lead to the syndrome called diabetes insipidus.

Hyperfunction of the Anterior Pituitary

Despite the fact that at least 5 important hormones (growth hormone, ACTH, FSH, LH, and TSH) are synthesized and secreted by anterior pituitary cells, there is a good correlation between structural abnormality and evidence of overproduction for only the first 2 of these hormones. In most cases of gigantism, there is an adenoma of the eosinophilic cells of the pituitary (Fig. 22–4), as there is in most cases of the adult form of excess growth hormone production, commonly called acromegaly. Excessive ACTH production causes a pattern of abnormalities collected together under the term Cushing's syndrome, named after the neurosurgeon who recognized the relationship to the adenoma of basophils of the pituitary. Oddly, overproduction of FSH, LH, and TSH are clinically rare, and tumors

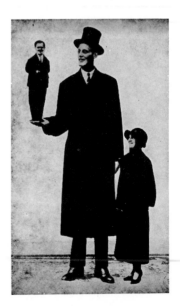

Fig. 22–4. This photograph shows the effect of hyperfunction of the anterior pituitary. The woman is of normal height and the giant could be suspected of having a growth-hormone secreting adenoma of the anterior pituitary.

responsible for their production have not been recognized. The occurrence of galactorrhea (milk secretion without pregnancy) is being found more frequently, and adenomas of prolactin-producing cells are seen often, thanks to newer diagnostic methods (radioimmunoassay) and to developments in the surgery of the anterior pituitary.

Acromegaly

This term designates the clinical syndrome that arises in adults when there is continuing excessive secretion of the growth hormone. The principal clinical manifestations and their frequency are outlined in Table 22–2. The principal significant abnormalities arise from growth within the pituitary of a clone of cells designated an adenoma. These cells appear to be eosinophilic on routine histologic examination in most cases. The patient with acromegaly produces only small amounts of growth hormone, but does it continually, unlike normal persons, whose growth hormone secretion is triggered by the many stimuli we have outlined. Sleep is the usual principal signal to growth hormone secretion, and the sleep need not be long. Thus the catnap or regular afternoon snooze has a valuable endocrinologic result. This only underscores the wisdom of our parents who used to insist on

Table 22–2.　Acromegaly: Frequency of Manifestations

MANIFESTATION	PERCENTAGE OF CASES
Enlarged sella turcica	93
Headache	85
Visual impairment	62
Secondary to growth hormone excess:	
Weight gain	39
Hypermetabolism	70
Excessive sweating	60
Impaired glucose tolerance	25
Clinical diabetes mellitus	12
Growth of flat bones	100
Prognathism	Common
Arthritic complaints	Common
Osteoporosis	Common
Soft tissue growth	100
Hypertrichosis	53
Pigmentation	40

an afternoon nap for all growing children, which we thought was only to give the parents some time away from looking after us.

Acromegaly is probably less often diagnosed than it might be, since, as with many insidious and slowly progressive disorders, the diagnosis does not become evident until the suspicion of its existence has crossed the mind of the consulting physician. This discovery is usually long after the patient has become symptomatic. Typically, this disorder of too much growth hormone in the adult appears in his or her 40's or 50's with headaches, sweating, weakness, fatigue and lethargy. These symptoms are all nonspecific in themselves. The presence of disturbances in vision should always suggest that the structures around the optic chiasm be investigated. Although x-ray studies of the pituitary fossa may be normal in up to one-quarter of acromegalics, most patients show abnormalities of the sella turcica, that small pocket in which the pituitary sits. In 1 study, 138 of 140 patients examined by x ray showed abnormalities!

The expression of acromegaly in the features and extremities of the unfortunate patient is memorable, as the accompanying photos demonstrate (Fig. 22–5), but the family, friends, and attending physician, as well as the patient, may all be oblivious to the slow changes that finally culminate in the coarsened facial appearance, prominent forehead, widened teeth, and change in hat size. A husky voice, a need for new gloves, and increasing deafness all may be signs of acromegaly. The prognosis of the untreated acromegalic is guarded, since many of them die with heart failure before the age of 60, for unknown reasons. One suggestion is that the constant secretion of excessive amounts of growth hormone requires unusual protein synthesis from heart muscle, and that this departure from normal leads to the increased size and eventual failure of this organ. Other complications of acromegaly are atherosclerosis, hypertension, and diabetes mellitus.

The diagnosis of the disease can now be easily confirmed by growth hormone assay (particularly of the cerebrospinal fluid) and treated by surgery to remove the adenoma, or with such new drugs as bromocriptine.

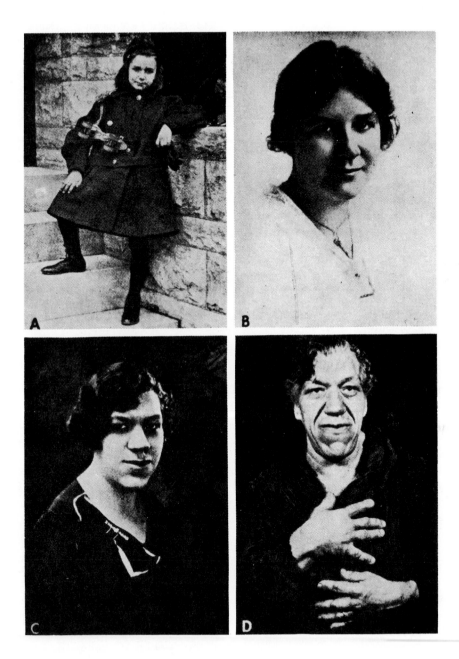

Fig. 22–5. The progression of acromegaly is illustrated in these photographs: *A*, normal, age 9 years; *B*, age 16 years with possible early coarsening of features; *C*, age 33 years, well-established acromegaly; *D*, age 52 years, end-stage acromegaly with gross disfigurement. (Clinical Pathological Conference. Am. J. Med., *20*:133, 1956.)

Prolactin Overproduction and Galactorrrhea

The result of hypersecretion of prolactin is milk secretion in individuals, either male or female. The hormone prolactin may have physiologic effects in addition to causing milk secretion, but we do not yet know what they are. Many persons, however, may have over-production of prolactin without milk production. The commonest cause of excess prolactin secretion is the presence of a chromophobe adenoma. Its appearance may be signaled by the involvement of the optic chiasm by the slowly growing tumor. The presence of an enlarged sella turcica is the warning to search for excess prolactin or growth hormone in the serum of the patient. However, in an era of drug therapy for every illness, real or imagined, another common cause of elevated prolactin levels and/or of abnormal milk secretion is the use of drugs that influence the hypothalamus (methyldopa, reserpine), or drugs such as monoamine oxidase inhibitors, phenothiazines, or estrogens. Thus the presence of an excessive amount of hormone in response to testing or the recognition of milk secretion may not, in fact, be due to a tumor.

Cushing's Disease

Although this subject is normally considered under diseases of the adrenals, since adrenal cortical hyperfunction is responsible for the excessive hormone production that leads to the signs and symptoms described by Harvey Cushing, he correctly ascribed the disorder to a functional basophil adenoma of the anterior pituitary. Thus the disorder should at least be mentioned as we consider disorders of hyperfunction of the anterior pituitary. For a further discussion of Cushing's disease and of Cushing's syndrome, we refer the reader to the sections on the adrenal in this chapter.

Hypofunction of the Anterior Pituitary

The pituitary may fail to produce hormones in 2 ways. The most common deficiency is called panhypopituitarism, since it is a deficiency of all the functions and may be caused by a variety of means, such as tumors that compress or destroy the gland from within or without, necrosis, or cysts. The less common deficiency is the absence of a single pituitary hormone, which is conventionally called monotropic deficiency. These deficiencies may be gonadotropic (usually both FSH and LH hormones are lacking, generally owing to a congenital deficiency of hypothalamic-releasing hormone). A lack of TSH may occur rarely; a lack of ACTH alone has been reported, but it is also rare and difficult to prove.

We might venture that the anterior pituitary is the only endocrine gland in which destruction by tumor is a significant or relatively common cause of hypofunction. The adrenal cortex and thyroid are rarely, if ever, so destroyed by the common metastatic tumors. The commonest cause of panhypopituitarism is compression by a tumor known as the chromophobe adenoma, discussed more completely in the chapter on the nervous system. Another tumor is the craniopharyngioma, a tumor of childhood, and the third commonest cause is metastasis, usually from breast or lung cancer.

Panhypopituitarism

There are some different clinical manifestations of panhypopituitarism, depending in part on the age of the patient (if it occurs before growth is completed, the person may be dwarfed), his or her sex, since menstrual irregularities may be the most prominent feature, or whether the pituitary function is lost gradually or suddenly.

The general rule for the deficiencies of hormone production, particularly when several hormones are lacking as in panhypopituitarism, is that the person may complain of some problem that is not obviously central to the loss of these several normal, human drives. Thus a male patient with panhypopituitarism may complain of being mistaken for a woman on the telephone, rather than complain directly about impotence. A peculiar apathy and listlessness of which the patient may not be aware may characterize panhypopituitarism. The woman may first recognize something is amiss when she has no menstrual period, owing to the lack of gonadotropic hormones (FSH and LH). The absence of growth hormone, thyroid stimulating hormone, and ACTH may go un-

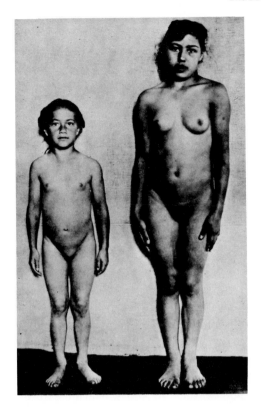

noticed, as these hormones lead more slowly to changes that may be nonspecific. The man may notice as his first complaint in addition to lassitude, weakness, and fatigue, a loss of sexual desire and function. Of course, if the cause of pituitary destruction is a tumor growing in the optic chiasm, the symptoms may not be referable to the loss of endocrine function, but rather to headaches and interference with vision.

One type of panhypopituitarism, pituitary dwarfism, occurs in children. The lack of hormone produces a mentally alert, normally intelligent, but small and sexually underdeveloped individual, who is much like a graceful and attractive child, and who never grows up, similar to Peter Pan (Fig. 22–6). This type of panhypopituitarism usually results from the presence of a cyst or tumor, which must be distinguished from a genetically determined dwarfism and from congenital hypothyroidism. The genetic dwarf has normal secretion of all hormones except growth hormone, whereas the cretin, or congenital hypothyroid, is condemned to subnormal mentality, and the appearance of the body remains infantile.

Simmond's disease is the term given to panhypopituitarism occurring in the adult, which results in the absence of all pituitary

Fig. 22–6. Hypophyseal infantilism. Girl on left, age 15, sexually infantile, next to normal sister on right, 2 years younger and fully matured. Striking example of pituitary dwarfism plus sexual infantilism. (Lisser and Escamilla: *Atlas of Clinical Endocrinology,* 2nd Ed. St. Louis, C. V. Mosby, 1962.)

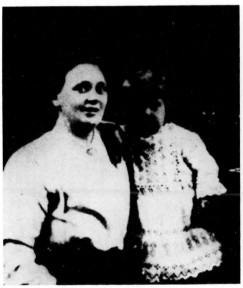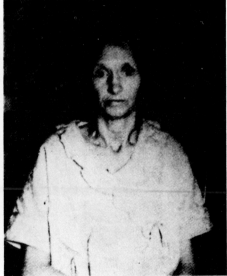

Fig. 22–7. The photograph on the left shows the patient with one of her children taken just before her last pregnancy. At this time she was 32 years old and weighed 140 lbs. The figure on the right was taken 9 years later following a pregnancy accompanied by a massive hemorrhage. Her weight at the time of this photograph was 85½ lbs. She died of pan-hypopituitarism 3 years later. These photographs were taken before the availability of replacement therapy.

Table 22–3. Average Size of Organs in Simmonds' Disease and Acromegaly Compared with Normal

BODY WEIGHT ORGAN	SIMMONDS' DISEASE (4 CASES) 95 LB. GM.	NORMAL GM.	ACROMEGALY (5 CASES) 194 LB. GM.
Heart	175	300	448
Liver	866	1500	2462
Kidney	89	155	247
Spleen	144	200	353
Pancreas	43	100	135
Thyroid	10	40	76
Adrenals (together)	6.4	12	26
Gonads	small	. . .	normal or large
Thymus	. . .	. . .	sometimes enlarged

secretions. The classic cause of this used to be the occurrence in young women of excessive blood loss at the time of delivery. The shock that accompanied this blood loss found a particularly sensitive target in the large, vascular pituitary of pregnancy, which may be 2 or 3 times normal size, and is particularly susceptible to hypotension. Sheean described the occurrence of panhypopituitarism in such young women (Fig. 22–7) and discovered that there was necrosis of the pituitary due sometimes to thrombosis and sometimes simply to ischemic necrosis. The onset of symptoms appeared insidiously during the postpartum period, and months and years later they were found to be changed persons, without thyroid or adrenal function (Table 22–3). Thus to the list of causes of panhypopituitarism, which include tumors (craniopharyngioma, chromophobe adenoma, metastatic tumor), cysts, granulomatous lesions such as tuberculosis and sarcoid, we may add postpartum necrosis, which carries the eponym **Sheean's syndrome.**

Posterior Pituitary

Any surgical trauma, inflammation, hemorrhage, or tumor may injure the posterior pituitary as well, and may interfere with the exquisite balancing mechanisms that control the tonicity of our blood plasma by regulating water and sodium absorption at the level of the kidneys. This regulation is effected through the secretion of the substance vasopressin. The posterior pituitary also secretes oxytocin. These hormones are synthesized and are secreted in the hypothalamus and are transported along axons that terminate in storage vesicles in the posterior pituitary. Any interference with this mechanism may lead to the syndrome of **diabetes insipidus,** which consists of polyuria (passing large volumes of urine, more than 2,000 ml per day) and polydypsia (the drinking of large volumes of water). This syndrome must be distinguished from the polyuria and polydypsia that accompany the presence of excessive serum glucose in diabetes mellitus and the occurrence of psychogenic water drinking.

ADRENALS

The adrenals are 2 small glands, each shaped like a cocked hat, 1 on either side of the aorta, located just above the kidney. Each adrenal consists of 2 parts, an outer portion or cortex, and an inner portion or medulla. These are not merely 2 parts; they are 2 different organs joined together, different in origin, in structure, in function, and in the diseases that visit them. The function of the adrenal gland is difficult to summarize. It does many things, but if one tried to generalize, one might say that it controls the body's adjustments to changes in posture by regulating the tone of blood vessels and the volume of blood, in conjunction with other organs such as the kidney and the heart. It also modulates the intermittent, rather than constant, intake of nourishment. It does this in conjunction with the liver. Finally, the adrenal gland acts as a storehouse for hormones that are used in times of great distress, such as hemorrhage, infection, and shock. The loss of these adrenal functions is a life-threatening phenomenon, as we shall see.

The cortex is essential to life, since, when it is removed, death occurs in a few days. For over 100 years, it has been known that patients with adrenal insufficiency often die from minor infections and stresses that patients with normal adrenals will survive. More than 20 different steroids with different types of physiologic action have been isolated from the adrenal cortex. Roughly, they may be divided into 3 general groups: (1) those that regulate salt and water metabolism; (2) those that regulate carbohydrate metabolism; and (3) those that modify sexual functions. For persons with a desire to memorize things easily, the 3 functions may be represented by the letter S, as salt, sugar, and sex. For the others, these categories are the mineralocorticoids, the glucocorticoids, and the androgenic hormones.

Mineralocorticoids. Aldosterone, produced by the cells of the more superficial layer of the cortex, is a hormone that governs sodium and chloride retention and potassium excretion, and thereby controls the amount of water retained in the body. The exogenous administration of aldosterone leads to edema and increase in body weight due to sodium retention. Persons with aldosterone-secreting tumors also complain of fatigue and show electrocardiographic abnormalities because of the depletion of potassium that accompanies sodium retention. Normal levels of aldosterone are essential for life, and the loss of aldosterone production contributes significantly to the syndrome of adrenal cortical insufficiency, known by the name of its discoverer, Addison.

Under normal circumstances, the production of aldosterone is regulated largely by the secretion of renin from the kidney. The small, specialized area of cells, called the juxtaglomerular apparatus discussed in the kidney chapter, detects pressure changes in the blood that perfuses the kidney. Any reduction in blood volume, for example as occurs in hemorrhage, results in decreased perfusion and, therefore, in decreased pressure. This reduction is perceived by the juxtaglomerular apparatus, and its response is the secretion of small granules containing a protein that is converted in the serum

and eventually results in increased aldosterone secretion from the adrenal cortex. Teleologically, this is a convenient means of retaining more salt and water, thus increasing the fluid volume that has been lost in the hemorrhage.

Glucocorticoids. Carbohydrate metabolism is regulated by a number of factors. Amino acids may be converted into glucose instead of into protein, raising the supply of serum glucose and contributing to the store of glycogen in the liver by the presence of glucocorticoids. Cortisone and hydrocortisone are produced by the inner layers of the adrenal cortex and are under the regulation of ACTH from the anterior pituitary.

Cortisone has been synthesized and available for over 30 years as part of the physician's armamentarium. In man, cortisone has an inhibitory effect on lymphoid tissue. Cortisone therefore suppresses the inflammatory response to practically all forms of injury. This anti-inflammatory reaction may relieve the pain and discomfort of inflammation, and is of value in noninfectious inflammation as exemplified by rheumatoid arthritis, but, unfortunately, whereas cortisone relieves the symptoms of disease, it does not influence the cause. It does not put out the fire, nor does it repair the damage after the fire. It could be thought of as providing the tissues with some kind of asbestos suit, which may itself be only temporary. We must remember that inflammation helps the body to mobilize its defenses against infection. When a patient is taking high doses of steroids, inflammation against bacterial invaders is also suppressed. The patient may appear well and show few signs of infection, although he may be experiencing a fulminating bacteremia. Cortisone is a two-edged sword that must be used with respect and understanding.

Androgens. These hormones tend to masculinize the body, to retain amino acids, and to enhance protein synthesis. Androgenic hormones are used (illegally to be sure, and unwisely in most cases) by weight lifters and those interested in increasing their body strength for questionable purposes. When androgens have been metabolized, the 17-ketosteroids are excreted in the urine. The breakdown products of androgens form the basis for the doping tests used at Olympic events, but they are also more commonly used in cases of virilism in which some disorders of the adrenal is suspected. Naturally, in adrenal cortical disease, the 17-ketosteroid levels will be low.

Medulla. The adrenal medulla is derived from the sympathetic nervous system. Unlike the cortex, its secretory products are epinephrine and norepinephrine. These substances have a direct effect on the smooth muscle in the walls of arterioles. They may also have an effect on glycogenolysis, liberating glucose from the stores of glycogen in the liver into the serum. In severe stress, such as rage or fear, surgical operations, or any life-threatening event, epinephrine is poured into the blood; in the words of Cannon, the person is prepared for "flight or fight" and may be enabled to perform extraordinary feats during this emergency.

Hypoadrenalism

Adrenal cortical insufficiency should be thought of in 2 general ways. First, it may be a medical emergency that, if not recognized, could result in the patient's death within hours. However, the commonest form is a chronic and insidious adrenal cortical insufficiency, which is often not recognized. The second general idea is that adrenal cortical insufficiency can either originate in the adrenals (and it is necessary for both adrenals to be involved), or it may be due to absence of the tropic hormone, ACTH, owing to destruction or disease of the anterior pituitary. We have come to talk about primary adrenal insufficiency—that originating in the adrenals, and secondary adrenal insufficiency—that which is not due to disease of the adrenals themselves, but rather to disease of the anterior pituitary (lack of ACTH) and which therefore causes atrophy of the adrenal glands.

Today, the causes of adrenal insufficiency are different from those recognized by Addison 130 years ago. They are also different from those recognized 50 years ago. The 3 most important causes of adrenal insufficiency in Addison's day were tuberculosis, tuberculosis, and tuberculosis. With the control of this disease, the most common finding in Addisonian patients now is a lymphocytic infiltration of the adrenal cortex with patches of fibrosis, seen in three-quarters of such patients. Two-thirds of these cases show immunofluorescent antibodies to an antigen derived from adrenal cell cytoplasm. These observations are interpreted as evidence for an autoimmune adrenalitis, the initiating cause of which remains obscure. We need not go into other associations that have been made with this discovery, such as the occurrence of autoimmune thyroiditis, but pass on to other causes of adrenal insufficiency before discussing their clinical manifestations.

Today, tuberculosis is still a significant cause of Addison's disease, but it probably accounts for chronic adrenal insufficiency

about only 1 case in 10. It used to be far and away the most common cause.

A third cause of chronic adrenal insufficiency is the atrophy that occurs with the long-term administration of exogenous corticosteroid for such disorders as arthritis and regional ileitis. The adrenal cortex becomes smaller and, if the steroids are withdrawn, the patient is unable to meet the normal requirements of hormone, which inability may precipitate a crisis. Alternate-day therapy with cortisone seems to be a way to attempt to resolve this atrophy. The cause of adrenal atrophy is called iatrogenic, naturally. There are also other instances in which there is no apparent reason for the adrenal failure, and we call those cases idiopathic. At present, autoimmune, tuberculous, and iatrogenic causes lead the list of causes of chronic adrenal failure.

The patient with **Addison's disease,** who is usually a woman, complains of weakness, loss of appetite, nausea, irritability, and orthostatic hypotension. These nonspecific symptoms are so universal that almost anyone might think that he has Addison's disease. However, 2 other observations should suggest the diagnosis as well as the appropriate laboratory examination to confirm the suspicion. Increased pigmentation of the skin occurs in almost all patients with primary adrenal cortical failure, since the feedback inhibition of the anterior pituitary is lacking. Owing to decreased cortisol production or lack of it, the anterior pituitary continues to secrete ACTH, and with it there is an excess of melanocyte-stimulating hormone, which causes the pigmentation. Of course, in cases of pituitary failure with secondary adrenal atrophy, the pigmentation does not occur. The second observation is the recognition of a low systolic and diastolic blood pressure. The person with Addison's disease may have a decreased blood volume and a loss of regulation of the normal responses that control blood pressure, because of the absence of the hormone that regulates salt and water retention. Thus hypotension and the sudden occurrence of life-threatening shock are all part of the syndrome of hypoadrenalism.

Acute adrenal cortical insufficiency is a problem with different causes and different clinical manifestations and implications. The person with adrenal insufficiency is in immediate danger of death. It is a medical emergency that often produces shock with prostration, hypoglycemia, and nausea and vomiting. Thus the explanation for the crisis may be confusing, because of the apparent gastrointestinal symptoms. Laboratory diagnosis is helpful, but the delay in waiting for the results of the serum sodium and potassium could be fatal. The appropriate treatment in cases of collapse from suspected acute adrenal cortical insufficiency is immediate administration of cortisol and other supportive measures.

The pathogenesis of acute adrenal cortical insufficiency is best understood in terms of 2 ideas. First, it may be superimposed on chronic disease, by which the adrenal cortical reserve has been eroded by chronic destruction and replacement or by atrophy of the gland. When a sudden challenge such as infection or a trauma occurs, the unfortunate patient has no ability to manufacture or to secrete supplemental steroids. Thus the crisis is due to a marked discrepancy between the need and the ability to respond. The second setting is the one in which the adrenal has been functioning normally, but is the site of sudden destruction. Most commonly, this phenomenon occurs because the highly vascular adrenal is the site of massive hemorrhage and necrosis. The causes of this pathologic process are usually septicemia, often from the meningococcus. This second type of insufficiency occasionally occurs with anticoagulant therapy, or after an operation. The name for this catastrophe is the Waterhouse-Friderichsen syndrome, named after the physicians who described death in cases of patients with meningococcemia, vascular collapse, and the presence of purpuric hemorrhages all over the skin.

Addison's disease, whether primary or secondary, can be managed today by replacement therapy. Daily oral doses of steroids can restore the metabolic equilibrium, just as insulin manages to restore the appropriate physiologic pathways in the diabetic. It is important, however, to remember that the patient with Addison's disease is still physiologically crippled and cannot adjust to increased demands for adrenal hormones as occur during infections or operations. Thus the dose needs to be adjusted to the circumstances. A medical alert card, bracelet, or notice greatly enhances his chance of survival in the event of an accident.

Hyperadrenalism

Hyperfunction of the adrenals may be either cortical or medullary. Many conditions have been described that result from the overproduction of 1, 2, or all 3 hormones. Each of the following syndromes represents an overproduction of a single hormone primarily.

Cushing's syndrome refers to the clinical features caused by excess glucocorticoid hormones, but it does not imply a particular cause. It may have already occurred to the thoughtful reader that the mere administration of cortisone may cause Cushing's syndrome, which is true and is probably the most common contemporary cause of this extraordinary change from normal. First, we shall consider the appearance of persons with this syndrome, and then we shall discuss the possible causes of it.

The clinical expression of Cushing's syndrome is unforgettable, as is seen in Fig. 22–8. A round, moon-shaped face, often with an acne-like eruption, and the presence of excess hair attract your attention at once. The body and trunk may be grossly exaggerated, compared with the thin, stick-like arms and legs. The presence of truncal obesity, a hump at the back of the neck, and purplish bruises are all classic findings on examining a patient with Cushing's syndrome. When the physician asks, the patient usually will speak of weakness, loss of strength, amenorrhea, impotence, and, sometimes, bone pain. Frequently, psychiatric symptoms are included. Weakness and diabetes mellitus are also part of the pattern. This pattern is unforgettable, and has many and complicated explanations, but it should suffice to attribute them to the excess of cortical hormone secretion.

Now the problem is to distinguish the different origins of this torrent of hormones. Since we know these hormones come from the adrenal cortex, a rare cause (10%) is the pres-

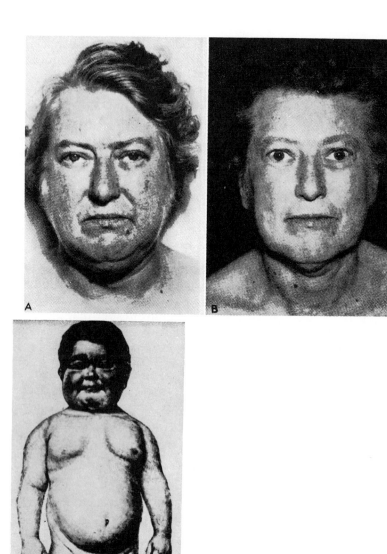

Fig. 22–8. *A,* Face of a patient with Cushing's syndrome due to bilateral hyperplasia of the adrenals. This 45-year-old patient underwent a two-stage bilateral total adrenalectomy. *B,* Disappearance of all signs and symptoms 8 months after the second adrenalectomy, during which period patient received complete substitution therapy. (A and B from Williams: *Textbook of Endocrinology,* 4th Ed. Philadelphia, W. B. Saunders, 1968.) C, Adrenal virilism in boy 4½ years of age.

ence of a tumor of the adrenal cortex. Even in this small number of cases, it is far more common for a benign tumor (adenoma) than for a carcinoma to produce Cushing's syndrome. A second and more common cause is Cushing's disease, which is the presence of an ACTH-secreting tumor in the anterior pituitary that stimulates the adrenal cortex to secrete excess amounts of hormone. The association of this basophil adenoma of the pituitary with bilateral adrenal cortical hyperplasia was described in the 1920's by Harvey Cushing, a neurosurgeon, and accounts for 80% of the cases of Cushing's syndrome (excluding iatrogenic causes and those rare cases of ectopic hormone production). This latter cause (ectopic hormones) is a much more recent discovery. It was observed that in a few cases of Cushing's syndrome, there was neither an adrenal tumor nor a basophil adenoma, and yet there was adrenal cortical hyperplasia in patients with carcinoma (frequently of the lung). Such tumors have now been shown to secrete ACTH or ACTH-like hormones, which achieve the same result, namely, excessive ACTH production, and to stimulate the adrenal to produce glucocorticoids in its own turn. Thus we have 4 significant causes of Cushing's syndrome: (1) iatrogenic administration of cortisone, (2) Cushing's disease, (3) adrenal tumors, and (4) ectopic hormones (lung).

Androgen excess (adrenal-genital hyperplasia) usually arises at any time between birth and early adolescence. The excess androgens tend to make little boys little men and little girls little boys. This syndrome is most often caused by a decrease in one of the enzymes leading to the production of cortisol. Therefore, low levels of cortisol feed back to the pituitary and adrenal synthesis is increased in efforts to achieve normal levels of cortisol. However, because of the partial block, many cortisol precursors are shunted into the synthesis of sex steroids.

This syndrome, with all its psychologic as well as physical ramifications, should be recognized because the whole pathway of overproduction of androgens can be turned off by giving the patient daily oral doses of cortisol.

Aldosteronism is an overproduction of aldosterone, the powerful mineralocorticoid produced by the most superficial layer of the cortex. Aldosterone serves to regulate fluid balance and the excretion of electrolytes; overproduction of this mineralocorticoid causes retention of sodium and increased loss of potassium. The biochemical picture of aldosteronism, then, is opposite to that of Addison's disease. The adrenal lesion is much more likely to be an adenoma than it is cortical hyperplasia or carcinoma.

The clinical picture (known as **Conn's syndrome**) is characterized by periodic, severe muscular weakness amounting to paralysis, by arterial hypertension, and by renal dysfunction. The serum potassium level is low, which explains the muscular weakness, whereas the sodium level in the blood is raised. The urinary aldosterone level is high. Surgical removal of the cortical tumor is followed by a dramatic and complete disappearance of the clinical signs and symptoms, including the hypertension.

The **adrenal medulla** is the second portion of this essential organ. The adrenal medulla is of neuroectodermal origin and consists of cells and tissue that stain with chromium salts. It is part of a system distributed throughout the body, principally along the arterial network, and its role is to modulate and to control, by endocrine means, the peripheral resistance. Epinephrine, a small molecule synthesized from tyrosine, is the principal vasoactive product of the adrenal medulla and other chromaffin tissues. It is of interest that the adrenal cortical hormones control the secretion and the liberation of the adrenal medulla indirectly.

The effect of epinephrine on the body is not limited to increasing peripheral resistance. It also increases the liberation of glucose from glycogen storage in the liver, inhibits release of insulin, and inhibits the synthesis of new glycogen in the liver. Epinephrine also directly affects the heart, increasing its rate and strength of contraction.

The principal effect of disease of the adrenal medulla is to produce excess epinephrine-like hormone. The tumor most commonly seen, although it is rare itself, is called a **pheochromocytoma.**

This is an important tumor to know about because it is a treatable cause of hypertension, it is sometimes hereditary, and it appears in association with other syndromes. However, most important is that the diagnosis can be difficult to make, because the presence of excess episodic or continuous amounts of epinephrine may be mistaken for other kinds of disease.

Most patients with pheochromocytoma have hypertension, sweating, palpitations, weight loss, and may appear with a chief complaint such as headache. In all patients with hypertension, pheochromocytoma should be suspected, only to be ruled out.

The diagnosis of these rare tumors can be guessed at from the clinical situation in which the patient may be able to evoke the hypertension and the secretion of norepinephrine and epinephrine. I (Huntington Sheldon) recall an instance in which the distressing episodes occurred when the patient bent his body sharply to one side; the adrenal mass was compressed on that side between the diaphragm and the kidney, and it squeezed out hormones like juice from an orange. Usually, the disease is one of many possible diagnoses and is established by laboratory findings of the catecholamines and their metabolic breakdown products in the urine. There are, in addition, challenge tests, using drugs that provoke the discharge of hormones from the adrenal (histamine, glucagon) or that block the effect of these pressor amines (Regitine (phentolamine)). Such pharmacologic experiments must be done with great care, with all the proper antidotes available, lest the blood pressure either skyrocket or disappear, leaving the patient at risk. Of course, direct (surgical) and indirect (radiologic) attempts to visualize the adrenal are also used.

There is an additional note about pheochromocytoma. We now recognize the increasing frequency of these tumors in families that have other endocrine tumors. In these instances, the pheochromocytoma is usually bilateral.

THYROID GLAND

The thyroid gland, shaped like a small shield, lies under the strap muscles of the

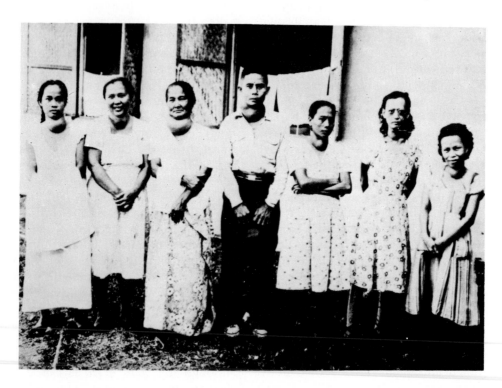

Fig. 22–9. This photograph shows a group of persons in the Philippines, all of whom demonstrate some thyroid abnormality. The large masses in the neck in 6 of the 7 persons are typical of nontoxic goiter. The seventh shows another abnormality characterized by the prominent exophthalmos and evidence of weight loss.

neck at the level of the larynx. When it becomes enlarged or nodular, it can be visualized or felt easily in most persons (Fig. 22–9). The cells that compose it are arranged in vesicles called follicles, surrounding a central lake of colloid, the storage form of the active material known as thyroxine, which is the only natural iodine-containing substance in the body. Each follicle of cells surrounding the colloid itself is enmeshed in a rich network of capillaries. From this network the amino acid tyrosine, which exists in most proteins, is continually extracted, iodinated, and sequestered in the form of a large molecule, thyroglobulin. When a person's energy requirements call for thyroxine, thyroid-releasing factor (TRF) from the hypothalamus stimulates the anterior pituitary to release the thyroid-stimulating hormone (TSH). This release, in turn, signals cells of the colloid follicles. They reach into their bank of colloid and withdraw from their savings account the active hormone, thyroxine, a small molecule that may contain either 3 iodine molecules (T3) or 4 iodine molecules (T4). This sequence of events, the uptake of iodine, its organification, and its subsequent release, depends on a number of enzymes, and different steps in the sequence may be blocked by drugs (thiouracil, lithium). More rarely, different enzymes may be congenitally absent. If iodine is absent from the diet, the important and necessary hormone is not made in adequate amounts, either; although the pathway is there, the essential iodine is not. The thyroid is unique among the endocrine glands in that it stores large amounts of hormone and releases it slowly. There is enough thyroxine in the normal adult gland for about 100 days. Thus there are several potential reasons for a lesion responsible for an inadequate amount of effective thyroid hormone: lack of iodine, blocked uptake, failure to manufacture thyroglobulin, or inappropriate release. These lesions can be thought of as being in the thyroid (primary failure), being in the anterior pituitary, or being in the hypothalamus.

What is the function of this hormone thyroxine? Without it, the body, and in particular the nervous system, fails to grow. In the adult, all the essential functions lose their normal tempo, and there is a slowing of the pulse of life, a coarsening of the features, and a general torpor which we shall discuss further under hypothyroidism.

The thyroid hormones, T3 and T4, are essential to maintain the cadence and tempo of normal metabolic processes in all tissues. Like the damper on the furnace door, thyroxine controls the draft or rate of oxidative metabolism. An excess of thyroxine uncouples oxidative phosphorylation and has the effect of a runaway furnace, burning up the patient with too rapid pulse rate, fever, increased respiratory rate, diarrhea. At the cellular level, mitochondria in all tissues from muscle to liver suffer from not having the correct amount of hormone. Without it, they cannot provide the normal amount of energy for cellular metabolism; with too much, they are like the out-of-control furnace just described.

During normal development in many forms of life, such as amphibia, thyroxine is the factor that initiates metamorphosis and enables liver cells to synthesize albumin, so that the amphibian can survive the transition onto land by having an intravascular pool of protein that protects the animal from immediate dehydration. Thyroxine starts the conversion from a fetal hemoglobin to an adult type, and initiates the remodeling that results in the development of limbs and in the resorption of the tail.

Exactly how thyroxine functions at the cellular level is a matter of dispute, but it is agreed that the hormone is essential for normal cellular health. One major function seems to be the stimulation of adenosinetriphosphatase (ATPase), which regulates sodium transport across cell membranes. Thus thyroxine directly affects cellular permeability and metabolism. A second observation is that there are thyroxine-binding sites in the nuclei of liver, kidney, and other cells, and the implication is that thyroxine also modifies the transcription of genetic information.

In the blood, thyroxine has been liberated from the colloid of the thyroid follicle and is bound to a serum protein, thyroid-binding globulin. A small fraction circulates free or unbound, and it is this fraction that is the active material. It seems that triiodothyronine (T3) rather than T4 is the more active form. We have methods today of measuring all these important substances: T3, T4, thyroid-binding globulin, thyroid-stimulating hormone, and thyroid-releasing factor.

Free or unbound T3 (8 to 10 times greater than T4 in normal serum) correlates most closely with the metabolic state of the person, rather than with the total concentration of T3 and T4. Thyroxine may be bound to thyroid-binding globulin, to prealbumin, or to albumin.

TSH, a glycopeptide secreted by the basophilic cells of the anterior pituitary, stimulates the thyroid follicle cells. Within minutes, these cells begin to reabsorb colloid from the follicle and to internalize it as colloid droplets, in which the thyroglobulin is broken down to release thyroxine, which in turn is liberated into the circulation. TSH stimulates the metabolism of nucleic acid and of protein; in fact, it stimulates all steps leading to the synthesis and secretion of thyroglobulin as well as its release. These effects can be seen histologically by the change from the normal cuboidal cells to tall columnar cells in the follicle following administration of this hormone. Conversely, in the absence of TSH, the cuboidal cells may become attenuated and may even appear squamous. Little activity takes place in these follicles.

TSH secretion, in turn, is regulated by thyrotropin-releasing hormone from the hypothalamus. There is a second antagonistic hypothalamic hormone that acts in the opposite way, but this process is more complex than we need to discuss here, except to indicate that the central nervous system control of these hormones, which in turn release thyroxine, underscores the possible effects of emotional and psychologic factors in governing our health. An example of such an effect is thyroid disease, which has been known to follow times of emotional turmoil and stress.

Hypothyroidism

The general term for a deficiency of thyroid hormone is hypothyroidism, regardless of the cause. The term **myxedema** is usually used to refer to the fully developed syndrome of this deficiency. Hypothyroidism is a systemic disorder affecting all tissues in the body, and it may be congenital or acquired. It may result from dysfunction of the thyroid gland itself, or from disease of the anterior pituitary or of the hypothalamus.

Congenital hypothyroid disease can be due to agenesis of the thyroid gland, to insensitivity of the thyroid gland and the thyroid-stimulating hormone, or to a variety of rare enzymatic defects, and the thyroid dysfunction may not necessarily be all or none. However, the significance of congenital hypothyroidism, whatever its cause, is that the failure to recognize the disorder in an infant condemns the child to imbecility. As we have said, all the tissues of the body (the central nervous system in particular) require thyroxine for normal growth and development.

The cretin is a dwarf physically and mentally. The mind, the skeleton, and the sexual organs do not develop. Like Peter Pan, the cretin never grows up, but he has none of Peter Pan's vivacity, because the vitalizing influence of the thyroid is lacking. He is a sad, old child. Osler described the cretin: "No type of human transformation is more distressing to look at than an aggravated case of cretinism. The stunted stature, the semi-bestial aspect, the blubber lips, retroussé nose sunken at the root, the wide-open mouth, the lolling tongue, the small eyes half closed with swollen lids, the stolid expressionless face, the squat figure, the muddy dry skin, combine to make the picture of what has been termed, the pariah of Nature" (Fig. 22–10).

In the adult, the disease **myxedema** begins usually without forewarning and may progress for decades before it is perceived as the pathologic pattern we now describe. Weakness, fatigue, lethargy, sleepiness, cold intolerance, menorrhagia, little appetite, but a gradual and steady increase in weight, may all suggest the disorder. The voice becomes deeper and husky, hair coarsens and may fall out, the skin becomes stiff and dry and the patient may become deaf. All of these changes may be mistaken for the decay of age.

The florid, full-blown case shows someone

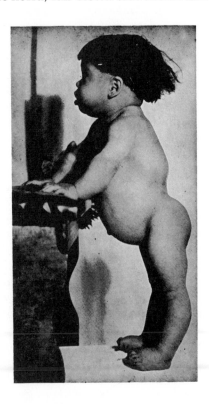

Fig. 22–10. A cretin.

with a dull, expressionless face (Fig. 22–11), who sits immobile, moving little and talking, if at all, with a lethargy that signals an effort for each word. It is as if the pendulum on life's clock were lengthened from a yard to a mile, and the ticking of time took an hour for each minute. There is periorbital puffiness, a swollen tongue that barely fits the mouth, and pale, dough-like skin that feels rough. The heart is enlarged and fails to function normally, the bowel dilates and accumulates stool, and the patient may lapse into coma.

One unusual complication of thyroid deficiency is called **"myxedema coma."** This rare phenomenon can be likened to the complication of hyperthyroidism called "thyroid storm." In myxedema coma, which usually has a serious prognosis because it has been overlooked as the underlying cause of the unresponsiveness, hypotension, hypothermia, hypoventilation, bradycardia, and convulsions, the suspicion of the diagnosis is the key to successful management. If the physician waits for laboratory tests to come back, the patient may be lost. The obese patient is the one in whom the suspicion should be raised, particularly someone in whom infection or trauma have occurred. A surgical procedure may precipitate this acute hypothyroid crisis,

which may be masked by the other things that are happening. A low basal temperature may be the feature that prompts the laboratory diagnosis, and the lifesaving treatment is intravenous administration of short-acting thyroxine.

The laboratory manifestation that best confirms the diagnosis is the elevation of the patient's level of TSH. This elevation occurs because the feedback loop in thyroxine is inhibited and fails to depress secretion of the stimulating hormone from the pituitary gland. Serum T4 is more reliable than T3 in this disease.

The explanation for all these changes is simple, in that thyroxine is not available to keep normal metabolism going, and every tissue suffers. There is a peculiar material that accumulates in the interstitial spaces and contributes to the coarsening of the skin and features, in addition to clogging up the larynx and heart and mechanically altering the structure and function of every organ, so that it does not move. Recently there is some evidence to support the idea that the edema derives from a disorder of the capillaries themselves.

Supportive treatment to manage the carbon dioxide narcosis and the administration of

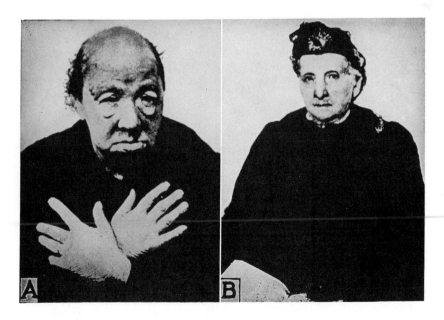

Fig. 22–11.   *A,* Myxedema of 20 years' duration; patient bedridden and imbecile. *B,* After treatment with thyroid extract; the same patient 30 years later, aged 94 years. (Harrington: *The Thyroid Gland—Its Chemistry and Physiology.* Oxford University Press.)

Table 22–4. Causes of Hypothyroidism

MECHANISM	CAUSE
Deficiency of TRH	Hypothalamic disease
Deficiency of TSH	Pituitary tumor or infarction
Thyroid destruction	Chronic inflammation
	Surgical ablation
	Radioiodine ablation
	Irradiation of the neck
	(usually for malignant disease)
Thyroid deficiency	Iodine deficiency
	(i.e., substrate lack)
	Iodine excess
	(i.e., interference with hormone release)
	Antithyroid drugs
	Biosynthetic defects

thyroxine rapidly reverse the progressive torpor and restore the patient to a normal state. The causes of hypothyroidism are shown in Table 22–4, and we shall consider here only the chronic and subacute inflammatory conditions, as the others seem self-explanatory.

Hashimoto's disease is probably the most common cause of hypothyroidism, except for iodine deficiency. This disorder would be better called chronic thyroiditis or chronic lymphocytic thyroiditis, since that is the nature of the lesion. Its cause may be debated by some, but the bulk of the evidence points to an autoimmune process. The disorder is far more common in women than in men (7:1), and can usually be perceived by the clinician as a diffuse swelling of the thyroid gland in a patient who may be hypothyroid. Nearly all such patients can be shown to have circulating thyroid antibodies. Biopsy of the thyroid shows marked lymphocytic infiltration with atrophy and loss of thyroid follicles. This process is progressive. It is of interest that the relatives of these patients frequently may have a history of thyroid disease, and they may also have antithyroid antibodies. Whether the disease arises from an earlier infection with some virus has not yet been shown. The patient with chronic lymphocytic thyroiditis is treated with thyroid replacement, and this is usually a lifelong requirement.

Hyperthyroidism

Excess circulating thyroid hormone arises from a variety of causes. The commonest cause is **Graves's disease** (70 to 90%), which goes by many names (e.g., toxic diffuse goiter). The second commonest cause is **toxic nodular goiter.** The third cause is a single adenoma or **toxic adenoma** of the thyroid. There are some other rare causes, and, except for the important concept that a pituitary tumor producing TSH has been reported, they are all so unusual as to be out of place here.

The clinical manifestations of hyperthyroidism usually begin in early adult life, more frequently in women (5:1), and the onset is often sudden and acute, sometimes following some serious emotional event or illness. The patient's complaints may vary, in that different presentations ranging from acute psychosis to muscle weakness to diarrhea alone are all well recognized. Perhaps the most common problem is a cardiac arrhythmia or palpitations. Sometimes the problem is heart failure.

The diagnosis is based on the classic physical findings: prominent, bulging eyes, a staring gaze, a diffusely enlarged thyroid gland, tachycardia, and marked fine tremor of the outstretched hands. The history is also classic: insomnia, irritability, frequent bowel

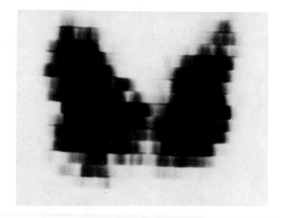

Fig. 22–12. This nuclear medicine scan of the thyroid gland shows the outline of the thyroid gland 24 hours after the adminstration of I¹³¹. In a hyperactive gland, the iodine is taken up rapidly and sequestered in the thyroid gland, as shown here.

movements, a good appetite but weight loss, and increased perspiration. She likes winter more than summer and cannot sleep with blankets. These observations leave little room for alternate explanations, especially when the pulse rate is 100 and there is a venous hum in the neck and a systolic murmur. Laboratory tests will confirm an elevated T3 and T4 level and an increased radioactive I^{131} uptake (Fig. 22–12). The serum cholesterol will be lower than normal. The basal metabolic rate is elevated, if the test is done. When the diagnosis is made, the problems begin, because the etiology of Graves's disease is poorly understood, and the correct treatment for the patient is a matter of debate and of individual consideration.

Graves's disease (toxic diffuse goiter) shows uniform enlargement of the thyroid follicle cells histologically (Fig. 22–13), and is diagnosed as we have indicated from the clinical pattern. Laboratory data will confirm the diagnosis. Whereas the etiology of the disease is a matter of current investigation, Mackenzie showed that the disease is mediated by an immunoglobulin antibody to the TSH receptor. This antibody stimulates increased production of thyroxine in an autonomous manner. The material present in the serum of many patients with Graves's disease has been called **long-acting thyroid stimulator (LATS).** The origin of this LATS appears to be the

lymphocytes of these patients, so the disease, like Hashimoto's disease, can be thought of as an autoimmune disorder. It used to be thought that excess thyroid-stimulating hormone was the offending agent, but this is not so in all but a few cases.

Exophthalmos in patients with Graves's disease is a serious and often complicated management problem. Its etiology is poorly understood, to put it mildly. The marked prominence of 1 or both eyes, with a staring gaze and a retraction of the lids, is an unforgettable sight. Examination of the retro-orbital tissues shows increased mucopolysaccharides, inflammatory cells, and connective tissue that collect to push the eye forward, often making it impossible to close the eyelids, and thereby exposing the cornea to abrasions and inflammation. The muscle weakness of the hyperthyroidism may contribute to difficulties with the eyelids. In the worst cases, exophthalmos can result in the loss of vision. The current view of this disorder is that it also is of autoimmune etiology, but that it is unrelated to the presence of LATS or TSH. It has been recognized that exophthalmos may occur by itself or with other endocrine disorders.

Toxic nodular goiter differs in several ways from Graves's disease. First, it occurs in persons who have had a goiter for many years, and in those who are older (40 to 65). Malig-

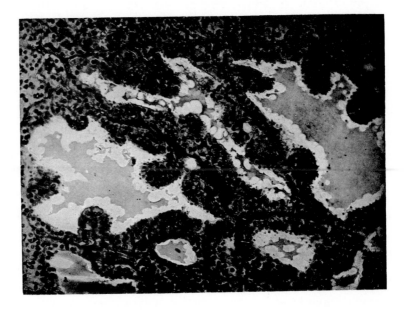

Fig. 22–13. Thyroid of Graves's disease undergoing involution under iodine treatment. The papillary processes are being withdrawn from the enlarged acini, and colloid is reappearing. Above and below there is still dense hyperplastic tissue. × 150. (Boyd: *Textbook of Pathology*. Philadelphia, Lea & Febiger.)

nant exophthalmos is rare, and the serum T4 levels are usually not markedly elevated. The radioactive iodine uptake level can be within the normal range. Finally, it is a diagnosis best understood by the statistic that it probably occurs in about 15% of all those with simple goiter. The best way to think of it is that it occurs within the gland that has undergone hyperplasia. After many years (and countless efforts), a group of thyroid cells have been able to free themselves from the controls imposed by the anterior pituitary and thus to function on their own, without regard for the inhibitory signals from thyroxine or stimulatory signals from TSH. To be sure of the diagnosis, a radioactive scan should show areas of increased uptake against the background of normal radioactive iodine uptake. In addition, the T3 level should be elevated.

Toxic adenoma is a single adenoma in the thyroid that produces symptoms of hyperthyroidism. The remainder of the thyroid gland is suppressed, as is production of TSH by the anterior pituitary, since the autonomous group of cells produces more T3 and T4 than the patient needs. Toxic adenoma is identifiable because there is only a single nodule in an otherwise normal or atrophied gland. This occurs naturally in a hyperthyroid patient. Radioactive scans confirm that the "hot" nodule is present (Fig. 22–14) in a gland that is physiologically depressed and yet responds to TSH. This can be done as a diagnostic test by giving TSH and by repeating the scan, which should now show an increased uptake in the thyroid around the hot nodule. The treatment of this cause of hyperthyroidism is uncomplicated, as either surgical removal of the nodule or the administration of radioactive iodine will cure the disease.

Whether the cases of hyperthyroidism should be treated with antithyroid drugs such as propylthiouracil, with or without the beta blocker propranolol, by subtotal thyroidectomy, or by radioactive iodine therapy is a matter of much debate and is beyond the scope of the present volume.

Before leaving hyperthyroidism, however, it would be well to comment on the hyperthyroid counterpart of myxedema coma, namely, **thyroid storm.** This condition is a

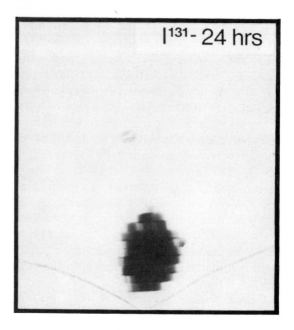

Fig. 22–14. This nuclear medicine scan of the thyroid following administration of I[131] shows the appearance of a hot nodule. The rest of the gland is suppressed.

severe, life-threatening extension of hyperthyroidism in which the symptoms become increasingly severe and incapacitating, with prostration, high fever, marked tachycardia, restlessness, and shock. Heart failure and possibly death may supervene. In short, it is the exaggeration of all we have been describing under the hyperthyroid state, and is usually seen as a complication of simple hyperthyroidism. The issue, of course, is to recognize it for what it is, and to treat it with emergency antithyroid drugs.

Goiter

This term is most confusing. It is typical of terms that have been used through the ages for different purposes, that are continually redefined and used, but that have different meanings for different people. Goiter is synonymous with enlargement of the thyroid gland and does not imply the reason for the enlargement. The enlargement is diffuse rather than nodular, and there are 3 forms of thyroid enlargement that can be recognized. First, as we have outlined, enlargement due to **Graves's disease,** which has been referred to also as diffuse toxic goiter. Second, as we have indicated in our discussion of chronic inflammatory disease of the thyroid, the gland may be diffusely enlarged, but the patient may be hypothyroid. **Hashimoto's disease** is an example of this condition. Third, the gland may be enlarged, and the patient may have normal thyroid function, or the patient may be hypothyroid. This diffuse enlargement is called *endemic goiter*, colloid goiter, or **simple nontoxic goiter.** We may understand it best as a hyperplastic response to a deficiency of iodine. The iodine deficiency may be due to different factors. It can be a relative lack because the body needs more iodine than is available from the diet, as occurs during periods of rapid growth. It may be due to inadequate amounts of iodine from the diet.

Endemic goiter typically appears in regions such as the alpine districts of Switzerland and the Himalayas, or the area of the Great Lakes in North America before the addition of iodine to salt and bread. The incidence of endemic goiter has been greatly diminished because of this supplement. In part of Ohio, a mass experiment was performed, giving the school children a small amount of iodized salt for 1 or 2 weeks twice a year, and by this simple expedient there was an astonishing reduction in the incidence of goiter in that community.

The symptoms of goiter are related to the local enlargement of the gland (Fig. 22–15) or to the long-term results of continuing inadequate ability to make thyroxine. Compression of the surrounding structures may cause difficulty in swallowing and noisy breathing.

The administration of iodine will make up for the dietary lack, and the gland may regain its normal small size. If the gland is massively enlarged, surgical removal may be appropriate.

Tumors of the Thyroid

This subject is of great interest for 2 reasons. The first is that 5% of the adult population have a nodule in the thyroid that can be felt by an examiner, and there is a remote chance that this nodule could be cancer. The other more likely possibility is that the mass represents a cyst or a benign, nonfunctioning group of cells, a benign adenoma. Of course, the nodule could be an inflammatory lesion. Unfortunately, there is no test other than a biopsy to establish the diagnosis.

The incidence of carcinoma of the thyroid is greater in persons who have a family history of such tumors, who have had irradiation to the neck, or who have a nodule that is either

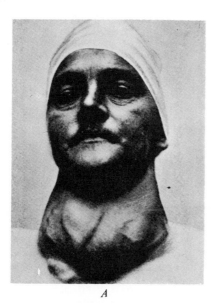
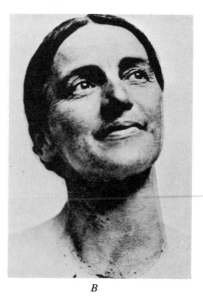

A   *B*

Fig. 22–15. *A,* Diffuse multinodular colloid goiter, showing the compressed veins and congested appearance of the face. *B,* Same patient 15 days after removal of the goiter. Note rapid relief of congestion of the veins of the face. (From de Quervain: *Goitre and Thyroid Diseases.* New York, William Wood & Co., 1924.)

hard or fixed, or is growing rapidly. The likelihood of the nodule's being cancer is small, but every case must be judged individually. It is of interest that whereas benign nodules are more common in women over 40 (10 times more frequent than in men), the incidence of cancer of the thyroid is twice as frequent in men.

The clinical signs of thyroid carcinoma are related to the type. The different types are not an important part of our discussion here. However, it is easy enough to delineate 3 general types, because they differ radically in their biologic behavior. Carcinoma of the thyroid may appear as a palpable mass or, as we have said, as a nodule that is either fixed or growing rapidly.

Of malignant tumors of the thyroid, the rarest, lethal type (5%) is an undifferentiated tumor that grows like wildfire and has a guarded prognosis, with a life expectancy of a year or less. The most common type of malignant tumor (60%) shows both follicular and papillary appearances on histologic examination. The better developed it is generally, the better the prognosis. This means a survival rate of 10 years for 70% of patients with well-differentiated carcinoma. The well-differentiated tumors respond to TSH and, if they are follicular, may take up radioactive iodine as well, allowing the physician both to suppress their function and to stimulate it, and to treat the tumor medically or surgically, or in both ways.

A few (15%) well-differentiated papillary carcinomas grow slowly and are compatible with a long survival rate for the patient. If you insist on having a tumor, this is probably the one to have.

A rare tumor, medullary carcinoma of the thyroid, only deserves mention because of its association with adenomas of other endocrine organs, and I refer you to other texts for a discussion of this disease.

PARATHYROID GLANDS

In the volume of endocrine romance, there are few more thrilling chapters than that which deals with the story of the parathyroids. For more than 70 years, these 4 tiny glands, each smaller than a lentil, have been identified, but their function was not understood. Normally, they lie in the neck, 2 on each side, behind the upper and lower poles of the thyroid gland. In 1925, Collip succeeded in preparing an extract of parathyroid glands that he called **parathormone**. Injection of this extract mobilized calcium and raised the serum calcium level. Normally the serum calcium is closely controlled between 9 and 11 mgs %. The route of calcium metabolism is absorption from the gut and deposition in the bone. Parathyroid hormone has been shown to affect the absorption from the gut, the resorption from the bone, and the reabsorption from the urine. Calcium is a divalent cation essential for function of all cell membranes, and it must be present in just the right amount. Medically, there are emergencies of both too much and too little serum calcium.

Parathyroid hormone acts directly to change the osteocyte into an osteoclast, which secretes a collagenase that breaks down the fully mineralized collagen and liberates both calcium and phosphate into the serum, as well as the hydrolytic products of the collagen breakdown. One can identify hydroxylysine or hydroxyproline excretion in the urine, as testimony to the lytic effect on bone of hyperparathyroid disease.

Serum phosphate, which normally ranges from 3 to 5 mg %, is also maintained in inverse proportion to the amount of serum calcium. Thus the product of the calcium times phosphorus is kept at a constant. Normally, the calcium/phosphorus ratio is maintained by intestinal absorption, renal excretion, and/or bone deposition or mobilization.

A second hormone that plays a role in calcium homeostasis was identified in the early 1960's, and this hormone has been called **calcitonin**. The role of this hormone seems analogous to that of glucagon in the pancreas, so that for the regulation of blood glucose levels we have 2 hormones, insulin and glucagon, and for the regulation of serum calcium and phosphate levels we have parathyroid hormone and calcitonin.

It is too complicated to describe the parathyroid hormone's mechanism on the absorption of calcium in the gut. The primary effect of calcitonin is to reduce the resorption of calcium from bone when the serum calcium level begins to rise. Calcitonin is an antihypercalcemic factor, and seems to be much more active in young, growing animals than in adults.

Hyperparathyroidism

This term is applied to any disorder in which an elevated level of effective parathyroid hormone occurs, and, as we shall see, its effect may be to raise the serum calcium under some circumstances. However, the serum calcium level may be normal or low. Hyperparathyroidism has been divided into 3 types: primary hyperparathyroidism, an excess that arises from an adenoma or hyperplasia of the parathyroid glands; secondary hyperparathyroidism, which represents an adaptive excess of parathyroid hormone in response to hypocalcemia, hyperphosphatemia, or, occasionally, hypomagnesemia; a third type of hyperparathyroidism is due to the ectopic production of hormones with parathyroid hormone-like activity.

Primary hyperparathyroid disease is due to a single or solitary adenoma occurring in 1 of the 4 parathyroids in 80 to 90% of cases. This adenoma is a clone of cells that have undertaken autonomous growth and secretion and are independent of normal control mechanisms. They synthesize and secrete excessive, active parathyroid hormone. There is no knowledge of any particular stimulus or cause for their growth or secretion, and, short of surgical removal of the enlarged, hyperfunctioning parathyroid adenoma, there is no satisfactory treatment.

Clinical patterns of hyperparathyroid disease range from the full-blown description by von Recklinghausen in 1891 of a patient with a deformed skeleton and bone pain, who showed cystic areas of rarefaction and fibrotic patches in the bone, owing to the extreme calcium loss, to the contemporary patient who is completely asymptomatic, but whose routine multiphasic analysis of serum turns up an elevated serum calcium. Generally, there are 2 patterns for patients with overt primary hyperparathyroidism. These patterns seem to relate to the size and duration of the hyperfunctioning gland. One group, like von Recklinghausen's patient, has bone pain and may even show collapse of vertebrae; these patients have high serum calciums and a short history of being ill; large adenomas are found at surgery. The second group, with smaller adenomas, have kidney stones and a longer history of illness with only modest hypercalcemia. We have always said that whenever kidney stones occur, a possibility that must be investigated is hyperparathyroid

disease, disappointing as it may be to uncover high serum calcium in fewer than 10% of patients with kidney stones.

A second cause for primary hyperparathyroidism is the presence of what is called **chief cell hyperplasia,** or four-gland enlargement. This variant is more perplexing, because it implies some regulating factor that is unidentified. Such patients may have lower parathormone levels than the solitary adenoma patients. Again, surgery is the treatment of the illness, leaving half of 1 parathyroid gland to maintain homeostasis.

In all patients with primary hyperparathyroidism, the symptoms may be vague and nonspecific. Weakness, weight loss, fatigue, and muscle atrophy, in addition to bone pain, gastrointestinal distress, pancreatitis, or kidney stones are common.

Hypercalcemia has come more and more to be the single finding around which the diagnosis of hyperparathyroidism revolves, and forces us to discuss the other causes of elevated serum calcium levels in order to avoid jumping to the conclusion that it is inevitably due to hyperparathyroid disease. Whereas more than 95% of patients with hyperparathyroidism have elevated serum calcium levels, there are other causes of a high serum calcium, as shown in Table 22–5. The serum calcium level is the product, as we have outlined, of reabsorption of calcium by the renal tubular cells from the glomerular filtrate (conservation), increased absorption from the gut

Table 22–5. Etiology of Hypercalcemia

Excess bone resorption
Hyperparathyroidism
Malignant tumors
Producing PTH
Producing other hormonal agents
Immobilization
Thyrotoxicosis
Excess absorption from gut
Sarcoidosis (other granulomas)
Vitamin D intoxication
? milk-alkali syndrome
? adrenal insufficiency
Excess renal reabsorption
? thiazide diuretics

(From Goltzman, D.: Parathyroid hormone and hyperparathyroidism: current concepts. Can. J. Surg., 21:285, 1978.)

of calcium (under Vitamin D control), and mobilization of calcium from bone (due to parathyroid hormone). In each of these mechanisms, parathyroid hormone plays a crucial role, as well as the other factors we have outlined.

Increased mobilization of calcium from bone that raises serum calcium levels occurs frequently in various neoplastic diseases, particularly in multiple myeloma. Occasionally, other cancers secrete ectopic parathyroid hormone, making the problem more complicated until the presence of the malignant neoplasm is recognized.

Hypercalcemia can represent a medical and surgical emergency when it rises above 18 mg %. The patient may lapse into coma, and emergency treatment should be instituted while preparing the person for the necessary surgical exploration of the neck to remove the functional parathyroid adenoma that causes the hypercalcemia.

Secondary hyperparathyroidism is an adaptive response of parathyroid hormone secretion. It occurs most commonly in chronic renal disease, in which the kidney is no longer able to excrete phosphate normally. Because of renal disease, the kidney may also have lost the ability to create the active form of vitamin D. In the absence of this vitamin, the gut absorbs less calcium than it would normally, thus contributing to a lower than normal calcium level. Either a low serum calcium or a raised serum phosphate level may act as a stimulus to the parathyroid glands to increase the secretion of parathyroid hormone. (It is well to remember the central homeostatic drive to keep the calcium times phosphate ratio constant.) Thus in chronic renal failure, it is common to find hyperplasia of all 4 parathyroid glands, but not necessarily elevated serum calcium. Rather, it is a normal serum calcium level in persons in whom one suspects a low serum calcium that suggests the diagnosis of secondary hyperparathyroidism. This situation represents the epitome of adaptation with respect to calcium homeostasis. Since the serum phosphate level is raised, it acts as a stimulus to the secretion of the parathyroid hormone which in turn calls out more calcium from the bone depot. The restoration of the serum calcium level (which had been low) toward normal repre-

sents a relative hypercalcemia in such patients with chronic renal failure. If the serum calcium level is abnormally high, and the serum phosphate level is, too, one occasionally finds metastatic calcification throughout the body.

Hypoparathyroidism

This deficiency of parathyroid hormone results in hypocalcemia. Of course, it is not the only cause of hypocalcemia, just as a high serum calcium level is not only attributable to excess parathyroid hormone. Most instances of hypoparathyroidism are the consequence of surgical operations of the neck, removal either of the thyroid or of the parathyroids. There are, in addition, rare disorders such as congenital pseudohypoparathyroidism, which we shall not consider.

The clinical pattern of hypocalcemia, whatever its cause, is interesting and important because of the ease with which the disorder may be treated. Numbness and tingling of the extremities and around the mouth are common complaints. Cramps of individual muscles, particularly in the hands and feet, are a result of inadequate calcium. Occasionally, convulsions occur. A host of nonspecific aberrations of thought, such as irritability, emotional lability, depression, are reported. To confirm the clinical impression of hypocalcemia, Chvostek's sign of twitching of the muscles about the mouth, nose, or eyelids can be evoked by tapping the facial nerve. Trousseau's sign (carpal spasm) occurs when a blood pressure cuff is inflated above systolic pressure for more than 2 minutes. These signs are testimony to the irritability of muscle and nerve in the absence of calcium.

Calcium replacement by oral or intravenous route is a readily available solution to the immediate problem.

These observations are called tetany, and this may also occur in other disturbances of calcium metabolism, such as in cases of alkalosis.

ISLETS OF LANGERHANS

The islets of Langerhans are small groups of cells scattered throughout the pancreas, in particularly large numbers in the tail. Together the islets of Langerhans constitute another endocrine organ. Their principal product is insulin, and their subsidiary product is glucagon. Recently, it has been shown that there are cells in the islets that also secrete somatostatin. Like other endocrines, there may be under- or overproduction of the hormones of these tissues. **Hypoinsulinism,** otherwise known as diabetes mellitus, has been discussed in an earlier section. Replacement therapy by insulin is the standard approach to this insufficiency.

Hyperinsulinism is caused by the presence of a tumor of the islets of Langerhans. This tumor is rarely malignant. More commonly, it is simply an adenoma with functional excess of hormone. The clinical pattern is distinctive, in that the person with an excess continuing secretion of insulin is continually hypoglycemic. This hypoglycemia leads to constant hunger, and that patient may not only be subject to hypoglycemia with fainting, convulsions, and loss of consciousness, but he also may be meeting his need by continuous feeding. Occasionally, a patient with insulinoma may be grossly obese. Today, the diagnosis of an insulinoma should be suspected whenever someone has convulsions, syncopal attacks, and/or a remarkable decrease in blood sugar level.

SYNOPSIS

Endocrine disorders can generally be considered to be instances of too much or too little secretion by respective endocrine glands. The anatomic lesions generally are functioning adenomas or hyperplasia of a particular type of cell, although there are rare examples of tumors of nonendocrine tissue that secrete substances with hormone-like activity.

Hyperpituitarism results in gigantism or acromegaly; hypopituitarism may appear as dysfunction of all the endocrine glands (thyroid, adrenal, gonads, etc.), or it may be symptomatic because of a particular dysfunction.

Benign and malignant tumors without endocrine function may occur in any endocrine gland.

Hyperadrenalism may result in Cushing's syndrome, Conn's syndrome, or the adrenogenital syndrome. Hypoadrenalism results in Addison's disease.

Hyperthyroidism and hypothyroidism each may have many causes.

The parathyroid gland's relation to calcium and phosphate metabolism is complex, and current views still do not explain the original stimulus to adenoma or hyperplasia.

The stimuli to adenoma and hyperplasia of the endocrine organs in general remain a riddle deserving more attention.

Terms

Hypophysis	*Pheochromocytoma*	*Androgen*
Growth hormone	*Goiter*	*Addison's disease*
Luteinizing hormone	*Hashimoto's thyroiditis*	*Cushing's syndrome*
Thyrotropin	*Hyperthyroidism*	*Myxedema*
Acromegaly	*Prolactin*	*Cretin*
Simmond's disease	*ACTH*	*Parathormone*
Mineralocorticoid	*Oxytocin*	*Calcitonin*
Glucocorticoid	*Vasopressin*	

FURTHER READING

Addison, T.: Disease of the suprarenal capsules. Lond. Med. Gaz., 43:517, 1855.

Allison, A. C.: Self-tolerance and autoimmunity in the thyroid. N. Engl. J. Med., 295:821, 1976.

Baxter, J. D., and Gunder, J. W.: Hormone receptors. N. Engl. J. Med., 301:1149, 1979.

Bergland, R. M., and Page, R. B.: Pituitary-brain vascular relations: A new paradigm. Science, 204:18, 1979.

Copp, D. H., et al.: Calcitonin. Endocrinology, 70:638, 1962.

Cushing, H.: The basophil adenomas of the pituitary body and their clinical manifestations. Bull. Johns Hopkins Hosp., 1:137, 1932.

DeLuca, H. F.: Vitamin D endocrinology. Ann. Intern. Med., 85:367, 1976.

Duncan, G. A., Hill, F. M., and Ezrin, C.: Acromegaly: a review of 100 cases. Can. Med. Assoc. J., 87:1106, 1962.

Etkin, W.: Logic versus imagination in an experimental analysis. Perspect. Biol. Med., 20:394, 1977.

Ezrin, C.: The pituitary gland. Ciba Found. Symp., 15:71, 1963.

Favus, M. J., et al.: Evaluation of 1056 patients. Thyroid cancer occurring as a late consequence of head-and-neck irradiation. N. Engl. J. Med., 294:1019, 1976.

Goltzman, D.: Parathyroid hormone and hyperparathyroidism: current concepts. Can. J. Surg., 21:285, 1978.

Guillemin, R.: Control of adenohypophysial functions by peptides of the central nervous system. Harvey Lect., 71, 1978.

Heath, H., III, Hodgson, S. F., and Kennedy, M. A.: Primary hyperparathyroidism: incidence, morbidity, and potential economic impact in a community. N. Engl. J. Med., 302:189, 1980.

Jones, H. W.: A long look at the adrenogenital syndrome. Johns Hopkins Med. J., 145:143, 1979.

Masi, A. T., Hartmann, W. H., and Shulman, L. E.: Hashimoto's disease: an epidemiological critique. J. Chronic Dis., 18:1, 1965.

McKenzie, J. M.: Does LATS cause hyperthyroidism in Graves' disease? (A review biased towards the affirmative.) Metabolism, 21:883, 1972.

Nelson, D. H., Meakin, J. W., and Thorn, G. W.: ACTH-producing pituitary tumors following adrenalectomy for Cushing's syndrome. Ann. Intern. Med., 52:560, 1960.

O'Malley, B. W.: Studies on the molecular mechanism of steroid hormone action. Harvey Lect., 72, 1978.

Ord, W. M.: On myxoedema: a term proposed to be applied to an essential condition in the "cretinoid" affection occasionally observed in middle-aged women. Med. Chir. Trans., 61:57, 1878.

Plotz, C. M., Knowlton, A. E., and Ragan, C.: The natural history of Cushing's syndrome. Am. J. Med., 13:597, 1952.

Utiger, R. D.: Treatment of Graves' disease. N. Engl. J. Med., 298:681, 1978.

Wilkins, L., Lewis, R. A., and Klein, R.: The suppression of androgen secretion by cortisone in a case of congenital hyperplasia. Bull. Johns Hopkins Hosp., 81:249, 1950.

Blood and Lymph Nodes

23

Half the secret of resistance to disease is cleanliness; the other half is dirtiness.—ANONYMOUS

The hematopoietic system includes the circulating blood, lymphoid tissue, and the system's site of origin, the bone marrow. For most purposes, the spleen is included in any consideration, and it is interesting that the liver may become the site of blood formation in some diseases, just as it is during fetal life. Whereas marrow of long bones is yellow and is partially composed of fat in adult life, in childhood it is red and full of active precursors of both red and white blood cells. One may regard the hematopoietic system as a tissue whose cells include the red blood cell series and white blood cell series, and the interstitial space is the plasma. Thought of in that way, the hematopoietic system is a large organ of from 4,000 to 8,000 grams depending on the size of the person. The normal liver weighs 1,200 grams and is the largest single organ of the body.

We may separate diseases of blood into 2 general categories; those of the red cells (erythrocytes), and those of the white cells (leukocytes). In both cases there may be too few cells (anemia for red blood cells, leukopenia for white blood cells), or too many (polycythemia for red blood cells, leukemia for white blood cells), but this classification is oversimplified.

We shall consider the normal structure and function of each of these elements before going on to discuss their diseases.

The **erythrocyte** is a biconcave disc without a nucleus. The shape has been a source of much discussion; like most successful packages, it does its job well, for a biconcave disc presents the largest interface between the surface of the cell and the plasma. This shape permits efficient absorption and release of gases. In health, there are 5 to 6 × 10^6 red blood cells per mm^3 in men, and 4.5 to 5 × 10^6 in women. The mature erythrocyte is derived in a sequence of steps from a primitive stem cell (erythroblast), which, in a monotheistic way, some believe to be the progenitor of all blood cells. This cell contains no hemoglobin, but as one line of differentiation takes place through **normoblasts** to **normocytes,** the ribosomes of this cell begin to make **hemoglobin,** that quintessential pigment of all animal forms. The normocyte loses its nucleus in man, becomes a **reticulocyte,** and then a mature erythrocyte, which lives for about 120 days under normal conditions.

The mature erythrocyte is easily deformed, which allows it to pass through narrow capillaries, and it has an average diameter of 8.4 microns, which can be used as a standard for estimating the size of other cells seen under the microscope. The normal erythrocyte appears uniformly stained with routine hematoxylin and eosin or Wright's stain, as distinct from abnormal erythrocytes, which appear in some of the congenital or acquired anemias. The erythrocyte is a simple bag of hemo-

Table 23–1.   Red Cell Values in Adults: Normal Range

	MEN	WOMEN
Red blood cells	5.11 ± 0.38	4.5 ± 0.36 × 10^{12}/l
Hemoglobin	15.5 ± 1.1	13.7 ± 1.0 g/dl
Packed cell volume	46.0 ± 3.1	40.9 ± 3.0 l/l
Mean corpuscular volume	90.0 ± 4.8	90.4 ± 4.8 fl
Mean corpuscular hemoglobin	30.2 ± 1.8	30.2 ± 1.9 pg
Mean corpuscular hemoglobin concentration	33.9 ± 1.2	33.6 ± 1.1 g/dl
Reticulocytes absolute	0.2 to 2.0	0.2 to 2.0 × 10^9/l

(From Brain, M. C.: (The anemias.) Introduction. In *Cecil Textbook of Medicine,* 15th Ed. Edited by P. B. Beeson, W. McDermott, and J. B. Wyngaarden. Philadelphia, W. B. Saunders, 1979.)

globin designed to transport this iron-containing pigment around and around, giving up oxygen in the microenvironment, taking on CO_2, only to release it later in exchange for oxygen. The living hemoglobin molecule is made of 574 amino acids in 4 chains, totaling 10,000 atoms with a molecular weight of 64,500. Each hemoglobin molecule can carry 4 molecules of oxygen at a time. It is estimated there are 280,000,000 hemoglobin molecules in each erythrocyte.

Recently, and told in a most enthralling way by Horace Judson in *The Eighth Day of Creation,* Max Perutz has been able to demonstate that the hemoglobin molecule changes its shape as it takes up oxygen and gives it off. This observation confirms the hypothesis of Monod that the conformation of proteins is directly related to their function, and that this structure/function relationship exists at the molecular level as well as at other levels of biologic action. Monod called hemoglobin an "honorary enzyme because it acts like one."

In the normal human adult male, there are about 15 grams of hemoglobin per 100 ml, and in the adult female there are about 14 grams per 100 ml. We estimate the amount of hemoglobin colorimetrically, and it is an easy and important clinical measurement to make. The second routine estimate of oxygen carrying capacity is the hematocrit.

Packed cell volume is measured by the **hematocrit.** Blood is drawn into a hematocrit tube, which is centrifuged until the cells are completely packed, and the result is read on the graduated tube. Newer

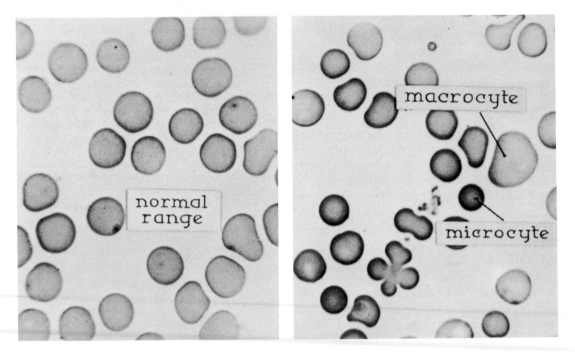

Fig. 23–1.   This photomicrograph shows the smear of normal erythrocytes on the left and erythrocytes with variable size on the right. A large red blood cell or macrocyte, and a small red blood cell or microcyte are both shown on the right. (From Ham, A.W.: *Histology,* 7th Ed. Philadelphia and Toronto, J. B. Lippincott, 1974.)

methods employed by hematology laboratories have a computer calculate the absolute and relative volume of red blood cells passing through a photoelectrically monitored microcolumn, The volume of packed cells is normally about 47% for males and 43% for females. Table 23–1 illustrates the normal range of cell volume for adults.

It must be emphasized that a well-stained blood smear, studied by an educated eye and brain, still affords one of the best means of arriving at an accurate hematologic diagnosis. The smear provides the observer with information as to the size and shape of the red cells, the concentration of hemoglobin in these cells, and the presence of nucleated cells and reticulocytes. The size and shape of the red cells demand special attention. Anisocytosis (variation in size) and poikilocytosis (variation in shape) are indications of disease. Anisocytosis is seen early in pernicious anemia, where poikilocytosis develops at a later stage and helps the physician to make the diagnosis. All these abnormalities tell us something of the functional activity of the bone marrow (Fig. 23–1).

The **leukocytes** or white blood cells number from 6,000 to 8,000 per cubic millimeter of blood. Large numbers, however, are trapped in unused capillaries, and as physical exertion causes great numbers of these capillaries to become opened, the leukocyte count shows a corresponding rise after exercise. Unlike erythrocytes, the white blood cells are not uniform in type, but are of several kinds, divided principally into 2 classes: those with granules and those without granules (called mononuclear cells). The **granulocyte** is a cell whose nucleus may have various forms, in comparison with the spherical nucleus of the lymphocyte and monocyte. In 1 variety, the granules are large and stain bright red with eosin; this type is known as the **eosinophil.** Eosinophils form only 2% of the total leukocyte count. The neutrophil or **polymorphonuclear leukocyte** (PMN), constitutes about 70% of the leukocytes, but this figure varies considerably. Another type has granules that stain blue, hence the name **basophil.** These types of cells are formed in the sinusoids of the bone marrow, in much the same way as the erythrocytes are formed, i.e., they go through immature stages before the adult form is reached. These stages are the **myeloblast** and the **myelocyte.** Granules appear for the first time in the myelocyte, and these cells are present in large numbers in the marrow, but they do not enter the blood stream under normal conditions. Polymorphonuclear leukocytes defend the body against bacteria by phagocytosis, a process discussed in connection with inflammation. PMN's in the blood are enormously increased in acute infections, because the depots in the bone marrow pour their reserve into the blood stream, and at the same time speed the rate of production. The function of eosinophils is uncertain, but their number may be markedly increased in allergic and parasitic conditions.

Lymphocytes form about 20% of the total leukocyte count. They are small, plain-looking cells, with little cytoplasm around the spherical nucleus. Large numbers of lymphocytes appear at a focus of chronic inflammation, some derived from the blood, others from the tissues. Lymphocytes have been divided into 2 classes, on the basis of their site of origin and their surface markers. We now recognize T cells (thymus-derived) and B cells (bursa-derived). These cells and their function have been discussed in the chapter on immunology.

Monocytes (large mononuclear cells), on the other hand, are actively phagocytic, and play an important part in the inflammatory process. In acute inflammation, they form the second line of defense, arriving later than the polymorphonuclear leukocytes and serving the useful purpose of scavengers. They are formed in the bone marrow and constitute about 8% of the leukocytes.

In a blood examination, the leukocytes may be examined in 2 ways: (1) leukocyte count and (2) differential count. The object of the leukocyte count is to estimate the total number of leukocytes, and to determine whether there is a leukocytosis (increase in the number). This useful procedure is simple and takes only a few minutes. In a differential count, several hundred leukocytes are examined, note being taken of whether each cell is a polymorphonuclear leukocyte, an eosinophil, a lymphocyte, or a monocyte. In this way, the percentage of the various cells is determined. In selected cases, this count may prove of great use. It is essential in the leukemias, where 1 or more white cell lines may predominate in blood.

Platelets are the third type of cell of the blood, but the last to have had their function recognized.

The electron microscope has revolutionized our concept of the platelet, which used to be regarded as an inert particle, structureless, and possibly an artifact. Now it is known to possess abundant metabolic equipment, microtubules, 3 types of granules, and 80 enzymatic activities.

The platelet is the first element to appear at a break in the lining of a blood vessel. Within 1 to 3 seconds, platelets adhere to the damaged wall, surely the promptest first aid we could imagine. By their adherence and agglutination, they initiate the coagulation cascade. And this is the element of the blood that we used to consider structureless, without function, and possibly an artifact.

Blood Groups. That the red cells of a person may clump together when mixed with blood of many others, with fatal results if transfusion is done, is old knowledge. The modern era was inaugurated in 1900 by Landsteiner of the Rockefeller Institute, who showed that all persons can be divided into 4 major blood groups, depending on the reaction of the serum of 1 on the red cells of another. Red blood cells and serum of each person are perfectly adapted to one another, but the cells of 1 person may be incompatible with the serum of another.

When 2 bloods are incompatible, the red cells from the donor clump together (agglutinate) in the serum of the recipient, owing to the presence of agglutinins in the serum of the latter. The incompatibility lies in that, in human blood, the red cells contain either no antigens or 1 or both of 2 antigens, known as A and B, which may produce agglutination, whereas the serum contains corresponding antibodies or agglutinins known as beta or anti-B and alpha or anti-A. Under natural conditions, an antigen and its corresponding agglutinin cannot be present simultaneously in the same blood. If, however, blood containing antigen A or B is introduced by transfusion into a person whose blood contains the corresponding antibody, agglutination occurs. Moreover, hemolysis as well as agglutination of the transfused red cells may occur. This hemolysis is the real danger of the blood transfusion, because blood breakdown products dam up the kidney and lead to renal failure.

Depending on the presence of the 2 antigens, the blood of all persons can be divided into 4 great groups, known as O, A, B, and AB. Group O contains no antigen, group A contains A antigen, Group B contains B antigen, and group AB contains both A and B antigens (Table 23–2). As group O contains no antigen, it does not react with the blood of other groups, even though they contain agglutinins. Persons belonging to this group are therefore called universal donors because their blood is compatible with that of any of the 4 groups. Fortunately, this is the largest group, comprising over 40% of persons. A person in any group may receive blood from anyone in the same group. The AB group, having no agglutinins in the serum, is a universal recipient, just as we have seen that group O, having no agglutinogens in the red cells, is, or used to be, regarded as a universal donor. The term "universal" unfortunately ignores the Rh factor, to be discussed.

The specific antigens and agglutinins (antibodies) are hereditary, a fact that is sometimes made use of in cases of disputed parentage. Agglutinins in the blood of a child must also be present in at least 1 of the parents. If the blood group of 1 parent and the child is known, in certain cases the group of the other parent can be determined.

The suitability of a donor is determined by 2 methods, known as grouping (or typing) and matching (or cross-matching). The blood group to which someone belongs can be decided by testing his red cells against serum from both a known group A (which contains anti-B agglutinins) donor and a known group B (which contains anti-A agglutinins) donor, and by noting whether any agglutination occurs. When the cells and serum of the prospective donor have been cross-matched for ABO blood group against the serum and cells of the patient, there still may be incompatibility. One factor we have not yet accounted for is the **Rh factor,** so called because it was first discovered in the blood of the **rh**esus monkey. About 85% of persons possess this factor or antigen, so they are said to be Rh-positive, whereas 15% lack the antigen and are Rh-negative. Anti-Rh agglutinins are not normally present in the serum, but may be formed in Rh-negative persons following transfusion by Rh-positive blood. Thus the first transfusion of Rh-positive blood into an Rh-negative person will **not** cause a reaction, because there are no antibodies yet. After this transfusion, the Rh-negative person will begin to synthesize antibody to this new antigen he has just encountered. The next time he receives an Rh-positive transfusion, the antibodies will attack the donated blood and cause a transfusion reaction. Today, all persons who donate or receive blood are "typed" with regard to the Rh factor, as well as A, B, and O; so this type of transfusion reaction is rare.

Rh factor may prove to be a menace in another and more subtle way. An Rh-positive father can transmit the factor to the fetus. If the mother is Rh-positive also, maternal and fetal bloods are compatible. If the mother is Rh-negative, the 2 bloods are incompatible and, should they mix, a transfusion reaction will occur. Normally, the placenta prevents blood from mixing; nutrients and wastes pass through thin membranes. At birth, however, tearing of the placenta may result in the entry of some fetal blood cells into the maternal system. The mother then begins to form anti-Rh antibodies. The first child is already born and is safe. However, in subsequent pregnancies, the now present anti-Rh antibody is small enough to pass through placental barriers and into the fetal circulation. The result is intrauterine hemolysis and hemolytic anemia or erythroblastosis fetalis

Table 23–2.   Determination of Blood Groups

Cells agglutinated by serum from a known:		Person belongs to:
Group A	Group B	
No	No	Group O
No	Yes	Group A
Yes	No	Group B
Yes	Yes	Group AB

(see Fig. 6–19). The reason for this name is that the most striking feature of the blood, apart from the anemia, is the presence of great numbers of nucleated red cells or erythroblasts. These calamities due to primary Rh immunization of the Rh-negative, child-bearing woman can now be prevented by an injection of anti-Rh gamma globulin by the third day after delivery, according to Bowman and Chown. It will be evident to the reader what a major advance this represents.

The novelist speaks of the life blood's ebbing away. The phrase is hardly an exaggeration, for it is the blood that carries to the innumerable cells of the body their requisites for life, namely, food and oxygen. Without sufficient blood, the cells are both starved and asphyxiated. As a severe loss of blood is so injurious, it is natural that the injection of blood from another person should be correspondingly beneficial. When this injection is made, it is called transfusion of blood.

The chief value of transfusion is replacement of blood after a severe, acute hemorrhage, when it is truly a lifesaving procedure. Transfusion is also useful for combating shock following surgical operations, especially those associated with much loss of blood, as in operations on the brain. Repeated transfusions are sometimes used in the treatment of chronic anemias with a low red cell count and in severe infections.

Unfortunately, it is not possible to use the blood of all and sundry for the purpose of transfusion. It should be clear that the blood of some persons carries agents such as the hepatitis virus.

If the bloods of the donor and the recipient are incompatible, there may be immediate signs of shock, as evidenced by restlessness, pallor, shortness of breath, feeble rapid pulse, and fall in blood pressure. There may also be a more delayed type of reaction, marked by chills, fever, pain in the back, jaundice, and the presence of hemoglobin in the urine. These delayed symptoms are all due to the breaking down of the red blood cells. About 40% of the patients showing these symptoms of hemolysis make a complete recovery. In the remaining 60%, symptoms of renal failure develop in the course of a week (because the kidney attempts to excrete blood breakdown products, but cannot; it becomes overloaded and shuts down), there may be complete suppression of urine, and the patient dies in convulsions or coma. From a consideration of these facts, it is evident how important it is to prevent reactions to transfusions, and how necessary are the preliminary laboratory tests to determine the question of blood incompatibility. It is essential that blood for cross-matching be correctly and adequately labeled, so that there can be no doubt about the identity of the person from whom it was collected. For many purposes, particularly in the treatment of shock, blood plasma can be used instead of whole blood. As the plasma contains no red cells, the question of incompatibility does not arise, and the dangers of using unsuitable blood

are thus avoided. Plasma has a great advantage over whole blood in that it can be dried, and can be kept in the dry form for an indefinite period, but, unfortunately, it may be contaminated with hepatitis virus.

For the purposes of this chapter, we divided disorders of the red blood cell series into considerations of too little (anemias) and too much (polycythemias). We then consider platelet disorders and abnormalities of coagulation. Finally, we turn to disease of the lymphoid system: namely, increase in circulating white blood cells (leukemias), and infiltrations of the lymphoreticular system (lymphomas).

ANEMIAS

Anemias are defined as a "decrease in the amount of hemoglobin in a given volume of whole blood." This reduction can be due to a decrease in the number of red blood cells in a given volume, or it may be due to a decrease in the amount of hemoglobin per red blood cell. It may also, much more rarely, be due to a decrease in the amount of blood, as in acute blood loss. The basic defects can be understood best in terms of (A) defects in synthesis of components of the red blood cell, (B) increased destruction of the red blood cell, or (C) loss that is greater than synthesis. Anemia should not be regarded as a disease, but

Table 23–3. Anemias: Morphologic Classification

1. Macrocytic (MCV 93 mm³)
   a) Megaloblastic erythropoiesis (deficiency of vitamin B_{12} or folic acid)
   b) Liver disease and obstructive jaundice
   c) Reticulocytosis
2. Normocytic
   a) Acute blood loss before reticulocytosis
   b) Hemolytic anemia when not associated with spherocytosis
   c) Anemia of chronic disease
3. Microcytic and hypochromic
   a) Iron deficiency
   b) Thalassemia
   c) Sideroblastic anemia

(From Brain, M. C.: (The anemias.) Introduction. In *Cecil Textbook of Medicine*, 15th Ed. Edited by P. B. Beeson, W. McDermott, and J. B. Wyngaarden. Philadelphia, W. B. Saunders, 1979.)

rather as evidence of a disease, which can reside in a red blood cell, or can be caused by some other abnormality.

Any consideration of anemias is complicated by the existence of so many different causes that some conceptualization of the problem is the only way to deal with the vast number of possibilities. Two general attempts to classify anemias as morphologic and as etiologic are shown in Tables 23–3 and 23–4. Neither of these classifications is the complete answer, any more than other attempts to impose schemes of organization on biologic phenomena satisfy all people. The advantage of recognizing both classifications is that often recognition of the anemia is made on examination of the smear, and the approach to diagnosis is facilitated by using a cross-reference.

Table 23–4.   Anemias: Etiologic Classification

I. Principally caused by impaired production
  A. Disturbances of the proliferation and differentiation of stem cells
    1. Aplastic anemia
    2. Anemia of chronic renal failure
    3. Endocrine deficiency (pituitary, thyroid, adrenal, or testicular hormones)
  B. Disturbances of proliferation and maturation of differentiated erythroblasts
    1. Defective DNA synthesis (vitamin B_{12}, folic acid, and metabolic defects in purine and pyrimidine metabolism)
    2. Defective hemoglobin synthesis
      a. Deficient globin synthesis (thalassemia)
      b. Deficient heme synthesis (iron deficiency)
    3. Protein malnutrition
    4. Anemia of chronic disease
    5. Myelophthisic anemias due to bone marrow infiltration
II. Principally caused by increased rate of destruction
  A. Intrinsic or red blood cell abnormalities
    1. Membrane disorders
    2. Congenital or inherited enzyme deficiencies
    3. Disorders of hemoglobin
  B. Extrinsic or extraerythrocytic abnormalities
    1. Plasma factors
    2. Physical factors
    3. Chemical or toxic agents
III. Anemia of blood loss (acute or chronic)

(From Brain, M. C.: (The anemias.) Introduction. In *Cecil Textbook of Medicine*, 15th Ed. Edited by P. B. Beeson, W. McDermott, and J. B. Wyngaarden. Philadelphia, W. B. Saunders, 1979.)

We shall consider the different types of anemias after we reflect on the signs and symptoms common to all anemias.

The first fact that emerges from any experience with patients who are truly anemic is the extraordinary variability of their symptoms. The significant majority of these patients may have no appreciation of any physiologic disability. The reason for this unawareness is that anemias usually evolve over months and years, and the gradual development of the significant decrease in hemoglobin may be so insidious that adaptive mechanisms completely compensate for concentrations of hemoglobin as low as 6 grams (normal 14). We have seen several elderly patients with hematocrits of 15% (normal 45%) who are totally without symptoms at rest, and for whom the physiologic embarrassment of shortness of breath is credited simply to old age. The awareness of a gradual loss of oxygen-carrying capacity goes unnoticed, particularly in the aged and sedentary patient. Severe blood loss, on the other hand, is accompanied by other alarming symptoms, and the anemia is usually of less significance than such problems as shock, collapse, dyspnea, or the appearance of blood in the stool or vomitus.

Typically, however, anemia causes nonspecific symptoms of decreased oxygen in the tissues: weakness, fatigue, shortness of breath on exertion, pain in the chest, awareness that the heart is beating rapidly (palpitations), irritability, headache, and light-headedness, all of which can be caused by other diseases, and most of which are often misinterpreted.

The physical examination of an anemic patient may show only the pallor of the mucous membranes, although this may be inconspicuous and overlooked. In some anemias (pernicious anemia, iron deficiency, or those with other systemic disease, e.g., uremia), there may be telltale skin manifestations such as peculiar lemon yellow tint to the skin (as in pernicious anemia), or a greenish appearance (as used to be seen in iron deficiency). In some other hematologic diseases, in which anemia is only part of the process because there is a general loss of cellular elements, there may be petechial hemorrhages or bruising when the platelets are diminished in number, but we are digressing.

For the purposes of this discussion, anemia will be grouped into 4 categories: normochromic and normocytic (normal size and color); hypochromic and microcytic (reduced color and size); hemolytic; and macrocytic.

Normochromic, Normocytic Anemias

The easiest form of anemia to understand is that in which there simply is not enough blood because of blood loss. The clinical patterns of this blood loss are shown in Table 23–5 and are appropriate and consistent with the volume of the loss. We do not ordinarily regard this situation as an anemia, because usually the explanation is obvious and it does not represent a puzzle to be solved, as many anemias usually do.

One of the commonest and most difficult clinical problems to solve, however, is the presence of a **normochromic** (normal amount of hemoglobin per cell), **normocytic** (normal and regular size of red blood cells) anemia in a person who may have a number of predisposing causes. The traditional explanations offered for the occurrence of this simple chronic anemia are: decreased life span of the erythrocytes, a failure of the bone marrow to compensate for the mild hemolytic process, or an impairment of iron release from the reticuloendothelial cells. Each and all of these lead to failure in maintaining the normal numbers of red blood cells. This disorder is seen usually in persons with 1 of the following: infection, arthritis, liver disease (cirrhosis), endocrine disorders, cancer, or renal failure. Because the anemia is often mild, and the underlying disease is severe, emphasis is on the management of the underlying disease. If treatment is successful, the anemia usually disappears.

Another cause of normocytic, normochromic anemia is malnutrition in which protein deficiency is a serious component. Worldwide, anemia is of great economic importance, especially in those parts of the world where protein is in short supply and is often unavailable for growing children.

A third, but much more general, cause for this type of anemia is the failure of the bone marrow to produce all cellular elements. This disease is called **aplastic anemia** and it may occur without apparent cause, or it may be related to exposure to chemical agents, drugs, infections, or be associated with such diverse etiologies as invasion of the bone marrow by cancer (myelophthisic).

Whereas the etiology of aplastic anemia in simplest terms is interference with the normal maturation and development of the pluripotent hematopoietic stem cell, resulting in a decreased number of red blood cells, white blood cells, and platelets, the mechanism by which this occurs is not entirely clear.

For those cases in which aplastic anemia can be traced to drug or medical treatment (x rays), the mechanism is interference with DNA synthesis. The best-studied example of this mechanism has been cases in which aplastic anemia followed the use of chloram-

Table 23–5. Clinical Manifestations of Acute Blood Loss

VOLUME OF BLOOD LOST		
% OF BLOOD VOLUME	ML	CLINICAL MANIFESTATIONS
10	500	Usually none; rarely vasovagal syncope
20	1,000	Few changes supine; upright or with exercise, tachycardia and mild hypotension are often present
30 to 40	1,500 to 2,000	Marked postural hypotension and tachycardia; central venous pressure, cardiac output, and arterial blood pressure are reduced; pulse is thready; skin is cold and clammy; thirst, air hunger, headache, and syncope are frequent
50	2,500	Severe shock, often leading to death

(From Brown, E. B.: Acute hemorrhagic anemia. In *Cecil Textbook of Medicine,* 15th Ed. Edited by P. B. Beeson, W. McDermott, and J. B. Wyngaarden. Philadelphia, W. B. Saunders, 1979.)

phenicol, an invaluable drug for a few infections that was widely and indiscriminately used as a panacea when it was first introduced.

Regardless of its etiology, aplastic anemia has been treated successfully with bone marrow transplants. The greatest success has occurred when there is an HLA-compatible sibling donor of the same sex.

Normochromic, normocytic anemia is diagnosed in the laboratory by finding simply too few normal red blood cells, as distinct from the other types of anemias (hypochromic, microcytic, and macrocytic), in which the appearance of the red blood cells suggests the diagnosis. Aplastic anemia is diagnosed by the paucity of all elements and not just of the red blood cells (pancytopenia).

Hypochromic, Microcytic Anemias

The commonest cause of anemia, worldwide, is **iron deficiency,** because of the increased iron loss due to intestinal parasites coupled with inadequate dietary intake. In much of the world (Asia, Africa) more than half the adult population may suffer from serious iron-deficiency anemia. Estimates range from 60% of pregnant women to 30% of all women, and 5% of all men. The reason for the difference is monthly loss of blood in the menses, coupled with the requirements for fetal iron during pregnancy. Repeated pregnancies and excessive menstrual loss are great drains on the body stores. A prolonged milk diet for children fails to supply them with iron. In the western world, inadequate meals of young mothers and hidden gastrointestinal bleeding in men of all ages are additional common causes that contribute to this particular type of anemia.

Iron-deficiency anemia is most easily diagnosed by finding small, poorly stained red blood cells on a good smear of peripheral blood. The red blood cells show variation in size (anisocytosis) and shape (poikilocytosis). A calculation of the mean corpuscular volume and of the mean corpuscular hemoglobin concentration show these values to be low. These values can be determined by knowing the number of red blood cells, the hemoglobin concentration, and the hematocrit. The mean corpuscular volume (MCV) is $\dfrac{\text{Hct}}{\text{RBC number}}$, which

gives a number that normally ranges between 80 and 105 μ^3. It is spuriously elevated with some of the newer counting methods because of trapping of serum, so that the value should be suspected from the examination of the smear.

The mean corpuscular hemoglobin concentration (MCHC) is determined by dividing the hemoglobin by the hematocrit. It is normally between 32 and 33 grams per ml and is never elevated. Values of less than 30 grams per ml indicate iron deficiency, and the mean corpuscular volume is usually less than 80.

Two other determinations to confirm the suspicion of iron deficiency as a cause of anemia are the plasma iron concentration and the total plasma iron-binding capacity.

When someone has been either losing iron or taking it in inadequate amounts, the next thing that happens is mobilization of iron stores from such cells as the reticuloendothelial system in the liver. When these iron stores have been used up, a signal is given to the small intestine to increase the rate of iron absorption. As the iron requirements for the biosynthesis of hemoglobin (and myoglobin, particularly in growing children) increase, the plasma iron concentration falls. The concentration of the serum protein responsible for transporting iron (transferrin) increases and the saturation of this protein by iron is decreased. When the demand for iron is not met, blood cells are liberated into the peripheral blood smear that show this lack; they are distorted and contain too little hemoglobin.

Iron is an essential element in man largely for its role in hemoglobin and myoglobin maintenance and production. With increased loss, as in bleeding from a peptic ulcer, decreased intake, or extra requirements (pregnancy), there may be insufficient iron to complete each new erythrocyte hemoglobin complement. This lack may be visible in the red blood cell itself, which appears as a pale, small shadow of its normal self. This manifestation of iron deficiency is a late result of the process, because the body, in its wisdom, tends to use up all the other stores before it circulates a physiologically unfit cell.

The symptoms of this type of anemia are no different from those of the previous types; they begin insidiously and are nonspecific. The tiredness, shortness of breath on exertion, headache, light-headedness, palpitations, and irritability are all part of the syndrome. Physical findings may show pallor alone, and the diagnosis is made only by laboratory examination of the smear and calculation of the indices. The treatment is twofold: short-term, to treat the anemia if necessary, even by transfusion, and to replace iron (by simple salts such as ferrous sulfate or ferrous gluconate). Second, to determine and treat the underlying cause of the iron deficiency, be it nutritional or bleeding.

Macrocytic Anemias (Megaloblastic)

The term megaloblastic (Greek *megas*, large, and *blastos*, germ) or macrocytic is used because the common abnormality is gigantism of all proliferating cells, most obvious in examinations of the smear of the peripheral blood, but also exfoliated cells of the gastrointestinal and genitourinary tract. The defect common to all these cells is delayed synthesis of DNA.

Macrocytic anemias are caused by inadequate ingestion of factors on which DNA synthesis depends (**folic acid and vitamin B_{12}**); inadequate absorption (due to interference with factors in which B_{12} depends for absorption, intrinsic and extrinsic); or increased requirement, excretion, or destruction of these factors.

A poor diet, such as strict vegetarianism, in which there are no sources of vitamin B_{12}, or long-term alcoholism, in which no folic acid is available, or simple poverty will often lead to macrocytic as well as other types of anemias. A gastrectomy or invasion of the stomach by cancer will bring about macrocytic anemias, just as atrophy of the gastric mucosa, associated with autoimmune disease, is a predisposing cause. **Pernicious anemia** is the name given to the particular type of macrocytic anemia that is due to deficiency of intrinsic factor, which is essential for B_{12} effectiveness. Pernicious anemia is a megaloblastic anemia caused by inadequate secretion of gastric intrinsic factor. This factor is a carrier that is secreted by the gastric mucosa and permits the passage of the large molecule of B_{12} across the mucosa of the ileum. Lack of carriers, for whatever reason, leads to B_{12} deficiency. This disease is age-related. It has a worldwide incidence of 1 per million at 1 year, 1 per 10,000

at age 10, 1 per 5,000 at age 35, and 1 in 200 at age 60. In some instances, there are circulating antibodies to intrinsic factor, which implies an autoimmune etiology for this disease. The discovery of intrinsic and extrinsic factors is an exciting chapter in medicine that took place in the 1920's.

Other causes of macrocytic anemias may occur if the small bowel is affected by disease, such as sprue, or by granulomatous lesions, or if the patient is taking drugs that impair normal mucosal renewal (e.g., methotrexate), or if the bowel has been resected. These conditions reduce absorption.

Another major cause is the competition for vitamin B_{12}, such as occurs with intestinal parasites or bacterial overproduction. The fish tapeworm (*Diphyllobothrium latum*) and the presence of loops of bowel that do not empty properly and in which bacteria grow abundantly (blind loop syndrome) are such examples.

It is important to remember that normal adult body stores of B_{12} last 3 to 6 years after absorption of B_{12} ceases. However, symptoms may not occur for 20 years or more after B_{12} is no longer ingested, because the body jealously guards its storehouse of B_{12} by continuing to reabsorb it from the bile.

Clinically, the symptoms are those of anemia in general, with the additional and

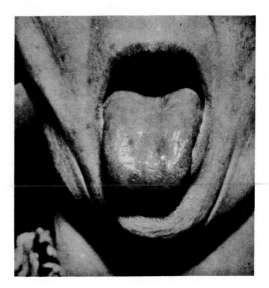

Fig. 23–2. Smooth tongue in a case of pernicious anemia. (Wintrobe, M.: *Clincal Hematology.* Philadelphia, Lea & Febiger.)

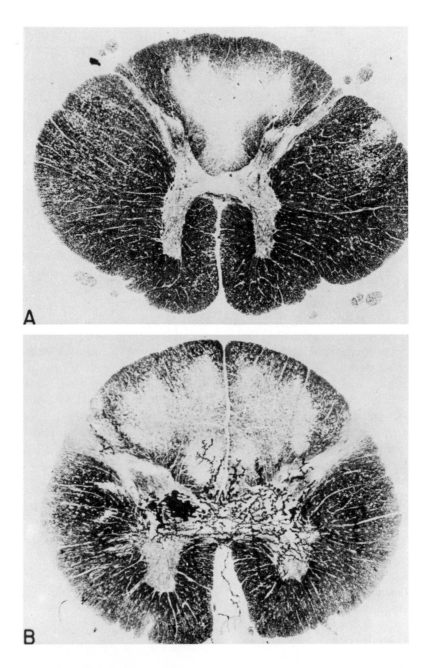

Fig. 23–3. These two photographs show sections from the thoracic and lumbar spinal cord of a patient dying with pernicious anemia in 1926, before treatment was available. The central pallor in the ascending and descending tracts of the posterior columns is typical of the irreversible neurologic lesions that accompany untreated pernicious anemia. (From Follis, R.H.: *Deficiency Disease.* Springfield, Ill., Charles C Thomas, 1958.)

important neurologic manifestations of B_{12} deficiency, such as parasthesias, numbness and tingling, and loss of vibration and position sense. I (Huntington Sheldon) once had a patient who was a musician in a local bar. His complaint was that his friends remarked how careless he had become in his piano playing. Because he also felt weak and in poor health, he came to the clinic, where he was diagnosed as having pernicious anemia (Fig. 23–2). Unsteadiness in walking and mental depression, and even paranoid ideas, may be part of the clinical pattern of pernicious anemia. This disease has also been called subacute combined degeneration because of the lesions seen in the spinal cord (Fig. 23–3).

One of the most important points in diagnosing macrocytic anemia is to distinguish between those anemias caused by folic acid deficiency and those due to B_{12} deficiency, because the neurologic changes of B_{12} deficiency may be irreversible. It is unwise to treat macrocytic anemia without clearly establishing the correct etiology. A patient whose lack of intrinsic factor causes his or her B_{12} deficiency would be on a monthly maintenance dose of B_{12} for life. B_{12} deficiency impairs myelin formation and is followed by axonal degeneration and finally destruction of the neuron.

The distinction between folate deficiency and B_{12} deficiency is made now by measuring serum levels of both B_{12} and folate, and it is wise to recognize that both deficiencies may occur in the same patient, for example, in an alcoholic with intrinsic factor deficiency. A more sophisticated warning is that when, for example, in pregnancy the folate level is low, this may have an effect also on the intestinal mucosa, thereby leading to malabsorption of B_{12}. Thus treatment with folic acid may be followed by a rise in B_{12} levels. The absorption of radioactive B_{12} is a useful diagnostic test.

Hemolytic Anemias

This is a large and heterogeneous group. A shortened life span of the red blood cells with resulting hemolysis, that is to say, lysis or solution of the red cells with liberation of the hemoglobin into the plasma, is the feature common to them all. The mechanism by which this process occurs may be 1 of 2 profoundly different types. In the first, the defect is hereditary, and in the second form it is acquired, being commonly caused by circulating antibodies. (These antibodies are frequently the product of autoimmune reactions.) Thus the red cell may either be born vulnerable or it may become so, owing to acquired external factors. In the congenital (hereditary) form, the fault lies in the red cells, whereas in the acquired form it lies in the environment. For this reason, removal of the spleen, the graveyard of the erythrocytes, may be beneficial in the congenital type of this disease. ACTH or cortisone may also benefit the acquired form. The 2 types are differentiated in the laboratory by means of the Coombs test, which is designed to show the presence of antibodies (agglutinins) absorbed to the surface of the red cells in the acquired, but not in the congenital, form.

We must also recognize that increased hemolysis does not necessarily result in anemia. Bone marrow activity may compensate for destruction of the erythrocytes. Under these circumstances, a person is said to have hemolytic disease, but not to suffer from hemolytic anemia, which only occurs when the bone marrow is unable to compensate for the shortened life span of the erythrocytes. The best single signpost of hemolytic anemia is a persistent increase to 5% or more in the number of reticulocytes (immature red blood cells). Other evidence of bone marrow overactivity is leukocytosis, nucleated red cells, and increased platelets.

The hereditary defect may involve abnormal red cells or abnormal hemoglobin. The outstanding sample of a red cell defect is spherocytic anemia; a corresponding example of hemoglobin defect is sickle cell anemia.

Congenital spherocytic anemia, as the name implies, shows a spheroidal shape of the erythrocytes in place of normal biconcave discs. Their shape is due to a defect in the phospholipid envelope, which in turn is responsible for the excessive red cell destruction or hemolysis.

The blood shows anemia, usually mild, but severe in crises. Two chief characteristics of the blood film are microspherulocytes and reticulocytes. A spherocyte is smaller than normal and spherical instead of biconcave. Reticulocytes are more numerous than in any other disease. In place of the usual 1%, they may comprise 20%. As biconcave cells become globular when placed in hypotonic saline solution, it is evident that the more spherical cells rupture more readily. Thus there is an increased fragility of the red cells when placed in a salt solution of a strength that leaves normal cells untouched. This is the basis of a laboratory test for spherocytic anemia.

The disease may remain latent for many years, although the fragility is there, hanging like the sword of Damocles over the head of the person carrying the defective gene. For some unknown reason, there may be occasional crises, in which there is increased blood destruction with attacks of pain in the region of the liver and the spleen. It has been suggested that the crises may really be due to an acute aplastic condition in the bone marrow with complete cessation of formation of red cells. This sounds good, but it explains nothing, for we are also ignorant as to the cause of the aplasia of the marrow.

Jaundice is the characteristic feature of the crises, although a mild degree of jaundice, often unrecognized, may be present all the time. Jaundice (French *jaune*, yellow) results from increased hemolysis, which produces an increase in circulating blood breakdown products, 1 of which is a pigment, bilirubin. It is, of course, the result of the increased fragility of the red cells, the actual destruction taking place in the spleen, which becomes enlarged, and which appears to assume a function of overactivity, known as hypersplenism. On this basis, splenectomy has become the recognized treatment for congenital spherocytic anemia, often with dramatic and satisfying results.

Sickle cell anemia is a genetic anomaly in the formation of the hemoglobin molecule; it has much in common with spherocytosis. Both conditions are hereditary; in both there may be active disease (anemia), or merely the hereditary fingerprints (spherocytes or sickle cells, as the case may be); and both are characterized by hemolytic anemia and by the appearance of large numbers of reticulocytes in the peripheral blood. A major difference is that the genetic defect in sickle cell anemia is largely confined to blacks (Fig. 23–4). It is transmitted as a dominant Mendelian charac-

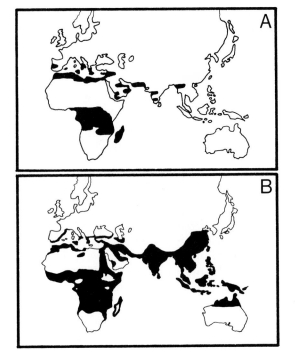

Fig. 23–4. These 2 maps show *A*, the distribution of sickle cell disease, and *B*, the distribution of malaria. One can superimpose maps *A* and *B* and identify the distribution of malaria and sickle cell disease in Africa. The sickle cell gene is not a significant part of the gene pool in Asia. Since the presence of the sickle cell trait (heterozygous) appears to confer some immunity to malaria, it is thought that the sickle cell trait is an evolutionary adaptation to malaria in the environment. (From Motulsky, A. G.: Metabolic polymorphisms and the role of infectious diseases in human evolution. Human Biol., 32:43, 1960.)

teristic by either sex. Sickle cell anemia is homozygous, the defective gene being inherited from both parents, whereas the **sickle cell trait** represents a heterozygous state. The biochemical defect is a substitution of one amino acid for another in the hemoglobin protein. This is the prototypic "molecular disease."

The blood presents a striking picture in the active phase of the disease. There is marked anemia as well as leukocytosis, and the blood smear shows an extraordinary change in the shape of the red cells, for large numbers of these are crescentic or sickle in form (Fig. 23–5). The serum is often deep yellow, owing to the great increase in bilirubin produced by hemolysis of the sickle cell.

In the latent phase, sickle cells are not present in the circulating blood, but they can be readily demonstrated in the presence of a decrease in the oxygen tension. When a wet film of the blood is made, to which a reducing substance (sodium metabisul-

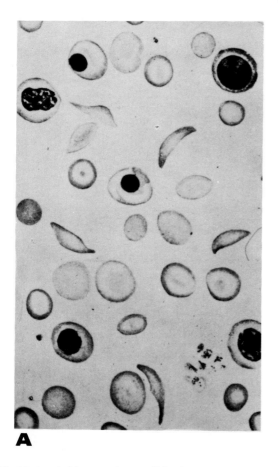
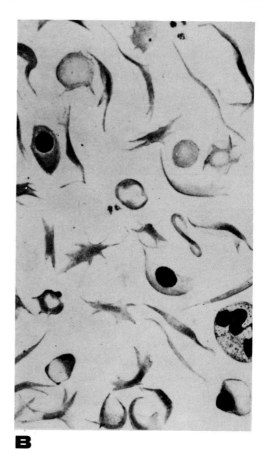

A   **B**

Fig. 23–5. *A*, this smear shows red blood cells, some of which are slightly distorted. *B*, following anoxemia, many cells appear to have an elongated sickle form with pointed ends. These cells cause the sickled erythrocytes to fill the capillary bed. (From Herrick, J.B.: Peculiar elongated and sickle-shaped red corpuscles in a case of severe anemia. Arch. Intern. Med., 6:517, 1910.)

fite) is added, many red cells will be found to have assumed the sickle form. The diagnosis is best made, however, from hemoglobin electrophoresis.

Acute crises occur in sickle cell anemia. Not only is the anemia intensified, but the patient suffers from attacks of abdominal pain that may be confused with acute appendicitis or with ruptured peptic ulcer. Infarcts of the spleen are common, owing to thrombosis in that organ. (The sickle cells have a tendency to stick in the capillaries, obstructing them and closing off a blood vessel.)

Thalassemia is another of the hereditary group of hemolytic anemias. The gene responsible for the defect in hemoglobin formation is distributed among the peoples of the eastern Mediterranean basin. For this reason, it has long been known as Mediterranean anemia or thalassemia (Greek *thalassa*, sea, i.e., the Mediterranean). The trait has now

been carried far and wide throughout the world by the migration of peoples. The hemoglobin defect results in a decreased life span of the circulating red cells.

The characteristic features of the blood smear are: (1) the great numbers of erythroblasts and (2) the presence of leptocytes of thin cells (Greek *leptos*, thin), oval cells, and target cells. Leptocytes are comparable to sickle cells, both being departures from the normal form of the red cell. Target cells have a central rounded area of pigment, surrounded by a clear zone with, further out, a thick, pigmented capsule. This appearance is responsible for the names target cells and Mexican hat cells. The most suggestive feature of the film is the presence of great numbers of immature, nucleated red cells, both normoblasts and megaloblasts.

The clinical features are: (1) a constant familial and racial incidence (most often in Greeks, but also in Italians and Armenians, and even more common in Africa than in the

United States), (2) a typical facial appearance, and (3) enlargement of the spleen. Thalassemia usually is evident in the first 2 years of life and sometimes in the newborn. The skin is yellow, the face mongoloid, the head enlarged, and abdomen prominent owing to the large spleen, and the stature stunted. There is a moderate or marked anemia, and a pronounced leukocytosis.

Many acquired hemolytic anemias are caused by extraneous agents. Among these may be mentioned chemical agents and drugs, bacterial toxins such as those of hemolytic streptococci, and the malaria parasite, which, as we have seen, specializes in destroying the red cells in which it resides.

In **hemolytic disease of the newborn**, the hemolysis with resulting anemia is caused by antibodies transferred across the placenta during pregnancy. As this disease has been thoroughly reviewed elsewhere in this text, it will be discussed here only briefly.

The simplest and best method of detecting the passive transfer of maternal antibody to the infant's circulation is to determine whether the infant's erythrocytes have been coated with antibody. This is demonstrated by the Coombs antiglobulin test. Hemolytic disease of the newborn occurs once in every 200 pregnancies worldwide and used to account for 2 to 3% of all neonatal deaths.

The clinical picture varies. The child may be born dead in a condition of extreme general edema or hydrops. About 7% of those who survive are mental defectives. Jaundice may or may not be present. The blood picture is that of congenital anemia and **erythroblastosis fetalis**, that is to say, with great numbers of nucleated red cells (erythroblasts), owing to compensatory activity of the bone marrow. The mortality rate formerly was 70 to 80%, but with modern treatment and prenatal care, the incidence has dropped markedly. Exchange transfusion was given at birth when there was evidence of disease, but now Rh immunization is the treatment of choice.

POLYCYTHEMIAS

The term polycythemia means an increase in the number of the cells of the blood, but in practice this increase applies only to the red cells.

Polycythemia vera, as the name indicates, is a true or primary increase in the number of red blood cells; its etiology is unknown. There is an infrequent but real association of polycythemia with tumors of the kidney. This observation is interesting because a hormone, **erythropoietin**, which stimulates the bone marrow, has been found in the kidney, but we are not sure which cells produce it. The role of the kidney in control of red blood cell numbers is further substantiated by the anemia that almost invariably accompanies chronic renal disease. Other explanations for anemia in chronic renal disease have been the suppression of bone marrow by the acidosis that occurs in uremia and the long-term blood loss that is sometimes seen.

In polycythemia, the red blood cells are greatly increased in number, usually from 7,000,000 to 10,000,000 per cubic millimeter. The blood volume is also increased, and the blood becomes viscid, owing to the burden of cells it carries. This predisposes a patient to thrombosis and infarction, particularly of the spleen, a frequent finding in polycythemia, whether it is primary or secondary. There is moderate leukocytosis, and occasional primitive red and white cells are present in the circulating blood. As might be expected, the bone marrow is markedly hyperplastic, so that the condition may be regarded as a type of neoplasia, being comparable to leukemia in this respect. Perhaps it is significant that occasional cases have changed from erythremia to leukemia of myelogenous type.

The clinical picture is striking, for the skin and mucous membrane of the mouth are red and the conjunctiva is bloodshot. The color is due to the increased number of red cells. The spleen is always enlarged. At autopsy, the visceral vessels are greatly distended and are often thrombosed. The disease may be treated and the blood volume may be effectively reduce by repeated venesection.

Secondary polycythemia is a compensatory increase of red cells in conditions of insufficient oxygenation, such as congenital heart disease, emphysema, and residence at high altitudes. It will be obvious that the condition is in no sense one of disease, but rather it represents a compensatory adaptation. There is no increase in leukocytes, a diagnostic point of value in distinguishing erythrocytosis from polycythemia vera.

HEMORRHAGIC DISORDERS

These disorders have been called by many names (bleeding disorders, purpuras), and have many causes, but the principle common to all is some perturbation in the mechanisms that normally control hemorrhage and maintain blood where it belongs, namely in the blood vessels. Bleeding disorders can result from such different causes as heredity, tumors, taking of drugs, or exposure to toxic chemicals. We shall consider first the normal hemostatic mechanisms, then heritable disorders characterized by bleeding, and finally a few assorted causes of increased bleeding tendencies.

Everyone knows that a characteristic of blood is its tendency to clot. This is one of the most important homeostatic mechanisms, for without the ability to clot, as we shall see, this essential juice of man oozes away from tiny nicks and scratches. Paradoxically, blood must be a liquid in order to circulate and it must rapidly become a coagulum in order not to be wasted.

Three different mechanisms are responsible for staunching the flow of blood when a vessel is severed, as in any traumatic injury. First, the blood vessel wall, which contains smooth muscle, will contract and narrow the orifice. There are abundant tales of severance of a limb after which arteries go into spasm and act as a virtual tourniquet. This is more likely to happen in small than in large arteries. When there is a disorder of small blood vessels, as occurs in scurvy, for example, all other hemostatic mechanisms are intact. However, bleeding may occur from slight trauma, and the application of a tourniquet, such as a blood pressure cuff, may lead to hemorrhages. This is called a positive tourniquet test. The second hemostatic mechanism is the formation of a platelet plug at sites of endothelial injury. When platelets are decreased in number in the peripheral blood (**thrombocytopenia**), the first signs of this abnormality may be the spontaneous appearance of

small hemorrhages in the skin (**petechiae**). The third hemostatic mechanism is coagulation proper. Before going on to consider the clotting mechanisms themselves, we shall digress for a minute to consider the platelet and its disorders.

Platelets. The normal platelet count is 150,000 to 400,000 mm^3 in the peripheral blood. One obtains an estimate of platelet numbers by examining a smear. A direct count is done with a particle counter or with a phase microscope. Platelets are formed in the bone marrow from large cells called megakaryocytes and represent fragmentation or subdivisions of these large cells. They are not complete cells in that they have no nuclei and cannot replicate, but they contain a number of compartments and are capable of a limited amount of protein synthesis. Currently, we regard platelets as performing 3 functions. The surface is covered with a mucopolysaccharide that is involved in adhesion. Platelets are the first line of defense in vascular injury and adhere to the lining of blood vessels whenever structures such as collagen and basement membranes are exposed to the circulating blood. Platelets also contain large numbers of membrane-bound granules that are released on contact with such an injured surface. These secretory granules have been shown to contain serotonin, catecholamines, and a heparin-neutralizing factor, as well as lysosomal enzymes such as acid phosphatase and cathepsins. Finally, there are many filaments and microtubules in platelets that enable the platelet to change its shape and to participate in clot retraction. Platelets live for about 10 days, and it is estimated that 80% of all platelets are in the circulation at any given time and that only 20% are in the spleen.

In addition to acting as a mechanical plug, the most important function of platelets is their release of a number of physiologically active substances when the platelets have become arrested on the wall of a blood vessel. The result of this release is the continued aggregation of platelets at the site of adhesion, and the progress of the coagulation process, which involves the conversion of fibrinogen to fibrin. Because platelet plugs stop bleeding from damaged capillaries, any deficiency in the number or function of platelets can be estimated by measuring the bleeding time. Conventionally, this is determined by the time it takes for bleeding to stop from 3 incisions 1 mm deep in the forearm. Bleeding time is normal in disorders of the coagulation system, but prolonged with a decline in the number of platelets and in disorders of platelet function. It is also prolonged when there is a total absence of fibrinogen. Table 23–6 illustrates the clinical distinctions between capillary and platelet deficiency and defects in the coagulation mechanism.

Table 23–6.   Differential Considerations of Bleeding Disorders

FINDINGS	DISORDERS OF COAGULATION	DISORDERS OF PLATELETS OR VESSELS—"PURPURIC"
Petechiae	Rare	Characteristic
Deep dissecting hematomas	Characteristic	Rare
Superficial ecchymoses	Common—large and solitary	Characteristic—small and multiple
Hemarthrosis	Characteristic	Rare
Delayed bleeding	Common—cannot maintain clot	Rare
Bleeding from superficial cuts and scratches	Minimal	Persistent, often profuse
Sex of patient	80 to 90% of hereditary forms only in males	Relatively more common in females
Family history	Common	Rare

Thrombocytopenia, or a platelet count of less than 100,000 mm³ often leads to bleeding, which may occur after an operation or trauma. When the count is less than 40,000, bleeding may occur spontaneously. The low platelet count may result from defective production, defective maturation, disordered distribution (sequestration), or accelerated destruction. Defective production can be due to direct injury to the bone marrow by drugs or chemicals, or it may be due to invasion of the bone marrow by carcinoma or lymphoma. With deficiency of B_{12}, for example, there may be a defective maturation.

Other conditions that lead to a decrease in platelets are disseminated intravascular coagulation (DIC), which captures platelets in thrombi aggregates, and a disorder of unknown etiology that usually leads rapidly to death, called thrombotic thrombocytopenic purpura (TTP).

Disseminated Intravascular Coagulation

This pathologic phenomenon was described relatively recently and has become a well-known entity in the last 20 years, although it is difficult both to diagnose and to treat. Because it may occur as a complication of many disorders, ranging from cancer to infections, as well as in many situations in which bleeding occurs (obstetrical or operative hemorrhage, allergic reactions), one should keep it in mind as a possible explanation for the hemorrhage's lack of response to first-line defense transfusions.

Disseminated intravascular coagulation (DIC) is characterized by abnormal clotting mechanisms and by generalized hemorrhage. As its name implies, there is an activation of the clotting mechanisms with the consequent consumption of fibrinogen and platelets and other coagulation factors of the circulatory system, particularly the capillary vessels. This activation is usually the result of triggering mechanisms, such as the presence of a large clot in the uterus, for example. The successful treatment of the underlying disorders (evacuation of the clot) will interrupt the vicious cycle of fibrinolysis and thrombosis. The sequence of fibrinolysis and thrombus formation leads to obstruction of the microcirculation by a fibrin meshwork. This fibrin meshwork, in turn, leads to the rapid breakdown of erythrocytes, due to the knife-like effect of the fibrin strands on red blood cells as they try to move through the partially obstructed capillary. To make the diagnosis, one should test for fibrinogen-fibrin degradation products (fibrin split products) in the laboratory, or see damaged red blood cells on the smear of the peripheral blood. Levels of less than 100 mg/100 ml of fibrinogen, thrombocytopenia (less than 100,000/mm³), and decreased coagulation factors V and VII all confirm this diagnosis. Treatment with heparin is sometimes successful, but the underlying disorder must be the principal target for the therapeutic efforts.

Coagulation Mechanisms

The coagulation system seems increasingly complex as we learn more about it.

One good way to look at the coagulation system is that it is a part of the host's response to injury. Many of the enzymatic relationships in coagulation are essential parts of the inflammatory or immunologic response to injury, and involve kinins, complement, and the fibrinolytic systems. Coagulation mechanisms can be viewed as having 2 main functions: to form fibrin, which mechanically blocks the flow of blood through ruptured vessels, and to produce thrombin, which stabilizes the platelet plug. Incidentally, thrombin also converts fibrinogen to fibrin. A number of proenzymes and proteins, called coagulation factors, participate in coagulation in addition to platelets and calcium. The simplest scheme of coagulation, which dates from 1928, is seen in Figure 23–6. This scheme anticipates the relationship of inactive substances to the activation of circulating plasma proteins. One can view the coagulation process as a series of limited cleavages of enzyme precursors. It is interesting that the cascade of reactions can also be viewed as a sequence of enzymatic conversions of substrate from an inactive state to an active one. Each conversion results in the production of a proteinase for the subsequent stage (Fig. 23–7). This process has the teleologic advantage of grading the response, so that it is not an all or none reaction, but it has the disadvantage of being complicated for study purposes.

The cascade of coagulation reactions can be divided into an intrinsic and an extrinsic pathway. These are defined by the fact that all coagulation factors necessary for the formation of a fibrin clot are present in the intravascular compartment in the intrinsic pathway, whereas the extrinsic pathway requires the addition of a tissue factor (from thromboplastin) to make the clot. As the diagram shows, calcium is essential, as are phospholipid surfaces.

If we are to consider any of the factors involved in the clotting mechanism, we should

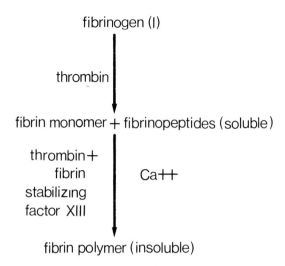

Fig. 23–6. This scheme shows the elementary, traditional coagulation mechanism, starting with fibrinogen at the top and ending with the insoluble polymers of fibrin at the bottom. Thrombin and calcium are shown as essential cofactors. (From Ratnoff, O.D.: Hemorrhagic disorders: coagulation defects. In *Cecil Textbook of Medicine*, 15th Ed. Edited by P. B. Beeson, W. McDermott, and J. B. Wyngaarden. Philadelphia, W. B. Saunders, 1979.)

start with fibrinogen. In order to simplify our consideration and to illustrate some of the principles outlined, we shall look at just 3 of the coagulation proteins: Factor I (fibrinogen), Factor II (prothrombin), and Factor VIII (antihemophilic factor). In addition, we should say a few words about vitamin K, because of its importance in this scheme. The reader is referred to other sources for more detailed accounts of each of the known factors in the coagulation scheme and their interactions.

Fibrinogen (Factor I) is a large protein (340,000 MW) with a small proportion of carbohydrate (3 to 5%) synthesized by the liver cells, with a half-life of about 5 days. The structure of this molecule has recently been elucidated, and it has been shown to consist of 2 halves, each consisting of 3 paired subunits. How this molecule is cleaved, what happens to the subunits after cleavage, and how polymerization into the indeterminately long but insoluble strands of fibrin (Fig. 23–8) is accomplished has not yet been deciphered and will be another chapter in molecular biology.

During conversion of fibrinogen to fibrin and its polymerization, an inactivating system precursor (of which there are many in normal blood) is incorporated into the growing clot. This substance, plasminogen, is normally kept in an inactive state

COAGULATION FACTORS

FACTOR	NAME
I	Fibrinogen
II	Prothrombin
III	Tissue thromboplastin, thrombokinase
IV	Calcium
V	Proaccelerin, labile factor
VII	Proconvertin, stable factor
VIII	Antihemophilic A factor (AHF), antihemophilic globulin (AHG)
IX	Antihemophilic B factor (AHB), plasma thromboplastin component (PTC), Christmas factor
X	Stuart factor, Stuart-Prower factor
XI	Plasma thromboplastin antecedent (PTA)
XII	Hageman factor, contact factor
XIII	Fibrin stabilizing factor, fibrinase

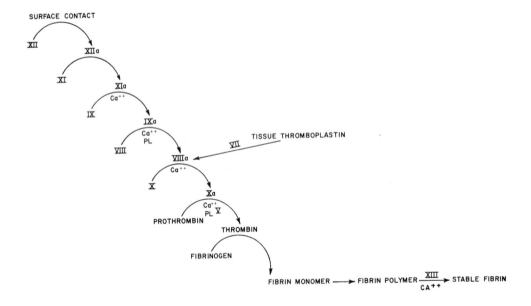

Fig. 23–7. This figure illustrates the cascade of clotting as we understand it today, including the intrinsic clotting mechanism, in which no extravascular components are necessary, and the extrinsic clotting mechanism, in which tissue factors play a role. (From Brown, B.: *Hematology: Principles and Procedures*, 2nd Ed. Philadelphia, Lea & Febiger, 1976.)

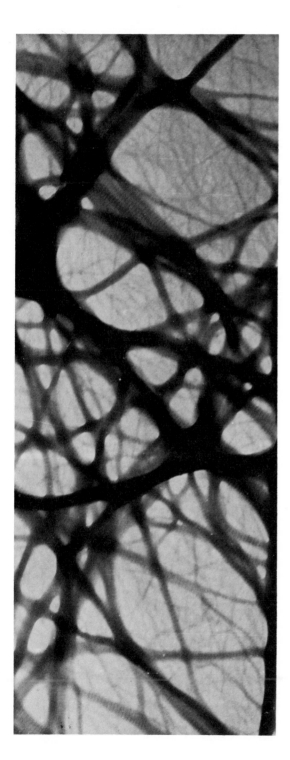

Fig. 23–8. This electron microphotograph shows the network of fibrin from a clot. This historic picture was taken by Dr. K. R. Porter in 1947 at the Rockefeller Laboratories.

by its own inhibitors, but in the clot it is sequestered or protected from these circulating inhibitory substances. Thus it comes to be activated to plasmin, which is a proteolytic enzyme. This substance, plasmin, is essential to the maintenance of the circulating system, rather as tow trucks are essential for the function of expressways, because plasmin digests fibrin and other products of coagulation. It is safe to say that we are all constantly forming clots at sites of minor injury and are constantly breaking them down again. This process of clot lysis results in degradation products that can be detected in the circulating blood. These may be called fibrin split products.

Prothrombin is a smaller (68,000 MW) proenzyme of interest, not only because on activation it becomes the highly active enzyme thrombin, but because the molecule has a calcium-binding region that is dependent on the presence of vitamin K. This molecule is also synthesized by liver cells and has a shorter half-life of about 3 days. We do not know whether the same liver cell produces prothrombin and fibrinogen, nor do we know precisely how these factors that regulate the production of essential coagulation proteins are controlled. Possibly, as for serum albumin, a decrease in the serum level of prothrombin stimulates liver cells to renewed synthesis of this protein.

The major importance of prothrombin lies in that it is a precursor of thrombin, which acts on fibrinogen. Normally, there is no thrombin in circulating blood. Thrombin can be produced either from the intrinsic source (prothrombin) or from the so-called extrinsic pathway, whose tissue components initiated its release. It is of relevance that blood may also coagulate when exposed to negatively charged surfaces, such as glass.

The third coagulation protein is a large molecule (in excess of 1,000,000 MW) and it includes at least 2 substances, in the absence of which serious uncontrolled bleeding results. These substances are **antihemophilic globulins**, the lack of which causes classic hemophilia.

This brings us to the hereditary coagulation disorders. The most common are classic hemophilia due to deficiency or defects in Factors VIII and IX, or Christmas factor.

Hemophilia is due to a deficiency of a normally functioning factor VIII. The serum contains this factor, but it seems to be unable to act appropriately. This disorder occurs in 1 out of 10,000 of the world population, and it is transmitted as a sex-linked recessive pattern appearing in males but not in females. Males with the disorder transmit the gene to all their daughters, and their sons are all normal. This diagnosis is suspected in families with the trait (see Fig. 4–10), but 30% of cases give no positive family history, suggesting this is a relatively frequent mutation. The most serious aspects of the bleeding tendency, apart from its life-threatening aspects following surgical operations or minor procedures (dental extraction), are bleeding into joints, which often results in destruction of the growing edges of bone and deformities of joints that do not heal.

A second hereditary disorder of the coagulation proteins is called **von Willebrand's disease**, and it is transmitted as an autosomal dominant. This, too, is caused by a Factor VIII abnormality, and, in addition, there is a defective serum protein necessary for normal platelet function. Thus such persons may have both disorders in platelet function and in their normal coagulation pattern. Transfusion of normal plasma has a markedly beneficial effect on these patients.

Vitamin K, as we have already described in Chapter 3, is essential for the normal biosynthesis of prothrombin and several coagulation factors (VII, IX and X). Recently, vitamin K has been shown to be involved in the biosynthesis of prothrombin by converting a precursor protein to active prothrombin.

Various tests to determine the presence or absence of the different factors have been used to separate one clinical disorder from another and to provide rational therapy for these hemorrhagic disorders. They are outlined in Table 23–7.

We can move on to consider another major category of diseases of the erythron, namely disorders of the white blood cell series: leukemias and lymphomas.

LEUKEMIA

This term was introduced by Virchow, and it literally means white blood. The term is applied to those disorders in which the normal growth and development of the white blood cells, either lymphocytes or granulocytes, are no longer ordered and controlled. This disorder is expressed in a rapid and excessive cellular proliferation. The leukemic cells are present in bone marrow and peripheral blood and may infiltrate other organs such as the liver or kidney. Characteristically,

Table 23–7.   Coagulation Tests

1. *Bleeding Time,* prolonged in patients with increased capillary fragility and/or inadequate platelet function. Examination of smear for platelets or direct platelet count is complementary information.

2. *Fibrinogen* content may be expressed in terms of highest dilution of plasma in which a clot may be seen after addition of thrombin, or as a directly estimated value. Greater than 100 mg/100 ml excludes fibrinogen deficiency as a cause of bleeding. Examples in which fibrinogen levels are decreased are disorders such as disseminated intravascular coagulation, thrombotic thrombocytopenic syndrome, and hemolytic-uremic syndrome. These disorders also have prolonged thrombin times.

3. *Thrombin Time.* Measurement of this time is required for fibrin clot formation when thrombin is added to plasma. Thrombin acts directly on fibrinogen. It is inhibited by fibrinogen degradation products and by heparin. Prolongation indicates either low fibrinogen content or presence of inhibitor.

4. *Prothrombin Time* is the time it takes fibrin to gel in plasma after calcium and complete thromboplastin have been added. The test involves VII, X, and V, prothrombin, and fibrinogen. Values are reported as percentage of control. Disorders in which it is prolonged are Vitamin K deficiency and hepatobiliary disease.

5. *Partial Thromboplastin Time* (PTT) depends on glass activation of factor XII. Partial thromboplastin is substituted. Both of these tests measure reactions in the intrinsic system, which depends on the combined activity of all coagulation factors except III, VII, and XIII. This test will be prolonged in most bleeding disorders, but is particularly valuable in von Willebrand's disease when all the other tests (PT, thrombin, fibrinogen) are normal.

the appearance of immature or "blast" forms of the white blood cells in the peripheral blood indicates the loss of the normal controlling mechanisms (whatever they are) and confirms the diagnosis. The white blood cell count may rise to hundreds of thousands per mm^3 compared with a normal of 7 to 10,000 mm^3. The patient may have uncontrollable hemorrhages and anemia, because the bone marrow is replaced by the neoplastic proliferation, thereby precluding the orderly progression of maturation that maintains the normal populations of red blood cells, white blood cells, and platelets.

Experience has shown that leukemias can be separated into different groups because of their biologic behavior, morphology, and response to therapy. Leukemias with mature cells in the peripheral blood, rather than blast cells, tend to have a more benign course.

There are a significant number of cases in which the number of cells in the peripheral blood is within normal limits, but immature forms are seen, indicating that the bone marrow examination will confirm the suspicion of leukemia. These cases are termed **aleukemic leukemia**. To make things more complicated, there are a few instances with excessively high white blood cell counts that turn out not to be leukemia at all, but rather a leukemia-like pattern (leukemoid reaction) to such other diseases as tuberculosis.

The etiology of leukemia (which can be considered another form of cancer) is of great interest because of a number of observations on leukemia in living forms other than man. To begin with, we should state that the etiology of human leukemias is not established. There are, however, 3 important associations with leukemia in man. In Down's syndrome (mongolism), in which there is an abnormal chromosome (trisomy 21), there is a remarkable increase over normal of acute leukemias, both myelocytic and lymphocytic. Radiologists and others exposed to radiation before significant protective measures were in use showed a tenfold increase in death from leukemia. Leukemia is increasingly apparent in persons treated with vigorous chemotherapy and immunosuppressive therapy for other disorders. None of these observations, put in the light of our ignorance of the etiologies of cancer in general, is overwhelming, but the data from observations on the incidence and transmission of leukemia in animals are more provocative.

Leukemias in such diverse species as chicken, mouse, cat, cow, monkey, and gibbon, are caused by RNA virus infection. Mice may transmit the virus vertically, that is, both parent and offspring may have leukemia, and, in some inbred strains, virtually every mouse develops leukemia. Whereas horizontal transmission, that is, passage from animal to animal, has been proved in several cases, this is not yet true for man. Although clusters of leukemia cases are reported in man, there are no clear-cut data to suggest either that leukemia is caused by a virus or that it is contagious.

We may divide the leukemias first into those types designated by the cell of origin.

Thus there are leukemias that are acute and chronic involving granulocytic (granulocytes) or myelocytic (immature white blood cell) elements, and acute and chronic leukemias involving lymphocytes. The 4 general types we shall consider briefly are thus acute lymphocytic, chronic lymphocytic, acute myelocytic, and chronic myelocytic leukemias.

Acute Leukemias

The clinical pattern of the **acute leukemias** differs somewhat from that of the chronic leukemias. The most common catastrophic indication of acute leukemia is an episode of hemorrhage in an otherwise normal child. Nose bleeds, bleeding from the gums, easy bruisability, and bleeding into the skin or gastrointestinal hemorrhage are common presenting findings. Failure to recover from an otherwise minor infection of the respiratory tract, urinary tract, or sinuses may be another prodromal episode, while the appearance of enlarged lymph nodes or splenomegaly are telltale signs of these blood dyscrasias. The crucial laboratory finding of blast cells on peripheral smear and an elevated white blood cell count confirm the clinical suspicion.

Acute leukemias, as the name implies, run a brief and hectic course. Persons so diagnosed seldom survive a year without treatment. Modern treatments, however, have altered this prognosis in many instances. The distinction between different subsets of acute myelocytic leukemia is beyond the scope of this book, but we should differentiate the acute myelocytic types from the acute lymphocytic leukemias, because the treatment and prognosis are different.

Acute myelocytic leukemia occurs in the Western world at a constant rate from birth to age 55, fluctuating slightly between 10 and 15 cases per million. After 55, this disease rises slightly in frequency. In contrast, **acute lymphocytic leukemia** has an incidence of 50 per million between the ages of 2 and 4 years. This rate halves in the next 4 years, and halves again to 10 per million until age 65, when it rises once more to about 15 per million. This pattern suggests an infectious etiology with the greatest susceptibility in early years, compared with patterns for acute myelocytic leukemia that could be interpreted as supporting a cumulative risk. The important fact is that over 85% of children with acute leukemia have the lymphocytic type, whereas over 80% of adults with acute leukemia have the myelocytic variety.

Fortunately, modern therapies offer the possibility of cure for acute lymphocytic leukemia with the use of vincristine and prednisone, and 85% of patients have remissions. The schedules of treatment are changing quickly, and it is hoped that successful management may change the outlook from this disease's grim pattern in the recent past.

Chronic Myelocytic Leukemia (Granulocytic, Myeloid, Myelogenous)

This variant of leukemia is rare below the age of 20 and accounts for about one-fifth of all leukemias in North America. It becomes more common to about the age of 60 and occurs at the rate of about 15 cases per million. The classic chief complaint may consist of such nonspecific symptoms as anorexia and weight loss with easy fatigability. Occasionally, an incidental blood count may turn up the diagnosis by revealing counts as high as 500,000 cells per mm^3. On physical examination, there may be a significantly enlarged spleen. The largest spleens in any disease occur in chronic myelocytic leukemia; it is not rare to find a spleen weighing 5 kilograms, and infarcts in these enlarged spleens may be the patient's original complaint (pain in the left flank) which alerts the physician to the diagnosis.

The etiology of chronic myelocytic leukemia is unknown, but 2 relationships are apparent. One is to known carcinogens such as ionizing radiation and benzene, and the other is to the presence of an abnormal chromosome. Eighty to 90% of patients with chronic myelocytic leukemia show an abnormality designated as a Philadelphia chromosome, which is a deletion of a long arm from chromosome number 22. This deletion is usually translocated to chromosome 9 rather than being lost. Patients with chronic myelocytic leukemia usually enter a phase called blast crisis, which is indistinguishable from acute leukemia.

During the chronic stage, anemia is the principal finding, and in remission, patients may be asymptomatic. One complication of this disease is the elevated uric acid and elevated uric acid excretion, which reflects the turnover of nucleic acids from the greatly increased number of white blood cells that are dying. With treatment and destruction of huge numbers of white blood cells, these uric acid levels may skyrocket, occasionally leading to uric acid precipitates in the tubules of the kidney and complete renal shutdown. One can anticipate a median survival of 3 years, with a range from 1 to 10 years. Paradoxically, this specific leukemia responds well to modern therapeutic regimens, but the survival time has not changed significantly in 50 years. The discovery that normal cells can repopulate the bone marrow and can replace the cells that possess the Philadelphia chromosome offers hope that newer methods of treatment may change these statistics.

Chronic Lymphocytic Leukemia (Chronic Lymphatic Leukemia)

This type of leukemia, characterized by the appearance of small lymphocytes in the peripheral blood, lymph nodes, and bone marrow, is compatible with a much better survival rate (median survival 6 years), and many cases live much longer, sometimes a quarter of a century. Often it is only the laboratory diagnosis that reveals the presence of this tumor in a patient who is receiving a routine examination for some other reason. Vague or nonspecific symptoms are typical, and sometimes enlarged lymph nodes or spleen suggest the diagnosis. Chronic lymphocytic leukemia accounts for 30% of leukemias and is unusual below age 45, but is nearly twice as common in men. There is no epidemiologic or other evidence to incriminate any of the agents we have mentioned earlier in the etiology of chronic lymphocytic leukemia. Ionizing radiation, carcinogens, and oncogenic viruses have not been shown to play any role in this disorder.

One might regard chronic lymphocytic

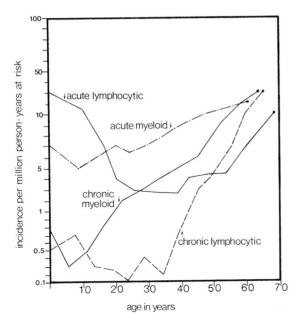

Fig. 23–9. This graph shows the frequency of the incidence of different types of leukemia in different age groups in cases per million person years. Acute lymphocytic leukemia has 2 peaks, 1 before the age of 20 and 1 after the age of 60. The incidence of chronic lymphocytic leukemia and of chronic myeloid leukemia both rise gradually toward the end of life. (From Upton, A.C.: Comparative aspects of carcinogenesis in ionizing radiation. Natl. Cancer Inst. Monogr., *14*:221, 1964.)

leukemia as the leukemic form of a well-differentiated lymphocytic lymphoma. Histologically, lymph nodes from patients with abnormal peripheral blood counts and smears cannot be distinguished from lymph nodes of lymphocytic lymphoma patients who have no peripheral blood abnormalities. Other organs, such as the liver and spleen, may be infiltrated, but massive splenomegaly is not characteristic. Immunologic abnormalities are a routine part of these disorders, and hypogammaglobulinemia is typical. This condition predisposes the patient to infections, which are a common and often terminal complication of chronic lymphocytic leukemia. Modern treatment is aimed at reducing the large numbers of lymphocytes. These 4 entities are compared in Figure 23–9.

Agranulocytosis

As the name suggests, this is a remarkable disappearance of the granulocytic series of leukocytes from the blood, with an accompanying drop in the total white cell count. The association of leukopenia with gangrenous lesions of the mouth is known as agranulocytic angina, the word "angina" in this sense meaning an acute inflammation of the throat.

Two groups of cases can be distinguished: (1) those occurring in persons who have been taking too much of some of the pain-killing drugs, particularly amidopyrine and the barbiturate series, i.e., chemicals containing the benzene ring; (2) cases in which no obvious cause can be discovered, although many industrial and household agents have been incriminated. The 2 factors, diminished leukocyte count and severe mouth infections, probably assist each other.

The disease often begins with the extraction of teeth. It is marked by fever, increasing weakness and fatigue, and sore throat. There may be extensive destruction of the gums and even the jaw, so that the teeth may fall out. Unfortunately, the victim, on account of the pain of the mouth lesions, may continue to take even larger doses of the drug. Such cases cannot fail to go on to a fatal termination, as the leukocytes fall to the vanishing point.

It is important to discontinue the use of any drugs that the patient may have been taking. The use of antibiotics has prevented the occurrence of serious infections in these cases, so that the patient's bone marrow will have a better chance of recovery from the damage done by the toxic drug.

DISORDERS OF THE LYMPH NODES AND RETICULOENDOTHELIAL SYSTEM

Lymphadenopathy or enlargement of a single lymph node or a localized group of nodes, such as along the side of the neck or in the armpit, is a frequent occurrence. Anyone with an infected tooth or a sore throat must have had the occasion to feel a mass where normally it was difficult to palpate any nodules. The causes of local or generalized lymphadenopathy form the final section of this chapter. A consideration of the normal structure and function of the lymphatic system has been outlined in Chapter 6, on the immune system. This section will go on to consider 1 or 2 inflammatory causes of lymphadenopathy, and will then offer a consideration of tumors of the lymphoreticular system, such as Hodgkin's lymphoma and lymphocytic lymphomas. We have considered Burkitt's lymphoma elsewhere, and the rarer diseases such as eosinophilic granuloma need not concern us in this text.

Infectious Mononucleosis

This is a self-limited disease of the lymphoreticular system characterized by sore throat, fever, swollen lymph nodes, generalized lassitude, and, sometimes, enlargement of the spleen. The diagnosis is established by examination of the peripheral blood smear, the demonstration of atypical lymphocytes, and the laboratory demonstration of heterophile antibodies (serum that will clump together sheep's red blood cells in high dilution). This last is the Paul-Bunnell test. The total white blood count may be elevated and the percentage of lymphocytes or mononuclear cells may be increased over normal. The absence of anemia and a normal platelet count are valuable suggestions that the lymph node enlargement is not due to leukemic infiltrate or malignant lymphoma.

Infectious mononucleosis is common among high school and college-age students; its incidence in the United States is more than 1,000 cases per 100,000 students per school year, indicating that one has a 1:100 chance of

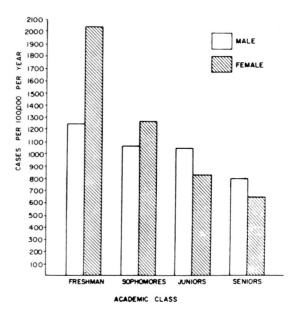

Fig. 23–10. Infectious mononucleosis attack rates, by sex and academic class, at 14 colleges, academic year 1969 to 1970. (From Brodsky, A.L., and Heath, C.W.: Infectious mononucleosis: epidemiologic patterns at United States colleges and universities. Am. J. Epidemiol., 96:87, 1972.)

acquiring the disease. Figure 23–10 shows the attack rate by sex and academic class at 14 colleges, and Table 23–8 shows the incidence of infectious mononucleosis during the 1969 to 1970 school year in these colleges.

Although it may be debated whether the Epstein-Barr virus is the causative agent of infectious mononucleosis, or whether it is merely associated with the disease, there is

Table 23–8.   Incidence of Infectious Mononucleosis at 7 Colleges and Universities by Race During the Academic Year 1969 to 1970

| SCHOOL | NUMBER OF CASES | | | UNDERGRADUATE POPULATION | | RATES/100,000/ SCHOOL YEAR | |
	WHITE	NONWHITE	UNKNOWN	WHITE	NONWHITE	WHITE	NONWHITE
Alaska	9			1,288	214	699	
Bryn Mawr	5	1		689	54	726	1,852
Emory	48		2	2,275	46	2,110	
Harvard	103	3	1	5,642	370	1,826	811
Oklahoma State	151	3		14,660	291	1,030	1,031
Purdue	248	3		14,612	4,404	1,697	68
Yale	67		7	4,295	195	1,257	
Total	631	10	10	43,461	5,574	1,452	179

(From Brodsky, A. L., and Heath, C. W.: Infectious mononucleosis: epidemiologic patterns at United States colleges and universities. Am. J. Epidemiol., 96:87, 1972.)

epidemiologic data from West Point, among other places, suggesting that infectious mononucleosis occurs with increased social contact, and in fact may be spread by intimate contact. It has been called the "kissing disease." Interestingly, spread among roommates seems infrequent, and implies that infectious mononucleosis patients need not be isolated as are hepatitis patients.

There is a further association that has come to light recently, relating infectious mononucleosis to acute leukemia, but the few cases reported to date are insufficient to establish any pattern. However, infection with the Epstein-Barr virus does suppress the immune response and suggests that the subsequent appearance of any lymphoproliferative disorder may be related to this phenomenon.

Sarcoidosis

It is difficult to know where the subject of sarcoidosis should best be discussed. It was first described more than 100 years ago, and yet we are still completely ignorant of its cause. The microscopic lesions are granulomatous in character, closely resembling those of tuberculosis, yet the nature of the condition remains obscure. The disease is endemic in regions of pine forests, such as the Scandinavian countries and the New England region of the United States, so that it has been suggested that pine pollen may be at least 1 etiologic agent that can excite the reaction characteristic of sarcoidosis.

The lesions are remarkable for the diversity of their distribution, the chief tissues involved being the lymph nodes, both superficial and deep, but the skin, spleen, liver, lungs, and many other organs may be affected. The disease lasts for months or years, with a tendency to fibrosis and healing. Usually there is an astonishing absence of symptoms. The microscopic appearance is that of circumscribed masses resembling miliary tubercles, and easily mistaken for these lesions.

Malignant Lymphomas

These are neoplasms of the lymphoreticular system. By lymphoreticular system we mean the lymph nodes, spleen, and their supporting structures. The idea of a lymphoreticular system is anatomically and physiologically difficult to defend, but easy to accept conceptually if one is not too critical. The lymphocytes (B and T cells in differing stages of activation) are well enough defined. It is the reticuloendothelial system that we find difficult. This system includes the connective tissue framework of lymph nodes and spleen and the macrophages of these organs, and includes the Kupffer cells of the liver and macrophages elsewhere in the body. Neoplasms of this system have been classified into 2 general groups: those of lymphocytes and those of the other cells. Tumors of the "other cells" often show large cells that look different from lymphocytes and have been designated Reed, Sternberg-Reed, or Reed-Sternberg cells, after their discoverers, Dorothy Reed and Carl Sternberg. Tumors that show these cells in abundance have been lumped together frequently under the eponymic heading of Hodgkin's disease. We shall talk about its subdivisions later. The other group is paradoxically called the non-Hodgkin's lymphomas. They are tumors of small lymphocytes.

During the last 25 years, it has become clear that our thoughts on the neoplasms of the lymphoreticular system were not only confused, but were usually primitive and often misleading. For example, it has become clear that some neoplasms may change in the same patient from a well-differentiated appearance (with a certain diagnostic term applied) to a much less well-differentiated appearance, with an entirely different prognosis, requiring a different diagnostic term in whatever nomenclature was used. This change usually also implied a different mode of therapy. Thus, in the old nosology, we used the term lymphosarcoma, whereas now we prefer to call such tumors lymphomas and to divide them into well-differentiated or poorly differentiated types, and to discuss whether they are lymphocytic, histiocytic, and T cell or B cell. The term reticulum cell sarcoma has largely been abandoned, but when it was used, it was applied to a histiocytic lymphoma.

A second and even more important change has come with the realization that the classifications of lymphoreticular disorders and our ways of thinking of them must be radically revised in light in our new knowledge of the structure and function of the lymphatic system. For example, 25 years ago, the distinctions between B and T lymphocytes had not been made, and the relationship between immunoglobulins and their cells of origin was just beginning to be uncovered.

One important recognition is that some of the large cells we observe with the light microscope are not histiocytes or macrophages, but are really activated lymphocytes. We now know that if lymphocytes are exposed to a particular plant-derived material (phytohemagglutinin), they become much larger than normal and look like reticulum cells. If cells are exposed to certain viruses (e.g., simian virus 40), they may become giant cells. In addition, there is epidemiologic evidence to support the association of at least 1 virus (Epstein-Barr) with 1 lymphoma (Burkitt's) (Fig. 23–11). This suggests that we could classify lymphomas on the basis of their cell of origin, and that it may be difficult to ascribe the tumor appropriately without some measure other than the appearance of the cells.

We shall consider here the 2 general problems of Hodgkin's disease and lymphocytic lymphomas (non-Hodgkin's lymphomas).

Hodgkin's Disease

This disease of unknown etiology is usually classified with disorders of the reticuloendothelial system. It frequently appears in young adults (20 to 40 years). In the Western world, there are an estimated 35 cases per million for white males and 25 cases per million for white females, with an annual death rate of 23 and 13 per million, respectively, although we may expect these figures to decrease, since new methods of treatment are having significant success. The disease has 2 incidence peaks, 1 between ages 15 and 34, and the other after age 50.

The disease announces its presence as a nonspecific malaise characterized by fever, anorexia, and enlargement of lymph nodes and, sometimes, the spleen and the liver (Fig. 23–12). Itching of the skin and bone pain following the intake of alcohol may be clinical clues to the correct diagnosis, which is established by histologic examination of the firm, rubbery lymph nodes. Sometimes, these lymph nodes are seen only on x-ray film of the mediastinum or are discovered at laparotomy in the abdomen, along the aortic chain.

The diagnostic features of Hodgkin's disease underline the controversies as to its etiology and classification. In the past, the

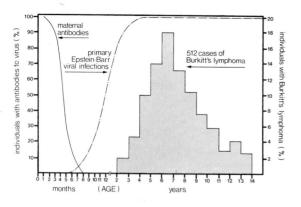

Fig. 23–11. This chart shows the relationship between the presence of maternal antibodies and infection with Epstein-Barr virus. The cases of Burkitt's lymphoma are shown in the bar graph. This indicates the latency between the primary infection and suggests a relationship between the Burkitt's lymphoma and previous Epstein-Barr infections. (From Henle, W., et al.: The Epstein-Barr virus. Sci. Am., *241*:48, 1979.)

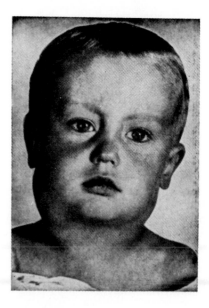

Fig. 23–12. Hodgkin's disease, showing enlarged glands in the neck.

disease was thought to be of infectious etiology because of the inflammatory cells that are present, of allergic nature because of the large numbers of eosinophils that are present, and as a neoplasm because of the bizarre cells and the relentlessly progressive course it used to run. Typically, a lymph node may show replacement of the germinal centers, usually full of lymphocytes, by a population of large pleomorphic cells. A large cell with a lobated nucleus, and sometimes 2 nuclei, has frequently been found among these pleomorphic cells. Although the cell is not pathognomonic of Hodgkin's disease, one always looks for it. Additionally, the lymph nodes may show areas of fibrosis and abundant eosinophils. In other cases, there may be bizarre cells with an absence of lymphocytes. The histologic appearance of this disease has been well correlated with the prognosis, which used to be uniformly poor. In earlier times, a few patients with Hodgkin's disease survived a decade; despite exacerbations and remissions, the disease was regarded as fatal.

Because of the marked difference in clinical behavior and in the histologic pattern of different cases of Hodgkin's disease, it was recognized long ago that these might be important distinctions for the management of the

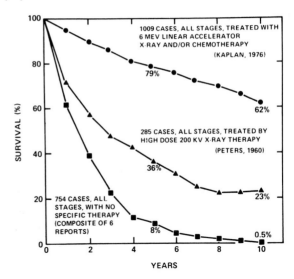

Fig. 23–13. These graphs show the survival of patients with Hodgkin's disease of all stages in 3 different therapeutic eras. The 62% ten-year survival of 1,009 cases treated with the linear accelerator x ray and/or drug therapy can be compared with 754 cases treated with no specific therapy. (From Kaplan, H.S.: Hodgkin's disease: multidisciplinary contributions to the conquest of a neoplasm. Radiology, *123*:551, 1978.)

disease. The more serious the disease, the greater the risks we are often willing to take to cure it. Fifty years ago, Hodgkin's cases were separated into 2 major categories, those called granuloma and paragranuloma, and those

Table 23–9. Histopathologic Classification of Hodgkin's Disease

TYPE	FEATURE	RELATIVE PROGNOSIS
Lymphocyte predominance	Abundant lymphocytic stroma; sparse Sternberg-Reed (S-R) cells	Most favorable
Nodular sclerosis	Nodules of lymphoid tissue of varying size, separated by bands of collagen and containing "lacunar" cell variants of S-R cells	Favorable
Mixed cellularity	More numerous S-R cells in pleomorphic stroma rich in eosinophils, plasma cells, fibroblasts, and lymphocytes	Guarded
Lymphocyte depletion	Paucity of lymphocytes; diffuse, irregular fibrosis in some instances; bizarre, anaplastic S-R cells usually numerous	Least favorable

Table 23–10. Staging of Hodgkin's Disease

Stage 0	No detectable disease.
Stage I	Disease limited to 1 anatomic region, or 2 contiguous regions on 1 side of the diaphragm (single lymph node or group).
Stage II	Disease in more than 2 anatomic regions, or in 2 noncontiguous regions on the same side of the diaphragm.
Stage III	Disease on both sides of the diaphragm, not involving more than the lymph nodes and spleen.
Stage IV	Involvement of any tissue or organ other than lymph nodes or spleen (e.g., bone, GI tract, lungs).
A:	Indicates the absence of generalized symptoms
B:	Indicates the presence of generalized symptoms such as fever, pruritus, bone pain.

designated unequivocal neoplasms. which were called sarcomas. Today, there is another characteristic, shown in Table 23–9 with the relative frequency and contemporary survival rates. These factors have changed markedly since the introduction of radiotherapy, chemotherapy, and staging (Fig. 23–13) (Table 23–10).

Non-Hodgkin's Lymphomas

As seen by the heading of this section, these neoplasms may be an assortment. However, they have in common their origin in cells of the immune system. They are not rare; an estimated 15,000 new cases were diagnosed in 1977 in the United States; this represents 2% of all cancer diagnoses in that country. They may occur at all ages and in both sexes; their etiology is not known. However, patients with genetic or acquired disorders of immune deficiency are clearly predisposed to these malignant neoplasms, and such patients include those who receive long-term immunosuppressive treatment for kidney grafts.

Contemporary classification of these neoplasms has arisen from the attempts by Rappaport and by Lukes to provide a clinically relevant approach based largely on the morphology of the tissue. This in turn depends on the characteristics of the cell population and the histologic pattern of the lymph nodes. It is common for most cases to be reviewed by more than 1 consultant, in attempts to standardize and maintain a constant diagnostic attitude to these often difficult-to-diagnose diseases. The histologic pattern is usually either nodular or diffuse; the diffuse pattern carries with it a poorer prognosis in general. The 4 general classifications of these lymphomas are outlined as follows:

Well-differentiated lymphomas appear most commonly after the fifth decade and are slowly progressive. The neoplasm is best viewed as the tissue component of chronic lymphocytic leukemia, and its histologic pattern is identical, being a diffuse infiltration of homogenous, small, well-differentiated lymphocytes. The patient's bone marrow is usu-

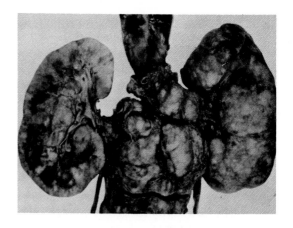

Fig. 23–14. Lymphoma. Great enlargement of lymph nodes along abdominal aorta with involvement of both kidneys.

ally involved by tumor, and the serum may show a single peak of abnormal gamma globulin. This disorder is currently regarded as a neoplasm of lymphocytes.

The clinical manifestations of this and other lymphomas are the presence of 1 or more enlarged lymph nodes, which may have been noticed for some time (Fig. 23–14). Fever and weight loss are not necessarily a prominent part of the pattern, but their presence alone may herald the development of these neoplasms. Involvement of the spleen, liver, and gastrointestinal tract (either stomach or small bowel) may cause the chief complaint. A high index of suspicion and a willingness to keep these tumors in mind in the differential diagnosis is often the only way a biopsy can be done early in the search for the cause of the general malaise in a given patient. Staging procedures, such as those used for Hodgkin's disease, have been useful in some cases, but in others their significance is debated. Chemotherapy and radiation therapy are currently effective; however, documented changes in survival rates are not yet available, as they have been for Hodgkin's disease.

Lymphocytic lymphoma, poorly differentiated, arises primarily in the lymph nodes and shows a considerable variation histologically, hence its name. This disease may be nodular or diffuse in adults. It carries a poorer prognosis than the well-differentiated type, and rarely progresses to frank leukemia in adults.

Histiocytic lymphoma used to be called reticulum cell sarcoma, because the cells were large and resembled reticulum cells rather than small lymphocytes. The cells are currently thought to be activated lymphocytes rather than macrophages by some, and are often difficult to distinguish from Reed-Sternberg cells, hence the difficulty in deciding whether the given case is Hodgkin's or non-Hodgkin's lymphoma. This disease occurs principally in adults and the older age groups and is first manifested by lymphadenopathy. There are 2 other types: a mixed histiocytic-lymphocytic type that usually resolves itself into histiocytic lymphoma, and an undifferentiated type that need not concern us here.

A complication of these lymphomas is anemia, as more than half the patients become severely anemic from involvement of their bone marrow, from hemorrhage, and from the response to therapy. Involvement of other systems, such as the meninges of the central nervous system and the liver, and occasionally organs adjacent to the lymphadenopathy (mediastinal structures), may be life-threatening because of mechanical interference, but infections, often of an unusual type such as fungal and viruses (herpes), frequently complicate the clinical course or cause death.

The short-term outlook for patients with non-Hodgkin's lymphomas has significantly improved during the last 10 years because of better use of various chemotherapeutic agents and radiotherapy, tools which have been used with much greater precision.

Multiple myeloma is a neoplasm of plasma cells and could be considered here. However, we discuss it in Chapter 25, to which the reader is referred.

SYNOPSIS

The common disorders of the hematopoietic system can be identified broadly as increased destruction, decreased production, or inherited disorders of the red blood cells (hereditary anemias) and proliferations of the white blood cells (leukemias). Less commonly, there are cases of increased production of red blood cells (polycythemias), or of decreased production of white blood cells and/or platelets (agranulocytosis, thrombocytopenia, aplastic anemia).

Laboratory examination (hematocrit, hemoglobin, red blood cell, white blood cell, and differential counts, and examination of the smear) generally reflects the function of the hematopoietic system.

Anemias may be regarded as due to inherited disorders, hemolytic disorders, as arising from increased blood loss (e.g., ulcers) or from decreased production (deficiencies of iron, folic acid, bone marrow depression). The symptoms are nonspecific; correct diagnosis depends on laboratory procedures.

Hemorrhagic disorders may have their origin in general depression of the bone marrow (leukemias, thrombocytopenia) or in disorders of clotting mechanisms (e.g., hepatic disease), and they may be inherited (hemophilia), acquired, or iatrogenic.

Leukemias can best be considered to be neoplasms of the white blood cell series, characterized by the presence of immature cells in the peripheral blood.

Diseases of lymph nodes and of the reticuloendothelial system commonly include inflammations, infections, and neoplasms (sarcomas). The origin and classification of tumors of the lymphoreticular system is controversial.

Terms

Erythrocytes
Normocytes
Reticulocytes
Hemoglobin
Hematocrit
Leukocytes
Myeloblasts
Megakaryocyte

Platelets
Hemolysis
Anemia
Polycythemia
Hemophilia
Purpura
Leukemia

Agranulocytosis
Leukopenia
Thrombocytopenia
Sarcoidosis
Infectious mononucleosis
Lymphoma
Hodgkin's disease

FURTHER READING

Editorial. Lymphokines: an increasing repertoire. Br. Med. J., *1*:62, 1978.

Adamson, J.W., et al.: Polycythemia vera: stem-cell and probable clonal origin of the disease. N. Engl. J. Med., *295*:913, 1976.

Bar, R.S., et al.: Fatal infectious mononucleosis in a family. N. Engl. J. Med., *290*:363, 1974.

Bodey, G.P.: Fungal infections complicating acute leukemia. J. Chronic Dis., *19*:667, 1966.

Bowman, J.M., and Chown, B.: Prevention of Rh immunization after massive Rh-positive transfusion. Can. Med. Assoc. J., *99*:385, 1968.

Brodsky, A.L., and Heath, C.W.: Infectious mononucleosis; epidemiologic patterns at United States colleges and universities. Am. J. Epidemiol., *96*:87, 1972.

Canadian Cooperative Study Group: A randomized trial of aspirin and sulfinpyrazone in threatened stroke. N. Engl. J. Med., *299*:53, 1978.

Carmel, R., and Johnson, C.S.: Racial patterns of pernicious anemia. N. Engl. J. Med., *298*:647, 1978.

Desforges, J.F., et al.: Hodgkin's disease. N. Engl. J. Med., *301*:1212, 1979.

Green, D.: General considerations of coagulation proteins. Ann. Clin. Lab. Sci., *8*:95, 1978.

Grufferman, S., et al.: Hodgkin's disease in siblings. N. Engl. J. Med., *296*:248, 1977.

Harker, L.A., and Slichter, S.J.: Platelet and fibrinogen consumption in man. N. Engl. J. Med., *287*:999, 1972.

Harris, J.W.: *The Red Cell*. Cambridge, Harvard University Press, 1970.

Herrick, J.B.: Sickle cell disease. Arch. Intern. Med., *6*:517, 1910.

Judson, H.: *The Eighth Day of Creation*. New York, Simon and Schuster, 1979.

Kaplan, H.S.: Hodgkin's disease: multidisciplinary contributions to the conquest of a neoplasm. (Erskine Memorial Lecture, 1976.) Radiology, *123*:551, 1977.

Klein, G.: The Epstein-Barr virus and neoplasia. N. Engl. J. Med., *293*:1353, 1975.

Lukes, R.J., and Butler, J.J.: The pathology and nomenclature of Hodgkin's disease. Cancer Res., *26*:1063, 1966.

Mann, R.B., Jaffer, E.S., and Berard, C.W.: Malignant lymphomas—A conceptual understanding of morphologic diversity: a review. Am. J. Pathol., *94*:105, 1979.

McIntyre, D.R.: Current concepts in cancer: multiple myeloma. N. Engl. J. Med., *301*:193, 1979.

Ratnoff, O.D., and Bennett, B.: The genetics of hereditary disorders of blood coagulation. Science, *179*:1291, 1973.

Reed, D.: On the pathologic changes in Hodgkin's disease with special reference to its relation to tuberculosis. Johns Hopkins Hosp. Rep., *10*:133, 1902.

Robboy, S.J., Colman, R.W., and Minna, J.D.: Pathology of disseminated intravascular coagulation (DIC). Hum. Pathol., *3*:327, 1972.

Suttie, J.W., and Jackson, C.M.: Prothrombin structure, activation, and biosynthesis. Physiol. Rev., *57*:1, 1977.

Wintrobe, M.M.: *Clinical Hematology*, 7th Ed. Philadelphia, Lea & Febiger, 1974.

Central Nervous System

24

The life unexamined is not worth living. —Osler

The nervous system may be arbitrarily divided into a central part, consisting of the brain and spinal cord, and a peripheral part, consisting of the nerves that carry motor messages from the brain and cord to the muscles and those that carry sensory messages from the skin and other parts of the body to the cord and brain. This chapter considers the central nervous system in the general context of those parts that are frequently involved by disease. For more details on the normal structure and function, and for information on the rarer diseases, the reader is referred to other sources.

STRUCTURE AND FUNCTION

The central nervous system altogether can best be considered as including: the skull and overlying skin, which are often subject to trauma; the coverings of the brain (the meninges), which often are involved by inflammation or hemorrhage; the blood supply to the brain (the arterial supply and venous drainage); the cerebrospinal fluid, which may be likened to the lymphatic circulation in the rest of the body; and the gray and white matter of the brain proper. Some disease processes are reflected particularly in one or another of these compartments, and it is wise to realize that each of these anatomic areas is subject to particular or peculiar diseases.

The brain proper consists of the cerebrum (right and left cerebral hemispheres), the brain stem, which connects the cerebrum with the spinal cord, and the cerebellum or little brain (Fig. 24–1). The cerebrum initiates motor impulses that pass to the muscles, receives sensory impulses from the periphery, and is the seat of thought and reason. The brain stem is composed of the midbrain, the pons, and the medulla, which is continued into the spinal cord. Through the brain stem pass the innumerable motor and sensory nerves; it also houses the groups of nerve cells from which arise the cranial nerves that pass to the eye, ear, face, and mouth. The cerebellum is concerned principally with coordination and with equilibrium, so that cerebellar disease is marked by incoordination and loss of equilibrium (ataxia).

The spinal cord is traversed by all the nerves going to and coming from the body. Those passing to the arm leave the cord in the upper or cervical region; those passing to the leg leave in the lower or lumbar region. The motor fibers from the brain terminate around nerve cells in the gray matter, which occupies the center of the cord, and from these motor cells a second set of fibers carries the motor messages to the muscles. The upper relay is called the upper motor neuron and is often injured in cerebral hemorrhage; the lower relay is called the lower motor neuron and is injured in poliomyelitis. Complete paralysis may be produced by destruction of either neuron, and by injury to the nerve cell or the nerve fiber that arises from it.

The central nervous system is composed of neurons and neuroglia (Figs. 24–2 and 24–3). **Neurons** are nerve cells, and nerve fibers that arise from them, which pass, sometimes for a long dis-

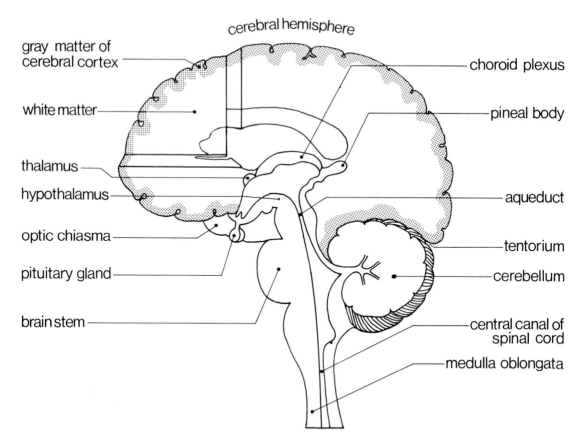

gray matter of cerebral cortex

white matter

thalamus

hypothalamus

optic chiasma

pituitary gland

brain stem

cerebral hemisphere

choroid plexus

pineal body

aqueduct

tentorium

cerebellum

central canal of spinal cord

medulla oblongata

Fig. 24–1. This schematic drawing illustrates the anatomic relationships of the various parts of the central nervous system. The cerebral hemisphere is partly removed to show gray and white matter; the adjacent ventricular space is shown. The cerebellum and brain stem and pituitary gland are all shown in proportional sizes. (Redrawn and adapted from Ham, A.W.: *Histology*, 7th Ed. Philadelphia and Toronto, J. B. Lippincott, 1974.)

tance, through the brain and spinal cord (Fig. 24–4). The motor nerve fibers (efferent) arise from nerve cells in the gray matter of the spinal cord and leave the cord by the anterior nerve roots to become the peripheral motor nerves. These nerve cells and their fibers are called lower motor neurons; they receive and respond to impulses coming from upper motor neurons (the motor cells in the brain and their descending fibers). Sensory impulses of various kinds are carried by the sensory nerve fibers (afferent), which enter the cord in the posterior nerve roots and pass up to appropriate centers in the brain. Here messages, on reaching our consciousness, give information concerning the outside world.

Nerve cells, of which there are some 10,000,000,000, have certain peculiarities that distinguish them from all other cells. Two of their most striking characteristics are their longevity and their great susceptibility to metabolic disturbances, most particularly loss of oxygen or glucose. Nerve cells can live for 100 years (compare this with

the short life of the polymorph), but they pay a heavy price for their relative immortality, because they cannot be replaced when they are destroyed. They have great metabolic activity, but on that account they require a constant, large supply of oxygen and glucose, so that the cells of the cerebral cortex cannot survive 10 minutes of anoxia at normal body temperature. A marked fall in blood sugar level also results in loss of consciousness.

Nerve fibers in the central nervous system consist of 2 elements: the axon, which conducts the nervous impulses, and the myelin sheath, which surrounds it (Fig. 24–5). In the peripheral nerves a nucleated sheath, the neurilemma, is added. The myelin sheath is made of many layers of insulation created by a special cell (Schwann's cell), which wraps itself around the axon. When a peripheral nerve is cut, the myelin breaks up into fine droplets, which eventually disappear as the material is phagocytosed (Fig. 24–6). This process is called demyelination and it is of particular significance in the central nervous system, where it constitutes the

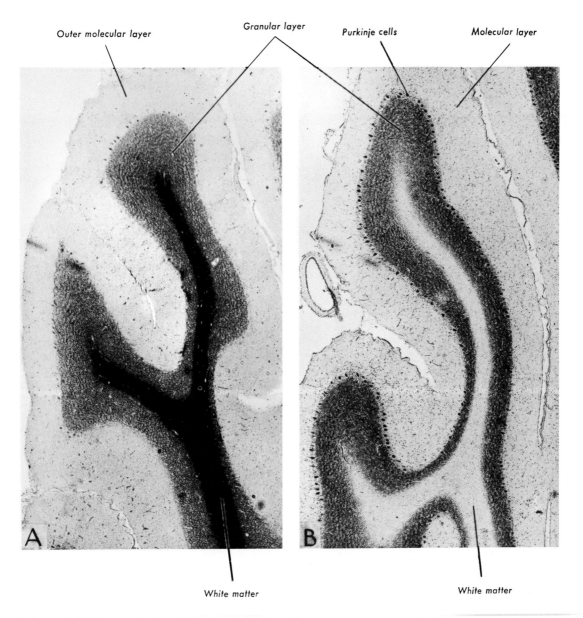

Outer molecular layer   Granular layer   Purkinje cells   Molecular layer

White matter   White matter

Fig. 24–2. *A and B,* The histologic section shows an area of the cerebellum prepared with two different stains. Neurons of the cerebellum are called Purkinje cells. (Courtesy of P. Bailey.)

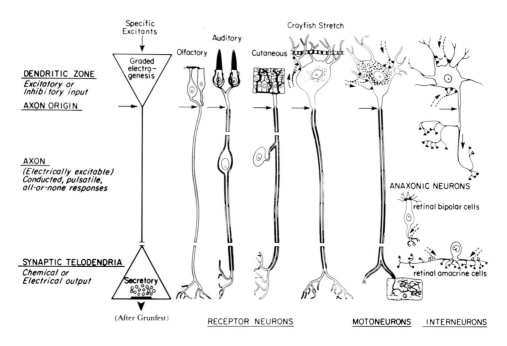

Fig. 24-3. The traditional selection of the mammalian motoneuron as the "typical neuron" has led to a misleading emphasis on the cell body as the focal point for analysis of neuron structure in functional terms—it being commonly assumed that dendrites must conduct toward and axons away from the cell body. The diagram presented here illustrates several variations in the position of the cell body in a number of receptor and effector neurons. A more important consideration in terms of function is the site of origin of the impulse. The location of the perikaryon in the neuron is not critical for the electrochemical functions of response generation, conduction, and synaptic transmission. The neuroplasm in the interior of the perikaryon is concerned primarily with the outgrowth and maintenance of the axon and dendrites and with metabolic functions other than membrane activity. (After D. Bodian.) (From Bloom, W., and Fawcett, D.W.: *A Textbook of Histology*, 9th Ed. Philadelphia, W. B. Saunders, 1968.)

principal feature of a group of so-called demyelinating diseases, of which multiple sclerosis is of special importance. When injury of this kind takes place, there is a response in the cell body of the neuron. This response can be seen with the light microscope and appears as a change in staining quality of the cytoplasm. The nucleus of this neuron may also be shifted to 1 side. This shift is called chromatolysis and is shown in Figure 24–7.

The nerve cells that send out motor impulses along nerve fibers and those that receive sensory impulses along corresponding fibers are situated in the gray matter of the brain, which is spread for the most part as a thin layer over the surface, to form the cerebral cortex. These cells are collected in groups known as centers or nuclei. The various centers are linked by bundles of fibers known as association fibers. In the performance of an action, many centers are associated, and when this is repeated many times, the nervous impulse appears to flow along the corresponding association paths with increasing ease. Some such mechanism may form the physical basis of habit. Every act, indeed every thought, serves to make these paths more

open and easily traversed. Every smallest stroke of virtue or of vice leaves its little scar. Nothing we ever do, in strict scientific literalness, is wiped out, but the tracks that are left are invisible to our current technology.

The interstitial tissue of the central nervous system has long been known as the **neuroglia.** *Glia* means glue in Greek, and the neuroglia was regarded as a kind of putty that served the humble purpose of holding together the more noble neurons. With ordinary stains, the interstitial elements appear for the most part as naked nuclei, but with gold and silver impregnation, the cells are seen to be provided with a forest of fibers. By the aid of these methods, it is possible to distinguish 3 types of cells in the interstitial tissue: (1) astroglia, (2) oligodendroglia, and (3) microglia.

The astrocytes, the cells of the astroglia, have peculiar processes called sucker feet, which are attached to the capillaries. For this reason, the astroglia is believed to be involved in the transport of water and electrolytes between the capillaries and the nerve cells. The repair of wounds in the brain is due entirely to the activity of the astrocytes, and

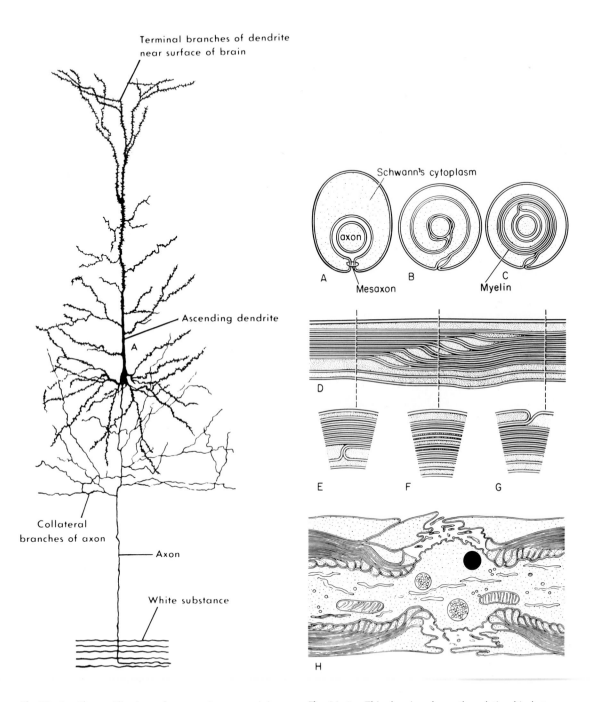

Terminal branches of dendrite
near surface of brain

Schwann's cytoplasm

axon

A

Mesaxon

B

C

Myelin

Ascending dendrite

A

D

E

F

G

Collateral
branches of axon

Axon

White substance

H

Fig. 24–4. The ramifications of a neuron's axon and dendrites are shown in this figure from a drawing done by the great Spanish neurocytologist, Cajal. (From Bloom, W., and Fawcett, D.W.: *A Textbook of Histology,* 9th Ed. Philadelphia, W. B. Saunders, 1968.)

Fig. 24–5. This drawing shows the relationship between the axon of the nerve and the Schwann's cell cytoplasm, which is wrapped about the axon and which constitutes myelin. (From Bloom, W., and Fawcett, D.W.: *A Textbook of Histology,* 9th Ed. Philadelphia, W. B. Saunders, 1968.)

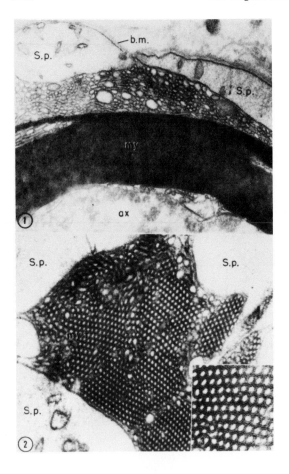

Fig. 24–6. This electron microphotograph shows the response of the myelin sheath to injury. This change is called Wallerian degeneration. The myelin sheath (my) which surrounds the nerve axon (ax) is the product of Schwann cell processes (s.p.), which have been wrapped around the axon as insulation. The outermost limit is the basement membrane (b.m.). After injury these lamellae of myelin break up into micelles of lipoprotein, as shown in the lower illustration. (From Thomas, P.K., and Sheldon, H.: Changes in the Fine Structure of Myelin During Wallerian Degeneration of Peripheral Nerve. J. Cell Biol., 22:715, 1964.)

come greatly swollen, their processes are withdrawn into the cell, and the cytoplasm is filled with droplets of disintegrating myelin, which they carry away and discharge into the nearest vessel.

The normal physiology of the brain may be altered by disease that affects principally the motor or sensory functions, or that affects intellect and behavior, or some combination of these. It is customary to speak of (1) "organic" disorders in which gross or microscopic lesions can be demonstrated, associated with interference with the supply of oxygen or carbohydrate to the brain or with abnormalities of cerebral enzyme activity, and of (2) "functional" disorders in which no such changes can be shown. It is becoming more and more probable that this distinction is due to inadequacy in our techniques for studying the brain. What in the past we have called mental disease and have stigmatized as insanity or madness is probably in most cases a biochemical disturbance of nerve cells that will be corrected in the future by pharmacologic means. Most of the popular tranquilizers act on the biochemical interactions between nerve cells.

Memory is the ability to receive a sensory impression, to retain it, and to recall it at the appropriate moment. Learning and memory are intertwined, and both may be lost because of disease and age.

This text is not an encyclopedia of disease, but it would be appropriate in the opinion of these writers to spend a few paragraphs on the serious problem of distinguishing diseases of the central nervous system for which we have reasonable explanations from those disorders of function for which the explanations are more difficult to determine.

It is important to recognize that disorders of function may range from gross disturbances such as coma to much more subtle derangements, which may be discovered only by careful neurologic assessment, by visual field testing, or by perceiving the changes in the personality over a long period. Mercifully, in many cases, the patient may be unaware of the changes that are occurring; disorders of the brain frequently provide their own anesthesia. However, for someone who is not a neurologist or psychiatrist, the most baffling problem may be to decide whether the impairment of function, such as a loss of recent memory, disorientation, lack of drive, difficulty in making decisions, impairment of judgment, and change in personality, is due to some treatable illness, or whether it is an irreversible disorder. In any case, the problem of how to manage the patient, who is

the gliosis seen in general paresis and other chronic inflammations of the brain consists of astrocytes and their fibers. Finally, it is from the astroglia that the glioma, the common brain tumor, takes its origin. The oligodendroglia is the largest group of the interstitial cells, but their function is still unknown, perhaps to the relief of the reader. The cells are smaller than the astrocytes, and they possess a small number of processes (Greek *oligos*, few). The microglial cells are tiny (hence the name) and are provided with numerous fine branching processes. These cells are the phagocytes or scavengers of the central nervous system, and, when called on to perform this function, they be-

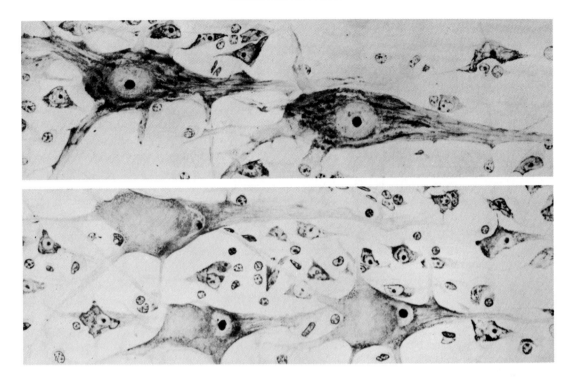

Fig. 24–7. Normal neurons in the upper drawing are to be compared with the lower drawing of neurons that show large pale areas rather than the stippled blue material known as the Nissl substance in the cytoplasm. This accumulation of eosinophilic material and shift of the nucleus to one side is called chromatolysis and is a morphologic sign of injury. (From Bloom, W. and Fawcett, D.W.: *A Textbook of Histology*, 9th Ed. Philadelphia, W. B. Saunders, 1968.)

often elderly, is difficult because depression, for example, may have a radically different prognosis and treatment from senile dementia. To clarify this area, it is worthwhile enumerating a few of the classic, organic brain syndromes and saying a word or so about each (Table 24–1).

For practical purposes, the term **neuroses** can be defined as including all those mental disorders that have no demonstrable organic basis, and in which the patient may have considerable insight and unimpaired reality testing. He does not usually confuse his morbid, subjective experiences and fantasies with ex-

Table 24–1. Simplified Classification of Mental Disorders

ORGANIC BRAIN SYNDROMES	FUNCTIONAL DISORDERS
Cerebral arterial sclerosis	Psychoses
Alzheimer's disease	Schizophrenia
Korsakoff's psychosis	Manic-depressive psychosis
Wernicke's psychosis	Neuroses
Senile dementia	Anxiety
Delirium tremens	Depression
General paresis of the insane	Phobia
Toxic psychoses from	Hysteria
Alcohol	Hypochondriasis
Drugs	Personality disorders
Heavy metals	
Slow virus diseases	
Kuru	

ternal realities. The patient's behavior may be greatly affected, although usually remaining within socially acceptable limits, but the personality is not disorganized. The principal manifestations of neuroses are excessive anxiety, hysterical symptoms, phobias, obsessional and compulsive symptoms, and depression. It is characteristic of many people that they may have episodes of decompensation, although they may have relatively adequate mental function. It is also characteristic that these persons respond inappropriately to stress. The age in which most neuroses are clinically apparent is between 25 and 45 years. There is no obvious difference between men and women, and over 80% of all patients with neuroses are both anxious and depressed.

Someone with a **psychosis** manifests a major disturbance of thinking, mood, and behavior to such a degree that he loses contact with reality. This interferes with the functions of sleeping and eating, with work habits, and with interpersonal relations. A neurosis, on the other hand, has been defined as "a benign episode of disordered mental function, with an exaggeration of the individual's personality."

A third category of functional disorder comprises those situations that have been called **personality disorders,** in which there is a long-term maladaptation of behavior that suggests an arrest or distortion of the development of personality. Such persons tend to blame others and seem to have little capacity for insight into reasons for their behavior. A final group of disorders without organic brain disease are those transient **situational disturbances,** e.g., a depressive reaction to grief. In concluding this rapid survey of functional disturbances, one might include those psychophysiologic disorders that at one time were called psychosomatic disorders, such as peptic ulcers, migraine, asthma, hypertension, and diseases such as ulcerative colitis, in which psychologic factors have been repeatedly seen to affect the patient.

A word or 2 may be devoted to schizophrenia in this discussion of the pathologic physiology of the brain, for it is a principal cause of chronic mental illness, and it is said to be responsible for more grave disability than any other illness in the whole of medicine. More than one-half of the beds for chronic disease in our hospitals are devoted to mental disorder, although the segregation of these beds in separate institutions conceals this fact from us. The frontier of the mind and its diseases remains one of the last to be pushed back in this day of incredible medical advances.

The word **schizophrenia** is derived from the Greek, meaning a divided mind, and it connotes a disconnection between thoughts and feelings on the one hand, and actions on the other. It manifests itself most often between the ages of 15 and 25 years (hence the older name of *dementia praecox*), first by a gradual social withdrawal, followed by the development of all sorts of bizarre hallucinations. It involves a fragmentation, a breaking-up, of all the processes of thought and feeling that enable a healthy person to remain in touch with the world; it might be regarded as a cancer of the mind, gnawing into the very soul of the patient. What interests us in the present discussion is that similar hallucinations can be induced in a normal person by means of the so-called hallucinogenic drugs, as a result of which the volunteer subject may experience marked distortions of reality. The significance of these observations is that they suggest that a chemical abnormality in a brain that is structurally normal may result in a condition of temporary insanity.

Evidence to support this hypothesis has recently accumulated from 2 sources. First, a small group of schizophrenics have been given hemodialysis which exchanges retained molecules that are not excreted normally. Hemodialysis is usually given to patients with renal failure. Through serendipity, a schizophrenic patient in renal failure was found to be markedly improved after hemodialysis, and attempts to repeat this observation in other patients have shown surprisingly good results. The implication of this discovery is that there may be a biochemical substance exchangeable by dialysis that directly affects the ordered functioning of the central nervous system. Second, biochemical studies on a group of schizophrenics have shown that the amount of serotonin present in platelets is significantly different from the platelet serotonin in normal persons.

With the drugs now available, many victims of mental illness need not be sent to mental hospitals. Psychotherapy in the shape of psychoanalysis has proved its great value, but we should not let this exclude therapy with the aid of chemical agents. In our consideration of mental disease, it would appear that we must bring back the soma as well as the psyche, just as we saw that in our study of physical disease we must not concentrate too much on the soma to the exclusion of the psyche.

SYMPTOMS OF DISORDERS OF THE CENTRAL NERVOUS SYSTEM

Disorders of consciousness, of perception, and of response are the signposts of pathology of the nervous system, and a vocabulary of considerable size has evolved to specify particular dysfunction. Since this is not a text for neurologic disorders, we shall limit the introduction of new terms and refer the reader to other sources.

Consciousness, the most obvious benefit of the nervous system, can be equated with responsiveness, and its pathologic alterations can be divided into several levels. **Lethargy** is a state of torpor or drowsiness that can have many causes, ranging from hypothyroidism and toxic states to an intracranial hemorrhage, which is simply pressing on the cerebral hemispheres. **Stupor** is a further step, in which the person is asleep, but can be aroused by appropriate stimuli, usually painful. However, he will return to the somnolent state after withdrawal of the stimulus. This state is an exaggeration of the previous level and suggests progression. More toxins, such as barbiturates, or increasing damage, such as extension of a hemorrhage or progression of an infection, are the classic causes of stupor. **Coma** is the state in which the patient is unresponsive except to the most painful stimuli, and in which the responses are limited to a reflex withdrawal. The higher cortical functions are absent in coma, which again may be due to trauma, metabolic disorders such as unmanaged diabetes mellitus, or toxic agents. **Convulsions** and seizures are another symptom of disorder in the central nervous system.

Brain death is the final and, currently, a most controversial level of damage to the central nervous system because of its legal, moral, and ethical implications. As we outlined earlier in this book, it is difficult to define death, and we have leaned heavily on the concept of irreversible change in cells and in tissues in earlier considerations, but most were directed at tissues and did not imply the death of the thinking being.

The Harvard criteria for defining irreversible coma or brain death include several points:

1. The inability to respond to or to perceive any type of stimuli indicating loss of the higher centers, the cortex, and the thalamus.
2. No spontaneous respiration or movement after 3 minutes off a respirator.
3. Absence of postural reflexes with fixed, dilated pupils and absence of swallowing, yawning, and vocalization.
4. Flat electroencephalogram for at least 10 minutes.
5. Repeat testing within 24 hours showing no change.
6. No evidence of hypothermia or of central nervous system depression.

To put these technical matters in another way, several states have enacted laws, one of which reads as follows: "A person will be considered dead if, in the announced opinion of a physician, based on ordinary standards of medicine in a community, there is the irreversible cessation of spontaneous respirations and circulatory functions. If artificial means of support preclude a determination that these functions have ceased, a person will be considered dead if, in the announced opinion of a physician based on ordinary standards of medical practice in the community, there is the irreversible cessation of spontaneous brain function."

We can now pass on to some other considerations.

The brain and spinal cord are enclosed in 2 bony cases that are continuous with each other, namely, the skull and the spinal column. They are therefore unable to expand when they become swollen with blood or as the result of inflammation, and the increased tension causes headache, that most common symptom. There is an ingenious mecha-

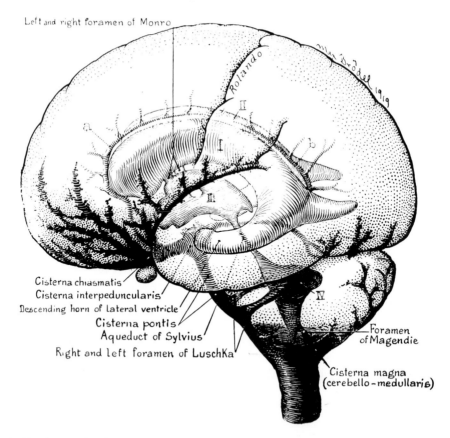

Left and right foramen of Monro

Rolando

Cisterna chiasmatis
Cisterna interpeduncularis
Descending horn of lateral ventricle
Cisterna pontis
Aqueduct of Sylvius
Right and left foramen of Luschka

Foramen of Magendie

Cisterna magna (cerebello-medullaris)

Fig. 24–8. In this schematic the relationship of the **ventricular system** to the central nervous system is shown in darker ink. This ventricular system receives fluid that is elaborated and circulated slowly from the different chambers and liberated onto the surface of the brain. The cerebrospinal fluid acts as a hydraulic cushion and also provides a second circulation similar to the lymphatic system.

nism that serves to take up some of the temporary increases of pressure that may occur inside the skull. This mechanism is the **cerebrospinal fluid,** which bathes the brain and in which the organ is suspended as in a water bath. This fluid not only covers the brain, but also passes down the spinal canal outside the spinal cord. There is far more spare space in the canal than in the cranial cavity, so that when the brain becomes swollen, the fluid flows out into the spinal canal, providing a much-needed safety valve. Cerebrospinal fluid is produced in a series of cavities in the interior of the brain known as the cerebral ventricles (Fig. 24–8).

From 1 of these (the fourth ventricle) it escapes by tiny openings in the roof of the ventricle to reach the exterior of the brain, the subarachnoid space, through the walls of which it is absorbed into the blood stream. The subarachnoid space with its contained fluid passes down outside the spinal cord to the third portion of the sacrum, whereas the cord ends at the level of the first lumbar vertebra; in its lowest portion, the sac contains only fluid. That is the site used to obtain samples of this fluid for

study. There is a constant flow out of the ventricles into the subarachnoid space. Should the openings in the roof of the fourth ventricle become blocked, the fluid accumulates and distends the ventricles, pressing the brain against the skull with serious results, a condition of hydrocephalus (Figs. 24–9 and 24–10).

The spinal fluid can be withdrawn by the simple procedure of lumbar puncture; a hollow needle is passed into the spinal canal between 2 contiguous vertebrae in the lumbar region, below the point where the spinal cord ends, and the fluid that escapes is collected. This procedure is a valuable means of diagnosis in diseases of the nervous system, for the fluid is a mirror in which are reflected many of the changes that may be affecting the brain and spinal cord (Table 24–2).

The changes that the cerebrospinal fluid undergoes in conditions of disease, and the diagnostic value of such changes as revealed by laboratory examination, will be better appreciated after these disease conditions have been discussed.

One structure still remains to be described, that

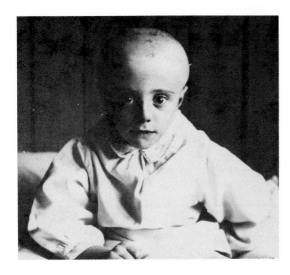

Fig. 24–9. This photograph shows a young child with **hydrocephalus** at the turn of the century. The increased girth of the skull is due to the increased accumulation of fluid within the ventricular system. Frequently, this is due to a blockage in the cerebrospinal fluid circulation, which does not absorb the fluid that is secreted and leads to the thinning and atrophy of the substance of the brain. (The Evans Collection, Osler Library, McGill University.)

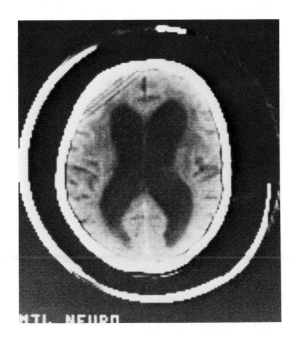

Fig. 24–10. This CT scan shows a remarkable increase in the size of the cerebral ventricles. This increase is typical of *hydrocephalus.*

is, the membrane or rather membranes that cover the brain and cord, just as the pleura covers the lungs and the peritoneum the abdominal organs. These membranes are known as the meninges, of which there are 3, the dura mater, the arachnoid mater, and the pia mater. The dura is a tough membrane that lies in the cranial cavity and the spinal canal. The pia clothes the brain and cord like a glove, and the arachnoid like a mitt; there is, therefore, a space between these membranes, and that space, known as the subarachnoid space, is occupied by the cerebrospinal fluid.

It may be of interest to know that dura mater is derived from the Latin *durus,* hard, and *mater,* mother, while *pia* means soft. To the ancients the meninges were the "mother" membranes. Hence Shakespeare's phrase, "nourished in the womb of pia mater." The ancients were not aware of the existence of the arachnoid, which means spider-like.

It is unwise to separate, for the purpose of this chapter, many varieties of disorders because the list becomes unnecessarily long. However, it is important to understand that some central nervous system disorders are developmental or congenital, that is, **childhood disorders.** Anencephaly, which is incompatible with life, and hydrocephalus, together with spina bifida and limb defects, can be listed here.

The most serious disorders may, however, be those in which the intellectual endowment is less than desirable, and attempts to catalog mental retardation are always controversial. A person with an IQ of less than 20 is usually referred to as an idiot, 20 to 50 an imbecile, 50 to 70 a moron, and over 70 but under 100 has many names. Other severe disabilities such as autism and major epilepsy, or inborn errors of metabolism that go unrecognized, cannot be discussed here.

VASCULAR DISEASE OF THE CENTRAL NERVOUS SYSTEM

For every 100 persons with any form of cerebrovascular disease, 40 will be permanently disabled and 10 will be institutionalized.

The most frequent diseases of the brain are the result of vascular disturbances. The word apoplexy comes from the Greek meaning a striking down, i.e., a seizure or stroke. It is an

Table 24–2.   Examination of Cerebrospinal Fluid

TESTS	NORMAL	BACTERIAL MENINGITIS	TUBERCULOUS MENINGITIS	VIRAL MENINGITIS	NEOPLASTIC MENINGITIS	PRIMARY CEREBRAL NEOPLASM
Microscopic examination	No cells	Many polymorpho-nuclear leukocytes early in course	Moderate increase in lymphocytes	Moderate increase in lymphocytes	Increased mononuclear leukocytes	Normal, or a few extra lymphocytes
Smear	No bacteria	Often bacteria are seen on gram stain	With prolonged search, acid-fast bacilli are often found	Negative	Malignant cells may be seen on cytology examination	Negative
Protein	15 to 45 mg/100 ml	Very high	Very high, may form "pellicle"	Elevated, usually not very high	Similar to tuberculosis	Normal or slightly high (very high with acoustic neuroma)
Glucose	About 20 mg less than blood	Very low	Moderately low	Normal or increased	Usually low	Normal
Chloride	120 mEq/L	Low	Very low	Normal	A little reduced	Normal

old term, for the condition was described by Hippocrates. To Galen it was "a sudden loss of feeling and of movement of the whole body, with the exception of respiration." The victim was believed to be struck down by some external force, as by the act of one of the gods. The word apoplexy is now seldom used in medical practice, rather the term stroke is used, particularly when the cause of the loss of sensation and motor function is not known. What are known as minor strokes, "little strokes" or "strokelets," are characterized by fleeting attacks of faintness, localized paralysis, aphasia (loss of speech), and visual disturbance. The attacks are so temporary that they are accompanied by no structural damage, and are apparently a manifestation of temporary cerebral anoxia, due to a combination of cardiac failure and cerebrovascular narrowing. They are spoken of as transient ischemic attacks, abbreviated as TIA.

A great change has taken place in our thinking regarding vascular disease in the central nervous system. The term "stroke" used to be synonymous with cerebral hemorrhage, and certainly a massive hemorrhage gives a classic picture. We realize, however, that the general term "stroke" cloaks our ignorance, and that the causes of loss of consciousness may be due to either ischemia (thrombosis) or hemorrhage. The term stroke is sometimes used interchangeably with "cerebrovascular accident," which hides an equal degree of ignorance. Ischemia most commonly is due to thrombosis, but it may also be due to embolism. The main arteries carrying blood to the cranial cavity are (1) the internal carotids in the neck, and (2) the vertebral arteries that arise from the subclavian at the root of the neck and pass upward in the vertebral canal. Revolutionary changes in the medical and surgical treatment of strokes demand accurate localization of the cause of the ischemia by means of cerebral angiography, using radiopaque material and radiographic technique.

The clinical picture of "cerebrovascular accident" varies within the widest limits. It may take the form of a violent assault, in which the patient collapses as if felled by an ax and is deprived of sense and motion. However, the most frequent type involves only a slight defect of speech, thought, motion, sensation, or vision; consciousness is not lost, and some degree of recovery is nearly invariable. It is obvious that the former type is likely to be caused by massive cerebral hemorrhage, the latter type by thrombosis. Ischemia is at least 4 times as common as hemorrhage, and carries with it a much graver prognosis.

Cerebral Hemorrhage. With advancing years, the arteries in the brain tend to narrow and become brittle (Fig. 24–11). If at the same time the blood pressure is raised, there is danger that one of the brittle arteries will burst. Even in the absence of hypertension, massive hemorrhage may occur in an area of softening produced by vascular occlusion. The effect will naturally depend on the site of the hemorrhage and also on the extent. The most common position is, unfortunately, that part of the brain where the motor nerves to the body are gathered together into a comparatively small space before passing down the spinal cord. Here, hemorrhage easily destroys these nerves, the motor impulses are cut off from the muscles, and the side of the body (face, arm, and leg) supplied by the side of the brain affected is paralyzed, a condition known as hemiplegia. Should the patient survive, the paralyzed arm and leg gradually become flexed and assume a characteristic appearance. As the motor nerves from 1 side of the brain cross to the opposite side before passing down the cord, it follows that hemorrhage on the right side of the brain will be followed by a left-sided hemiplegia, and vice versa. The speech center in right-handed persons is on the left side of the brain, so that hemorrhage on the left side will destroy the nerve fibers that go to the organs of speech, producing a condition of speechlessness or aphasia, in addition to a right-sided hemiplegia.

Cerebrovascular accidents seldom produce sudden or instantaneous death, because the part of the brain in which they most often occur contains no vital centers. "Sudden" death is nearly always due to sudden heart failure or to pulmonary embolism. But if the hemorrhage is large and close to the ventricles, it may rupture into those cavities in the course of a day or so, a complication that is sure to prove fatal (Fig. 24–12). On the other

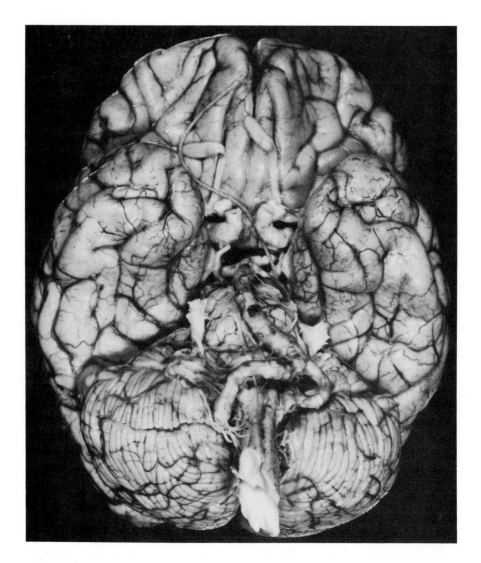

Fig. 24–11.   At the base of the brain the vertebral basilar arteries and internal carotids can all be seen to be markedly distorted by **atherosclerosis**. (McGill University, Department of Pathology Museum.)

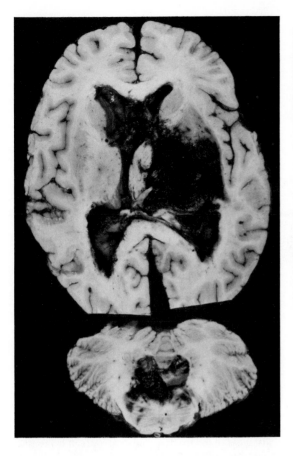

Fig. 24–12.   This section through the cerebral hemispheres of an adult brain shows **intracerebral and intraventricular hemorrhage** extending from the right lateral ventricle as far as the fourth ventricle (shown in the section through the cerebellum in the lower portion of the picture). Such a destructive hemorrhage will cause death, usually by compression of the brain stem due to the increase in intracerebral pressure. (McGill University, Department of Pathology Museum.)

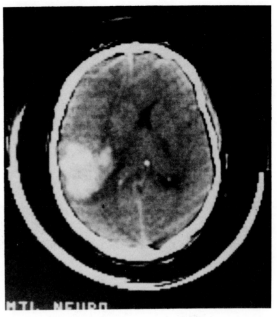

Fig. 24–13.   This CT scan shows the presence of a dense mass in the left cerebral hemisphere. Note that the pineal gland has shifted to the right, the ventricular system on the left is obscured, and the right ventricular system is moved to the right because of the space-occupying lesion.

hand, if the hemorrhage is small, the amount of damage to the brain is correspondingly limited, and only the arm or the leg may be affected. The blood is gradually absorbed, and the patient may make a good recovery, with only a slight disability in the affected limb. The signs of intracerebral hemorrhage—headache, vomiting, hemiparalysis, decreasing consciousness, and rapid respirations—are normally not preceded by warning signs, as in ischemic attacks. In 15 to 20% of patients who survive the first few days with no progression, attempts to prevent further loss of function may restore the patient to a useful life.

One might mention the difference between intracerebral (Fig. 24–13) and cerebellar hemorrhage, because the latter carries with it a vastly different prognosis, and strong indications for intervention are present in the case of any cerebellar hemorrhage.

Of course, there is always the danger of another hemorrhage later, a danger that hangs suspended over the patient's head like the sword of Damocles, but may never fall. The thought faculties are not necessarily interfered with. Pasteur did some of his best work after a small cerebrovascular accident.

Thrombosis. This is the most common cause of cerebral ischemia, comprising probably 50% of all cases. Atherosclerosis is the primary lesion; it causes narrowing of the lumen, the occluding thrombus being added at a late stage to produce ischemia. The main site of obstruction is not in the brain, but in the extracerebral vessels, often in extracranial vessels, more particularly the internal carotid in the neck and the vertebral artery. Diagnosis of occlusion, and in particular the exact site of the occlusion, can be established with certainty by cerebral angiography (Figs. 24–14

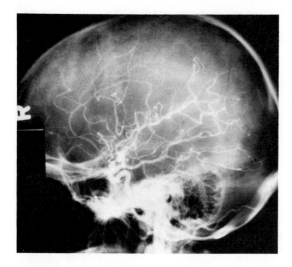

Fig. 24–14. This cerebral angiogram shows the lateral view of filling of the left carotid and its branches.

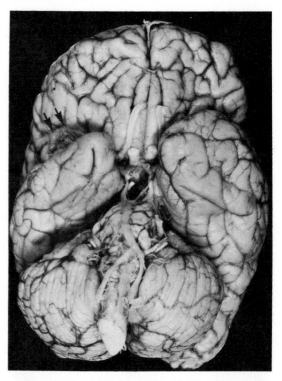

Fig. 24–16. This photograph shows (at arrows) the loss of substance of the right temporal lobe. Such **ischemic necrosis** and atrophy are common. They are symptomatic when functional areas of the brain are involved. (McGill University, Department of Pathology Museum.)

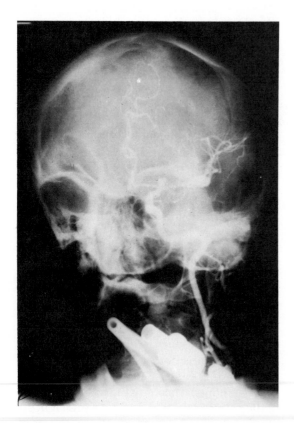

Fig. 24–15. This cerebral angiogram shows the anterior view of the distribution of the branches of the cerebral arterial tree.

and 24–15). Excision of the occluded segment of the artery and anastomosis or insertion of an arterial or synthetic graft may yield gratifying results in selected cases. This development would have been impossible to imagine only a few years ago. The lesions are infarcts followed by cerebral softening with eventual liquefaction or the formation of a cyst (Fig. 24–16).

The clinical picture varies with the site of the vessel occluded and with the size of the area of brain affected. It would be fruitless to give a detailed description here. Neurologic symptoms may take several days to develop. Compare this with the cerebral hemorrhage, in which the period is measured in minutes or at most in hours, or with cerebral embolism, in which the period is so short that it cannot be measured. There is a tendency for the occlusion to develop while the patient is asleep or within an hour of arising; a hemorrhage is likely to develop during waking hours of activity. The occlusion that is due to embolism may, of course, occur at any time.

Cerebral Embolism. The third cause of cerebrovascular accidents is embolism to the smaller cerebral vessels within the brain. The embolus most often arises from the left side of the heart, either from a vegetation on the mitral or aortic valve or from a thrombus in the appendix of the left atrium, or from a mural thrombus that has formed in the left ventricle at the site of a myocardial infarct. The embolus usually passes into the left carotid artery and is most likely to lodge in the middle cerebral artery. The accompanying paralysis may be extensive. Cerebral embolism is distinguished from other accidents by the extreme suddenness of the onset of symptoms, with complete development in 10 to 30 seconds and a total absence of warning.

Intracranial Hemorrhage

Hemorrhage is described in relation to the meninges, and may be extradural, subdural, or subarachnoid, or it may occur within the substance of the brain (see Fig. 24–17).

Extradural hemorrhage is a condition in which blood pours out between the skull and

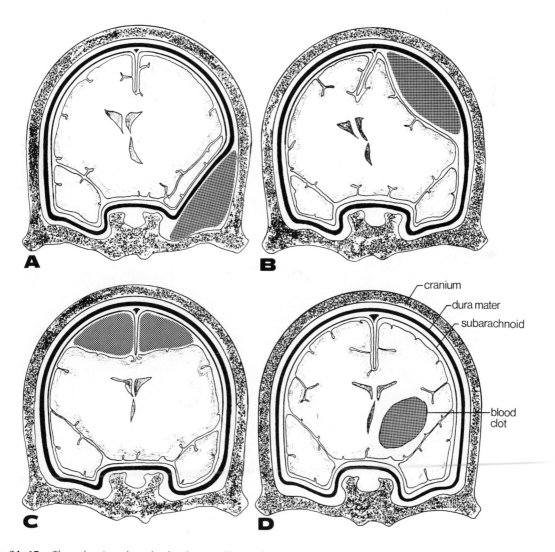

Fig. 24–17. These drawings show the distribution of hemorrhages into the various spaces of the brain. *A* shows an *extradural* hemorrhage. Note the presence of the skull and the displacement of the dura. *B* shows a *subdural* hematoma. Note the displacement of the brain substance. *C* shows a *subarachnoid* hemorrhage. *D* shows an *intracerebral* hemorrhage (From Gilbert, E.F., and Huntington, R.W.: *An Introduction to Pathology.* New York, Oxford University Press, 1978.)

the dura mater. It is commonly caused by bleeding from the middle meningeal artery. This artery lies in contact with the inside surface of the skull in the region of the temple, and is liable to be torn by a hairline fracture of the skull in this region. The condition is readily diagnosed because the patient is first stunned by a blow to the skull; he then recovers consciousness and appears to be all right for a few hours—this is known as the "lucid interval;" at the end of that time the patient becomes dull, drowsy, and finally loses consciousness again, owing to the increasing pressure of the blood that is accumulating between the skull and the brain outside the dura mater. The condition must be diagnosed, for by immediate operation the collection of blood can be removed, the bleeding vessel tied, and the life of the patient saved. There is no blood in the cerebrospinal fluid at lumbar puncture, because the thick dura mater intervenes between the bleeding vessel and the cerebrospinal fluid.

Subdural hemorrhage is most frequently venous in origin, not arterial, and in this respect it differs fundamentally from extradural and subarachnoid hemorrhage. The condition is much more common than extradural hemorrhage, and it is of great importance because the life of the patient depends on a correct diagnosis, which is easily missed. The cause is a blow in the frontal or occipital region (e.g., knocking the head against a shelf or door in the dark) that injures the cerebral veins passing into the subdural space. The blood clot so formed is converted into a kind of cyst, which may increase in volume. There is thus a continually increasing pressure on the underlying brain with the production of symptoms similar to those of a brain tumor. The confusing feature is that weeks may intervene between the relatively slight injury

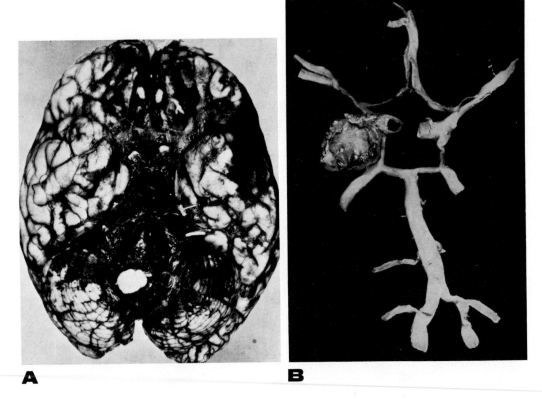

A   **B**

Fig. 24–18. *A,* This photograph of the base of the brain shows the staining of the surface of the inferior aspect of the cerebellum, brain stem, and the cerebral hemispheres by fresh blood. This is a **subarachnoid hemorrhage** which commonly results from the rupture of an aneurysm. (McGill University, Department of Pathology Museum.) *B,* Aneurysm of circle of Willis. The aneurysm, which is of unusually large size and still unruptured, arises from the internal carotid artery. The location adjacent to a bifurcation is characteristic. (University of Alabama Medical School.)

to the head and the development of cerebral symptoms, so that the injury may have been forgotten.

Intracranial hemorrhage of the newborn, a common cause of death, is a variety of subdural hemorrhage. The hemorrhage is due to injury during delivery that tears the cerebral veins crossing the subdural space to enter the longitudinal sinus. Death may occur in a few hours or in the course of a day or so. If the child survives, paralytic and other symptoms may develop later.

Subarachnoid hemorrhage is hemorrhage into the subarachnoid space between the arachnoid and the pia mater (Fig. 24–18A). Blood in large amount will be found in the cerebrospinal fluid at lumbar puncture. Such hemorrhage occurs when the surface of the brain is torn by a fracture of the skull, or it may be due to rupture of an aneurysm of an artery that lies beneath the arachnoid at the base of the brain (Fig. 24–18B). This condition, which is not uncommon in young people, was usually fatal in the past, but modern neurosurgery has made it possible to deal with the aneurysm and to arrest the hemorrhage. Perhaps it is well to note that hyperten-

sion is the most important common predisposing cause to hemorrhage in the central nervous system, regardless of its location.

Today, the availability of computer tomography (CT) (Fig. 24–19) for intracranial disease has made the diagnosis and management of vascular disease infinitely safer for the patient and easier for the neurologist and neurosurgeon.

Trauma

This subject may be considered in connection with cerebral hemorrhage, because the essential danger of this condition is laceration of the surface of the brain with accompanying hemorrhage. The fracture may involve the upper part of the skull, or vault, or the base of the skull. The latter is by far the more serious, and is apt to prove fatal, if not properly treated. The fracture itself is of little moment, although it may open into the ear or nose, causing bleeding from those organs. There is nearly always an accompanying laceration of the base of the brain, with rapidly developing edema of the structure. Some of the most important vital nerve centers essential for life, those for the heart and for respiration, are situated in this part of the brain, and the increasing pressure on these centers caused by the edema may prove fatal. At the same time, there is an accumulation of cerebrospinal fluid in this region that increases the pressure further. It is evident that the most urgent need is to reduce the pressure inside the skull before the vital centers become paralyzed, and this is done most rapidly and effectively by creating burr holes (trephining, just as the ancients used to do). Since this method of treatment has been introduced, the mortality in cases of fracture of the base of the skull has been greatly reduced.

INFECTIOUS DISEASE OF THE CENTRAL NERVOUS SYSTEM

Inflammatory disease in the central nervous system is generally due to infectious agents and, fortunately, is much less common today than in yesteryear. One may look on infectious diseases of the central nervous system as diffuse or localized, or classify them accord-

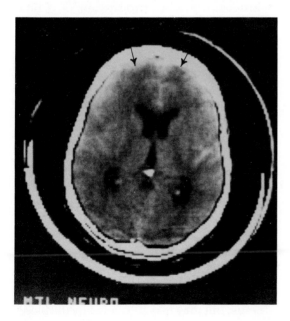

Fig. 24–19. This CT scan shows the presence of dense material over the surfaces of the frontal poles (arrows). This is interpreted as the CT scan appearance of a *subarachnoid hemorrhage*.

ing to their etiology (bacterial, fungal, viral, or protozoal). We shall consider local infection first, then meningeal disease, and, finally, viral and spirochetal infections.

Abscess of the Brain

The microorganisms that cause abscess of the brain may come from a focus of infection in the skull or may be carried by the blood stream from a distance, but by far the most common local source used to be the middle ear or mastoid sinus, which was so often the site of infection. Antibiotic therapy has now given us control of this condition. The infection spreads inward and causes abscess formation in the adjacent part of the brain. Another source of danger is infection in the frontal and other air sinuses that communicate with the nose. Here the abscess is likely to be in the frontal part of the brain. If the infecting organisms come from a distance, the most common source is an abscess or other septic process in the lung. Indeed, a danger of abscess of the lung is the formation of a secondary abscess in the brain. Figure 24–20 shows the CT scan image of multiple abscesses in the brain of a 50-year-old patient

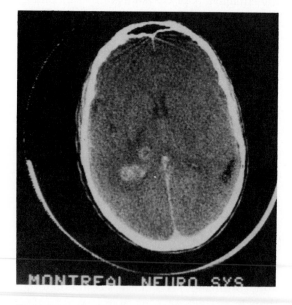

Fig. 24–20. This CT scan shows the appearance of 2 dense, small areas in the left posterior cerebral hemisphere. This is compatible with a diagnosis of *cerebral abscess*.

with bronchiectasis. The diagnosis was not made until too late for effective treatment.

Clinical Pattern. The symptoms of abscess of the brain are apt to be misleading. It might be imagined that a collection of pus in so delicate a piece of machinery as the brain would cause a violent disturbance, but the reverse is the case. Many parts of the brain are what are called silent areas, that is to say, a lesion of that part produces no characteristic symptoms, and this is particularly true of those parts in which an abscess is likely to occur. Moreover, the inflammation is usually of a quiet rather than a violent character. For these reasons, the abscess may give rise neither to "localizing symptoms" nor even to those indicating infection. Instead, the clinical picture will be that of gradually increasing intracranial pressure, which may suggest a tumor instead of an abscess. Suspicion, however, will be aroused by the coexistence of middle-ear and mastoid infection, inflammation in the frontal sinus, or lung abscess.

Remarkably good results may follow the drainage of a brain abscess, provided the operation is performed by a surgeon who knows what he or she is doing, but there is always danger of the infection's reaching the meninges, with the production of a fatal meningitis. This complication may now be avoided by the use of antibiotics.

Meningitis

We have already seen that the brain and spinal cord are covered by membranes or meninges, inflammation of which is called meningitis. Many organisms may cause meningitis, but the common ones are meningococcus, streptococcus, pneumococcus, and tubercle bacillus. The first 3 organisms are pyogenic or pus-forming bacteria, so that the diseases they produce are acute in type; the tubercle bacillus is less violent in action and more difficult to diagnose.

The streptococcus and pneumococcus reach the meninges from the middle ear or the frontal sinus, but they may be carried by the blood stream from distant parts, especially the lung. The meningococcus comes from the cavity of the nose or throat. Meningitis may assume an epidemic form, with many cases developing in a single locality or in many places throughout the country. Such epidemic meningitis is always due to the meningococcus. The infection is spread by carriers, who harbor the organisms in their throat, but who do not themselves develop infection of the meninges. The term cerebrospinal meningitis is often applied to the meningococcal type, but the other forms of the disease are also cerebrospinal, in the sense that the meninges of both the brain and the spinal cord are inflamed.

Tuberculous meningitis is in a class by itself. It has none of the acuteness of the other forms of meningitis and used to be the most uniformly fatal, with a mortality of 100%. The hopeless outlook has dramatically changed in recent years by the use of chemotherapy.

At autopsy, the subarachnoid space is filled with an acute inflammatory exudate in the meningococcal, streptococcal, and pneumococcal forms (Fig. 24–21), so that the brain and cord are covered with yellow pus. In tuberculous meningitis, however, there is only a thin, milky-white layer in which tubercles may be distinguished with difficulty.

Examination of the cerebrospinal fluid obtained by lumbar puncture usually establishes the diagnosis, including the type of bacterial infection. When normal cerebrospinal fluid is removed, it is as clear as water, and the pressure is so low that it flows out drop by drop. In meningitis, owing to the pyogenic bacteria, the fluid is turbid, because in reality it is thin pus. When the fluid is examined under the microscope, it is found to be crowded with polymorphonuclear leukocytes (pus cells) and to contain varying numbers of the bacteria responsible for the infection. In tuberculous meningitis, the spinal fluid is only slightly milky or may be almost clear, for as the inflammation is less acute, the cells are much fewer in number and are for the most part lymphocytes. The level of protein is

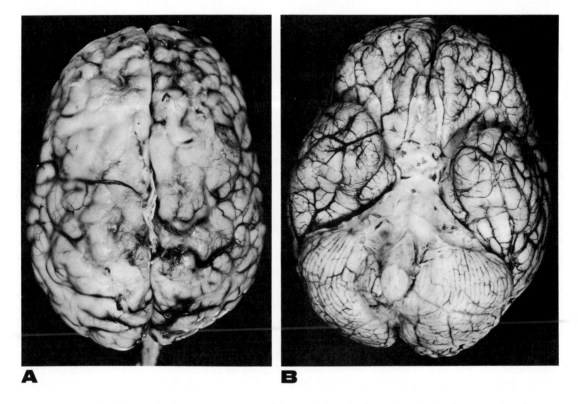

A   **B**

Fig. 24–21. *A,* This photograph of the superior aspect of the cerebral hemispheres of the brain of a young child shows the purulent exudate that is typical of **purulent meningitis**, caused by a variety of bacteria. This pus may occlude the circulation of the cerebrospinal fluid and lead to hydrocephalus. (McGill University, Department of Pathology Museum.) *B,* This photograph of the inferior aspect of the brain shows the disposition of an inflammatory exudate around the brain stem, pons, and cerebellum that is typical of **tuberculous meningitis.** (McGill University, Department of Pathology Museum.)

increased, the sugar level is decreased and sometimes disappears, and the level of chloride is low. This last is the most valuable of all the chemical tests, for no other condition gives a really low chloride reading. The demonstration of tubercle bacilli is the conclusive proof.

Syphilis of the Nervous System

Among the most tragic manifestations of syphilis are those due to infection of the central nervous system in cases untreated by penicillin. A peculiarity of these lesions is that they do not develop for many years after the original infection; it may be 10, 15, or even 20 years later. The patient may have been without symptoms for years, even may have almost forgotten that he ever had syphilis. Various parts of the nervous system may be attacked, so that the symptoms may be varied, but only 2 clearly-cut clinical pictures or diseases will be described here. The first of these is general paresis or general paralysis of the insane, the second is tabes dorsalis or locomotor ataxia.

General Paresis. The name is descriptive, for it implies not only a weakness of the muscles, but also a general weakening of all the faculties of the mind. The even more sinister "general paralysis of the insane" describes the final state of the patient. The spirochetes of syphilis are scattered widely throughout the brain and produce multiple areas of inflammation, together with destruction of the nerve cells and nerve fibers. As a result of this destruction, the brain atrophies and wastes away, becoming much smaller than normal. This wasting particularly affects the cerebral cortex in the frontal region, that is to say, the part of the brain concerned with the highest functions of the mind. The areas concerned with muscular movements and with sensation are also involved.

Clinical Pattern. The symptoms of the disease are as diverse as the lesions are widely disseminated. The first indication that all is not well is a deterioration of the higher qualities of the mind. The moral sense is impaired, and there is a weakening of the faculties of judgment, reason, and self-control. Delusions of grandeur lead to domestic and fi-

nancial difficulties, for if a man believes that he is worth millions and orders motor cars and grand pianos in corresponding amount, it is not conducive to domestic happiness. The structure of the mind crumbles, and the final stage is that of childishness and complete dementia. All these changes are due to destruction of the nerve cells in the cerebral cortex. Tremors are highly characteristic; they involve the face, lips, and tongue, so that the speech becomes thick and indistinct, and the hands are tremulous. These tremors are due to lesions in the motor centers. The sensory centers are also involved, so that sensibility is dulled and pain may hardly be felt. The pupil of the eye no longer contracts when exposed to bright light, although it still does so when the eye looks at a nearby object, a condition known as the Argyll Robertson pupil. Convulsive seizures followed by unconsciousness are common. The weakness of the muscles implied in the name of the disease becomes extreme. In the end, the patient is not only mindless but helpless.

The cerebrospinal fluid shows changes that are of great importance, because they allow the physician to make an early diagnosis at a time when treatment may arrest the progress of the disease. The cells of the fluid, particularly lymphocytes, are increased in number, especially at the beginning of the malady. The protein level is increased, but far more significant is that the Wassermann test on the fluid is positive, showing that the patient is suffering from syphilis of the central nervous system. The colloidal gold reaction gives a significant paretic curve.

Tabes Dorsalis. The word tabes means a wasting away, and as the lesion in this syphilitic disease of the spinal cord is a wasting of the posterior or dorsal part of the cord, the condition is called tabes dorsalis. In the dorsal columns of the cord run the nerves that carry the sensation of position, called muscle sense and joint sense. When these are lost, the patient is no longer certain of the position of his legs, so that he becomes unsteady or ataxic in his locomotion.

Anyone wishing to read a description of the onset of the symptoms of tabes by a master of literature should look up Kipling's wonderful little story, "Love o' Women." There is no muscular weakness, for the lesion is confined to the sensory nerves, but the power of muscular coordination is gradually lost, so that the patient is unable to make his legs do what he wants them to do. Things are not so bad as long as the patient has the assistance of sight, but in the dark he is completely at sea. The ordinary person walks by faith (without watching the ground), but the tabetic walks by sight. He walks with legs wide apart to increase stability, and is unable to stand with feet together and eyes closed without swaying or falling (Romberg's sign). To the trained eye, the tabetic can be recognized at once as he walks down the street, by his peculiar wide-based gait and by the way he throws his feet out and brings them down with a slap.

Other sensory disturbances are sudden, severe shooting pains passing down the legs, known as lightning pains, and occasional attacks of abdominal pain and vomiting, called gastric crises, which may be mistaken for acute appendicitis. There is loss of the knee-jerks, i.e., lack of response when the tendon below the knee-cap is tapped, loss of the normal contraction of the pupil to light (Argyll Robertson pupil), as in general paresis, and gradual wasting of the optic nerve, optic atrophy, with corresponding impairment of vision. The cerebrospinal fluid shows the same changes as in general paresis, so that its examination is of the greatest help in diagnosis. Again, in this form of central-nervous-system syphilitic infection, penicillin is the best method of treatment and may often arrest the progress of the condition and relieve many of the symptoms.

If the reader should ask why the *Treponema pallidum* attacks the brain in 1 patient and the spinal cord in another, there is at the present time no answer.

At any rate, both diseases are much less prevalent today than they were 25 years ago.

Viral Diseases

Many known viruses can attack the central nervous system, sometimes setting up an inapparent infection, not infrequently meningitis or nonparalytic poliomyelitis, less often encephalitis. Viruses with a special affinity for the nervous system are called neurotropic and cause some of the most serious diseases of that system, such as poliomyelitis and rabies. There is another group of common, febrile viral diseases (measles, chickenpox, smallpox, vaccinia), in which injury to the nervous system occurs on rare occasions.

Encephalitis is the characteristic disease caused by virus as contrasted with meningitis (caused by bacteria). Clinically, encephalitis causes symptoms of headache and coma, whereas meningitis is normally recognized by the stiff neck and other signs of meningeal inflammation. Viral encephalitis constitutes a group of diseases, some of which are epidemic. Any detailed consideration of this group is beyond the scope of this book, but 1 or 2 members may be mentioned. Lethargic encephalitis, also called "sleeping sickness," appears in epidemic form at long intervals and sweeps across the world. In an epidemic that I (William Boyd) studied in Winnipeg in 1919, the patient was dull, lethargic, and somnolent. He would lie like a log in bed with drooping lids or closed eyes, sunk in a stupor that no external stimuli could penetrate, the dim rushlight of reason hardly flickering. About 20% of these cases subsequently develop some degree of postencephalitic paralysis agitans or Parkinsonism, a condition of generalized rigidity of the face and body that is described later in relation to Parkinson's disease. Equine encephalitis, as its name indicates, is a viral disease of horses that appears in epidemic form. Farm workers may also fall victim to it. Human infection is probably due to mosquitoes, which convey the infection from horse to man, although this connection has not been proved. Wild birds may act as the reservoir hosts of the virus. Secondary encephalitis may occur as a complication following one of the common viral fevers, usually measles, more rarely mumps and chickenpox. Finally, postvaccinal encephalitis must be mentioned, in which, in rare instances, a severe form of encephalitis follows vaccination for smallpox.

Poliomyelitis or infantile paralysis is an acute infectious disease of the spinal cord and brain caused by a filterable virus (poliovirus) and chiefly affecting children. Most of the infections are clinically inapparent and go unrecognized. Today, we have a vaccine, and the disease has virtually disappeared from North America.

There is no more dramatic and deadly example of viral infection than **rabies**. Its practical significance is that when a person has been bitten by a dog suspected of being rabid, microscopic examination of the animal's brain will show whether or not the fingerprint of rabies, the Negri body, is present in the nerve cells, and preventive lifesaving inoculation can be begun at once, if necessary. Finally, as in poliomyelitis, we are now beginning to practice preventive vaccination, yet this practice was introduced by Pasteur with complete success for the prevention of rabies more than 100 years ago.

Herpes is a viral disease characterized by the formation of small vesicles. The name is derived from the Greek word meaning to creep. There are 2 distinct forms: (1) herpes zoster or shingles, in which the vesicles follow or creep along the distribution of a sensory nerve, and (2) herpes simplex, in which there is no such distribution. An attack of the former is followed by lasting immunity, but in the case of the latter, there is no immunity. A puzzling feature is that the eruption is always unilateral, running in a zone (zoster) as far as the middle line, being preceded by neuralgic pains, which in old people may be persistent and severe. The virus appears to be identical to that causing chickenpox, the spread in the latter case being by the blood stream, whereas in zoster it is along the nerves. Herpes simplex is the common form of herpes, usually on the lips as a complication of infective fevers, pneumonia, and even the common cold, so that it is best known as a "cold sore." This virus seems to be carried in cells of the epidermis and only becomes evident when such stimuli as sunlight or fever call it out to create lesions.

There is, in addition, a group of "degenerative" or chronic neurologic diseases that have been suspected of having a viral etiology, but of a different kind from the acute viral disease already discussed.

A **"slow" viral infection** is that in which the virus fails to cause acute disease, the host fails to clear the virus, and the result of the virus-host interaction evolves slowly, producing clinical signs and pathologic changes. The term was introduced in 1954 from studies on disease in Icelandic sheep. Slow viral infections differ from latent infections in that the virus can be isolated in a "slow" infection.

The concept of an infectious etiology for a group of diseases that have in common (1) infection in a single species, (2) a long period of latency (months or years) between the possible infection and manifestation of this disease, (3) slow progression of the disease, and (4) limitation of the disease to a particular part of the nervous system, has been developed clearly during the last 2 decades, largely from studies on a disease of New Guinea cannibals (kuru), who relished eating the brains of their enemies and suffered the consequences. A model of this "slow virus" disease has been found in sheep in Scotland and Iceland, and human diseases of the nervous system have been transmitted to chimpanzees. Most recently, there are reports of transmission of a rare disease (Jakob-Creutzfeldt) from 1 patient to 3 others by electrodes contaminated with slow virus. This process is mentioned here not only because of its particular interest (the number of cases of kuru, Jakob-Creutzfeldt disease, and multifocal leukoencephalopathy is small), but also because of the concept that there can be such an agent and such a different type of response to an infectious agent. The strong evidence in favor of the existence of "slow virus disease" now draws attention to other diseases of unknown etiology and should direct your thinking to reconsider some of the processes that seem so mysterious in tissues other than the nervous system.

DISEASE OF UNCERTAIN ETIOLOGY

It is easy to group many of the diseases of the central nervous system under such headings as traumatic, vascular, and infectious. In these instances, we have a good idea of the etiologic agent involved and of the meaning of the pathologic changes. Unfortunately, there remains a heterogeneous collection of conditions of unknown etiology, referred to vaguely as degenerative diseases of the nervous system. From this collection it seems justifiable to consider at least 1 group, known as the demyelinating diseases.

The essential feature of a demyelinating disease is destruction of the myelin sheaths and relative sparing of the axons, nerve cells, and neuroglia. Although we are ignorant as to the etiology and pathogenesis of the demyelinating diseases, several explanatory hypotheses have been put forward. Some of these diseases are genetically determined, and the myelin is abnormally formed. Others of these disorders are acquired, and the myelin is probably normal. The latter group comprises mostly adult diseases and is more prevalent than the former.

Multiple Sclerosis

This disease is the most common of these disorders, and if we spend more time on it, it is because of its fascinating epidemiology and current attempts to discover its etiology. First, we shall describe the disease. The condition is also known as disseminated sclerosis. It is a chronic disease of the nervous system characterized by remissions and relapses and by the presence of patches of demyelination associated with sclerosis or hardening, scattered diffusely thoughout the gray and white matter of the brain stem and spinal cord. Nerve fibers in the white matter degenerate and are replaced by glial scar tissue (Fig. 24–22). The disease runs a fluctuating, but usually progressive, course that affects various portions

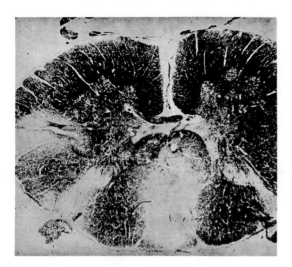

Fig. 24–22. Multiple sclerosis. There are irregular asymmetrical patches of degeneration in the posterior and lateral columns. (Weigert's myelin stain.) × 8.

of the nervous system at different times. The plaques we have described show dead glial cells and loss of myelin that may have occurred at widely differing times.

Clinical Pattern. The disease, common among young adults in the western world, occurs usually at about age 30. In those instances in which the signs and symptoms suggest the diagnosis in a patient who is a child, or who is over 50 years old, the diagnosis is probably not correct. The disease is most frequent in the high latitudes, occurring in western Europe, the northern United States, southern Canada, New Zealand, and southern Australia. Five per cent of the cases are familial, usually occurring in siblings. Cases occurring in husbands and wives have also been reported. Epidemiologic studies of migrant populations show that those persons carry a low susceptibility from a low susceptible area when they move into an area of higher frequency. One study done in Israel indicated that persons immigrating there before their fifteenth year had the same liability for the disease as native Israelis, but those immigrating after 15 years of age had the same propensity for the disease as people in their country of origin. The incidence of the disease in northern areas ranges from 50 to 80 per 100,000 population.

The patient is often a young man, who sees a physician because of the sudden onset of impaired vision that may progress to complete blindness in 1 eye, followed by partial or complete restoration of vision. Permanent blindness may come on again months later. Tingling or numbness in the extremities and transient urinary incontinence or frequency are also important hallmarks of the disease. Intention tremor, a stiff gait, jerky eye movements, and a peculiar, staccato speech always suggest involvement of the central nervous system by this disorder. The most important general criteria are the evidence of multiple signs in different parts of the central nervous system and their recurrence at different times. Considering the nature of the disease, it has often been noted that the patient seems inappropriately cheerful. The prognosis is guarded, because it is well recognized that the patient may live for many years despite the insidious progression of the disease.

The lesions of glial proliferation and demyelination are often bilateral, but not symmetrical, always central and never peripheral, and the explanation for the remissions and relapses are the presence of edema that resolves and the compensatory plasticity of alternate neurologic pathways. It is also likely that demyelinated axons may still conduct, or that remyelination may occur.

Examination of the cerebral spinal fluid may show no abnormality, although in many cases there is a mild lymphocytosis and an increase in protein. These changes may be absent in the advanced stage of the disease.

The etiology of multiple sclerosis remains unclear. Because gamma globulin is present in plaques, it has been suggested that the disease may be of immune origin; because patients with multiple sclerosis and their relatives belong most frequently to HLA groups 3 and 7, a hereditary etiology is spoken of; because coastal-dwelling fish eaters have a lower incidence of the disease than animal eaters at the same latitude, diet has been implicated; and because antibodies to measles virus are present in most patients, an infectious etiology has frequently been suggested.

A most interesting study has been recently reported from the Faroe Islands, which lie between Norway and Iceland at latitude 62

north and longitude 7 west. They are a semi-independent unit of the Kingdom of Denmark with a population of 41,000 in 1976.

As shown in Figure 24–23, there was an epidemic of multiple sclerosis on these islands in which new cases appeared in 1943 and disappeared, with 1 exception, by 1960. The explanation for this epidemic lies in that British troops occupied these islands from 1940 to 1945. The number of soldiers was as great as 8,000, bringing the ratio of outlanders to islanders to 1 in 3. The diet of the Faroese seemed generally unchanged during the war, and possible explanations for the epidemic may be sought in classic causes such as the introduction of toxins or infectious diseases. The hypothesis is put forward that the epidemic is due to an infectious disease. It is of great interest that during this same period, the chief veterinarian of the islands reported that canine distemper was pandemic during the war and absent before the British occupation. Since 1956 or 1957, there has been no further distemper among dogs on these islands. The concurrence of the 2 epidemics suggests a relationship. Whether the virus of canine distemper can indeed lead in susceptible populations to multiple sclerosis is an unproven but provocative idea. The notion that such an infectious agent requires time to

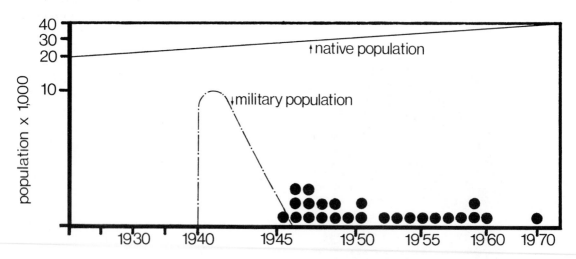

Fig. 24–23. This graph shows the presence (black dots) of cases of multiple sclerosis between 1945 and 1970 in the Faroe Islands. Each dot represents a single case. The native population rose during the period of 1920 to 1970 from 20,000 to 40,000, as shown on the top line. The military population resident on the islands arrived in 1940, with approximately 10,000 soldiers, and decreased over the next 5 years. Note the temporal relationship between the multiple sclerosis epidemic and the visit of the army to the islands. (From Kurtzke, J.F., and Hyllested, K.: Multiple sclerosis in the Faroe Islands: I. Clinical and epidemiological features. Ann. Neurol., 5:6, 1978.)

induce its effects, and that not all persons exposed will respond with a clinically apparent manifestation of disease, is important. It is of interest that other relationships of rare neurologic disorders to viral infections are being proven, as we have discussed in the section on slow virus, and as is apparent in sclerosing subacute pancephalitis syndrome, in the high proportion of antimeasles antibodies in such individuals.

Parkinson's Disease

Also known as "the shaking palsy," this disease is a chronic, nonkilling, but profoundly disabling degeneration of the brain. The clinical picture was drawn in 1817 by Parkinson with the hand of a master. The classic triad of symptoms is rigidity, tremor, and an attitude of flexion. The rigidity involves all the voluntary muscles, until, in an extreme case, the unhappy sufferer becomes as rigid as a block of marble. This rigidity gives the face the familiar "Parkinsonian mask." The tremor affects the fingers and hands, giving a cigarette-rolling movement.

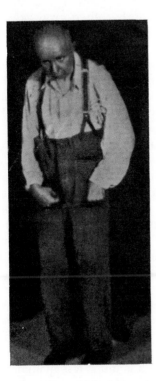

Fig. 24–24. Parkinsonism. (Grinker's *Neurology*, Charles C Thomas.)

Curiously enough, it is present when the part is at rest, disappearing for a few moments with movement, thus justifying the term "shaking palsy," and differing from the "intention tremor" of multiple sclerosis. The whole attitude is that of flexion. The head is flexed on the chest, the body is bowed, the arms and wrists are flexed, the knees are bent, and the forward-leaning posture enforces steps that are short and almost running, so that an advanced case of the disease can be diagnosed at a glance (Fig. 24–24).

In most cases, major changes are found in the nerve cells of the corpus striatum, consisting of the globus pallidus and substantia nigra in the midbrain. In the primary form, there is marked disappearance of the large, pale motor cells of the globus pallidus, whereas in the secondary form, the degenerative changes are in the substantia nigra, with loss of melanin in the pigmented cells and also of the neurohormonal transmitter dopamine, of which dopa is a precursor. The dopamine stores in the basal ganglia are depleted. There is a correspondingly low content of dopa in the urine. The essence of the condition is an enzyme defect. The most recent method of treatment is the daily intramuscular injection of dopa in the form of L-dopa, a derivative. This treatment results in a dramatic improvement in both the appearance and the behavior of the patient through reversal of the crippling effects of the disease. The disease used to be a rarity, but since around 1920 it has become much more common. This increased incidence may be because the viral agent of the encephalitis epidemic damaged the subthalamic cells, but not to a sufficient degree to produce clinical symptoms. The passage of the years or possibly some kind of delayed-fuse action brought the submerged disturbance to the surface. If this idea is correct, Parkinson's disease will, happily, soon become a rarity once more.

TUMORS OF THE CENTRAL NERVOUS SYSTEM

We have already seen that the brain is composed of 2 types of cells, the nerve cells and the neuroglial cells. Tumors of the brain only arise from and are composed of neuroglial cells and therefore are called gliomas. Not uncommonly, a tumor grows from the meninges, which cover the brain, and is therefore called a meningioma (Fig. 24–25). There is a fundamental difference between these 2 types of tumor, for the meningioma is a benign tumor that is encapsulated and merely presses on the brain, whereas the glioma is a malignant tumor that infiltrates the brain and is not demarcated from it in any way. Table 24–3 lists the incidence of intracranial and intraspinal tumors in a given period.

Two points might be added to this brief summary. (1) It is evident that intracranial tumor may be intracerebral or extracerebral. The intracerebral tumors are the gliomas and metastatic carcinoma, as well as a few rarities that will not be mentioned. The extracerebral tumors are the meningiomas, tumors of the acoustic nerve, pituitary tumors, and craniopharyngiomas, which arise from the remnants of the epithelial tract from which the pituitary is formed. (2) The reason that intracerebral tumors are gliomas rather than nerve cell tumors is that glial cells, particularly astrocytes, are capable of unlimited mitotic division, whereas the adult nerve cells live on, but are incapable of multiplying. Cells

Table 24–3.   Incidence of Intracranial and Intraspinal Tumors at Boston City Hospital, 1900 to 1930

Total no. of autopsies	10,592	
Total no. of tumors	1,458	
Tumors of other organs	1,270	
Intracranial and intraspinal tumors	188	(12.7%)
Gliomas	81	(43.1%)
Pituitary adenomas	6	(3.2%)
Sheath tumors	22	(11.7%)
Meningioma	18	
Acoustic neuroma	4	
Metastatic tumors	29	(15.4%)
Blood vessel tumors	6	(3.0%)
Congenital tumors	8	(4.3%)
Granulomas	19	(10.1%)
Spinal cord tumors	4	(2.1%)
Unclassified	13	(7.1%)

From Wintrobe, M., et al.: *Harrison's Principles of Internal Medicine*, 7th Ed. New York, McGraw-Hill, 1974.

that are not capable of division cannot give rise to neoplasms.

Although **gliomas** are malignant by virtue of their infiltrative power, they vary greatly in their degree of malignancy, and although some are rapidly growing and kill the patient in a few months, others grow slowly, and the patient may live for many years, especially if he receives skillful surgical treatment. Moreover, gliomas do not form metastases or secondary growths in other parts of the body as most malignant tumors do, probably because the tumor cells fail to escape from the interior of the skull.

There are many different kinds of glioma, but only 4 will be described. Of these 4, 2 occur principally in the adult, namely, glioblastoma multiforme and astrocytoma; 2 occur in children, namely, medulloblastoma and ependymoma. The glioblastoma multiforme is a highly malignant tumor occurring in middle life and is usually found in 1 of the cerebral hemispheres (Fig. 24–26). The margin is ill defined, so that the surgeon may have great difficulty in knowing where the tumor ends and the normal brain begins (Fig. 24–27). It is highly invasive and is likely to kill the patient in the course of a few months. The astrocytoma is much less malignant, and the average time of survival after operation is 6 years. It may occur in any part of the brain,

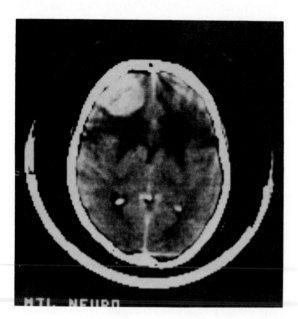

Fig. 24–25.   This CT scan shows the presence of 2 meningiomas impinging on the frontal lobes.

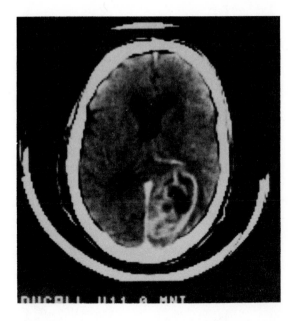

Fig. 24–26. This CT scan shows a large cystic space in the posterior cerebral hemisphere of the right side. Notice the slight displacement of the ventricular system. This is interpreted as cerebral tumor.

but in children the common site is the cerebellum. The cerebellar tumor in children is usually completely benign. The medulloblastoma is a highly malignant and rapidly growing tumor in the roof of the fourth ventricle in the midline of the cerebellum (Fig. 24–28). The prognosis of this tumor of children is therefore the very opposite of that of astrocytoma. The ependyoma is the rarest of the 4. It usually occurs in children and in the same location as the medulloblastoma. It is, however, much less malignant than that tumor.

A nearly always benign tumor arising from the meninges covering the brain, a **meningioma** is a common form of intracranial neoplasm. Although benign, it may obviously kill the patient in due time by virtue of its intracranial position and by the pressure it exerts on the brain, unless the tumor is removed. The meningioma is usually much firmer than the glioma, and it is adherent externally to the dura. As it presses on the brain from the outside, it forms a deep bed for

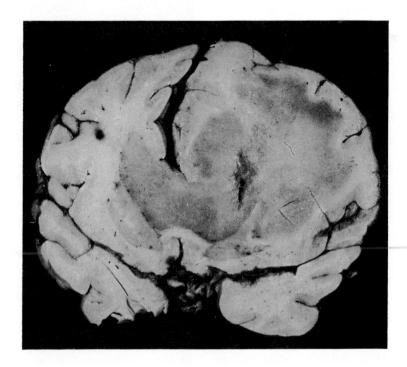

Fig. 24–27. Glioblastoma multiforme, showing massive infiltration of right and left frontal lobes. (University of Alabama Medical School.)

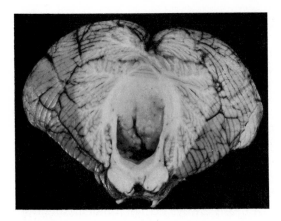

Fig. 24–28. This section through the fourth ventricle shows the cerebellum and whitish material that protrudes into the lumen of the ventricle. This is a **medulloblastoma**. (McGill University, Department of Pathology Museum.)

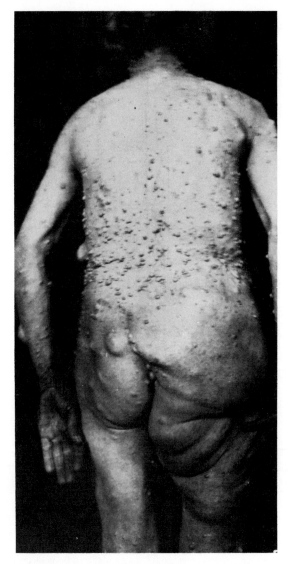

Fig. 24–29. This photograph, taken at the turn of the century, shows a number of warty protrusions all over the body, characteristic of **neurofibromas**. It has been remarked that "if you need to examine more than one of these growths you do not know what it is." Multiple neurofibromas, described by Von Recklinghausen, are benign tumors. (The Evans Collection, Osler Library, McGill University.)

itself, from which on the autopsy table it can readily be lifted out. In the operating room, things are much less simple, for there is danger of severe or even fatal hemorrhage from large vessels that pass between the highly vascular overlying bone and the tumor. Local changes in the skull may be of great help in diagnosis. In about 25% of cases, there is bony thickening of the skull over the tumor that can be detected radiographically and sometimes even by physical examination.

Acoustic nerve tumor is another intracranial tumor that is much more closely related to meningioma than to the gliomas. It grows from the eighth cranial nerve at the angle between the pons and the cerebellum and forms a firm, round, well-encapsulated tumor. It presses on the nerve supplying the muscles of the face as well as on the acoustic or auditory nerve. The principal symptoms are therefore facial paralysis and deafness on 1 side. It is important to realize that the tumor is benign, so that, when removed surgically, there is no chance of its return. Peripheral nerve tumors also occur. One of the more common is a neurofibroma, illustrated in Figure 24–29.

One additional tumor worth mentioning is a congenital tumor, called a craniopharyngioma, that may remain clinically silent until middle or old age. Visual field loss at any age should suggest the presence of this growth, which is frequently calcified (98% in chil-

dren) and is visible on roentgenograms (Fig. 24–30). Symptoms of increased intracranial pressure, headaches (86%), and vomiting (74%), and such eye signs as papilledema, optic atrophy, and strabismus, all are classic findings. Surgical excision has become technically easier and carries the best chance of recovery for the patient.

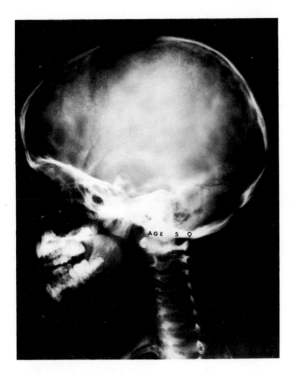

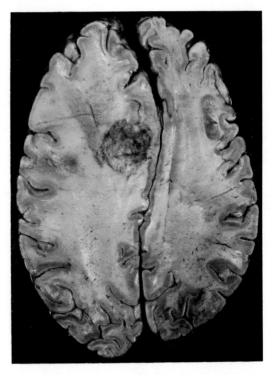

Fig. 24–30. This skull film shows the presence of calcification in and around the base of the skull. This is the classic sign of the presence of craniopharyngioma.

Fig. 24–31. This section through the cerebral hemispheres shows a round discolored nodule that has caused a shift of the midline structures from the left to the right and an increase in the size of the left cerebral hemisphere. This space-occupying lesion is typical of a **metastatic** tumor to the brain. Such metastases commonly come from lung, breast, or kidney carcinomas. (McGill University, Department of Pathology Museum.)

When a diagnosis is made of tumor of the brain, the doctor has to bear in mind the possibility that the tumor may be a metastatic carcinoma (Fig. 24–31). In such cases, by far the most common tumor that metastasizes to the brain is bronchogenic carcinoma, constituting 30 to 40%; 15% come from cancer of the breast, kidney, and gastrointestinal tract (colon, rectum). The tumors are usually multiple rather than single, and on this account the clinical picture may be perplexing. To add to the confusion, the signs and symptoms may be entirely cerebral, with the primary tumor remaining silent. This situation is particularly likely in the case of bronchogenic carcinoma.

Clinical Pattern. The symptoms of a brain tumor may be divided into 2 groups, the first general and the second localizing. The general symptoms are due to the increased intracranial pressure produced by the mass of new tissue inside the skull and are more or less the same in whichever part of the brain the tumor is situated. The chief of these symptoms is headache, which may become excruciating in intensity. The cerebrospinal fluid pressure is greatly increased. Vomiting may be marked in the later stages, but is often absent. The pressure on the optic nerves produces swelling of the termination of these nerves in the eye, a condition called optic neuritis, followed by optic atrophy, which can be recognized when the retina of the eye is viewed with the ophthalmoscope.

The localizing symptoms are naturally varied, because they depend on the site of the tumor in the brain. If the motor centers are involved, there will be weakness of the muscles of the face, arm, or leg. If the sensory centers are affected, there will be corresponding disturbance of sensation. Involvement of the special senses, such as sight or hearing, will point to the areas concerned with these functions (Fig. 24–32). It is for this reason that these symptoms are known as localizing, be-

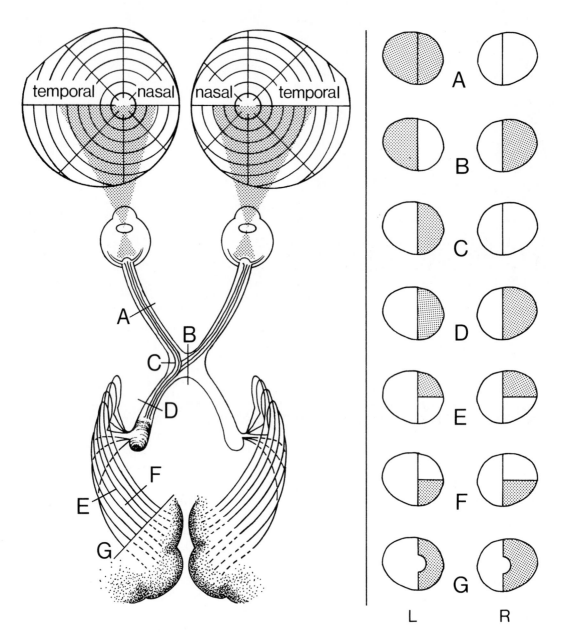

Fig. 24–32. The drawing on the left illustrates the radiation of the visual fields through the optic nerves at the decussation to the posterior lobes of the cerebral hemispheres. Lesions A, B, C, D, E, F, and G cause the abnormalities of vision shown on the right. Lesion A, for example, shows complete blindness in the left eye. (From Thorn, G.W., et al. (Eds.): *Harrison's Principles of Internal Medicine*, 8th Ed. New York, McGraw-Hill, 1977.)

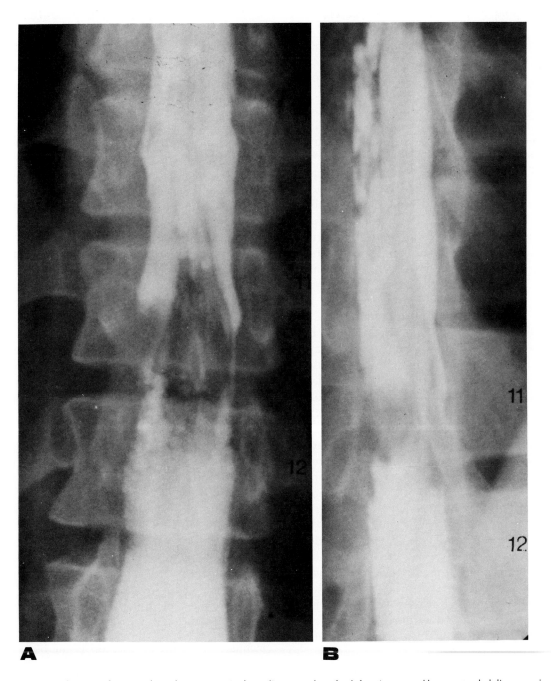

Fig. 24–33. These **myelograms** show the presence in the radiopaque dye of a deformity, caused by a protruded disc, seen in both the anteroposterior *(A)* and lateral *(B)* views.

cause, by a careful analysis of these disturbances, the physician is able to determine the exact location of the tumor, and the surgeon is then able to open the skull at the correct spot, where he will have access to the lesion. Unfortunately, there are extensive regions of the brain known as silent areas, so called because lesions of these areas do not give rise to any localizing symptoms. If the tumor was situated in a silent area, it used to be impossible to determine its exact location, impossible even to decide on which side of the brain to operate.

The radiologist may provide invaluable information in the diagnosis and localization of intracranial tumors. Gases that are radiolucent when introduced into the subarachnoid space, and thus into the cerebral ventricles, outline the ventricles and indicate the site of a tumor that may distort that outline. The use of radiopaque oil in the spinal canal also localizes protruded intervertebral discs (Fig. 24–33), tumors, and obstructions to the free flow of fluids. This study is called myelography. Of particular value is angiography, which consists of injecting a radiopaque oil into the cerebral circulation. By this means, the outline of the tumor may be indicated even in those lesions that do not distort the ventricles. The procedure is of special importance in the case of intracranial aneurysms and other vascular anomalies. However, these methods have now largely been supplanted by the use of computer tomography. This vastly expensive tool has revolutionized diagnosis of lesions.

If the reader would like to get a vivid idea of what it is like to be a patient with a brain tumor, he should read *A Journey Round My Skull*, by the distinguished Hungarian novelist, Frigyes Karinthy, who himself was the patient. The rather terrifying description of the operation under a local anesthetic is perhaps somewhat highly colored.

The treatment of brain tumors is discouraging, but by no means hopeless. If the tumor can be located, much or all of it may be removed. In the case of meningioma, a complete cure may be expected. With the gliomas, it is much more difficult for the surgeon to know whether he has removed all the tumor, so that there is great danger that some of it

may be left behind and that the growth will recur. But even if a cure cannot be assured, several years of comfort and comparative health may be added to the patient's life. Perhaps the most important advice for the patient with a brain tumor is to choose the right surgeon.

INCREASED INTRACRANIAL PRESSURE

Regardless of the cause, which ranges from the presence of hematoma, abscess, tumor in the closed box of the skull, to the effects of poisons such as lead or barbiturates, or metabolites, as in hepatic coma, to the serious problem of anoxia, the swelling of the brain may lead quickly to irreversible damage or death by compression of venous return, or by herniation and ischemic necrosis of the brain stem.

Headache, visual disturbances, slowing of the heart rate, and progressive loss of consciousness all suggest that there is increasing intracranial pressure. One great dilemma in these cases is whether to establish the diagnosis by direct measurement of the cerebrospinal fluid pressure with the cerebrospinal tap (thereby running the risk of precipitating herniation of the brain) or to use the physical signs such as papilledema or protrusion of the optic nerve and to institute therapy directed towards reducing the swelling. Such therapy will include the use of mannitol, anti-inflammatory agents such as cortisone, hypothermia, and decompressive surgical procedures.

CEREBROSPINAL FLUID IN DISEASE

The normal spinal fluid is as clear as water, contains sugar and chlorides, no protein, less than 5 lymphocytes per cubic millimeter, and no polymorphonuclear leukocytes. In acute meningitis (see Table 24–2), the vessels in the inflamed meninges allow the constituents of the blood to pour into the fluid, so that it contains much protein and great numbers of polymorphonuclear leukocytes. The fluid is therefore purulent and turbid. The bacteria feed on and destroy the glucose, so that it is reduced in amount. Bacteria are found in smears of the pus and in culture. Tuberculous meningitis, which is much less acute, gives different spinal fluid readings. The fluid is clear or only slightly milky, as it usually contains less than 100 cells per cubic millimeter, most of which are lymphocytes. The protein (globulin) is only moderately increased, and the glucose is correspondingly diminished. The most characteristic findings are a marked diminution in the chloride level and the presence of tubercle bacilli in the smears.

In suspected brain tumor, the spinal fluid may be examined for tumor cells. These are much more likely to be found in secondary carcinoma than in glioma, although in the latter condition there may be a marked increase in the lymphocyte count. The use of the millipore membrane filter gives better results than the conventional sedimentation methods. In spinal cord tumors, which resemble intracranial tumors and are not considered here, the spinal fluid may show the "compression syndrome" if the canal is blocked. Below the obstruction, the characters of the fluid are as follows: (1) massive spontaneous coagulation, (2) xanthochromia or yellow coloration of the fluid, (3) marked increase in the protein, (4) no corresponding increase in the cells. The exact site of a spinal cord tumor may sometimes be determined by the intraspinal injection of Lipiodol followed by radiography (Fig. 24–33). It is evident that lumbar puncture can be of value in the diagnosis of suspected spinal cord tumors.

SYNOPSIS

In considering diseases of the central nervous system we include: the skull, the meninges, the blood supply, the ventricular system, as well as the anatomic subdivisions of the cerebrum, cerebellum, and brain stem.

Obstructions to circulation of the cerebrospinal fluid may be due to congenital, inflammatory, or neoplastic disease.

Cerebrovascular disease may be due to rupture and hemorrhage of branches of the arterial tree or to thrombosis and occlusion of the arterial or venous system. Embolization may also cause infarction, but much less frequently.

Hemorrhage inside the skull most commonly results from trauma, hypertension, or rupture of an aneurysm. It may be localized to the extradural, subdural, or subarachnoid space, or it may occur within the substance of the brain or in the ventricular system.

Infections of the central nervous system are most commonly caused by pyogenic bacteria, tuberculosis, syphilis, or viruses. They may be localized (abscesses) or generalized (meningitis, encephalitis).

Demyelinating diseases (e.g., multiple sclerosis) are of unknown etiology, but recent evidence points toward "slow viruses" as an etiologic factor.

Tumors of the central nervous system are most commonly metastatic from the lung or other organs. Primary tumors arise from glial cells or from the meninges.

Terms

Hydrocephalus   *Subarachnoid hemorrhage*   *Demyelinating disease*
Hemiplegia   *Intracerebral hemorrhage*   *Gliomas*
Extradural hemorrhage   *Meningitis*   *Meningioma*
Subdural hemorrhage   *Encephalitis*

FURTHER READING

Adams, R.D., and Sidman, R.L.: *Introduction to Neuropathology*. New York, Blakiston, 1968.

Blackwood, W., and Corsellis, J.A.N. (Eds.): *Greenfield's Neuropathology*, 3rd Ed. London, Edward Arnold, 1976.

Constantinides, P.: Pathogenesis of cerebral artery thrombosis. Arch. Pathol., *83*:422, 1967.

Edelman, G.M., and Mountcastle, V.B.: *The Mindful Brain: Cortical Organization and the Group-Selective Theory of Higher Brain Function*. Cambridge, M.I.T. Press, 1978.

Engel, W.K., et al.: Myasthenia gravis. Ann. Intern. Med., *81*:225, 1974.

Gajdusek, D.C.: Slow infections with unconventional viruses. Harvey Lect., *72*, 1978.

Guillemin, R.: New endocrinology of the brain. Perspect. Biol. Med., *22*:S74, 1979.

Jennett, H.B., and Plum, F.: Persistent vegetative state after brain damage. Lancet, *1*:734, 1972.

Kety, S.S.: The biological roots of mental illness: their ramifications through cerebral metabolism, synaptic activity, genetics, and the environment. Harvey Lect., *71*, 1978.

Kurtzke, J.F., and Hyllested, K.: Multiple sclerosis in the Faroe Islands: I. Clinical and epidemiological features. Ann. Neurol., *5*:6, 1979.

Maugh, T.H.: Multiple sclerosis: two or more viruses may be involved. Science, *195*:768, 1977.

Sabin, T.D.: The differential diagnosis of coma. N. Engl. J. Med., *290*:1062, 1974.

Seligman, S.J.: The rapid differential diagnosis of meningitis. Med. Clin. North Am., *57*:1417, 1973.

Shenkin, H.A., and Bouzarth, W.F.: Clinical methods of reducing intracranial pressure: role of the cerebral circulation. N. Engl. J. Med., *282*:1465, 1970.

Snyder, S.H.: Opiate receptors in the brain. N. Engl. J. Med., *296*:266, 1977.

Terry, R.D.: Dementia: a brief and selective review. Arch. Neurol., *33*:1, 1976.

Ward, J.I., et al.: *Haemophilus influenzae* meningitis: a prospective national study of secondary spread in household contacts. N. Engl. J. Med., *301*:122, 1979.

Zacks, S.I.: *Atlas of Neuropathology*. New York, Harper & Row, 1971.

Musculoskeletal System

Parents are the bones on which children sharpen their teeth. —USTINOV

All our activities, except for the single act of thinking, depend on the integrity and interaction of elements of the locomotor system— muscles, bones, and joints—which have raised us from the primordial slime. This chapter is concerned with the structure, function, and common disorders of each of these elements.

BONE AND CARTILAGE

Normal Structure and Function

A bone is not a dead thing. It is true that it is impregnated with minerals, which gives it its rigidity, but the bone itself is just as much alive as the heart or the brain. It consists of cells surrounded by a modified fibrous tissue saturated with salts of calcium phosphate, in which there are spaces or interstices, which are particularly numerous at the ends of the bone. In the center of the shaft of the bone there is the medullary cavity, filled with bone marrow, which manufactures red blood cells and the leukocytes (Fig. 25–1). This cavity is active in the long bones of young, growing people, but becomes replaced by fat after the

age of 20. Lining the medullary cavity and interstices are cells called osteoblasts, whose function is to form new bone. In normal bone, there are also larger cells, giant cells, containing several nuclei called osteoclasts. They are concerned with removal, instead of formation, of bone. There is considerable evidence to support the idea that the osteoblasts are converted to osteoclasts under the stimulus of parathyroid hormone, as if these cells were the custodians of a bank of calcium and phosphate where they can function either as depositors or as withdrawers.

During childhood and adolescence, the bones grow in length. This they do entirely by virtue of a layer of cartilage at each end of the bone known as the epiphyseal apparatus (Fig. 25–2). When a child grows up, this cartilage becomes calcified and converted into bone, after which no more growth is possible. Bone responds to growth hormone secreted by the anterior pituitary. When this gland becomes overactive in early life as a result of a pituitary tumor, the growth of the epiphyseal cartilage is speeded up and the person becomes a giant. Gigantism is not possible once the cartilage has become converted into bone. Conversely, if the pituitary is insufficiently active, growth ceases and the person remains a dwarf. However, whereas there is only 1 cause of gigantism, there are many causes of dwarfism (Fig. 25–3). Indeed the study of

591

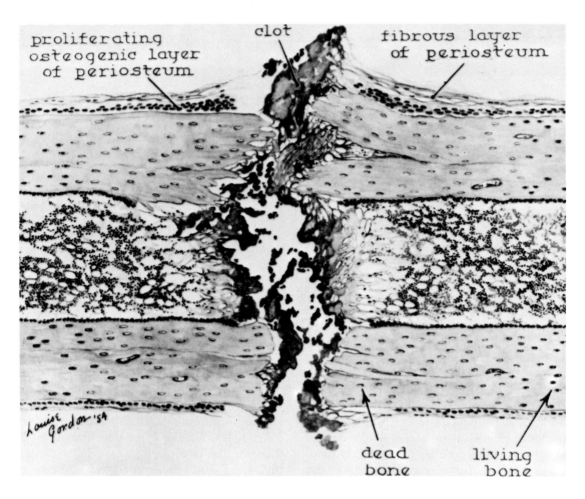

proliferating
osteogenic layer
of periosteum

clot

fibrous layer
of periosteum

dead
bone

living
bone

Louise
Gordon '54

Fig. 25–1.   This drawing shows a **fractured bone.** In the center of the bone is the marrow cavity. The drawing illustrates the relative proportions of the periosteum, living bone, marrow cavity, and hemorrhage in the area of fracture. (From Ham, A.W., and Harris, W.R.: In *Bourne's Biochemistry and Physiology of Bone.* New York, Academic Press.)

dwarfism is extensive; to discuss it here is out of the question.

A bone must grow in thickness as well as in length. Increase in thickness is brought about by the periosteum (Fig. 25–4), a fibrous membrane that closely covers the bone and contains osteoblasts on its deep surface. It is through the periosteum that the superficial part of the bone receives its blood supply, so that anything that injures or removes the periosteum threatens the health and even the life of the bone.

We have said that the epiphyseal cartilage is at the end of the bone, but this is not strictly true. It is separated from the actual end of the bone, i.e., the joint surface, by a small piece of bone known as the epiphysis. The epiphyseal cartilage therefore intervenes between the shaft of the bone and the epiphysis. Many of the most important diseases of

bone (inflammation, tuberculosis, sarcoma) commence in this region of the bone on one or the other side of the epiphyseal cartilage.

Calcium is stored principally in the bones, which contain 99% of the total body calcium as well as 90% of the phosphorus, combined with calcium in the form of calcium phosphate. In bone, the calcium phosphate crystals are deposited within the collagen fibril. One unanswered question is why bone collagen calcifies and other collagens normally do not.

The small amount of calcium that is not in the bones plays a vital role in most physiologic functions, for it affects enzyme activity, cell membrane permeability, cardiac rhythm, and neuromuscular excitability. A fall in the level of serum calcium may produce tetanic contractions and death. Serum calcium and phosphorus maintain a delicate inverse

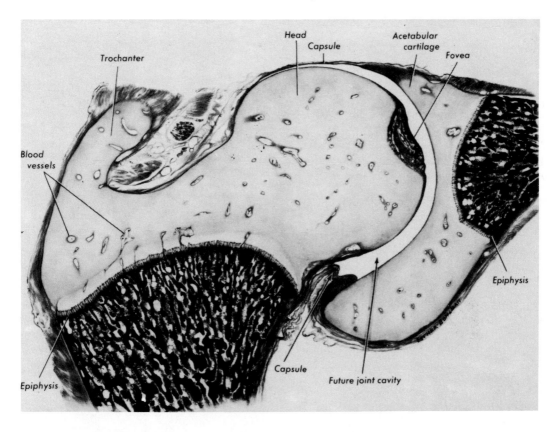

Fig. 25–2. This photograph illustrates the epiphyseal apparatus and the head of the femur, its synovial space and capsule, and the acetabular cartilage of the hip. (From Bloom, W., and Fawcett, D. W.: *A Textbook of Histology,* 10th Ed. Philadelphia, W. B. Saunders, 1975.)

equilibrium with each other: when one goes up, the other goes down. A minor change in serum calcium results in a major disturbance of health, but a change in phosphorus causes only a slight disturbance.

The metabolism of calcium and phosphorus in relation to bone must be considered as a whole. When we speak of calcification, we mean of course the deposition of calcium phosphate and not merely calcium. Calcium and phosphorus metabolism is influenced by many different factors, such as parathormone, the hormone of the parathyroid glands; vitamin D, which controls absorption of calcium from the small intestine and absorption and excretion by the kidneys; and such hormones as estrogens, androgens, adrenal corticoids, thyroxin, and those of the anterior pituitary. When the complexity of the entire mechanism is considered, it becomes a matter of surprise that anyone has normal bones.

Osteoblasts, when multiplying rapidly, produce the enzyme alkaline phosphatase, which hydrolyses organic phosphate compounds, altering the local calcium-phosphate balance and resulting in the precipitation of calcium salts in the soft tissues. The phosphatase level of the serum may be raised either in excessive bone formation or in bone destruction, for in both of these phenomena, increased osteoblastic activity comes into play.

Metabolic Bone Disease

As with other systems, there are a variety of pathologic processes that may affect the tissue in question. Because bone is composed of 3 basic elements—the cells (osteocytes, osteoblasts, and osteoclasts), their product, the protein matrix (collagen), and the inorganic salts (hydroxyapatite), which impregnate the collagen—we can imagine several areas where lesions may occur. In theory, at least, there can be inadequate dietary intake of calcium and phosphate, there can be disorders of

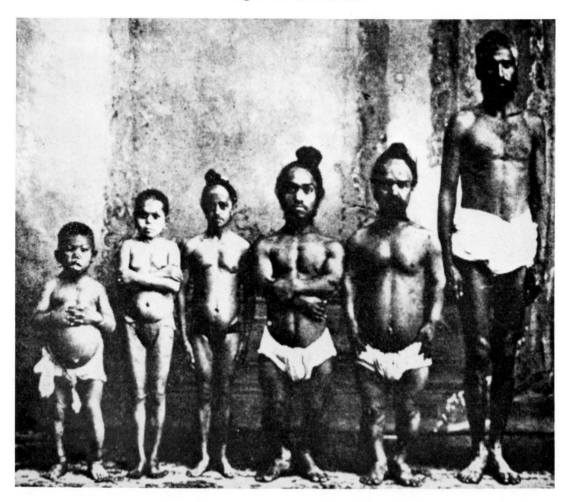

Fig. 25–3. This photograph shows a normal male on the right and three types of **dwarfism.** On the extreme left is a child who has failed to grow because of congenital absence of the thyroid gland (cretin). The next pair of dwarfs have entirely normal proportions but are half normal size. The next pair on the right show disproportionately short extremities but normal size trunk and head.

the collagen and its ability to initiate and to maintain calcification, and there may be disorders of the bone cells that result in decreased synthesis of collagen or other defects such as enzyme disorders. This, naturally, is not the entire list of possible problems, but it gives one a simple way of looking at metabolic bone disease.

The most common form of metabolic bone disease is called **osteoporosis,** or osteopenia, because the bones appear diminished in structure, as if the steel skeleton of a bridge or building had been heavily rusted and its mass severely decreased. However, osteoporotic bone is only diminished in amount. It is otherwise normal, having normal matrix and

mineralization. This generalized disorder of the whole skeleton is seen commonly in those over 60; in fact, it is estimated that half the women over 60 in North America have osteoporosis, compared with the 35-year-old population. This diagnosis is most often made radiologically by comparison with bone of normal people. It is a quantitative, morphologic diagnosis, most easily seen in the vertebrae and pelvis, and is common in elderly persons or in those who have been bedridden for any length of time. It is to be expected in patients who have been given exogenous adrenal corticosteroids. The pathogenic mechanism common to all these processes is presumably inhibition of the

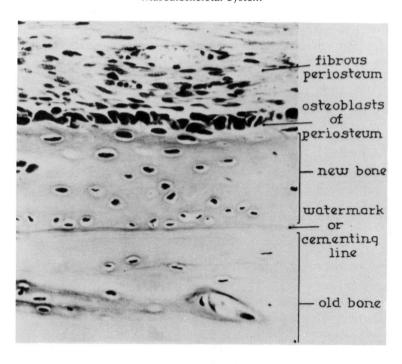

fibrous periosteum

osteoblasts of periosteum

new bone

watermark or cementing line

old bone

Fig. 25–4. This photograph shows the microscopic appearance of the periosteum, of osteoblasts, of osteocytes, and of an area of new and old bone. (From Ham, A.W.: *Histology,* 7th Ed. Philadelphia and Toronto, J. B. Lippincott, 1974.)

normal collagen synthesis, although we acknowledge that the etiology of osteoporosis is unknown. Osteoporosis also occurs in the bones of a leg or an arm that has been placed in a cast, while the remainder of the skeleton continues to maintain a normal appearance. The stimuli to normal bone growth and development are both local and general, and so we can generalize that bone, like all our other tissues, constantly adapts to the demands placed on it. The serum enzymes and ions related to bone integrity are all normal (alkaline phosphatase, calcium, phosphorus), a feature that distinguishes osteoporosis from osteomalacia.

In summary, osteoporosis or **osteopenia** may be due to (1) senility or aging, for which the causes are related to protein metabolism; (2) atrophy or disuse, as in the single limb that is in a cast, or in the limbs of a paraplegic, or in the bedridden; (as an aside, one of the major biochemical problems of the astronauts was calcium loss—what role does gravity play in the maintenance of our skeletal system?) (3) gonadal deficiency; (4) adrenocortical hormone excess, whether endogenous or

exogenous, as in patients with rheumatoid arthritis who are given steroid hormones or in those who have Cushing's disease.

The most common complications of osteoporosis are fractures of the femur or other weight-bearing bones such as the vertebrae. These fractures may be major or only visible with the most careful inspection. Management is often directed to improving protein metabolism, physiotherapy, and occasionally administering anabolic steroids.

The second generalized metabolic bone disease is that in which there are inadequate amounts of mineral in the bone. This is called **osteomalacia** in the adult and **rickets** in the child or person who is still growing. The name implies softening (*malakia,* Greek for soft). This can be due to an inadequate dietary intake during infancy or at any time, but the minimal requirement of the child is much more crucial than that of the adult, who has already built up a large store of calcium and phosphate. There are, however, other causes of rickets in addition to dietary deficiency. For example, there are rare cases of hereditary rickets, such as hypophosphatasia, and vitamin D-resistant rickets (inborn errors of metabolism), in addition to the better-known form caused by vitamin D deficiency.

We shall consider rickets more completely as it is an interesting and important disease, particularly for those in northern climates.

Rickets is a form of osteodystrophy completely different from those already considered, because it is a manifestation of a vitamin deficiency. We have already seen that the chief mineral constituents that impart rigidity to the bones are calcium and phosphorus, combined in the form of calcium phosphate. These substances are absorbed from the food and deposited in the bones. If they are not present in the food in sufficient amount, the bones remain soft and are easily bent.

Vitamin D is important to proper calcification. The ordinary food of a child usually contains a reasonable amount of calcium and phosphorus, but may be lacking in vitamin D. This vitamin is necessary for the proper absorption of calcium and phosphorus from the intestine, and in its absence, no matter how abundant the minerals may be in the food, the body is unable to use them, and rickets will result. Vitamin D is a fat-soluble vitamin, in contrast to some of the other vitamins that are water-soluble. It is therefore contained principally in fatty foods, although it is also found in certain vegetables.

The causes of rickets are deficiencies in some of the factors necessary for the proper calcification of bone. The fault may lie in the quality, not the quantity, of the food. A child may be starved and emaciated but show no signs of rickets, whereas a plump baby may show marked rickets. The disease is much more common in artificially fed infants than in those who are breast-fed. Owing to the absence of light, rickets is more common in large, smoky cities and during the winter months. All the factors are included in the statement that rickets is a disease of the slums of large cities in countries that get little sunshine.

The symptoms are partly connected with bones, partly systemic. The disease is one of infancy and early childhood (6 months to 2 years), a period at which there is the greatest demand for calcium and phosphorus by the rapidly growing bones. The softened bones

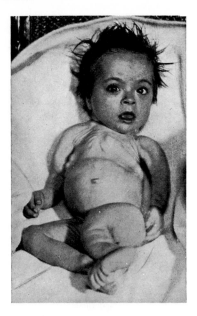

Fig. 25–5. Rickets, showing large forehead, deformed chest, curvature of arms and legs, and pot belly.

become deformed, especially those that bear the weight of the body (Fig. 25–5), and backward curvature of the spine develops (kyphosis). The head is large and square. The sternum is pushed forward (pigeon-breast), and a series of nodules develops at the anterior ends of the ribs called the rickety rosary. Nodular swellings are formed at the wrists, knees, and ankles. The most serious deformity is a narrowing of the inlet of the pelvis, which in the female may make normal delivery impossible in later life. Among the other signs and symptoms are sweating, restlessness, and flabbiness of the muscles, often giving the child a "pot belly." The serum phosphorus is markedly decreased.

Treatment consists in making good the deficiencies that may have been present. Cod liver oil was an old and well-proved remedy. An abundance of sunlight is desirable. Sunlight loses its ultraviolet rays when passed through window glass, for the short-wave rays are screened out by the glass. Special lead-free glass may be used in the nursery, or the child may be exposed to the light of a lamp capable of producing ultraviolet rays, such as the mercury vapor lamp or the carbon arc lamp.

Trauma

Trauma as a pathologic entity has already been considered in Chapter 3. However, a specific paragraph dealing with injury to bones is warranted, because of the frequency with which this occurs at all ages.

A fracture may occur without the skin's being torn; this is a simple fracture. If the broken ends of the bone project through the skin, the condition is a compound fracture. The great difference between the 2 types of fracture is that in the compound fracture there is danger of infection from the skin or air, which in the days before antisepsis and antibiotics often proved fatal. Compound fractures and battlefield wounds before the middle of the twentieth century were life-threatening. A greenstick fracture in children is a crack rather than a frank break of the pliable bone; it has been likened to the injury to a branch caused by bending a green twig. The relation of a pathologic fracture to some unrelated cause of weakening of the bone (carcinoma) has already been mentioned. Fractures of the skull are of particular importance, because even a minor crack may tear one of the numerous meningeal arteries that run in relation to the inner surface of the skull, with the possible development of a dangerous, or even fatal, meningeal hemorrhage.

The importance of fractures, generally speaking, is the extent to which the adjacent tissues are damaged or devitalized (hemorrhage), the extent of the systemic reaction (shock), the immediate complications (fat and other emboli), and the long-term complications (lack of union and loss of function). Naturally, the damage will depend on the areas of bone involved and on the nature of the injury. It is safe to say that current treatment emphasizes the use of immediate reduction and restoration of the patient to an ambulatory condition as soon as possible.

Infections of Bone

Although bone infections are much less common today, they require a few paragraphs.

The word **osteomyelitis** means inflammation of the bone (osteitis) and of the bone marrow (myelitis) (Fig. 25–6).

The inflammation is usually caused by gram-positive cocci, which generally gain access to the body through the skin, causing a boil, and are then carried to the bone by the blood stream. The disease is essentially one of children and adolescents in whom the bone is still growing, and it is 3 times as common in boys as in girls, probably because the former are more liable to trauma. As growth takes place only in the region of the epiphyseal cartilage, and as this is the part most abundantly supplied with blood vessels, it follows that the disease affects the end of the bone, usually on the side of the epiphyseal cartilage next to the shaft. Injury to bone is a common accessory factor, because this disease is apt to cause rupture of a small vessel, and the circulating staphylococci are able to settle down in the blood clot and grow rapidly. The injury may be a twist or a direct blow. The bones most frequently affected are the femur, tibia, and humerus.

The lesion begins as an abscess of the bone. As the result of acute inflammation, pus is produced and tends to spread down the medullary cavity and outward to the surface. When the pus reaches the surface, it raises the periosteum from the bone, and it may spread along the surface for a considerable distance. As it is from the periosteum that the bone receives a considerable proportion of its blood supply, it follows that a large area of the shaft may become devitalized and die. Such a piece of dead bone is called a sequestrum (Fig. 25–7), and in the course of time this becomes separated from the living bone by the action of the osteoclasts. The inflamed periosteum is stimulated to form a thick layer of new bone, which surrounds the sequestrum. In the new case, there are a number of openings through which purulent discharge escapes from the interior. One of the most serious results of the inflammation is thrombosis of the vessels in the marrow. The thrombi become heavily infected with staphylococci, and they may break down and be carried by the blood to the lungs and other organs, where they set up multiple abscesses.

From what has been said, it is apparent that osteomyelitis tends to be both a local and a

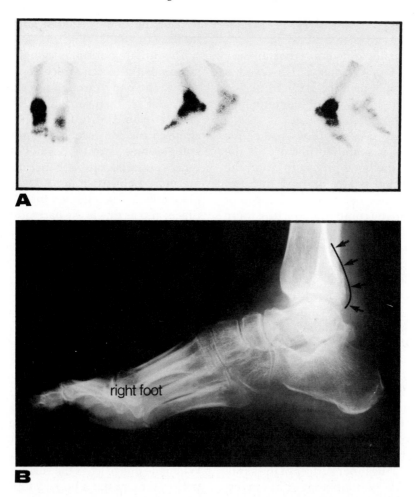

Fig. 25-6. *A,* This bone scan of the ankle in three views shows increased uptake (dark areas), which is consistent with osteomyelitis. A Gallium 67 scan would confirm that this case was due to inflammation. *B,* This conventional radiograph shows changes of periosteal elevation and inflammation at the arrows. This sign is typical of osteomyelitis.

general infection; the symptoms are therefore both local and general. The local symptoms are pain and tenderness at the end of a long bone, often in the region of the knee, together with heat, redness, and swelling—the classic signs, in short, of acute inflammation.

The general symptoms are those of any severe acute infection, i.e., high fever, chills, rapid pulse, marked leukocytosis, and the presence of bacteria in blood culture.

Fortunately, the entire picture of osteomyelitis has been changed since the introduction of antibiotic therapy. The only treatment for this disease used to be to open up the bone surgically, so as to allow the pus and the infecting organisms to escape. The condition is now treated by medical means, and if the

diagnosis is made early and correct treatment is started at once, the widespread bacterial infection described in the preceding paragraphs will be prevented. It is evident also that if the patient is properly treated, there will be no development of a sequestrum or of sinuses.

Tuberculosis of bone, like osteomyelitis, is a chronic disease. Like the acute disease, it affects the ends of the bones, but begins in the epiphysis much more frequently than does osteomyelitis. The bones most often attacked are the long bones of the arms and legs, the bones of the wrist and ankle, and the vertebrae. As in the case of acute osteomyelitis, the region of the knee (lower end of femur and upper end of tibia) is a common site.

The lesion consists of a slow destruction of the end of the bone, not a wholesale destruction, but a nibbling here and there, giving the bone a worm-eaten appearance, a word that implies dry rot. If the disease begins in the shaft, the epiphyseal cartilage is gradually eaten away and the epiphysis is invaded. From the epiphysis, whether it is infected primarily or secondarily, the disease spreads to the articular cartilage, which is eroded bit by bit, until the articular surface comes to be formed by the diseased and roughened bone.

Tuberculosis of the spine, also known as Pott's disease, used to be a frequent occurrence in children, although it may also occur in the adult. The disease affects 1 or more vertebrae, which it slowly destroys, just as the ends of the long bones are destroyed. The pressure from above causes the softened vertebrae to collapse, with resulting deformity of the spine, so that the child develops a "humpback." It is possible that Quasimodo, the hunchback of Notre Dame in Dumas's famous novel, had tuberculosis as a cause of his deformity (Figs. 25–8 and 25–9). A more serious result is pressure on the spinal cord, with the gradual production of paralysis of

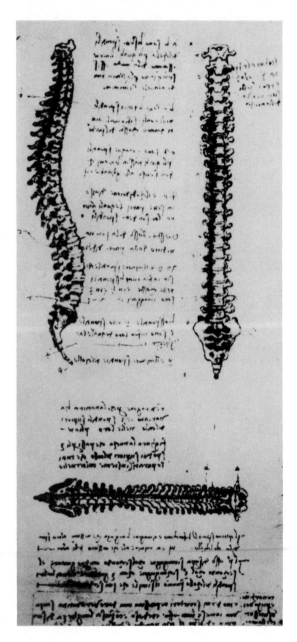

Fig. 25–7. This radiograph shows diffuse destruction of bone with periosteal reaction and an area of decreased density surrounding a single, dense bony island. This island is a "sequestrum" of necrotic bone, seen within a focal area of destruction. This is typical of osteomyelitis.

Fig. 25–8. These drawings by Leonardo da Vinci show the normal lateral curves of the thoracic, lumbar, and sacral spine.

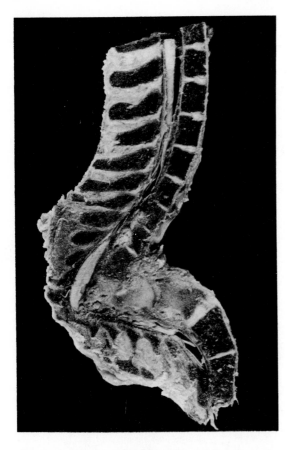

Fig. 25–9. This spine shows marked angulation, due to the presence of *tuberculosis* (Pott's disease). (McGill University, Department of Pathology Museum.)

the legs. A tuberculous or cold abscess may develop, the peculiarity of which is that it tends to spread along the psoas muscle, which passes from the lumbar part of the spine to the upper end of the femur. This psoas abscess, as it is called, will therefore appear in the groin as a soft swelling which may easily be mistaken for a hernia.

Whichever joint is affected, be it the wrist, the knee, or the joints of the spine, the first symptoms will be limitation of movement. This is natural, because no one moves a diseased joint more than is absolutely necessary. If the disease starts in the bone, symptoms do not appear until the joint is also involved, unless there is a place where the periosteum is close to the surface, as in the tibia, or shin. The joint is swollen, owing to tuberculous swelling of the synovial membrane. The affected limb tends to be shorter than the normal one, partly because of the bone destruc-

tion, but mainly because the epiphyseal cartilage, which is responsible for growth in the length of the bone, is killed. When the articular cartilage is destroyed and the roughened ends of the bones come in contact, pain develops. There may be no pain during the day, because the muscles around the joint contract and prevent movement from occurring. But when the child falls asleep, the muscle watchdogs are no longer on guard, and the joint may be moved, causing intense pain, so that the child wakes with a start and a cry. These pains are therefore known as "starting pains" or "night pains." For a long time, the patient may show none of the general symptoms of tuberculosis such as fever or loss of weight.

It is hardly necessary to add that modern antibiotic therapy has completely altered this picture, but one should be aware that there has been a resurgence of tuberculosis in many persons who have received steroids.

Legg-Perthes disease is the most common of a group of lesions known as aseptic or ischemic necrosis of bone. In Perthes disease, the lesion is confined to the head of the femur, but in other members of this group (known by other men's names), the epiphyses in a variety of bones are involved. The lesions are of clinical importance not because they cause any marked disability, but because they are so easily mistaken for bone tuberculosis. In all cases, the lesions represent a quiet necrosis of bone, aseptic and nonbacterial in character, and apparently due to ischemia, which develops for some unknown reason.

Perthes disease usually occurs in boys between the ages of 5 and 10 years. There is often a history of recent injury. The bone in the center of the epiphysis is fragmented, so that it may resemble fragments of mortar. As a result, the head of the femur becomes flattened and splayed. When healing occurs, the fragments coalesce and the bone regains some of its structure, but the flattening is permanent. The roentgenogram is absolutely characteristic, and it is by this means that a final diagnosis is made. The earliest symptom is a limp, accompanied by little or no discomfort. The condition must be distinguished from early tuberculosis in a child.

Syphilis of bone used to be a disease of great importance, but modern chemotherapy has changed a common type of lesion into a rarity, so that we may dispose of the subject with welcome brevity. It differs from tuberculosis in the following respects: (1) it affects the shaft of the long bones rather than their ends, (2) the joint is seldom involved, and (3) osteosclerosis with new bone formation is much more prominent than osteoporosis or rarefaction. Destruction of the bones of the nose and hard palate used to be common, so that the bridge of the nose fell in at the root (saddle-nose), and there might be a large perforation of the palate. It may avoid embarrassment to remember that not every saddle-nose is caused by syphilis.

Salmonella infections of bone in children are unusual; however, they seem to occur with some frequency in patients with sickle cell disease. The reason for this is unknown.

Tumors of Bone and Cartilage

We have already seen that bone is a complex structure composed of bone cells, periosteum, cartilage, marrow, and blood vessels. Tumors of various kinds may arise from any of these elements. For the purpose of this brief outline, however, bone tumors may be divided into primary and secondary, while the primary tumors may again be divided into benign and malignant.

Primary tumors. These may be benign or malignant. The 3 chief benign tumors are osteoma, chondroma, and giant cell tumor. The osteoma and chondroma are similar, the former consisting of bone cells and the latter of cartilage. Both are hard tumors that usually arise at the end of a long bone, although they may occur in practically any bone in the body. Being benign, they are localized and usually remain small, but occasionally they grow to a great size. When removed, they show no tendency to recur.

Giant cell tumor develops in children and in young adults, usually before the age of 30 (Fig. 25–10). It occurs principally at the ends of long bones, and the common location is the knee. It is highly destructive locally, but does not cause metastases or kill the patient. It consists of a soft, red, hemorrhagic mass, which greatly distends the bone and almost completely destroys it. This gives the highly char-

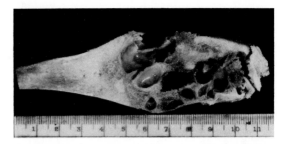

Fig. 25–10. Shown here are the large cystic spaces characteristic of **giant cell tumor** of bone. (McGill University, Department of Pathology Museum.)

acteristic roentgenographic picture of large bubbles separated by thin strips of bone. The tumor gets its name from the many giant cells that are seen in the microscopic section.

The 3 chief primary malignant tumors of bone are osteogenic sarcoma, Ewing's tumor, and multiple myeloma.

Osteogenic sarcoma is the most common of the 3 tumors. It is a disease of young persons between the ages of 10 and 30 and is rarely seen after the age of 50. The location is similar to that of giant cell tumor, namely, at the ends of the long bones, usually in the region of the knee joint. The tumor expands the end of the bone, so as to give it a "leg of mutton" appearance (Fig. 25–11). The periosteum is lifted from the bone by the tumor, and spicules of new bone are laid down, which radiate outward from the central mass, giving a characteristic "sun ray" effect in the roentgenogram. Spread takes place by the blood stream, and metastases often appear first in the lungs. Secondary growths in other bones are rare; multiple bone tumors suggest Ewing's tumor in the young and multiple myeloma in the middle-aged.

Ewing's tumor occurs at an earlier age than does osteogenic sarcoma, usually between the ages of 5 and 15. It is rarely seen after the age of 30. It involves the bone much more diffusely than does osteogenic sarcoma, giving rise to a uniform thickening. The tumor does not begin at the end of a bone. One of the more striking features of the disease is that, as the tumor progresses, other growths become apparent in many widely distant bones, particularly the flat bones, such as the scapula, sternum, vertebrae, and skull. The roentgen-

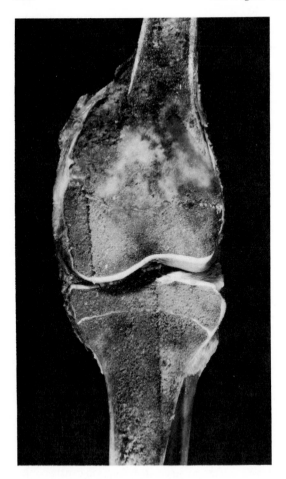

Fig. 25–11. Shown in the center of the upper field is a whitish mass replacing the normal marrow cavity. This is an **osteogenic sarcoma,** a primary malignant tumor of bone. Note the increase in size of the bone in this area. (McGill University, Department of Pathology Museum.)

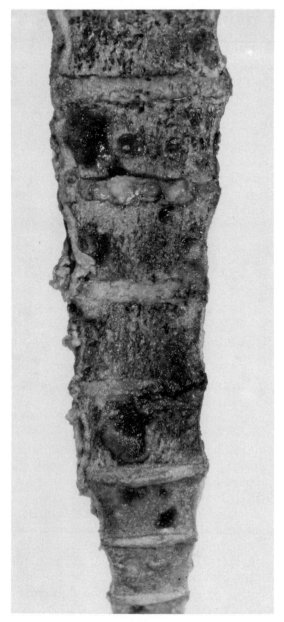

Fig. 25–12. This photograph shows the gross appearance of several vertebral bodies separated by intervertebral discs. The normal trabecular pattern has been replaced by currant-jelly reddish material, typical of **multiple myeloma.** (McGill University, Department of Pathology Museum.)

ogram shows diffuse involvement of the greater part of the shaft. There is a combination of bone formation and bone destruction; formation in the early stage, destruction later. The new bone on the surface may present a laminated appearance in the film, like the layers of an onion. One of the most striking characteristics of the tumor is its response to radiation; it may melt away like a lymphosarcoma, only to return later.

Multiple myeloma, also known as plasma cell myeloma, is composed of plasma cells, but these cells are responsible for one of the most important characteristics of the tumor (Fig. 25–12). As the name myeloma suggests, this is a tumor of bone marrow rather than of bone. It is usually multiple, and by the time

the patient comes to the doctor, a large number of the flat bones may be involved (Fig. 25–13). The age incidence is in striking contrast to that of Ewing's tumor; 80% of the cases occur after the age of 40 years. Huge amounts of calcium may be freed from the bones, with resulting high serum calcium

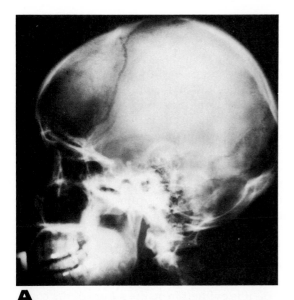

A

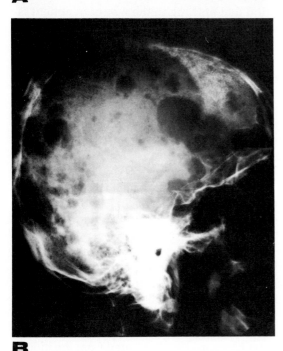

B

Fig. 25–13. *A,* This routine lateral roentgenogram demonstrates the appearance of a normal skull in lateral projection. *B,* This film shows the multiple "punched-out" lytic lesions consistent with a diagnosis of multiple myeloma or of metastatic tumor.

levels and deposits of calcium in the kidneys, so that pathologic fractures are common. Marrow aspiration shows tumor cells in the sternal marrow, even though there is no other evidence of a tumor. Recently, combined

chemotherapy and radiation have dramatically extended the life span of patients in whom this diagnosis has been established.

Plasma cells normally produce gamma globulins, so it is only natural that a neoplasm of cells should produce these and related globulins in excess quantity. The total serum proteins are raised to 10 mg or higher, and there is a marked inversion of the normal albumin-globulin ratio, owing to the great overproduction of gamma globulin by the tumor cells. In addition, there may be a copious excretion in the urine of a unique protein, the Bence Jones protein, which was recognized in the urine over 100 years ago. It appears as a cloud when the urine is heated to 55°C, disappears at 85° or on boiling, but reappears on cooling. The reason it is found in the urine and not in the serum is that its molecular weight is only half that of albumin, so that it can readily escape from the blood into the urine through the glomerular filter. It must be noted that Bence Jones protein is present in the urine in less than 50% of cases of myeloma, so that its absence does not mean that the patient is not suffering from the disease. Renal failure may occur in the later stages, and may be so severe as to lead to uremia and death. This may be because large numbers of renal tubules may be blocked by casts of abnormal protein, and the calcification already alluded to cannot improve the functional capacity of the kidneys.

Treatment of malignant bone tumors consists in surgical removal at the earliest possible moment, in the hope that metastases may not yet have occurred. Radiologic examination of the lungs must first be made, because if secondary growths are found in these organs, no treatment is of any avail. Some forms of sarcoma respond well to x-ray treatment,

Table 25–1. Estimated New Cases and Deaths From Some Cancers in 1974 (U.S.)

	NEW CASES	DEATHS
Sarcoma of bone	1,900	1,900
Thyroid carcinoma	7,900	1,150
Hodgkin's disease	7,100	3,500
Small intestine carcinoma	2,200	700
Lip carcinoma	4,000	225

and the tumor may disappear for a time, but the relief is only temporary, and sooner or later the tumor will recur. In general, as illustrated in Table 25–1, the prognosis for malignant tumors of bone is poor.

Secondary Tumors. Metastatic tumors of bone are carcinomas, the tumor cells coming from a cancer in some other organ. The most common forms of cancer that are likely to metastasize to bone are cancer of the breast, lung, prostate, and kidney (Fig. 25–14). The metastatic tumor destroys the bone, and the first indication of its presence may be the occurrence of a fracture from a trivial injury. Other evidence of the presence of a tumor in bone may be pain, of a constant and gnawing kind, or chemical evidence, such as the presence of elevated serum alkaline phosphatase or calcium. The bones commonly affected are the ribs, vertebrae, sternum, and skull (the flat bones), and the upper end of the femur and humerus. In all these bones, the marrow is of the red variety and is therefore well vascularized, and so it is natural that the blood-borne tumor cells will be arrested at these sites. It is evident from the nature of the condition that nothing in the way of treatment is of any avail.

Miscellaneous Bone Diseases

A condition known as **osteitis fibrosa cystica** (von Recklinghausen's disease) is characterized by highly porous and decalcified bones, which may be much deformed and curved, sometimes with the formation of bone cysts and spontaneous fractures of the rarefied bone. The decalcification is a manifestation of hyperparathyroidism, usually due to an adenoma, but occasionally to hyperplasia of the parathyroid glands, a condition that has already been described. The calcium removed from the bones appears in the blood, so that the serum calcium rises from 10 mg/100 ml to 15 or 20 mg, and the serum phosphorus is correspondingly low. The calcium may be deposited from the blood into the kidneys, giving shadows in the x-ray film, or it may form a single stone in the kidney.

Fibrous dysplasia of bone is readily confused clinically with osteitis fibrosa, but the pathogenesis of the 2 conditions is entirely different. Fibrous dysplasia is not related to hyperparathyroidism, but, as the name implies, is a congenital anomaly in the development of bone, with the formation of fibrous swellings that replace the bone and that give rise to deformities such as those of osteitis

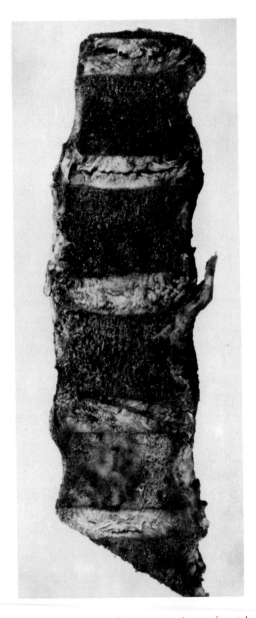

Fig. 25–14. Shown in this gross specimen of vertebral bodies and intervertebral discs is the replacement of the vertebral body in the lower portion of the picture by a firm, white tissue characteristic of **metastatic carcinoma** from the prostate. (McGill University, Department of Pathology Museum.)

fibrosa. There is no disturbance in the serum calcium and phosphorus.

Paget's disease is otherwise called osteitis deformans; it is a common asymptomatic radiologic finding in elderly people, estimated to be present in 10% of all those over 60 years of age. It is twice as common in men as in women, and it is usually clinically recognized because of pain in the back, hips, or pelvis. The full-blown case of this disease of unknown etiology may have deafness, increasing head size (Fig. 25–15), headaches, neuromuscular signs and symptoms, and heart failure. The diagnosis is established by radiologic and serum alkaline phosphatase determinations. Urinary hydroxyproline determinations may be elevated as the disease progresses.

The explanation for these manifestations, although we do not know the cause of the disorder, is that there is an increase in bone cell activity, beginning perhaps with increased osteoclastic resorption, followed by the increased laying down of new bone (Fig.

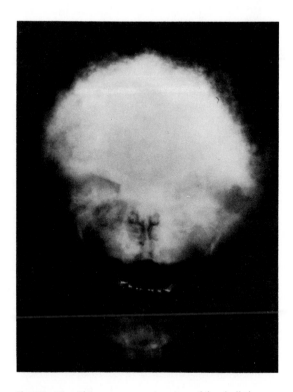

Fig. 25–15. This anteroposterior view of the skull shows a marked thickening of the cranial vault with densities typical of Paget's disease of the skull. This is called a leonine appearance.

25–16). This resorption and new bone formation proceeds rapidly with a change in the normal pattern of bone collagen and with the development of new vascular channels. The increased vascularity results in fistula formation, requires an increased cardiac output, and results in an increase in the temperature of the skin over the affected bones.

The complications of Paget's disease are structural deformities that may cause compression of spinal and cranial nerves and of the spinal cord, and the cardiovascular complications of heart failure following on the increased cardiac output, and finally, malignant change in the new bone. Osteogenic sarcomas are rare enough, but a patient with Paget's disease is at increased risk of developing this cancer.

JOINTS

Structure and Function

A joint is a structure of peculiar delicacy, and one that responds only too readily to injurious stimuli. When we consider the amount of stress and strain, not to mention abuse in sports, to which the joints are subjected in a long life, it is little wonder that disease of the joints is among the most common of clinical disorders. Man was not originally designed to stand upright, and so it is natural that the weight-bearing joints, in particular those of the lower limbs and vertebral column, should be among the principal sufferers.

A joint consists of 2 articular surfaces: a capsule or strong, fibrous structure, which joins the 2 ends of the bone together, and a synovial membrane, which lines the capsule and produces an oily fluid that lubricates the articular surfaces and ensures the smooth working of the mechanism. It now seems that the presence of lubricant and the health of the joint depend in some measure on the activity to which the joint is subject. Rather than having a totally destructive effect on joints, it seems more likely that moderate, regular exercise is beneficial, because it causes exchange of fluid between the underlying cartilage and the joint fluid. Any or all of these structures may be damaged by disease.

The Arthritides

Arthritis is a general term for inflammation of the joints, and we may arbitrarily divide all

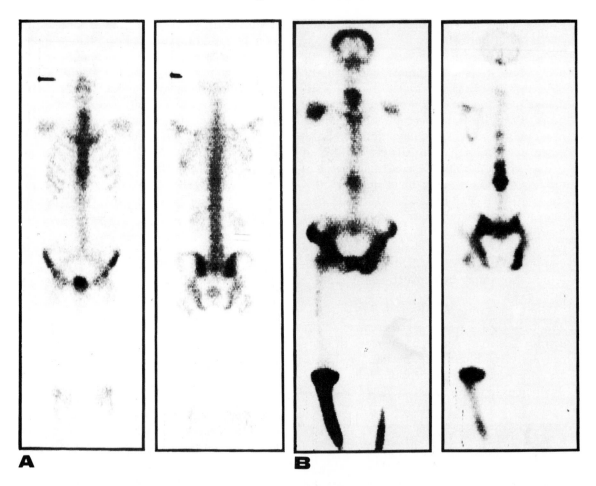

A   B

Fig. 25–16. *A,* This nuclear medicine scan, using technetium 99m methylene diphosphonate, which is a calcium-seeking agent that localizes in areas of active bone turnover, displays no skeletal abnormalities. The first scan of each pair shows the anterior bones, the second scan shows the posterior bones. *B,* This bone scan, using the same technique, shows increased uptake with areas of expansion of bone, particularly in the right lower limb and pelvis, typical of the appearance of Paget's disease.

inflammations of joints into acute or chronic forms.

Pyogenic or suppurative arthritis used to be the most important form of acute arthritis; bacteria were introduced through a wound, or spread to the joint from a bone that was the seat of acute osteomyelitis. Antibiotic therapy has now pushed this complication into the background. Gonorrheal arthritis, formerly an occasional complication of acute gonorrhea affecting many joints, has also passed into the realm of the forgotten, as the result of the present adequate treatment of the infection with penicillin in the acute stage of the disease. Rheumatic arthritis is the acute nonsuppurative arthritis of rheumatic fever. There is an acute synovitis with excess of tur-

bid fluid in the joint. Extreme tenderness is characteristic of the swollen and acutely inflamed joint. The inflammation usually undergoes complete resolution, but some permanent stiffness occasionally may persist. Traumatic synovitis is a good example of acute nonsuppurative arthritis, the inflammation being confined to the synovial membrane (acute synovitis), with no destruction of tissue and therefore no permanent stiffness. The synovial membrane is swollen, juicy, and congested, while the synovial fluid is increased in amount and cloudy.

The chronic arthritides are more common and disabling and we shall mention several types. Tuberculous arthritis used to be more common than it is today.

Tuberculosis of the joints is a disease of children and is usually secondary to tuberculosis of the adjacent bone, a subject that has already been considered. When it occurs in an adult, it is more likely to be primary in the synovial membrane, the infection having been carried by the blood stream from some distant focus. The synovial membrane may be even thicker and more voluminous than in rheumatoid arthritis, so that it may fill the entire cavity. The fluid is usually scanty, but highly fibrinous, so that it contains flakes of fibrin that may develop into foreign bodies known as melon-seed bodies or rice bodies. The destruction of the articular surfaces that may develop and the resulting clinical picture already have been described in connection with tuberculosis of bone, and will not be discussed here.

Rheumatoid Arthritis. This widespread,

tragic, and crippling disease is perhaps the second most common form of chronic arthritis. It is a chronic inflammatory condition that particularly affects the small joints of the hands and feet, although the larger joints may be affected later (Fig. 25–17). The condition usually occurs in women between 20 and 40 years of age. Rheumatoid arthritis is one of the greatest causes of disability in the north temperate zones, and it has been estimated that it is responsible for an annual loss of $200,000,000 in the United States. This is perhaps not remarkable when we consider that there are an estimated 2,000,000 persons who suffer from the disease in Canada and the United States, and that 200,000 are totally disabled.

ETIOLOGY. An enormous amount has been written about the cause of rheumatoid arthritis, a sure indication that little is known about

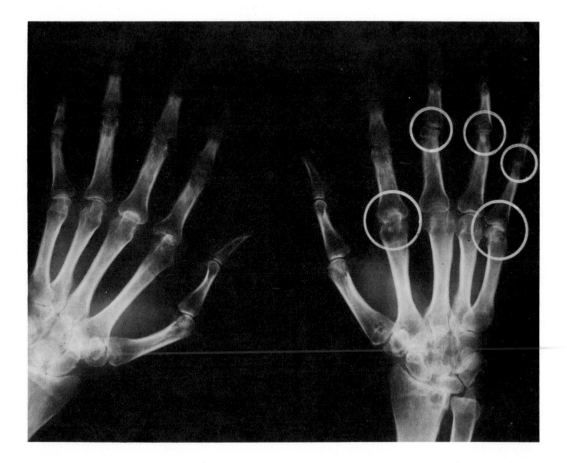

Fig. 25–17.   This conventional x-ray study of two hands shows narrowing of the metacarpophalangeal joints and of the proximal interphalangeal joints, with multiple erosions. This is consistent with the appearance of rheumatoid arthritis.

the subject. The most reasonable view appears to be that the arthritis is the result of a combination of minimal hematogenous bacterial infections with tissue hypersensitivity. The sensitization may be the result of a series of minor infections or a chronic focus that periodically discharges a few bacteria into the blood. At no time do the bacteria reach the joints in sufficient numbers to produce conventional lesions, but the tissues are constantly being sensitized, until finally 1 bacteremic episode culminates in a definite arthritis. Psychologic factors such as stress, operating perhaps through the adrenal cortex, seem to play a part. Marked and sometimes startling relief of the arthritic symptoms is common during the early months of pregnancy and is attributed to the increased availability of adrenal cortical hormones. This observation initiated the breakthough in the late 1940's that resulted in the biosynthesis of cortisone.

Laboratory tests support the idea of an immunologic pathogenesis. A specific agglutination reaction occurs when the serum of the arthritic patient is added to a suspension of a variety of particles. At first, the red blood cells of sheep, coated with tannic acid and sensitized with human gamma globulin, were used, but more recently a suspension of latex particles mixed with gamma globulin has been used. Only a drop of serum is needed, a positive latex fixation test being indicated by an agglutination of the particles visible to the naked eye. The latex particles simply act as inert carriers of gamma globulin, and the same is true of the coated red blood cells. The reaction seems to be due to the presence of a rheumatoid factor in the blood, which has now been isolated and shown to be a macroglobulin antibody or antigen-antibody complex. By fluorescence microscopy, it has been demonstrated that the rheumatoid factor originates in the lymphocytes and plasma cells of the lymph nodes and the hypertrophied synovial membrane.

LESIONS. The synovial membrane is primarily affected, so that the disease might be called synovioarthritis in contrast to osteoarthritis, the other great form of chronic arthritis. The pathologic changes resemble in certain respects those of joint tuberculosis, although it attacks many joints instead of 1, and does not lead to destruction of the bone. There is the same swelling of the synovial membrane with the formation of pulpy masses or fringes and tags, which cause the joints to be enlarged, the same gradual destruction of the articular cartilage, the same interference with the function of the joint that finally results in complete disability and fusion of the joint surfaces. The most significant feature is the superabundance of lymphocytes and plasma cells, suggesting the immunologic character of the process. The periarticular soft parts share in the inflammatory swelling and edema. The ligaments become softened and absorbed, thus contributing to the deformities that form so distressing a feature of the end picture of the disease. Subcutaneous inflammatory nodules may be found in the neighborhood of the affected joints, particularly in the arms (Fig. 25–18). The course of the disease is marked by curious remissions and exacerbations, and at any stage the progress may be arrested. However, as in tuberculosis, the injury to the joint is permanent, and the hands and feet are twisted, gnarled, and crippled for life (Fig. 25–17). On this account, and because of its commonness, the disease is of great economic importance, since it is a disease of great morbidity but small mortality; it cripples, but does not kill.

SYMPTOMS. The symptoms are pain and swelling of the joints, together with increasing stiffness and disability. In the later stages, the joints become distorted and deformed. During the exacerbations, the patient often suffers from mild fever, malaise, anemia, and sweating.

TREATMENT. During the acute phase of the rheumatoid disease, rest is of great importance, together with methods of physiotherapy that help to restore function and particularly to prevent crippling deformities. The maintenance of correct posture of the joints involved provides for the maximum of function when the acute process subsides. Relief of pain with mild analgesics is necessary in most cases. The use of cortisone and ACTH in rheumatoid arthritis has proved beneficial in many cases. This treatment is accompanied by relief of pain, decrease in swelling, and increase in movement of affected joints. Un-

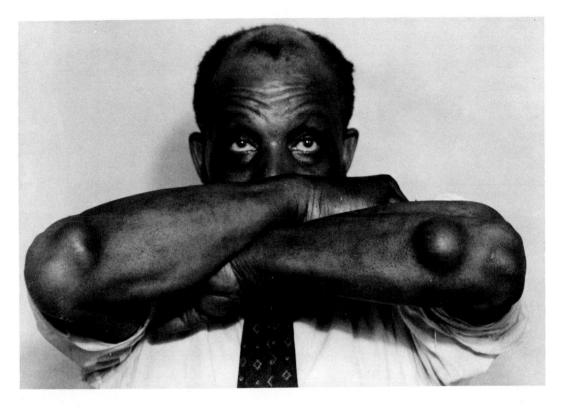

Fig. 25–18. This photograph shows large nodules on the ulnar surfaces of both elbows. These are typical **rheumatoid nodules,** although in this instance they are somewhat larger than usual. (McGill University, Department of Pathology Museum.)

fortunately, in many instances this improvement is not maintained after the drug is stopped.

Ankylosing spondylitis is an unusual variant of rheumatoid arthritis, and the name means stiffness of vertebral joints. Although rheumatoid in character, it differs from rheumatoid arthritis in that it has a high male sex incidence and a negative serologic reaction for the rheumatoid factor. The articular cartilage is destroyed, fibrous adhesions develop, and eventually bony fusion occurs with calcification of the intervertebral discs. The condition begins in the sacroiliac joints and spreads slowly upward, ending with extreme rigidity, which may justify the term poker back. In early cases, the roentgenogram shows a fuzziness of the apposed surfaces of the bones, followed by calcification and later ossification of the vertebral ligaments (Fig. 25–19). In exceptional cases, there are lesions of the aortic valve and ascending aorta. It is a particularly tragic disease, because so often it affects young people.

Osteoarthritis. Probably the most common type of arthritis, osteoarthritis is the term applied to a degeneration of articular cartilage and bone, so that it might well be called degenerative arthritis. In this it differs from rheumatoid arthritis, which is primarily an inflammation of synovial membrane, and indeed it differs from that condition in almost every respect. Thus it is as common in men as in women; it is a disease of the later period of life; there are no general symptoms; the large joints are commonly involved, often only 1 joint, particularly the hip; and there is no true ankylosis or fusion between the articular surfaces. The small joints of the hands and feet may also be involved, the knuckles becoming greatly swollen and knobby (Fig. 25–20).

The lesions are primarily atrophic, followed later by localized hypertrophy. The articular cartilage undergoes degeneration and softening, so that it is gradually worn away, until the underlying bone is exposed. There is atrophy of the central part of the bone, so that much of the head and neck of the femur may

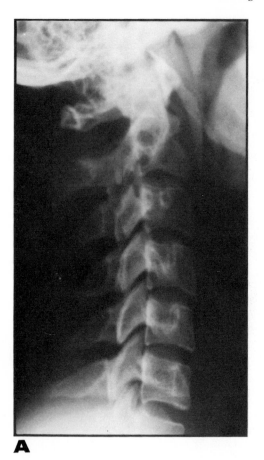

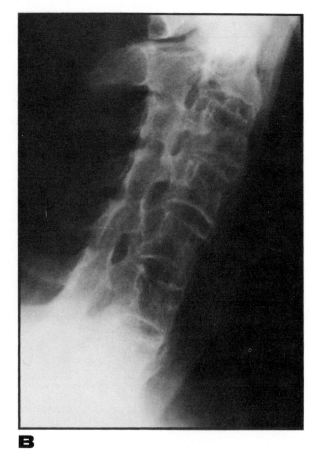

A   **B**

Fig. 25–19. *A,* This roentgenogram demonstrates a normal cervical spine in lateral projection. *B,* This demonstrates the bamboo spine appearance of *ankylosing spondylitis,* due to calcification in the anterior spinal ligaments and to fusion of the posterior joint spaces.

disappear. The peripheral part of the cartilage has a much better blood supply than the central area, and overgrowths of cartilage, which resemble candle drippings, develop at the edge of the articular cartilage, a condition known as lipping of the joint. These cartilaginous excrescences tend to become ossified, so that the atrophied head of the bone is surrounded by a ring of bony excrescences, which may gravely limit movement and form a striking feature in the roentgenogram. Thinning of the intervertebral discs is also a feature of diagnostic importance in the film.

The etiology of osteoarthritis is obscure. It is a degenerative condition in which the aging process, probably associated with local ischemia, plays a leading part. If a joint is continually exposed to trauma, as in a trade or in professional athletes, it may show the char-

acteristic changes. The condition may indeed be described as "wear and tear" arthritis.

Lesions of the Intervertebral Discs

When we consider the important joints of the body, we are apt to forget the intervertebral discs (Fig. 25–21), and yet there is perhaps no part of the body in which strain and movement are so constant, and in which impairment of movement, especially when associated with pain, so cripples the full enjoyment of life. Owing to man's upright position, the discs are subject to constant strain for which they were not originally intended, so that degeneration in later life is more common than in any other organ, with corresponding loss of the normal cushioning function.

The nucleus pulposus is the essential part of

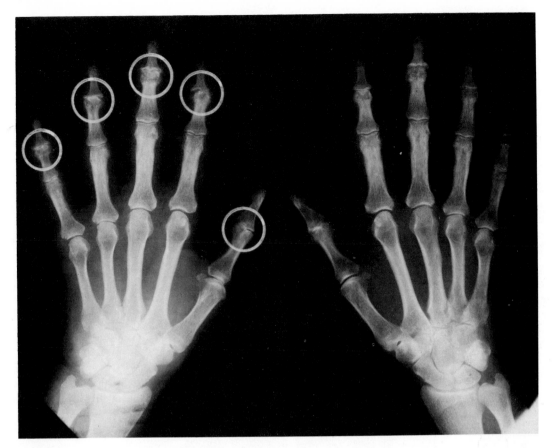

Fig. 25–20. This routine x-ray study of the hands shows narrowing of the distal interphalangeal joints with multiple erosions and subarticular sclerosis. This is consistent with erosive *osteoarthritis*.

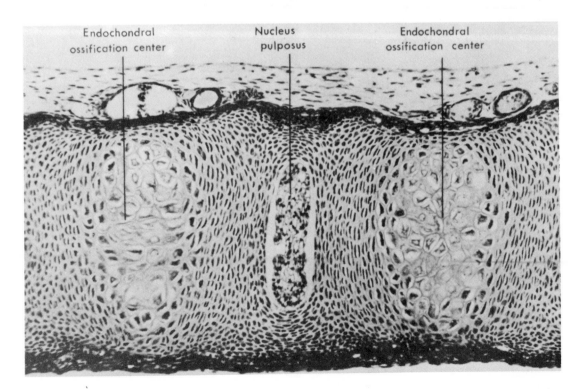

Endochondral ossification center   Nucleus pulposus   Endochondral ossification center

Fig. 25–21. This histologic preparation shows the appearance of the ossification center and the nucleus pulposus in sections of a developing vertebral column. (From Bloom, W., and Fawcett, D.W.: *A Textbook of Histology*, 10th Ed. Philadelphia, W. B. Saunders, 1975.)

the disc, and plays the chief role in pathologic changes. It is a highly elastic, semifluid mass compressed like a spring between the vertebral surfaces. In youth, it presents a marked elastic turgor, depending on the fluid content of the tissue. With age, this turgor gradually diminishes, and it is completely lost in various degenerations.

An intervertebral disc may protrude or herniate into the vertebral canal and press on the spinal cord or stretch the nerves. This is the condition known popularly as "slipped disc." Protrusions occur at the sites of the maximum anterior spinal curvature, that is to say, the region between the fourth lumbar and first sacral, and between the fifth and seventh cervical vertebrae (Fig. 25–22). The cause of the protrusion varies. Most common is trauma, either sudden, as in fall from a height, or repetitious, as in heavy labor that involves lifting. The turgid nucleus pulposus is confined by a circular band of fibrous tissue, the anulus fibrosus. When this tissue is torn or degenerates, the disc is forced backward into the canal. In many cases, no cause can be suggested.

The chief symptoms are low back pain and sciatica or pain passing down the back of the leg along the course of the sciatic nerve, symptoms that carry little threat to life, but they may interfere greatly with living. In addition to the sensory disturbances, there may be severe spasm of the muscles of the back, causing marked disability. It is possible to localize the lesion accurately by clinical observations in over 75% of cases. Excision of the protruded disc is required in only a small proportion of cases.

TENDONS

The tendons in which the muscles terminate are nonvascular and therefore are relatively immune to inflammation, but the ten-

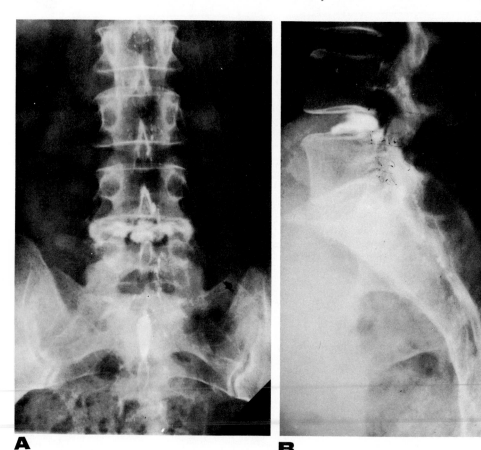

A   **B**

Fig. 25–22. *A*, This shows an anteroposterior view of the spine following a myelogram. *B*, This shows a lateral view. Here the myelogram demonstrates a protruded intervertebral disc.

don sheath in which they move, especially at the wrist and ankle, is often inflamed. Suppurosynovitis may result from spread of infection from a septic process in the fingers. Tuberculous tenosynovitis is marked by the formation of tuberculous granulation tissue, which causes a "white swelling" such as that seen in tuberculosis of a joint. Traumatic tenosynovitis is the most common form, occurring in piano players, in typists, and in other persons whose tendons are subjected to excessive use. Fibrin is laid down on the surface of the tendon and the wall of the sheath, so that crackling is felt when the tendon is used.

Ganglion is a cystic swelling that develops in connection with a tendon sheath. The common site is the back of the wrist. It is attached to the outer surface of the tendon sheath and begins as a proliferation of the connective tissue of the sheath, which undergoes mucoid degeneration, with the formation of numerous small cysts that eventually fuse to form a large cyst filled with soft mucoid material.

A bursa is a sac lined by synovial membrane, containing viscid fluid and situated at points where friction would otherwise develop, usually close to a joint. Those with an interest in words may care to know that bursa is derived from the Latin word meaning a purse, from which comes our bursar, the man who holds the purse. Traumatic bursitis is usually caused by chronic and repeated irritation (housemaid's knee, student's elbow), but occasionally it is due to a blow. A common site is the region of the shoulder, involving the subdeltoid and subacromial bursae (subacromial bursitis), with pain most marked on motion, so that the arm is not moved and a "frozen shoulder" results. The bursa is distended with serous fluid (hydrops). Tuberculous bursitis usually takes the form of hydrops with melon-seed bodies, or the bursa may be filled with granulation tissue.

MUSCLE

Structure and Function

Muscle is the largest single kind of tissue in the human body (Fig. 25–23). It is a unique organ in that it is capable of converting chem-

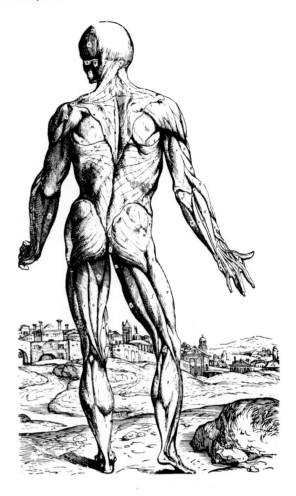

Fig. 25–23. This drawing by Leonardo da Vinci shows the major muscles of the back in man.

ical energy into mechanical work; it can fine-tune a violin or lift a thousand pounds. The elements of skeletal muscle are structural proteins that respond to a well-organized set of chemical pathways, arranged in neat packages. The unit of skeletal muscle is called the motor unit and consists of a single motor neuron located in the spinal cord with its axons distributed to the muscle fiber, where the connection is called the neuromuscular junction, or motor end-plate (Fig. 25–24). Muscle fibers are cylindrical, elongated cells that extend from points of attachment (tendons), usually bridging joints. Each muscle fiber has 1 or many nuclei, an intricate cytoplasmic membranous system (which provides a surface across which ions flux), mitochondria in large numbers that provide the ATP, and a system of myofibrils (Fig. 25–25).

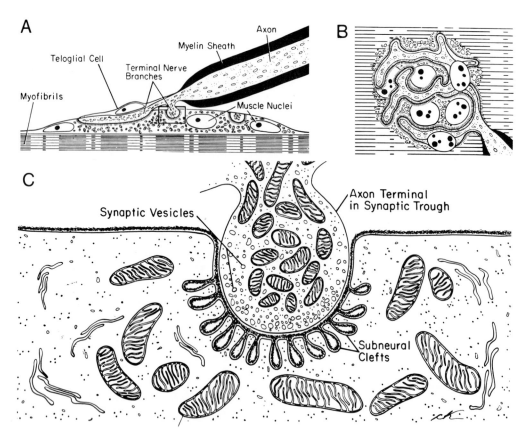

Fig. 25–24. These drawings show the appearance of a neuromuscular junction. (From Bloom, W., and Fawcett, D.W.: *A Textbook of Histology,* 10th Ed. Philadelphia. W. B. Saunders, 1975.)

Most skeletal muscle contains approximately equal amounts of 2 types of fibers arranged in a mosaic pattern, but each type belongs to 1 motor unit (Table 25–2). Until 1978, it was believed that the fiber types in a given muscle were genetically determined, and that marathon runners or sprinters were born, not made, because the proportion of red or white muscle fibers were fixed. Recent experiments have shown that fiber types in muscle can be shifted from white to red by physical training. It has been known for a longer time that muscles respond to demand by adapting to meet the demand; in skeletal muscles, this is more clearly seen in the response of the weight lifter's muscles, which show an increase in the numbers of myofibrils. Endurance runners, on the other hand, show that their muscles adapt by increasing the number and size of mitochondria. A third type of adaptation is a change in the cytoplasmic enzyme systems with respect to their content of a variety of enzymes. A training program will enable muscles to use substrate more efficiently. Glycogen may be made more rapidly and calcium may be more easily transported. A fourth adaptation is the vascular supply to skeletal muscle; there is considerable evidence that increased training creates a microvascular bed that enhances oxygenation to the muscle. And, finally, we know that just as bone loses its mass with disuse, muscle atrophies remarkably quickly if it is not used. There is no such biologic phenomenon as hoarding or saving your strength; the unused muscle wilts like a cut flower on a hot summer day.

Thus we have at least 4 different levels at which muscle may be affected by disease:

(a) loss of motor neuron that leads to denervation atrophy;

(b) interference with conduction or disuse that leads to atrophy;

(c) interference with neuromuscular junc-

SKELETAL MUSCLE

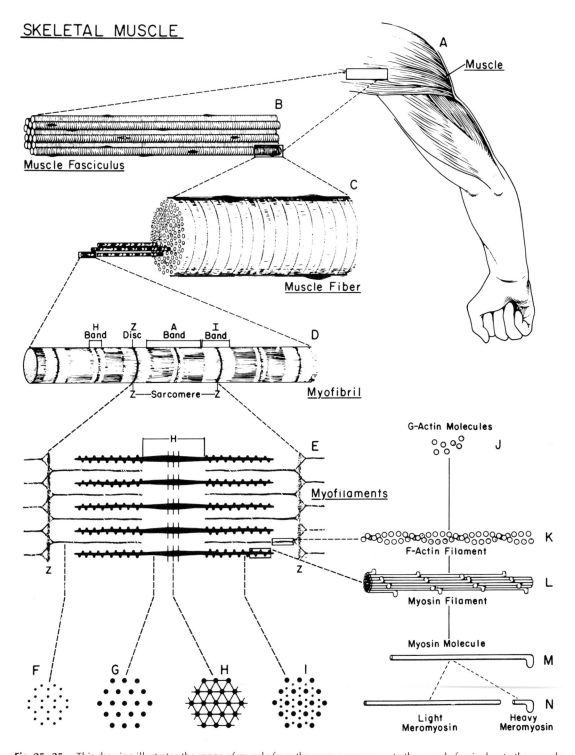

Fig. 25–25. This drawing illustrates the range of muscle from the gross appearance to the muscle fasciculus, to the muscle fiber, to the muscle myofibril, to the myofilaments, and, finally, to the myosin and actin molecules. The cross sections are shown in F, G, H, and I. (From Bloom, W., and Fawcett, D.W.: *A Textbook of Histology*, 10th Ed. Philadelphia, W. B. Saunders, 1975.)

Table 25–2.   Muscle Fiber Types

	SLOW (RED)	FAST (WHITE)
Mitochondrial enzymes (SDH)	High oxidative capability	Low oxidative capability
Creatinine phosphokinase		
mMoles/min/g protein	13.1	16.6
Lipids	High Content	Low Content
Glycogen enzymes (Phosphofructokinase)		
mMoles/min/kg	9.4	20.0
Capillary supply	++++	+++

(Adapted from Saltin, B., et al.: Fiber types and metabolic potentials of skeletal muscles in sedentary man and endurance runners. Ann. N. Y. Acad. Sci., *301*:3, 1977.)

tion function that leads to loss of strength (myasthenia gravis);

(d)   primary disease of the muscle cell itself (storage disease or acquired disease, as in alcoholic myopathy).

A few additional points may be mentioned. Potassium affects muscle metabolism. Both too little potassium (hypokalemia) and too much potassium (hyperkalemia) will cause paralysis of muscle. Transaminase (glutamic-oxaloacetic transaminase, abbreviated GOT) is an enzyme present in greatest concentration in cardiac and skeletal muscle. Destruction of this tissue results in a liberation of the enzyme into the serum, and an estimation of the transaminase serum level is a valuable test for determining the presence and extent of such injury, more particularly in myocardial infarction. Muscle is unusually adaptable to training. Nowhere is there better evidence of the general concept that many diseases are disorders of adaptation. Muscle responds to different stimuli by modifying its structure to meet the demand, provided the stimuli are within normal limits and recur sufficiently frequently to permit adaptation to take place. This is the basis for all sports training. It would be unwise for us to consider more than 1 or 2 of the many obscure diseases that may involve the muscles and tax the resources of the physiotherapist.

The general term myopathy is often applied to muscle disease. Unfortunately, this term is used casually, and it is not clear in many instances where the lesion lies, if indeed we know. This term may be applied to any disease or syndrome in which the patient's symptoms and/or physical signs can be at-

tributed to pathologic, biochemical, or physical changes occurring in the muscle fibers or in the interstitial tissues of the voluntary musculature.

Hereditary myopathy, an example of which is **muscular dystrophy,** is a rare group of diseases of muscle characterized by progressive muscle wasting and weakness, accompanied, for a time at least, by a paradoxical increase in muscle size. Histologic features of muscle affected by these diseases include variations in fiber size, some fiber necrosis, and phagocytosis of muscle fibers with replacement by proliferating connective tissue and fat. Muscular dystrophy disease generally begins in childhood, shows a marked familial tendency, and attacks only males, but it is transmitted only by females. The large muscles of the hip and, later, the shoulder, are chiefly affected. In striking contrast to some other diseases of muscle, for example, myasthenia and myotonia, the dystrophies show change in muscle structure. The biochemical lesion of the muscular dystrophies seems to be a loss of storage of creatine by the affected muscle that can be detected as an increased loss in the urine. The serum transaminase level is raised, especially when there is much pseudohypertrophy of the muscles. This observation suggests, then, that the disease is located in the cytoplasmic membranes of the muscle cell and is genetically determined.

For over 100 years, sporadic cases of episodic muscle weakness or paralysis, often occurring at night and improved by exercise, have been recognized and are called periodic paralysis. We now know that they may be traced to disorders of potassium, and there are at least 3 different types: 1 with high, 1 with low, and 1 with normal serum potassium levels. The familial cases appear to be inherited as an autosomal dominant with complete penetrance. Central core disease, another rare disorder characterized by muscle weakness, can be traced to a cellular disorder in which there is an absence of the normal sarcoplasmic reticulum in the muscle cells. However, both these disorders are so infrequent that it is exaggerating their importance even to mention them.

From a clinical viewpoint, a decrease in muscle mass is an important problem, but it is difficult to quantify, unless there is a normal opposite limb or side for comparison. From a patient's point of view, one of the most common serious symptoms is weakness, although it may be generalized and not have its origin in the muscular system itself. This is a problem for the careful questioner to solve. However, atrophy of a muscle or of a group of muscles, as we have said, may have its origin at several different levels in the hierarchy of musculoskeletal function.

Inflammation of Muscle

When a young adult without previous training engages in strenuous athletic exercises such as running, jumping, or kicking a football, or in long marches, he or she may rapidly develop firm swelling, aching pain, and paralysis of the muscles in front of the tibia. In its milder form, this is known to athletes and their coaches as "shin splints." A more severe form, in which the affected muscles actually become necrotic, carries the more academic title of the anterior tibial syndrome. It is believed that the strenuous exercise of an untrained muscle liberates excess quantities of metabolites, which lead to swelling of the muscle, and that this swelling, in turn, causes pressure, first on the veins and later on the arteries, resulting in ischemic necrosis. It is now clear that such extraordinary work as running the marathon or skiing the 85 km Vasaloppet cross-country ski race may cause reversible metabolic injury to muscle that can be recorded in abnormalities of serum enzyme levels (e.g. creatine phosphokinase). The gradual increase in intensity and dura-

tion of such work, as with appropriate training, which cannot be done in days or weeks but only in months and years, to allow adaptive change to take place, decreases this risk.

Volkmann's contracture usually occurs in young persons and affects the muscles of the forearm. It is commonly associated with the pressure of splints or a tourniquet or with hemorrhage resulting from a fracture. Within a few hours of the injury, burning pain develops in the hand or forearm, followed by contracture of the fingers, which become fixed in the flexed position. This is an example of ischemic necrosis or infarction of the muscle, the ischemia being caused by arterial spasm resulting from injury to the vessel wall.

There are 2 kinds of ossifying myositis, or **myositis ossificans,** in which bone is formed in the muscle. Traumatic myositis ossificans is a common condition that may result from repeated injury to a muscle or from a single severe injury, especially when accompanied by hemorrhage. There is a danger that the lesion may be mistaken for an osteogenic sarcoma of bone invading the muscle. Progressive myositis ossificans is fortunately a rare progressive disease, which commences in childhood and slowly kills the patient. Soft swellings develop in the muscles, which are gradually converted into bone, until the body is finally enclosed in a bony sheath that makes breathing impossible.

There are other causes of inflammatory disease in muscles such as parasites and disorders of the immune system. Trichinosis is a relatively common muscle disease in the world, caused by the larvae of the round worm *Trichinella spiralis*, which is ingested in uncooked meat. The larvae have a predilection for muscle rich in cytochrome and seem to migrate selectively to the heart, extraocular muscles, and diaphragm, but they may be found in all muscles. These organs may also be the focus of our attention because they are crucial to our well-being. As with many diseases, the symptoms are directly related to the numbers of parasites, and muscle pain is the outstanding feature. The presence of large numbers of eosinophils in the peripheral blood, together with a history of eating raw pork, hamburger, or bear meat, will point to the correct diagnosis. Today, skin testing helps with the diagnosis, which should always be suspected when the eosinophil count is elevated.

Treatment is directed to alleviating the inflammatory response, and steroids are used. There is some evidence that at least 1 Arctic expedition foundered because the castaways all became severely infected with the trichina after eating polar bear.

Dermatomyositis is a collagen vascular disease in which inflammatory muscle disease may be the principal clinical complaint, and, as are the others of this group, it is attributed to an autoimmune disorder.

Miscellaneous Muscle Disease

Myasthenia gravis, with its ominously descriptive name, is characterized by great weakness or rather fatigability, most marked in the muscles of the face, which is blank and expressionless, but shared to a lesser extent by all the voluntary muscles. After the muscle has been used a few times, it rapidly loses its power of contraction, only to regain it as rapidly with rest. In extreme cases, the limbs are so weak and easily fatigued (myasthenia) that they can hardly be lifted. This is not the same as paralysis.

The cause of the condition remains unknown, despite the enormous amount of work that has been devoted to the problem. No morphologic lesions to explain the astonishing weakness can be found in the motor nerve cells, the nerves, or the muscles they supply. It is presumed that there is some defect at the myoneural junction (Fig. 25–24), where the nerve enters the muscle fiber, perhaps a biochemical abnormality that blocks the transmission of the nerve impulse to the muscle. Normally, the chemical substance acetylcholine is released at the myoneural junction when impulses are passed across it, and this substance is believed to stimulate the muscle fiber to contract. The enzyme cholinesterase is normally present and destroys whatever acetylcholine remains after the contraction is effected. It has been suggested that in myasthenia gravis there is either an overabundance of cholinesterase or too little acetylcholine. Treatment consists of the use of drugs antagonistic to cholinesterase. Neostigmine is by far the most useful drug during acute attacks. In many cases, there is hyperplasia or a neoplasm of the thymus gland in the neck. What this association means is unknown, but in occasional cases, surgical removal of the thymus has been attended by dramatic improvement.

Passing reference may be made to the myotonias in spite of their rarity, because the condition is the reverse of myasthenia. As the name indicates, there is an increase of muscle tone, with the result that there is prolonged contraction of a muscle after cessation of the stimulus, the fibers being unable to relax. When a movement is repeated a number of times, the muscles warm up, and normal contraction and relaxation may then occur.

Muscle Tumors

Despite the fact that there are over 600 separate muscles in the human body and muscle tissue may account for more than 40% of the body mass, muscle tumors are extraordinarily rare. The only one worth mentioning is the **rhabdomyosarcoma,** and it occurs most frequently in the lower extremities. The diagnosis is made by the identification of cells with striations. The treatment is radical excision. The five-year survival rate is less than 10%; therefore these are tumors that we do not like to diagnose.

SYNOPSIS

Bone is composed of cells, matrix, and mineral. It depends on hormones, diet, and physical activity for its well-being.

Osteoporosis, osteomalacia, and rickets are important metabolic disorders of bone.

Osteomyelitis and tuberculosis are significant infectious diseases of bone.

Osteogenic sarcoma, giant cell sarcoma, multiple myeloma, and Ewing's tumor are important primary tumors of bone, but metastatic cancer from breast, prostate, and lung are more frequent.

Different types of arthritis (inflammatory, traumatic, degenerative) are an economically important cause of chronic disability.

Muscle diseases are of diverse etiologies, and, in comparison to the mass of muscle tissue in the body, these disorders are remarkably rare.

Terms

Osteoblast	*Rickets*	*Tenosynovitis*
Osteoclast	*Osteomyelitis*	*Muscular dystrophy*
Osteocyte	*Osteogenic sarcoma*	*Myasthenia gravis*
Osteoporosis	*Arthritis*	*Rhabdomyosarcoma*
Osteomalacia	*Osteoarthritis*	*Myopathy*

FURTHER READING

Editorial: Pathogenesis of osteoarthrosis. Lancet, 2:1131, 1973.

Adams, R.D., Denny-Brown, D., and Pearson, C.M.: *Diseases of Muscle,* 3rd Ed. Hagerstown, Md., Harper & Row, 1975.

Barker, D.J.P., et al.: Paget's disease of bone in fourteen British towns. Br. Med. J., 1:1181, 1977.

Drachman, D.B.: Myasthenia gravis. N. Engl. J. Med., 298:136, 1978.

Furukawa, T., and Peter, J.B.: The muscular dystrophies and related disorders. J.A.M.A., 239:1537, 1978.

Harris, J.B.: Muscular dystrophy and other inherited diseases of skeletal muscle in animals. Ann. N.Y. Acad. Sci., 317, 1979.

Keiser, H., et al.: Clinical forms of gonococcal arthritis. N. Engl. J. Med., 279:234, 1968.

Nordin, B.E.C.: Clinical significance and pathogenesis of osteoporosis. Br. Med. J., 1:571, 1971.

Orlander, J., et al.: Low intensity training, inactivity, and resumed training in sedentary men. Acta Physiol. Scand., 101:351, 1977.

O'Sullivan, J.B., and Cathcart, E.S.: The prevalence of rheumatoid arthritis. Ann. Intern. Med., 76:573, 1972.

Sinkovics, J.G., and Plager, C.: Bone sarcomas: clinical experience. Can. J. Surg., 20:542, 1977.

Siris, E.S., et al.: Paget's disease of bone. Bull. N.Y. Acad. Med., 56:285, 1980.

Care of the Patient

26

One of the first duties of a physician is to educate the masses not to take medicine. —OSLER

This text has thus far concerned itself with diseases and their causes. In this chapter, we digress slightly, in order to examine disease and its ramifications in real life. We look at disease from the point of view of the diseased person and his caretakers; from the perspective of care of the patient. This is a large subject; indeed, the care of the patient is the fundamental reason for the existence of the medical and paramedical professions. This care covers the diagnosis and treatment of disease, preventative and palliative measures, hospitalization, home care, rehabilitation, and support of many kinds.

THE PATIENT

Each patient is unique, with a unique personality and past experiences. How he reacts to health professionals and how they react to the patient will vary, depending on these characteristics: age, the nature of the problem, his resources, personality, and how the patient feels. Naturally, the characteristics of the caretakers, the institutions, and the patient's culture are important in this relationship.

The patient may be more than 1 person. If a man recovering from an open heart operation needs counseling on when and how to resume his sex life, then he and his wife may become a "group" patient. If a child is dying, the whole family may become a patient. This concept is especially important in psychiatry, since family dynamics are often involved in a patient's disease process. All these persons require patience and understanding.

Many different persons are involved with most patients. Some are professional: physicians, nurses, physiotherapists, occupational therapists, pharmacists, speech therapists, social workers, clergymen, to name a few. Others are not professional, but may nevertheless be even more closely involved; they are the relatives and friends of the patient. A recent study showed that the most important emotional support the patient received in hospital was from other patients, not from the medical staff.

BECOMING A PATIENT

When a patient arrives at the physician's office, the first step is taken in the patient's care, which is to attempt to establish a diagnosis. In order to do this, the physician employs 3 different disciplines of the science and art of medicine. These are: (1) history taking, (2) physical examination, and (3) laboratory investigations.

History taking elicits the patient's description of what is presently wrong, and how the symptoms have changed or developed since he first realized that something was wrong. The history taker then asks questions that he considers to be relevant to the complaint, as well as questions about the patient's general health, past history, and family history.

The medical history serves 2 important functions:

It describes the chronology of the patient's troubles and reveals the pattern of the disorder. It is said that the physician can make the diagnosis from the history in more than half the cases seen. In addition, the clues given in the history will allow the examiner to focus on specific organ systems during the physical examination.

The history represents the patient's first contact with the health professional. It is during this initial meeting that a working relationship is established between the patient and the medical profession. The rapport, or lack of it, established in the initial interview often affects the subsequent relationship.

Taking a good history is a most difficult task (particularly if the patient is confused, delirious, vomiting, or unconscious). It demands all the skill, insight, and patience of the physician, and often it is the most valuable of all the examinations.

One oft-forgotten purpose of history taking is to establish confidence between the patient and physician that can permit subsequent examination of a more direct and intimate kind, and will permit the examination to be less threatening because of the confidence that has grown out of the dialog during history taking. Some modern physicians are too harried and hasty, and they forget the great therapeutic value of the interview and its importance in securing the cooperation of the patient, since, after all, it is during this phase of the relationship that the patient reveals his troubles and in his own way describes the disease. Osler used to say, "Listen to the patient. He is telling you the diagnosis."

Physical examination means the employment of what used to be called the 5 senses, more particularly, sight (inspection), touch (palpation), and hearing (auscultation). Of these, inspection appears the easiest, yet it distinguishes the really skilled from the ordinary observer; palpation of the abdomen, breast, and other parts reveals much to the sensitive, educated fingers. Auscultation involves the use of a stethoscope. Smell also plays a role in diagnosis, but has often been superseded, as have these other modalities, by modern laboratory methods.

We might distinguish objective data from subjective impressions in the physical examination. It is customary to measure temperature (with a thermometer) rather than to estimate it, to measure the blood pressure (systolic and diastolic, usually in both arms), to count the pulse (for a minute to determine whether it is regular or irregular), and to count the respirations. These are called the **cardinal signs** and provide a most valuable guide to the general health or severity of illness of the patient, as well as frequently pointing the way to disorders of a specific system.

Modern science has vastly extended the range of the unaided senses. A wide variety of fiberoptic scopes, radiologic techniques, and machines such as the electrocardiograph have revolutionized diagnosis. (Some of these have been described in detail in Chapter 3.) All of them represent extension and amplification (rather than replacement) of our special senses, by amplifying the sounds or the sights, by permitting us to look into otherwise hidden places, or by translating from 1 sense to another.

Laboratory examinations. It is in the field of laboratory examination of material from the patient that modern medicine has made the greatest leap forward, involving an incredible development of new methods, particularly those that are biochemical. Laboratory methods, which were first developed in connection with research, are quickly applied to the patient.

The explosive development of new methods of laboratory investigation during recent years is responsible for a natural tendency to place undue reliance on these techniques as opposed to the more traditional clinical methods outlined. It is well to recognize the limitations of laboratory procedures, as well as their considerable value. The data are compiled by fallible human beings, who are as liable to errors of technique and of interpretation as are all persons. Mistakes may be made by those responsible for the collection and labeling of the material to be tested. Finally, it must be remembered that the normal figure for any given chemical value is variable from 1 person to another, just as height and weight vary. Moreover, we must recognize that even emotions can influence biochemical processes, although these processes are controlled by enzyme systems, ultimately under the direction of genes.

These modern diagnostic tools have been of invaluable assistance, but we must be careful not to rely too heavily on them for another reason; no diagnostic machine can yet replace the human nervous system. The unaided human senses can accomplish more than any machine. Richard Selzer provides a fascinating example of diagnosis using only the human senses in his book, *Mortal Lessons*. This procedure is described at the end of Chapter 3 and is worth reviewing.

From the pattern of the history, the physical examination, and the laboratory data emerges a set of possible explanations for the fever, or the pain, or the jaundice of the patient. This list of possibilities is called the **differential diagnosis** because a number of different disease processes may explain the patient's particular symptoms and signs. It is the responsibility of the physician to put on his thinking cap and to construct such a list, and then to decide which additional tests might make the diagnosis more certain, or which therapeutic trial he should embark on in managing the patient's discomfort.

THE HOSPITAL

The modern hospital is an institution that houses secondary and tertiary care facilities. (The initial contacts that a patient has with the health care system, e.g., primary family physician, constitute primary care; secondary care usually refers to specialties, e.g., surgery, and tertiary care is comprised of subspecialties, e.g., plastic or neurosurgery.) As specialties have developed from technologic advancements, the hospital, and in particular the university teaching hospital, has become as essential way of dispensing sophisticated diagnostic procedures and therapies. However, this process has created some disadvantages for the care of the patient. Often, the patient feels alienated from the medical staff because of the size of the institution. Much too often, the referring family physician (if the patient is lucky enough to have one) does not have admitting privileges to the institution and is made to feel an outsider or a bother by busy house staff. The referring physician may have valuable information about the patient and his medical history and should be encouraged to visit the hospital to discuss the patient. This is particularly important if the patient's mental status was compromised on arrival at the hospital, casting doubt on the completeness and accuracy of the history obtained at that time. If the primary physician is not associated with the hospital, it is rare that he and his patient's new physicians meet. The patient's care, at worst, may become fragmented and discontinuous, and, at best, repetitive in the inquiry. This situation is unfortunate, but is not in itself serious. What is serious, however, is that often no member of the normal house staff fills the role of interpreter of medical care, which the primary physician has previously assumed. In fact, no member of the house staff assumes complete responsibility for the patient; he or she becomes the part-time patient of several physicians, and the full-time patient of none. Thus the patient is left without anyone in direct control, or responsible for his care, to whom the patient can communicate his wishes and fears, and without a single person who communicates the results of diagnostic procedures and the prognosis of the disease.

The alienation that the patient experiences can corrode the keystone of the medical profession—the physician-patient relationship. Without it, the modern advances of medicine cannot be used. The failure to keep appointments and the refusal to take prescribed medicine are common symptoms of alienation. The most obvious symptom is the exponential rise in the number of malpractice suits, which in themselves further erode the physician-patient relationship.

When several physicians become involved in 1 case (as is frequent), another result is that the concept of the patient as a whole person disappears. The cardiologist is concerned with the patient's heart, the endocrinologist with the patient's hormones, the gastroenterologist with the gastrointestinal tract. The whole patient is lost in the mass of component parts, like the loose pieces of a jigsaw puzzle. This problem stretches beyond medicine and into the specialties of health care: physiotherapists, dietitians, pharmacists, and so on, each of whom is preoccupied with his own piece of the puzzle. The nursing staff may become the patient's most important contact under this circumstance, since nurses are with the patient 24 hours a day and are aware of all other professional contacts and actions, medical and paramedical.

Teamwork and emphasis on team effort and collaboration represents an attempt to rectify this situation, to put the pieces of the puzzle together. In some psychiatric institutions, the psychiatrists, psychologists, social workers, and nurses meet regularly as a team to discuss the patients they all see. Together, they pool their information, create a total picture, and establish a team strategy for dealing with the patient's problems. At least 1 general hospital has tried this same approach, including doctors, nurses, physiotherapists, and pharmacists on their teams. One result has been a significant reduction in medication errors. However, whether they work as a team or not, all the professionals involved are concerned with the patient and do their utmost to promote his recovery.

Medicine certainly has changed from the cramped office occupied by the kindly, graying physician so often sketched by Norman Rockwell on the cover of the *Saturday Evening Post*. However, the patient still expects the concern for the individual captured in Rockwell's drawings, and it is still the goal of members of the health team. Today, the care of the patient must include the most up-to-date diagnostic and therapeutic regime suited to the situation, but the concern typified by the "old-fashioned M.D." should not be substituted with modern technology, but rather, should remain the basis of care.

Nursing. When the patient is safely in bed, the nurse becomes the most important member of the team concerned with his care. There are endless services by which the nurse ministers to the patient's comfort and contributes to his eventual recovery. If he is to receive rest, both physical and mental, which we have already seen to be so essential, it is the nurse who is best qualified to provide it.

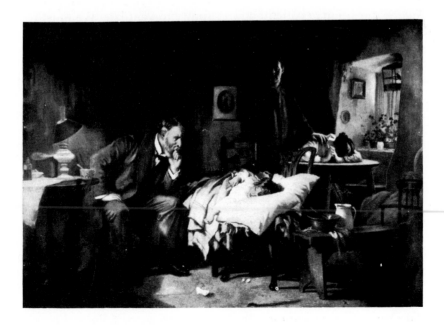

Fig. 26–1. The Doctor. (Luke Fildes.)

The nurse must exercise keen observation of the patient, together with accurate recording of any changes in the symptoms and physical condition, including the functioning of the bowel and bladder. A broad cultural education with knowledge of past and current events, enabling the nurse to converse with and interest the patient, is a valuable asset. Together, the nurse and the physician form the fundamental basis of the medical team. If the nurse fails to record and to communicate the details of the patient's function accurately, brilliant diagnosis and skill on the part of the attending physician can in no way make up the lack. The degree to which the nursing staff recognizes the needs of the individual patient is often reflected in the success and reputation of the hospital as a whole. In 1 particular neurologic institute, the quality of the nursing care alone materially increased the surgeons' success and decreased the postoperative complications. The physician and nurse must work together as a team with successful communication in both directions.

Mental Health. Being sick is rarely a pleasant experience, and being hospitalized can be difficult and threatening for some persons. When a person becomes a patient, he is usually required to give up certain rights, such as privacy, dignity, self-destiny, and independence. Those who pride themselves on these values may find the transition to patienthood harrowing, and may even become "management problems." A managment problem is a two-way street—the patient behaves in a way that is inconvenient for the staff, and vice versa.

Treatment. Medical and paramedical treatments are far too numerous and complicated to be described here. However, a few general measures and the subject of drugs are worth our attention, because they apply to most patients. Two important measures taken to promote comfort and recovery are rest and diet. The greatest physicians are Dr. Rest and Dr. Diet.

Perhaps **rest** is the most important single therapeutic measure in combating disease. A sick animal does this by instinct, when it crawls into the bushes and lies low. It is difficult to explain on scientific grounds the exact manner in which rest helps the sick person. All infections are benefited by rest, which may be general or local. An example of the value of local rest is afforded by immobilization of an infected hand by a splint or a sling. By this means, upward spread of the invading organisms along the lymphatics as a result of muscular movements is reduced to a minimum. Another example of local rest to an organ is the use of light diets or predigested foods for gastrointestinal disorders.

It is important, however, to remember that rest is not simply a state of inactivity, of freedom from toil. There must be rest of the mind as well as of the body, relaxation and freedom from unnecessary worry. Mental fatigue is often more harmful than physical fatigue and more difficult to relieve. Sometimes the best way of resting a tired person is by changing from mental work to recreation through physical activity. The patient's worries and anxieties can often be relieved by an alert and concerned medical staff who are willing to spend time with the patient. Often the anxieties about a surgical procedure can be alleviated or ameliorated by a detailed explanation of what is to be expected. Too often, however, tranquilizers—the omnipotent Valium and Librium—are prescribed without first making efforts to discover the source of the anxiety. The patient may also have more nonmedical concerns and may need an opportunity to ventilate. We must remember that, in all probability, a patient's normal resources for ventilation are inaccessible now that he is in the hospital. Inconvenient visiting hours and lack of privacy may prevent the patient from using friends and relatives for this purpose. In these cases, it is important for the staff to be alert and available to listen. Often it does not matter who is the listener, whether nurse, doctor, clergyman, or the cleaning lady, so long as he knows how to listen.

Rest can be overdone, especially in the aged. When the octagenarian takes to bed for too long, he may never be able to get out of it again. Prolonged disuse of an organ inevitably leads to deterioration of function, to be followed sooner or later by disintegration of structure. The dangers of prolonged rest in bed, particularly for the elderly, have been summarized as follows: "Look at the patient lying in bed. What a picture he makes with the blood clotting in his veins, the lime draining from his bones, the scybala stacking up in his colon, the flesh rotting from his seat, the urine leaking from his distended bladder, and the spirit evaporating from his soul." Prolonged bed rest has been much over-prescribed.

Correct **diet** is assuming a position of ever increasing importance in the treatment of disease, as well as in the preservation of health. This illustrates the need for an expert dietitian in a well-organized hospital. Proteins are traditionally the principal source of material for the maintenance and repair of tissues. Such maintenance and repair may be specially needed in febrile and other diseases in which there is marked breakdown of tissue. Intravenous hyperalimentation is assuming a greater and greater role in the management of severely ill patients. Vitamins and minerals, such as iodine, calcium, and iron, are obviously vital in the treatment of dietary deficiency diseases. Low-protein diets are equally important in the treatment of liver and kidney disease, in which the diseased organs are unable to excrete harmful protein or metabolites properly. Low-sodium diets are frequently prescribed for certain types of cardiovascular disease (e.g., hypertension) and edema, associated with retention of sodium, which holds fluid in the tissues.

On the nurse rests the responsibility of seeing that the patient eats the prescribed diet; he must report to the doctor if the patient does not do so. The regulation of fluids may be as important as the regulation of food. When there is much fluid loss, which may be due to vomiting or diarrhea, that loss must be made up. Conversely, when the tissues are water-logged, as in myocardial failure, the intake of fluid must be diminished.

Drugs. These agents have many different functions, and any specific drug may have several functions. Drugs put people to sleep, lower their blood pressure, and cure their bacterial infections. Human life from conception to death is influenced by drugs. Needless to say, they play a tremendous role in therapeutics, but, unfortunately, they are not without their side effects. They tend to be like the curly haired girl in the nursery rhyme— when they are good, they are very, very good,

but when they are bad, they are horrid. The side effects of drugs (or drug reactions) tend to fall into 1 of several categories.

EFFECTS DUE TO THE DRUG ITSELF. Many drugs have well-known side effects, and these are considered before the drug is prescribed. For example, some of the antineoplastic agents result in temporary baldness. In the treatment of leukemia, this is obviously a minor consideration. The patient is forewarned and, though distressed, quickly warms his head with a wig or a hat.

AN IDIOSYNCRATIC DRUG REACTION. Many drug allergies fall into this category. These are reactions that are known to occur, but that occur rarely and unpredictably in any given person. Penicillin allergy is an example. The importance of any allergy is to inform the patient of its existence, so that the drug will not be administered again inadvertently.

Improper dosage can be caused by the patient or the physician, but most commonly by both. For example, if a depressed patient takes too many sleeping pills in a suicide attempt, the fault lies with the patient. However, the physician is not blameless; he prescribed either a large number of tablets or a drug known to be a potentially suicidal agent.

A prescription is often written but not explained fully to the patient, and improper dosages are taken through misunderstanding. Often, the "dose," though generally correct, is wrong for a given patient. For example, a drug excreted by the kidney must be reduced in a patient with impaired renal function. It is, therefore, obligatory for the physician to look for evidence of renal failure in a patient to whom he wishes to give the drug.

DRUG INTERACTION. A not unusual event in any medical clinic is the arrival of a patient carrying a large shopping bag filled with unlabeled syrups, pills, and suppositories, which are the legacy of several generations of physicians at several hospitals. The patient is usually still taking a small percentage of the medication regularly, and often takes more as the condition worsens. Each drug alone might be of benefit (as it no doubt was when prescribed), but together the drugs worsen the patient's medical problems or create new ones. As the saying goes, too many cooks spoil the broth. Sometimes the problem is not the interaction per se, but rather, indiscriminate drug combinations. The classic case usually cited is antibiotic therapy. When a patient is hospitalized with septicemia, the patient's blood is cultured and he is given several antibiotics immediately. The culture results return in 2 days, and the antibiotics are adjusted once the organism is isolated. However, sometimes the adjustment is not made, because cultures were not taken or because of faulty reasoning (the patient is getting better and no one wants to change the antibiotics). Organisms that are resistant to the prescribed antibiotics then grow, and the patient is left with unusual bacteria, fungi, or problems against which the usual antibiotics are obviously ineffective.

PLACEBO EFFECT. In many situations, non-specific drugs are given for the purpose of helping the patient to have a night's sleep or to allay anxiety, and these drugs may in all honesty be directed at relieving the patient's symptoms. However, the mere action of giving a pill has a large positive effect on many patients because of our only too human trait of suggestibility. The readiness to believe is common. One professor sprayed water around a classroom and told the students to raise their hands as soon as they detected an odor. Seventy-three per cent of the class signified that they smelled the odorless water. In Latin, placebo means I shall please, and it is currently used in the medical context of a medicine given to suggest that treatment is being given, when the pill may in reality be of little or no benefit. Although placebos are used occasionally in clinical trials, one should not underestimate the important effect of faith in the practice of medicine. It is well recognized that inert medications and minor nostrums may provide relief to the patient, and this is testimony to the faith, confidence, and trust that the patient has in his caretakers.

Prevention. The most effective "treatment" of any disease clearly is its elimination through prevention. Immunization against bacterial and viral diseases is the obvious example. Other preventive measures are just as important, though not as obvious. Prenatal classes and visits, diet counseling, screening for inborn errors of metabolism in newborns, and visual and auditory testing are other examples.

Basic research fits into the category of prevention, although its application is often not apparent until several years after discoveries have been made. In the late 1940's, a pragmatist might have argued that government funding should be channeled into portable iron lungs and special treatment centers for poliomyelitis victims. However, basic research in tissue culture paved the way for the isolation of the virus that caused polio and the development of a vaccine. In retrospect, the funding of the research has paid for itself many times over in actual money saved in the treatment of polio victims, let alone the saving in human suffering. The opportunities for basic undirected research must be maintained despite economic recession.

Modern theories of prevention include a popular notion that healthy habits can keep someone alive by avoiding the common causes of premature death—cancer, heart disease, and stroke. However, it should be kept in mind that we really do not understand the pathogenesis of all diseases, and thus our prevention rationale may not be as valid as we think. It is only theory, arising out of **association** of disease with life-style, not demonstrated causality. As Lewis Thomas has said in *On Magic In Medicine:*

"The popular acceptance of the notion of Seven Healthy Life Habits, as a way of staying alive, says something important about today's public attitudes, or at least the attitudes in the public mind, about disease and dying. People have always wanted causes that are simple and easy to comprehend, and about which the individual can *do* something. If you believe that you can ward off the common causes of premature death—cancer, heart disease, and stroke, diseases whose pathogenesis we really do not understand— by jogging, hoping, and eating and sleeping regularly, these are good things to believe even if not necessarily true. Medicine has survived other periods of unifying theory, constructed to explain all of human disease, not always as benign in their effects as this all is likely to be....

"Nobody can say an unfriendly word

against the sheer goodness of keeping fit, but we should go carefully with the premises."

PREPARATION FOR DISCHARGE

At a certain point in the patient's progress, the patient, the physician, and the staff who have been active in his care begin to think about discharge from the hospital. Discharge-related questions arise: What is this patient's home like? What kind of situation will he return to? Will the family be able to care for the patient if he needs it, and cope with any problems that will arise? A patient, for example, may be left with an open wound; some operations on the bowel involve incisions that are not sewn up because of the danger of fecal contamination. Instead, the wound is packed with gauze that is changed and washed frequently, and the incision is allowed to heal from the bottom up (healing by second intention). This takes much more time, so the patient will take a large wound-care problem home. Who would help with this? In addition, any person who has experienced a major operation requires about 6 weeks before his energy level returns to its preoperative level.

Helping the patient and the family prepare for discharge can be an important part of care of the patient. We shall take the example of a young child who has just been hospitalized and is a newly diagnosed diabetic. Preparing this child's parents for homecoming involves many hours of teaching by physicians, nurses, and dietitians. The parents must learn how to care for their child at home, how to give injections, how to monitor their child's insulin requirements, how to recognize crises such as insulin shock, how to juggle the new diet and nutritional regime so that the child eats the right number of calories, and somebody must make sure that they understand and retain this information. This is additionally difficult because the parents are bound to be anxious, perhaps too anxious to learn.

A first hospitalization for alcoholism-related problems affords another kind of discharge problem. When discharged, the patient may well be returning to a home situation that seems guaranteed to make him ill again. Here, the social workers of the hospital become involved. If some attempt has been made by the staff to examine the patient's problem, rehabilitation and suitability for self-help groups such as Alcoholics Anonymous should be discussed. Alcoholism is a topic frequently avoided and regarded as hopeless by hospital staff. It certainly will be hopeless if no attempts to alter the situation are made. However, on the chance that this and other difficult psychosomatic problems have some solutions, it is the responsibility of the staff to investigate.

The patient may not be discharged to his home, but to a rehabilitation center. Rehabilitation may have already begun in the hospital through physiotherapy, occupational therapy, and related disciplines. These play a fundamental role in helping the patient to regain the use of a disabled or impaired body part, so that he can return to a former level of functioning as quickly as possible.

Finally, if the patient will require any home services, these should be arranged before discharge.

HOME CARE

Care of the patient has not finished when the patient leaves the hospital. Indeed, for many, it has only just begun. Professional concern, given on a regular basis, is of tremendous value to the patient and the family, who may know little about medicines, dressings, and peculiar new symptoms. Each new problem is likely to send them spiraling into chaos, unless they know someone they can trust and can call on when necessary.

Caring for a sick person at home can be difficult for the family. One big problem is isolation; our health care system is simply not set up to care for patients at home, so patients and their families tend to become isolated from the medical community in many instances. Any elderly person who is disabled or weak, in pain, or unaccustomed to being awake for more than a half-hour obviously finds the task of coping impossible at times. The elderly desperately need physicians who make house calls. It is unfortunate that home care, which is infinitely cheaper than institutional alternatives, is rendered so difficult by the present North American system. (It is also unfortunate for the physician that he does not visit the home, because this means that the patient can be far more easily depersonalized on arrival at the hospital).

Home care of any bedridden patient can be a monumental job. The patient must be kept clean, as mobile as possible, guarded from pressure sores, fed, hydrated, medicated; urination and defecation must be closely monitored, and, most important, the patient must be kept comfortable. At home, there are no shift changes and no days off. There is no dietary staff to prepare special diets, there are no physiotherapists with expertise in exercise, no nurses constantly present to monitor medication and symptoms (unless at tremendous expense, which few can afford).

However, there are resources for patient care, and it is up to the family to locate these and to exploit them fully. Visiting nurses are invaluable and available in most communities; visiting physiotherapists are also available in some places. If the patient is lucky enough to have a family physician, he can always be reached by phone, though perhaps not for urgent problems. Many pharmacists are taking an active role in the use of medicines and are usually happy to discuss drugs and their uses and side effects. If there is a clergyman, he can also be a valuable resource. He may know much about what the community has to offer, and more important, he may be able to counsel both patient and family. In some communities, there are services that provide homemakers, "sitters," and then there are special organizations that provide information and help, such as the American Cancer Society, the National Hospice Association, and others, which can be found in the classified telephone directory under "Social Service Organizations."

TERMINAL CARE

Terminal care refers to the care that a patient receives while dying. It is a separate category because it has its own special problems, some of which represent the greatest challenges of medicine and life.

Before we deal with terminal care, we must define what we mean by terminally ill. How do we know when a patient is terminally ill? Obviously something is indicated from signs and symptoms, or from tissue diagnosis, which may fall into an identifiable pattern. The first question the physician must ask is: Do the patient's symptoms reflect the terminal phase of the disease, or do they result from a different, treatable condition? For example, a patient may be treated for colonic cancer and recuperate, and for several months have no symptoms. When he reappears at the hospital with abdominal pain, it will probably be assumed that cancer has recurred. If the patient goes into shock two days later, he may be assumed to be terminally ill, but it could be a ruptured appendix, an incarcerated inguinal hernia, or some other treatable condition. For this reason, it is crucial that the patient have a complete physical examination and history. It still happens occasionally that a patient who is assumed to be terminally ill dies or is withheld treatment for a condition that, on autopsy, is found to have been treatable (and unrelated to the assumed terminal disease).

The terminal patient has been defined as someone nearing death from progressive, unrelenting illness that cannot be arrested or reversed in our present state of knowledge (or ignorance). The physician should investigate the symptoms to convince himself that this is indeed the case. Having reached this decision, several issues need to be dealt with, and some of these will be discussed here.

1. What does the patient know about the condition, and how does he feel about it? All staff members need to know the patient's state of mind, otherwise care becomes uncoordinated and based on the wrong assumptions. The easiest way to discern this information is for the physician to ask the patient what he understands about the illness. This provides the patient with the opportunity to tell the physician, directly or indirectly, how much he wants to know. Usually he will ask questions, and these should be answered simply and truthfully.

It has often been noted that dying patients know that they are dying, even when told little or nothing about their condition. For most people, the truth dawns gradually, even when they do not ask and are not told. Some do not wish to discuss it, and we should respect their wishes. Even terminally ill children, who are frequently told nothing, come to know that they are dying. The various stages through which they learn this—through watching their distressed parents and relatives, frequent hospitalization, discussions with other sick children, and finally watching a fellow patient die of the same disease—have been outlined by Myra Bluebond Langner in her book *The Private Worlds of Dying Children.* This fact is a good reason for dealing with these patients truthfully; lying to them will only give rise to doubts, disbeliefs, and erosion of trust between staff and patient. This can be far more devastating than the truth.

Once the patient knows or suspects that he or she is dying, he may have any of several reactions, which have been well documented in recent years. Common emotional responses outlined by Kübler-Ross include denial, anger, bargaining, depression, and acceptance. An understanding of these responses will greatly help those professionals who deal with dying patients. Hinton has found that about one-quarter of patients in 1 study show acceptance and positive composure to their fate. They will comment that they are dying, and that they have had good lives. They speak positively of this feeling of consenting to life's ending. About one-quarter acknowledge that they are dying, with slight regret, but no distress. One-quarter are distressed, and one-quarter say little or nothing about it. Acceptance was found to be more common in the elderly, and those with young children were more likely to discuss the fact that they were dying.

2. How can the patient be made comfortable? There are some who consider that physical, mental, and spiritual comfort for those who are terminally ill can best be accomplished in the home or in a hospice, and adherents to this view are increasing. The term "hospice" once referred to a house or shelter, usually kept by a religious order, that provided rest for pilgrims and strangers. Today, however, it refers to a special kind of care for the dying. The hospice concept of care is to make the patients physically and mentally as comfortable as possible, with dignity and as much joy as possible. Hospice care may be given in a regular hospital, where some have installed palliative care units for this purpose, or in a special hospice care facility run by specially trained professionals.

Death is frequently associated with pain in the lay mind, but this is not necessarily the case. Should the patient suffer pain, however, there is no reason why he should not be totally relieved of it. The cause of the pain must be ascertained, and treatment directed at the cause. The use of narcotics to treat intractable pain in the dying is commonplace today. At times, physicians and nurses are overconcerned about tolerance with these drugs, and out of caution provide less relief than is needed. Risk of tolerance is real, but that should not be a barrier to the use of narcotics in terminal care. Tolerance is far better than the alternative, whereby the patient becomes incapacitated with pain in his greatest hour of need.

Skilled nursing care can provide a great deal of comfort for the dying patient. Careful positioning and attention to hygiene and physiologic functions can prevent many uncomfortable complications. Attention to psychologic needs and flexibility on the part of the nurse can also bring great comfort. Above all, the patient should feel that the staff are doing their utmost and that they will not abandon him.

3. When should life-support or heroic measures be withdrawn? Efforts to preserve life become unethical at a certain point in the patient's progress, and outright useless toward the end; but exactly what constitutes a heroic measure, and when it should be withdrawn, and who sanctions the withdrawal, can become complicated issues.

Most persons feel that this should be the patient's decision, and, as a result, many states have enacted laws providing for "living wills"—legal documents that give patients their right to refuse heroic measures when in a terminal condition. The patient's autonomy has been thought to be the best way of insuring that any actions taken are strictly in the interest of the patient. Thus the patient decides, and the doctor carries out his wishes. However, it is not always so simple. Jackson and Youngner have described 6 problems that can greatly complicate the heroic-measures decision:

(a) Ambivalence of the patient. The patient may oscillate between allowing life-supporting procedures and forbidding them. In this case, the staff does not know which of the patient's wishes to honor.

(b) Depression. The patient may refuse life-supporting therapy because he is depressed and has given up. However, if the depression lifts (for example, if temporary discomforting symptoms pass) he may request therapy.

(c) Refusal of life-support may, like an attempted suicide, be a plea for help and attention.

(d) The patient may refuse treatment out of fear, realistic or not, of the treatment.

(e) The wishes of the family and those of the patient may conflict. For example, the patient may state that he wishes life-supporting therapy to continue, and then may lapse into a delirious state from which he cannot communicate. The family may wish at this point that no heroic measures be taken. Whose wishes should be honored?

(f) The staff may assume that a comatose patient with a terminal and painful condition would not want heroic treatment, when in fact this may not be the case.

Detailed examination of the patient's rationale for this decision, and discussion with the family at the time of the decision, may help to avoid some of these situations.

4. How is the patient's family coping? The family should be fully informed of the patient's progress. If they are kept in the dark, they may become anxious, and this anxiety may be manifested as hostility towards everyone and everything connected with their dying relative. They should also have opportunities to express their own feelings. Guilt, frustration, and fear are all intermingled with grief, and someone should let them know that these feelings are normal, and that the staff understands. Finally, they need to have some indication of the patient's life expectancy, but this should not be too specific, and they need to be forewarned about possible new developments in the patient's course.

In conclusion, it is not our purpose here to outline all aspects of care of the patient, but merely to put disease into the perspective of the patient and his caretakers. Disease does not appear in isolation; its diagnosis and treatment may be greatly compounded by the psychosocial circumstances of the sufferer. We talk frequently of such concepts as the compliance of the patient, the will to live, the difficult personality, and stress, all of which we suspect influence the development and outcome of disease. Health professionals who deal with disease must usually cope with far more than disordered structure and function of a particular organ. We would be remiss in not drawing to the attention of the reader that disease is not only an abstraction, but also that it exists in reality in the form of persons who need help.

FURTHER READING

Bordley, J., III, and Harvey, A.M.: *Two Centuries of American Medicine.* Philadelphia, W. B. Saunders, 1976.

Crichton, M.: *Five Patients, The Hospital Explained.* New York, Alfred Knopf, 1970.

Dubos, R.J.: *Mirage of Health: Utopia's Progress and Biological Change.* New York, Harper and Row, 1959.

Engel, G.L.: The care of the patient: art or science. Johns Hopkins Med. J., *140*:222, 1977.

Fries, J.: Aging, natural death, and the compression of morbidity. N. Engl. J. Med., *303*:130, 1980.

Gardner, J.J., and Ouimette, R.: A nurse-physician team approach in a private internal medicine practice. Arch. Intern. Med., *134*:956, 1974.

Gillum, R.F., and Barsky, A.J.: Diagnosis and management of patient noncompliance. J.A.M.A., *228*:1563, 1974.

Groves, J.E.: Taking care of the hateful patient. N. Engl. J. Med., *298*:883, 1978.

Hinton, J.: *Dying.* New York, Penguin Books, 1972.

Ingelfinger, F.J.: Health: a matter of statistics of feeling? N. Engl. J. Med., *296*:448, 1977.

Jackson, D.L., and Youngner, S.: Patient autonomy and "death with dignity." N. Engl. J. Med., *301*:404, 1979.

Langner, Myra B.: *The Private Worlds of Dying Children.* Princeton, Princeton University Press, 1978.

Lasagna, L.: *The Doctor's Dilemmas.* New York, Harper & Bros., 1962.

Osmond, H.: God and the doctor. N. Engl. J. Med., *302*:555, 1980.

Prado De Molina, M.: The confrontation with death. Am. J. Psychoanal., *36*:261, 1976.

Rosenbaum, E.: *Living With Cancer.* New York, Praeger, 1975.

Smith, D.L.: *Medication Guide for Patient Counseling.* Philadelphia, Lea & Febiger, 1977.

Toynbee, P.: *Patients.* New York, Harcourt Brace and Jovanovich, 1977.

Weed, L.L.: *Medical Records, Medical Education and Patient Care.* Cleveland, Case University Press, 1969.

Epilogue

Ignorance is not so damnable as humbug, but when it prescribes pills it may happen to do more harm. —G. ELIOT

The study of disease is the sum of our attempts to comprehend man's illness. It is challenging, constantly changing, and endlessly fascinating. It ranges from retrospective estimates of epidemics to prospective observations of tumor response to new therapy. It is more than the history of a man and his illness. The interplay of genetics and environment is puzzling in our attempts to understand who becomes sick. The forces behind the evolution of illness in mankind are as perplexing as remission in a disease of unknown etiology. It is fashionable to write of molecular disease, as if by naming the biochemical lesion we understand why pain arises in a particular place. The study of disease must include an awareness that diseases change as we study them, both in the patient and in the world at large. The importance of our knowledge of disease is an ability to predict what will happen in the individual and in society and to prevent illness where we can. We should recognize that the symmetry and order we see may really be a product of our vision rather than the result of a divine plan. Our comprehension of disease, indeed, may be our paradigm imposed on nature. We see what we wish to see.

The parsimony of William Occam, that a single explanation is better than several explanations, has led us for the last 80 years to teach that disease has single causes. This theory may be more appealing than it is truthful. In this text we have attempted to display the varied expressions of illness and to underscore the variety of ways in which we look at disease. So often, manifestations of illness are portrayed in a specialized way because of the special interest of the observer.

We should like to conclude this volume by urging the reader to return once more to a general point of view, to look with a critical eye at our attitudes to illness and at what we think are truths about disease.

Prefixes and Suffixes

An appreciation of the meaning of Latin and Greek prefixes and suffixes serves to make obscure and forbidding medical terms easy to understand and therefore far more interesting. Some of those more commonly used in the subjects we have been considering are given. To make the subject more living, the reader may care to put together the prefix and suffix in such words as hematemesis, pathogenesis, osteomalacia, dyspnea, and menorrhagia.

PREFIXES

a- without or not: *achlorhydria*, absence of hydrochloric acid.

acro- extremity: *acromegaly*, large extremities.

adeno- gland: *adenitis*, inflammation of a gland.

an- without: *anuria*, suppression of urine.

ante- before: *antemortem*, before death.

anti- against: *antitoxin*, antagonistic to a toxin.

arthro- joint: *arthritis*, inflammation of a joint.

auto- self: *autolysis*, self-dissolution.

bio- life: *biology*, study of living things.

chol- bile: *cholecystitis*, inflammation of the gallbladder.

cyst- bladder: *cystitis*, inflammation of the bladder.

dia- through: *diarrhea*, a flowing through.

dys- difficult, bad: *dysmenorrhea*, difficult menstruation.

en- in, into: *encapsuled*, enclosed in a capsule.

endo- within: *endometrium*, lining of the uterus.

entero- intestine: *enteritis*, inflammation of the intestine.

epi- upon, outside: *epidermis*, outer layer of the true skin.

ex- out of: *exostosis*, bony growth from surface of bone.

hem-, hemo- blood: *hemoglobin*, coloring matter of red blood cells.

hetero- dissimilar: *heterophile* antibody, having affinity for antigen other than that for which it is specific.

homeo- similar: *homeostasis*, stability of normal body states.

hydro- water: *hydrothorax*, fluid in the pleural cavity.

hyper- above, excessive: *hyperacidity*, excessive acidity.

hypo- deficiency or beneath: *hypoacidity*, deficient acidity.

hyster- uterus: *hysterectomy*, excision of the uterus.

infra- below: *infraorbital*, beneath the orbit.

inter- between: *intercellular*, between cells.

intra- within: *intracellular,* within cells.
leuko- white: *leukocyte,* a white blood cell.
macro- large: *macrocyte,* an abnormally large red blood cell.
mal- bad: *malnutrition,* poor nutrition.
mast- breast: *mastitis,* inflammation of the breast.
mega- great: *megacolon,* enlargement of the colon.
melan- black: *melanin,* a black pigment.
men- month: *menses, menstruation,* monthly blood flow from uterus.
micro- small: *microcyte,* an undersized red blood cell.
myo- muscle: *myositis,* inflammation of muscle.
myx- mucus: *myxedema,* mucinous edema.
necro- death: *necrosis,* death of cells.
neo- new: *neoplasm,* a new growth or tumor.
nephr- kidney: *nephritis,* inflammation of kidney.
oligo- few: *oliguria,* scanty urination.
osteo- bone: *osteomyelitis,* inflammation of bone.
para- beside: *paramedical,* having a secondary relation to medicine.
peri- around: *pericardium,* the membrane around the heart.
phago- to eat, devour: *phagocyte,* a cell that devours bacteria.
phleb- vein: *phlebitis,* inflammation of a vein.
polio- gray: *poliomyelitis,* inflammation of gray matter of spinal cord.
poly- many: *polycythemia,* excess in number of red blood cells.
post- after: *postmortem,* after death.
pro- before: *prophylaxis,* measures taken to prevent disease.
pseudo- false: *pseudopodia,* false feet of astroglia.
pyo- pus: *pyosalpinx,* fallopian tube filled with pus.
syn- together with: *syndrome,* a constant complex of symptoms.
xantho- yellow: *xanthochromia,* yellow coloration of the cerebrospinal fluid.

SUFFIXES

-angio, vessel; *lymphangiitis,* inflammation of a lymph vessel.
-algia, pain; *neuralgia,* pain involving nerves.
-ase, designating an enzyme: *amylase,* a starch-splitting enzyme.
-cele, a protrusion: *meningocele,* a hernial protrusion of the meninges.
-centesis, perforating or tapping: *thoracentesis,* aspirating fluid from the thorax.
-chole, bile: *acholic,* without bile.
-ectasis, dilate: *bronchiectasis,* dilatation of the bronchi.
-ectomy, excision: *tonsillectomy,* removal of a tonsil.
-emesis, vomit: *hematemesis,* vomiting blood.
-emia, blood: *anemia,* deficiency of red blood cells.
-esthesia, sensation: *anesthesia,* absence of sensation.
-genesis, generation of: *pathogenesis,* generation of disease.
-iasis, a process, especially a morbid one: *amebiasis,* state of being infected with amebae.
-itis, inflammation of the part named: *appendicitis,* inflammation of appendix.
-lith, stone: *phlebolith,* calcified body in a vein.
-lysis, to dissolve: *autolysis,* self-dissolution.
-malacia, softening: *osteomalacia,* softening of bone.
-megaly, large: *splenomegaly,* enlargement of spleen.
-odynia, pain: *pleurodynia,* pain in the region of the pleura.
-oid, like, resembling: *mucoid,* like mucus.
-oma, tumor: *osteoma,* a tumor of bone.

-osis, full of: *amyloidosis,* full of amyloid.

-ostomy, mouth: *gastrostomy,* to make an artificial opening into the stomach.

-otomy, cut: *gastrotomy,* to cut into the stomach.

-pathy, disease: *neuropathy,* any nervous disease.

-penia, poverty: *thrombocytopenia,* decrease in the thrombocytes or blood platelets.

-phila, affinity for: *eosinophil,* leukocyte staining with eosin.

-plasia, to form: *hyperplasia,* overgrowth of tissue.

-plegia, paralysis: *hemiplegia,* paralysis of one half (side) of the body.

-pnea, breath: *dyspnea,* difficult breathing.

-ptosis, falling: *visceroptosis,* falling of abdominal viscera.

-rhagia, bursting forth: *menorrhagia,* profuse menstruation.

-rhea, flow: *diarrhea,* abnormal flow from bowel.

-sclerosis, hardening: *arteriosclerosis,* hardening of the arteries.

-stasis, standing still: *hemostasis,* arrest of circulation.

-trophy, nourish: *atrophy,* wasting.

-uria, relating to urine: *anuria,* absence of urine.

Index

Page numbers in *italics* indicate illustrations; those followed by t indicate tables.

COMMON NORMAL LABORATORY VALUES

HEMATOLOGY

	"Classic Units"
Complete Blood Count (CBC)	
Hemoglobin, Male	13.5–18.0 g/ml
Female	12.0–16.0 g/ml
Hematocrit, Male	42–52%
Female	37–47%
Erythrocyte count, Male	4.6–6.2×10^6/mm^3
Female	4.2–5.4×10^6/mm^3
Leukocyte count	4,000–10,000/mm^3
Erythrocyte sedimentation rate,	
Male	1–13 mm/hr
Female	1–20 mm/hr
Reticulocyte count	0.2–2.0%
Platelet count	150–400×10^3/mm^3
Prothrombin time	70–100%
Immunoglobulins—Normal Range	
IgE	15–800 IU/M
IgD	0.3–40 mg% (mean 3 mg%)
IgG	750–1900 mg%
IgA	150–470 mg%
IgM	50–260 mg%

ROUTINE URINALYSIS

Test	Normal	Possible Significance
pH	5–9	relative to diet and medication
Protein	<15 mg/dl	nephritis/nephrosis
Glucose	<33 mg/dl	diabetes mellitus
Ketones	<5 mg/dl	carbohydrate deprivation
Blood	<0.0015 mg/dl	genitourinary bleeding
Bilirubin	<0.05 mg/dl	liver function tests and
Urobilinogen	0.1–1.0 Ehrlich Unit	clarification of jaundice
Nitrite	<0.075 mg/dl	bacteriuria
Specific gravity or	1.008–1.030	relative concentration of the urine
Osmolality	500–1,500 mOsm/24 hrs	
Microscopic		
—WBCs	$<0.13 \times 10^6$/24 hrs	infection
—RBCs	$<0.65 \times 10^6$/24 hrs	genitourinary bleeding
—hyaline casts	<2,000/24 hrs	nephritis

CLINICAL CHEMISTRY

	"Classic Units"
Amylase	70–300 IU
Bilirubin	0.1–1.1 mg/dl
Blood gases pH	7.35–7.45
P_{O_2}	80–105 mmHg
P_{CO_2}	34–45 mmHg
Calcium	8.5–10.5 mg/dl
Chloride	99–107 mEq/L
Creatine phosphokinase (CPK)	20–100 IU
Creatinine	1–1.8 mg/dl
Folate (serum)	3–15 ng/ml
Glucose (fasting)	65–100 mg/dl
Iron	60–160 μg/dl
Iron binding capacity	250–400 μg/dl
Lactic dehydrogenase (LDH)	80–200 IU
Lipids: cholesterol	150–300 mg/dl
triglycerides	20–150 mg/dl
total lipids	450–1000 mg/dl
Phosphatase: acid	<0.7 U/L–11 IU
alkaline	30–85 mU/L
Phosphorus, inorganic	3.0–4.5 mg/dl
Potassium	3.7–5.5 mEq/L
Protein: total	6.0–8.0 g/dl
albumin	4.0–4.8 g/dl
globulin	2.0–3.2 g/dl
Sodium	137–148 mEq/L
Serum glutamic-oxaloacetic transaminase (SGOT)	10–30 IU
Uric acid	3.5–7.5 mg/dl
Magnesium	1.5–2.5 mg/dl
Copper	70–140 μg/100 ml
Blood urea nitrogen (BUN)	10–20 mg/dl
Creatine: whole blood	3.0–7.0 mg/dl
plasma	0.4–0.8 mg/dl

NORMAL ENDOCRINE VALUES

	"Classic Units"
Adrenocorticotropic hormone (ACTH)	20–100 pg/ml
Cortisol: 8 AM	15–29 μg/100 ml
4 PM	5–20 μg/100 ml
midnight	1.5–10 μg/100 ml
Growth hormone	<5 ng/ml
Insulin (fasting)	7–20 μU/ml
Thyroxine	5–11 μg/dl
T-3 uptake	25–35%
Triiodothyronine	70–210 ng/dl
Thyroid-stimulating hormone (TSH)	<8 μU/ml
Catecholamines: epinephrine	0–0.5 μg/L
norepinephrine	0–1.0 μg/L
Aldosterone: recumbent	3–16 ng/100 ml
ambulant	4–31 ng/100 ml
Progesterone: male	0.1–0.9 ng/ml
female follicular	0.2–0.7 ng/ml
luteal	1.7–30 ng/ml
menopause	0.04–0.33 ng/ml
Testosterone: male	273–1200 ng/100 ml
female	26–130 ng/100 ml